AF577296

Atlas of Vertebral Angiography

MUTSUMASA TAKAHASHI, M.D.

Professor and Director, Department of Radiology
Akita University School of Medicine, Akita, Japan

UNIVERSITY PARK PRESS BALTIMORE AND LONDON
IGAKU SHOIN LTD. TOKYO

Library of Congress Cataloging in Publication Data

Takahashi, Mutsumasa.
Atlas of vertebral angiography.

Bibliography: p.
1. Spinal cord—Blood-vessels—Radiography.
I. Title. [DNLM: 1. Angiography—Atlases. 2. Brain neoplasms—Radiography—Atlases. 3. Spine—Blood supply. 4. Vertebral artery—Radiography. WG17 T132a 1974]
RC406. EV3T34 616. 8′1′07572 73-19783
ISBN 0-8391-0681-5

PUBLISHERS
© First edition, 1974 by IGAKU SHOIN LTD., 5-24-3 Hongo, Bunkyo-ku, Tokyo.
Sole distribution rights for USA and Canada granted to
UNIVERSITY PARK PRESS, Chamber of Commerce Building, Baltimore, Maryland 21202
All rights reserved. No part of this book may be translated or reproduced in any form by print, photoprint, microfilm, or any other means without written permission from the publisher.

Printed and bound in Japan

To my parents,

Katsumasa Takahashi

and

Late Midori Takahashi

Foreword

Dr. MUTSUMASA TAKAHASHI is eminently qualified to write a book on vertebral angiography. He has received training in Diagnostic Radiology in Japan as well as advanced Fellowships in Vascular Radiology and Neuroradiology in the United States. A perusal of the literature will convince the reader of his expertise by the frequency of references to Dr. TAKAHASHI's contributions.

This book is ideally suited to the student who has completed his introduction to neuroradiology, including neuroanatomy, and is now ready for the challenges of difficult clinical material. The book clearly illustrates the changing concepts of posterior fossa diagnosis by vertebral angiography. This material illustrates the accuracy that is possible by vertebral angiography that was formerly thought possible only with pneumoencephalography and tomography.

The book should prove very valuable to the neuroradiologist who has completed his training and wishes to refresh his diagnostic acumen by reviewing a large amount of well organized clinical examinations. The breadth of this book allows a handy reference for comparison to current vertebral angiography problems.

WILLIAM N. HANAFEE, M. D.

Professor of Radiological Sciences
UCLA Center for the Health Sciences
Los Angeles, California, U. S. A.

Foreword

With the rapid development of neurosurgery, roentgenologic techniques are more frequently utilized in the investigation of neurological diseases. However, there have been few neuroradiologists in Japan to meet the demands of this field. Dr. MUTSUMASA TAKAHASHI was trained in general radiology, cardiovascular radiology and neuroradiology during five years at the University of Michigan, Stanford University and the University of California at Los Angeles. On returning to Japan in May, 1967, he actively participated in the development and progress of neuroradiology and vascular radiology in this country. Particularly, he has helped to develop transfemoral catheter techniques for cerebral angiography and has made numerous contributions to the scientific literature concerning the utilization of these methods. Dr. TAKAHASHI has laid a foundation for the rapid development of neuroradiology in Japan.

Vertebral angiography has now become more widely utilized than pneumoencephalography and ventriculography, but its real value in the diagnosis of posterior fossa lesions has heretofore not been established. This atlas contains numerous subtracted roentgenograms of high quality with their corresponding careful analyses and interpretations. By vividly presenting finely detailed angiographic findings the author has succeeded in demonstrating the advantages and limitations of vertebral angiography in diagnosing posterior fossa lesions.

The members and staff of the Department of Radiology of Kyushu University are indeed very proud of this book's being published at the international level, through the outstanding cooperation of the neuroradiology group headed by Dr. TAKAHASHI. It is a great honor for me to write the foreword for this text, for I believe this book will become an essential reference for physicians in the neurological sciences.

KEIICHI MATSUURA, M. D.

Professor and Chairman
Department of Radiology
Faculty of Medicine
Kyushu University
Fukuoka, Japan

Foreword

It was in 1931 that EGAS MONIZ's monograph "Diagnostic des tumeurs cérébrales et épreuve de l'encéphalographie artérielle" appeared with a preface by BABINSKI, who greatly appreciated this new idea of injecting radio-opaque media into the internal carotid artery for diagnostic evaluation of intracranial pathology. Since then, cerebral angiography has been widely accepted and further refined by many investigators and authors.

Until recently, however, pneumoencephalography initiated and developed by DANDY had been more generally utilized. This was because of early difficulties in accurate interpretation of angiographic findings and also because of the frequency and severity of untoward effects of this procedure and of the contrast media then used for opacifying the vessels. Neurologists, neurosurgeons and neuroradiologists have always desired more and more precise information, specific for vascular anatomy which was relevant to each case. And in recent years, rapid development of vascular surgery has made more keenly apparent, requirements of the neurosurgeon's ability to interprete accurately his findings. The continuing development of the radiologic equipments and contrast media has done much to relieve the original apprehension related to this method. Besides, by the continuing development of varied and improved injection techniques as well as the general accumulation of basic knowledge of normal and pathological vascular anatomy of the brain, much has been added which assists in obtaining a more precise evaluation.

Angiography, in contrast to other diagnostic methods, presents a factual representation of the vascular antaomy in its relationship to the brain, but, because of the many variabilities seen, can and does offer frequently puzzling findings which in turn lead us to erroneous conclusions despite the greatest care in interpretation. This present text, authored by Prof. TAKAHASHI has determined to present basic instructional guidelines to interpretation, supported by many illustrative clinical examples, and as such, will most certainly provide many important clues for correct and accurate diagnostic evaluations of our angiographic findings. Utilizing this text will also assist each of us who work in the field of neurodiagnostics, in ascertaining new and valuable considerations in angiographic interpretations.

Neuroradiology in Japan is still relatively recent in its development. However, Prof. TAKAHASHI is a neuroradiologist of international reputation, especially in the field of cerebral angiography, and is recognized as a pioneer in his specialty in Japan. Until March, 1972, Prof. TAKAHASHI was associated with the Department of Radiology of Kyushu University Hospital as a specialist in neuroradiology, and during this time, we were eyewitness to his diagnostic acumen. He continues as Professor of Radiology at Akita University since his appointment in 1972. With the completion of this practical, yet comprehensive text, Prof. TAKAHASHI avails his diagnostic insight to all that are seriously engaged in the field of the neurosciences, and I send him congratulations on his great work. It is my sincere hope that this text, written in English, will be widely read and utilized abroad as it will be in Japan, and I predict that someday it will be recognized as one of the classic texts on this subject.

KATSUTOSHI KITAMURA, M.D.

Professor and Chairman
Department of Neurosurgery
Neurological Institute
Faculty of Medicine
Kyushu University
Fukuoka, Japan

Preface

Although vertebral angiography has become an important diagnostic procedure, no comprehensive textbook or atlas dealing with this subject has heretofore been available. This text, which describes in detail the angiographic findings, is meant to satisfy this need. It was a painstaking task to present concisely the basic aspects of vertebral angiography for those concerned with interpretating vertebral angiograms. I have included our experience with vertebral angiography in the diagnosis of neurological diseases and emphasized the value of selective vertebral angiography in the diagnosis of intracranial tumors and vascular lesions. Special emphasis has been placed on the manner in which correct diagnoses can be made by assessing minor arterial and venous changes in the evaluation of posterior fossa tumors.

This atlas, though written and edited by me, is a product of the daily work of the staffs of the Departments of Radiology and Neurosurgery of Kyushu and Akita University Hospitals. The author gratefully acknowledges their cooperation and support. In particular, Hideo Irie, M.D., Professor Emeritus and the former Chairman of the Department of Radiology, Keiichi Matsuura, M.D., Professor and Chairman of the Department of Radiology, and Katsutoshi Kitamura, M.D., Professor and Chairman of the Department of Neurosurgery of Kyushu University, rendered invaluable support and assistance, for which I am sincerely thankful.

My special gratitude goes to William N. Hanafee, M.D., Professor of Radiology, University of California at Los Angeles, School of Medicine, my former teacher in neuroradiology, for his critical review of the text and for his valuable advice.

I am deeply indebted for the cooperation of my colleagues in radiology and would be remiss were I not to acknowledge specifically that of Drs. Toshio Okudera, Hisashi Kawanami, Takehiko Higuchi, Makoto Tanaka, Keikichi Mihara, Takao Toyama, Yoshiharu Tamakawa, and Takashi Kishikawa. Koichi Yamaguchi, M.D., Department of Radiology, Research Institute of the Brain and Blood Vessels, Akita, graciously allowed me to include several cases from his valuable collection. John Bentson, M.D., Department of Radiology, University of California at Los Angeles, School of Medicine, kindly reviewed the manuscript and gave many helpful suggestions.

I am grateful to Miss Noriko Haraguchi, my former secretary, and to Messrs. Motoo Mukoyama and Hiroshi Kubota, of Igaku Shoin Ltd., for their invaluable assistance in preparing the manuscript.

MUTSUMASA TAKAHASHI, M.D.

Professor and Director
Department of Radiology
Akita University School of Medicine
Senshu Kubota-machi, Akita, Japan

Contents

List of Cases

1

Introduction

Vertebral angiography has in recent years become a routine diagnostic procedure at many medical centers. It has been utilized in the investigation of the posterior cranial fossa, cervical regions and the posterior and basilar portions of the supratentorial structures as well as the diseases of the vertebrobasilar vascular system. In the diagnosis of posterior fossa tumors it has almost replaced pneumoencephalography, and ventriculography, at least, as the first diagnostic procedure.

In spite of its widespread use and acceptance, there does not appear to be a standard method which is widely employed. Among the various methods proposed in the literature, we have utilized several methods and arrived at the conclusion that selective vertebral angiography with the transfemoral or transaxillary catheter techniques produces consistently excellent results with low incidence of untoward effects. The value of this technique should be emphasized as widely as that of direct puncture vertebral angiography and retrograde brachial angiography.

Although the normal course and position of the arteries and veins of vertebrobasilar system have been established anatomically and radiologically, it has been rather difficult to make a positive diagnosis of tumors in this region. This is partly because the vascular displacement or deformation is so minimal that single vessels are rarely of definitive value in localizing tumors, requiring assessment of several vessels at the same time.

Table 1 Age and Sex Distribution of 485 Patients.

Age	Total	Male	Female
0–4	37	19	18
5–9	35	17	18
10–14	27	17	10
15–19	25	16	9
20–29	70	39	31
30–39	88	65	23
40–49	100	56	44
50–59	72	48	24
60–69	28	17	11
70–	3	2	1
Total	485	296	189

Five hundred and forty selective vertebral angiographies via the femoral and axillary arteries have been performed on 485 patients at the Kyushu University Hospital from July 1967 to March 1972. One patient was examined 4 times, 3 patients 3 times, 46 patients twice and the remaining 435 patients once. The age and sex of patients are shown in Table 1. Angiographic diagnoses of the patients are shown in Tables 2 to 5. Only the cases with surgical or clinical confirmation are included. At this institution vertebral angiographies were performed with or without combination of an-

Table 2 Angiographic Diagnosis of Infratentorial Tumors.

Diagnosis		
Cerebellar hemispheric tumor		*14*
Astrocytoma	6	
Hemangioblastoma	5	
Metastasis	2	
Intracerebellar cyst	1	
Tumor of the cerebellar vermis		*16*
Medulloblastoma	12	
Hemangioblastoma	4	
Brain stem tumor		*4*
Glioma	4	
Fourth ventricle tumor		*5*
Ependymoma	2	
Epidermoid tumor	2	
Papilloma	1	
Tumor of the cerebellopontine angle		*41*
Acoustic neurinoma	35	
Meningioma	2	
Abscess	1	
Fifth nerve neurinoma	1	
Metastasis	1	
Vascular tumor	1	
Tumors over the clivus		*9*
Nasopharyngeal tumor	6	
Chordoma	1	
Vascular tumor	1	
Multiple myeloma	1	
Other extracerebellar tumor		*7*
Tentorial meningioma	3	
Torcular meningioma	1	
Sigmoid sinus meningioma	1	
Extracerebellar cyst	1	
Eleventh nerve neurinoma	1	
	Total	*96*

giograms of the opposite vertebral, internal carotid, external carotid and common carotid arteries (Table 6). For vertebral angiography, various approaches have been utilized depending upon the anatomy of vessels, clinical need and condition of the patients (Table 7).

The purpose of this book is to present our material to emphasize the value of selective vertebral angiography as well as to illustrate how a correct diagnosis can be arrived by assessing minor arterial and venous changes.

Table 3 Angiographic Diagnosis of Supratentorial Tumors.

Occipital tumor		*9*
Metastatic tumor	5	
Meningioma	2	
Hemorrhage	1	
Astrocytoma	1	
Temporal and middle fossa tumor		*10*
Neurinoma of Gasselian ganglion	5	
Ependymoma	3	
Vascular tumor	1	
Epidermoid tumor	1	
Deep midline tumor		*10*
Thalamic tumors	6	
Hypothalamic tumors	2	
Glioblastoma of splenium	1	
Hematoma	1	
Pineal tumor		*13*
Pinealoma	10	
Teratoma	2	
Glioblastoma	1	
Parasellar and suprasellar tumor		*10*
Craniopharyngioma	6	
Pituitary adenoma	3	
Parasellar meningioma	1	
Intraventricular tumor		*7*
Oligodendroglioma	3	
Ependymoma	2	
Teratoma	1	
Meningioma	1	
	Total	*59*

Table 4 Angiographic Diagnosis of Vascular Diseases.

Aneurysm		*7*
Posterior inferior cerebellar artery	2	
Basilar bifurcation	2	
Junction of the vertebral arteries	1	
Origin of superior cerebellar artery	1	
Multiple	1	
Arteriovenous malformation		*20*
Supratentorial	17	
Infratentorial	3	
Arteriosclerosis		*3*
Stenotic and occlusive disease		*19*
Multiple progressive cerebral occlusions	7	
Posterior cerebral artery	3	
Superior cerebellar artery	1	
Basilar artery	1	
Vertebral artery	1	
Leptomeningeal collaterals to the occluded anterior and middle cerebral arteries	6	
Intracerebral hemorrhage		*2*
Pontine	1	
Occipital	1	
	Total	*51*

Table 5 Angiographic Diagnosis of the Remaining Patients.

Hydrocephalus and cerebral atrophy	17
Congenital anomalies	10
Spinal tumor	2
Cervical tumor	2
Cervical arteriovenous malformation	1
Normal	237
Unsuccessful	10
Total	279

Table 6 Types of Vertebral and Carotid Angiograms.

Vertebral angiogram	219
Vertebral and right or left carotid angiogram	193
Vertebral and bilateral carotid angiogram	118
Unsuccessful study	10
Total	540

Table 7 Techniques Used for 540 Vertebral Angiograms.

1)	Left vertebral artery via femoral artery	474
2)	Right vertebral artery via femoral artery	15
3)	Bilateral vertebral artery via femoral artery	12
4)	Right vertebral artery via right axillary artery	6
5)	Left vertebral artery via left axillary artery	3
6)	Left subclavian artery via femoral artery	14
7)	Right subclavian artery via femoral artery	2
8)	Bilateral subclavian artery via femoral artery	1
9)	Right subclavian artery via right axillary artery	3
10)	Unsuccessful study	10
	Total	540

2

History of Vertebral Angiography

Although MONIZ introduced carotid angiography in 1927, vertebral angiography had not been developed until 1933 when MONIZ and his associates advocated the technique of retrograde subclavian artery injection after surgical exposure of the subclavian artery. They injected 14 cc of thorotrast with temporary occlusion of the peripheral subclavian artery They demonstrated the carotid and vertebral arteries on the right and the vertebral artery on the left. SHIMIDZU in Japan (1937) evolved a technique of injecting contrast media into the subclavian artery percutaneously. The subclavian artery was punctured percutaneously on the pulsation of the artery. Seven to 8 cc of thorotrast were injected with compression of the axillary artery.

SJOQVIST (1938) was successful in injecting the vertebral artery at its entry into the costotransversal foramen of the sixth cervical vertebra following direct exposure of the vertebral artery. TAKAHASHI in Japan (1940) developed a percutaneous technique of injecting the vertebral artery just before its entry into the costotransversal foramen of the sixth cervical vertebra. This was the first percutaneous technique developed for direct puncture of the vertebral artery. However, the success rate was considerably lower because of associated technical difficulty. Therefore, the subclavian injection techniques after surgical exposure had been the most widespread method for visualization of the vertebrobasilar systems.

Percutaneous vertebral angiography, utilizing direct arterial puncture at the intervertebral spaces, has been developed independently by SUGAR et al. (1949), LINDGREN (1950), SANO (1950) and SUTTON and HOARE (1951). This technique has enjoyed a widespread use in visualization of the vertebrobasilar system because of lack of surgical procedure, shorter time required and technical simplicity. Success rate is relatively high, usually in the vicinity of 85 per cent. Therefore, this technique has still been in use at many medical centers.

In the meantime, various methods for vertebral angiography have been developed. AMELI (1952) developed a retrograde vertebral angiography with a percutaneous needle placed in the right common carotid artery while the distal carotid artery and the ipsilateral brachial artery are occluded mechanically. GOULD et al. advocated vertebral angiography by retrograde injection into the brachial artery in 1955. This latter technique has prevailed in many medical centers because of its simplicity and safety. The only drawback of this technique is superimposition of carotid and vertebral systems as well as decreased definition of the vascular beds. SHIMIDZU's percutaneous puncture of the subclavian artery was modified and improved with relatively frequent use until recently (BARBIERI and VERDECCHIA, 1957; AMPLATZ and HARNER, 1962).

First application of the catheter technique on the vertebral artery was introduced by RADNER (1947), who placed a catheter in the exposed radial artery and advanced to the orifice of the vertebral artery for injection of contrast media. This method did not receive widespread acceptance since the radial artery had to be sacrificed and the success rate was not high. HAUGE (1954) succeeded and further developed RADNER's technique. The transfemoral catheter technique was first developed by LINDGREN (1956), and elaborated by BONTE et al. (1958) and CRONQVIST (1961). This technique was considered at first to be applicable only in children and young adults. However, various authors emphasized the value of this technique in all age groups (NEWTON, 1966; TAKAHASHI et al., 1969 and 1970). HANAFEE (1963) and NEWTON (1963) developed selective catheter vertebral angiography by a transaxillary catheter, which is particularly useful in patients with marked atherosclerosis of the iliac arteries and thoracic aorta. These selective catheter methods are now considered to be most reliable, easy method of obtaining a consistently excellent definition of the vessels.

Since 1965 we have performed catheter vertebral angiography with transfemoral or transaxillary catheter technique. All the patients are examined at the first attempt by the transfemoral catheter technique. If this fails, the transaxillary catheter technique is utilized. In our hands, the catheter technique has produced consistently good results with low complication rate.

3

Techniques of Vertebral Angiography

PREPARATION OF PATIENTS, PREMEDICATION AND ANESTHESIA

The patient should be prepared for the examination psychologically. It is usually wise to explain the patient how the examination is performed. It may also be advisable to administer sedatives the night before the examination in apprehensive patients.

For premedication an adequate amount of barbiturates and atropine is sufficient and administered 30 minutes before the examination. Narcotics are not used unless the patient is very apprehensive.

The procedure is performed under local anesthesia in adults and children above 7 years of age. However, the direct puncture technique of the vertebral artery may be performed under general anesthesia. In infants and children below 7 years of age, general anesthesia is usually used. We have used ketamine intramuscularly in these patients for cerebral angiography with excellent results. Intramuscular administration in a dose of 5 mg per kilogram of body weight maintains adequate anesthesia for vertebral angiography. Maintaining dose of 2.5 mg per kilogram of body weight may be given as necessary.

Intradermal or intravenous test injections of contrast media may be used the day before the examination. We do not perform this type of sensitivity test, but inject 3 to 5 cc of contrast media through the catheter placed in the artery or vein on the radiographic table. Approximately 5 minutes should elapse without reactions before we can proceed to the angiographic examinations.

TRANSFEMORAL CATHETER TECHNIQUE

This is the method of selectively catheterizing the left or right vertebral artery by a catheter placed in the femoral artery. The catheter placement into the femoral artery is performed by an arterial cut-down or by the Seldinger technique (Fig. 1).

Various catheter materials have been used. The author has successfully used radio-opaque polyethylene catheters made by Becton-Dickinson Company (Fig. 2). Endhole polyethylene catheters with a "J" shaped curve tip (RPX 045H; O.D. 1.65 mm) are usually used in adults and children. Slightly larger catheters with "S"-shaped curve at its distal 12 to 15 cm (RPX 062H; O.D. 2.1 mm) may also be utilized in adults, especially in patients with atherosclerosis of the thoracic aorta and brachiocephalic vessels.

Under television fluoroscopic control the catheter is advanced into the aortic arch and the catheter tip is first manipulated into the left subclavian artery. This is easily done in young adults and children, since the vertebral artery forms a straight line with the proximal left subclavian artery and descending aorta. When the aortic arch and the brachiocephalic vessels are tortuous, the "S"-shaped catheters are preferably used to overcome the tortuousity at the origin of the subclavian artery. As soon as the catheter enters the subclavian artery, a test injection is performed to see whether the vessel is large enough to accommodate the catheter. Another test injection is performed following advancement of the catheter tip into the vertebral artery to the level of the fourth or fifth cervical vertebra and serial angiograms are obtained. If blood flow is slowed, the catheter should be withdrawn immediately into the subclavian artery, and a subclavian vertebral angiogram is performed or the right vertebral catheterization may be performed.

Catheterization of the right vertebral artery is some-

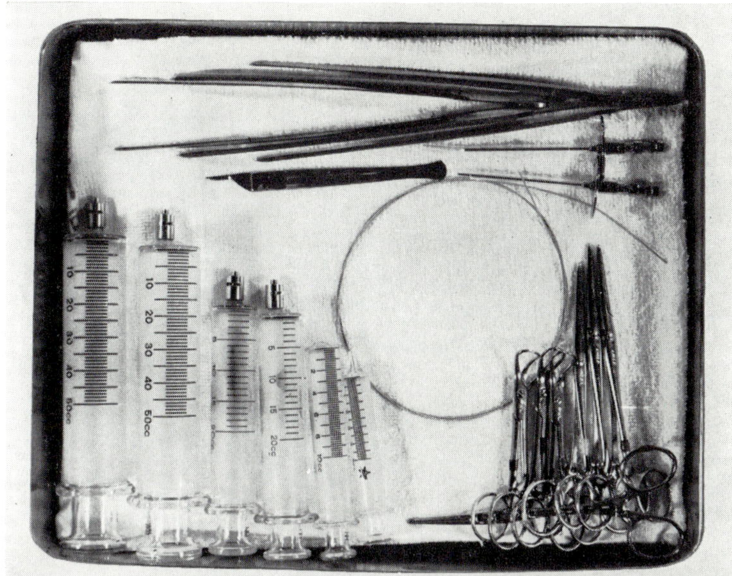

Fig. 1 Instruments for vertebral angiography by transfemoral and transaxillary technique.

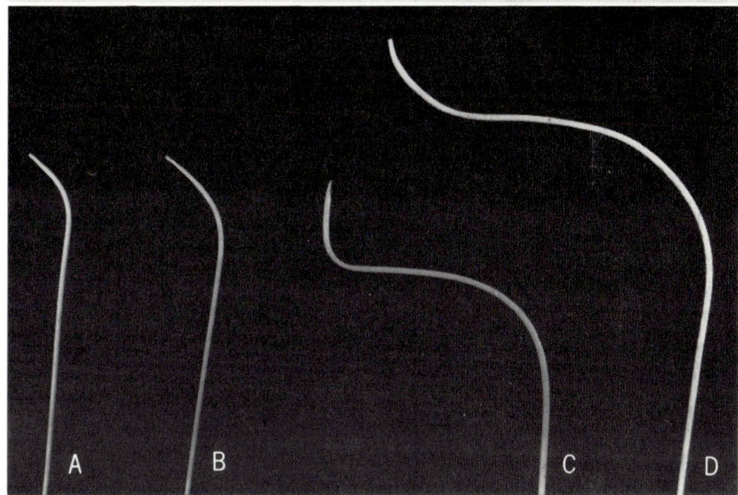

Fig. 2 Catheters used for transfemoral and transaxillary vertebral angiography. A and B: Endhole catheters with "J"-shaped curved tip (Becton-Dickinson RPX 045 H). C and D: Endhole catheters with "S"-shaped curve (Becton-Dickinson RPX 062H).

what difficult, since the catheter frequently enters the right common carotid artery at the bifurcation of the brachiocephalic trunk. Following placement of the catheter tip into the brachiocephalic trunk, the catheter or the leading guide-wire is advanced with the tip directing downwards. Then, the catheter tip is rotated superiorly at the vertebral orifice for selective catheterization of the right vertebral artery. The catheter may be advanced to the fourth or fifth cervical vertebra when blood flow is good.

Among the advantages of the transfemoral catheter techniques, a single arterial puncture allows a study of multiple cerebral vessels in addition to visualization of a vertebral artery. Excellent detail of the vascular bed is consistently obtained (Figs. 3, 4, and 5). This is particularly important in patients with subarachnoid hemorrhage and vague neurologic findings. In children this technique can be performed with relative ease and safety, and provides better definition of the cerebral vascular bed. Further advantages of this technique include less discomfort to patients, easy positioning of the head for filming, less exposure dose to the examiners and no local hematomas.

The main disadvantage of the catheter method is plugging of the vertebral artery. However, this can be avoided by careful manipulation of the catheter and test injections. The fact that the procedure requires a longer time and the examiner should be well trained may be a drawback of this technique. The unsuccessful studies are infrequent. Unsuccessful attempts are analyzed in our material (Table 8).

Table 8 Analysis of Unsuccessful Attempts at Vertebral Angiogram.

1) Left vertebral via femoral			
	Reason:	Tortuous artery	6
		Hypoplastic artery	3
		Vertebral spasm	1
2) Left vertebral via left axillary artery			
	Reason:	Tortuous artery	1
3) Right vertebral via right axillary artery			
	Reason:	Tortuous artery	2
		Total	13

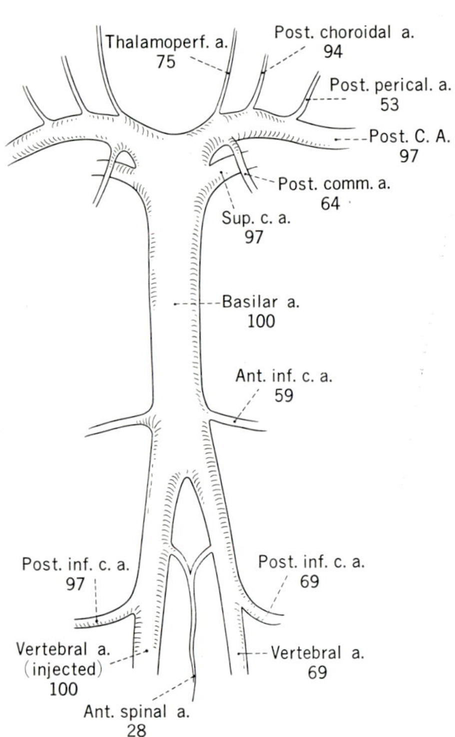

Fig. 3 Percentage visualization of the branches of the vertebrobasilar system.
Post inf. c.a. = Posterior inferior cerebellar artery. Vertebral a. = Vertebral artery. Ant. spinal a. = Anterior spinal artery. Ant. inf. c.a. = Anterior inferior cerebellar artery. Sup. c.a. = Superior cerebellar artery. Basilar a. = Basilar artery. Post. comm. a. = Posterior communicating artery. Post. C. A. = Posterior cerebral artery. Post. perical. a. = Posterior pericallosal artery. Post. choroidal a. = Posterior choroidal artery. Thalamoperf. a. = Thalamoperforate artery. (Through the courtesy of Journal of Neurosurgery. From TAKAHASHI et al., J. Neurosurg. 30: 722, 1969)

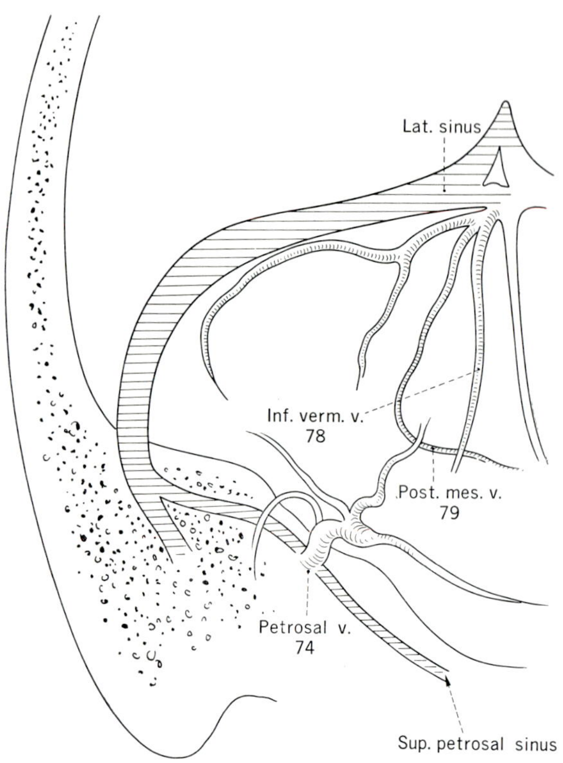

Fig. 4 Percentage visualization of the tributaries of the venous system in the Towne projection.
Lat. sinus = Lateral sinus. Inf. verm. v. = Inferior vermian vein. Post mes. v. = Posterior mesencephalic vein. Petrosal v. = Petrosal vein. Sup. petrosal sinus = Superior petrosal sinus. (Through the courtesy of Journal of Neurosurgery. From TAKAHASHI et al., J. Neurosurg. 30: 722, 1969)

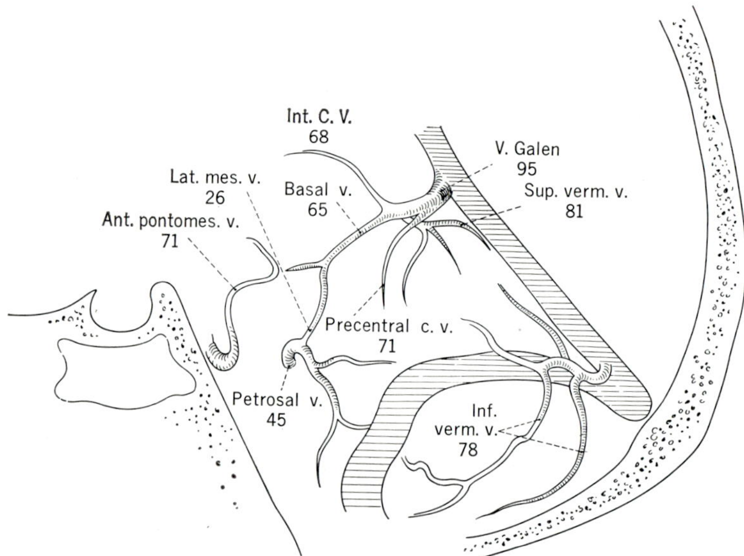

Fig. 5 Percentage visualization of the tributaries of the venous system in the lateral projection.
Int. C.V. = Internal cerebral vein. Ant. pontomes. v. = Anterior pontomesencephalic vein. Lat. mes. v. = Lateral mesencephalic vein. Petrosal v. = Petrosal vein. Precentral c.v. = Precentral cerebellar vein. Sup. verm. v. = Superior vermian vein. V. Galen = Vein of Galen. Inf. verm. v. = Inferior vermian vein. Basal v. = Basal vein or posterior mesencephalic vein. (Through the courtesy of Journal of Neurosurgery. From TAKAHASHI et al., J. Neurosurg. 30: 722, 1969)

TRANSAXILLARY CATHETER TECHNIQUE

A preformed "J"-shaped catheter (RPX 045H; O.D. 1.65 mm) is placed in the right axillary artery or proximal brachial artery and advanced into the subclavian artery. Following a test injection, the catheter tip is introduced into the vertebral artery with manipulation of the catheter. If blood flow is adequate in the vertebral artery, the catheter tip is advanced to the level of the fourth or fifth cervical vertebra and serial films are obtained. At our institution, this technique is the secondary procedure which is utilized in patients with unsuccessful vertebral angiograms via the transfemoral catheter technique. This may be used as a primary procedure in patients of older age group (usually above 60 years of age), when extensive atherosclerosis is expected to be present.

Some authors, using a subclavian catheter, have advocated injection of contrast media into the subclavian artery near the orifice of the vertebral artery (PYGOTT et al., 1959; TATELMAN and SHEEHAN, 1962). The non-selective technique can visualize the entire vertebral artery, but frequently provides poor definition of the intracranial vascular beds.

RETROGRADE BRACHIAL TECHNIQUE

This technique consists of insertion of a needle into the brachial artery, through which a bolus of contrast media is injected with a high pressure. The contrast media refluxes into the subclavian artery in the retrograde manner, thus visualizing the vertebral artery.

A needle is placed in the brachial artery just above the antecubital fossa, following percutaneous puncture or surgical exposure of the brachial artery. A needle No. 15 to No. 18 gauge is selected according to the size of the brachial artery. An 18 gauge needle is used for children, while larger needles are used for adults.

The injections are made as rapidly as possible with a pressure of 6 to 8 kg/cm^2 or its equivalent using a pressure injector. Twenty to 40 cc of contrast media are used for each injection. During the injection a tight turniquet or a blood pressure cuff inflated to above the systolic pressure is applied about the arm below the needle.

Among several advantages of this technique, the examinations can be performed easily and expediciously. The neck can be moved for positioning without fear of dislodging the needle. Disadvantages include superimposition of the carotid and vertebral systems, relatively poor definition of the vessels and larger amounts of contrast media required.

DIRECT PUNCTURE TECHNIQUE

This technique consists of insertion of a needle into the vertebral artery running through the costotransversal foramen.

Following adequate cleansing of the neck and hyperextension of the neck local anesthesia is well applied to the intervertebral foramen. The examiner's left fingers press down the area lateral to the upper margin of the thyroid cartilage and separate the carotid artery laterally and the trachea medially. Then, the transverse process of the cervical vertebra can be palpated. The needle is inserted about 1 cm medial to the transverse processes and between the upper and lower transverse processes. The needle is cautiously advanced along the anterior inferior margin of the transverse process with its tip pointing slightly laterally and superiorly. Entrance of the needle tip into the subarachnoid space should be cautiously avoided. As soon as the bony resistance is lost, the intervertebral foramen is entered with puncture of the vertebral artery. Since the needle passes through the anterior and posterior walls of the artery, it should be withdrawn slowly until good pulsatile spurt of arterial blood comes out. The needle is then advanced 4 to 5 mm. At this point, a polyethylene tubing is attached and serial films are obtained with injection of contrast media.

Short-bevelled needles are preferably used so that the bore of the needle entirely lies within the arterial lumen. Needles used are usually No. 17 or 18 gauge with an inner stilet (Fig. 6).

Advantages of this technique include rapidity and simplicity of the procedure in the experienced hands. Better vascular details may be obtained because of direct vertebral injection of contrast media. However, there are dangers of vascular spasm, occlusion and formation of arteriovenous fistulae. Among other disadvantages examiners should be well trained, general anesthesia is frequently required and there are always dangers of dislodging the needle for repeated injections. Success rate of this technique is in the vicinity of 80% to 90% even in the experienced hands.

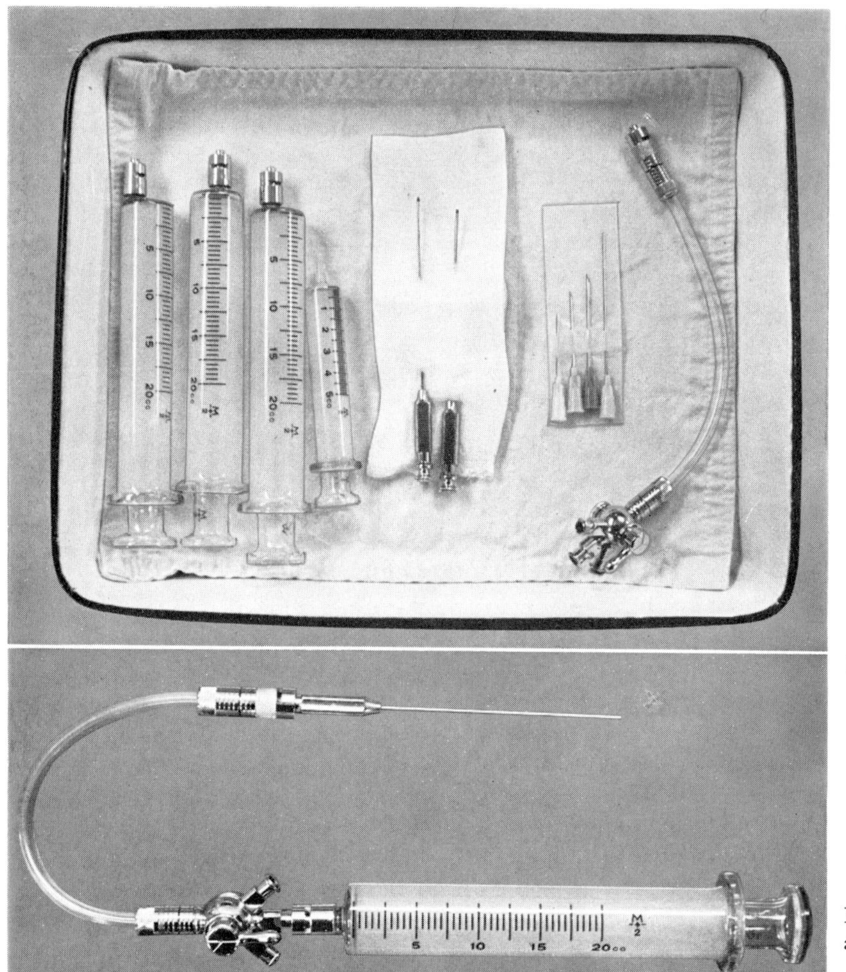

Fig. 6 Needle and instruments for vertebral angiography by direct puncture technique. A: Instrument set. B: Needle and syringe.

DIRECT PUNCTURE OF THE SUBCLAVIAN ARTERY

There are two routes for this technique: supraclavicular approach and infraclavicular approach.

The supraclavicular approach consists of inserting a needle through the supraclavicular triangle formed by the anterior scalenus muscle, the omohyoid muscle, and the upper margin of the clavicle. The needle tip is directed inferiorly, posteriorly and medially towards the pulsation of the subclavian artery. One of the drawbacks of this technique is a frequent complication of pneumothorax. In addition, the definition of the vascular beds is not excellent.

The infraclavicular approach was developed to minimize the complication rate of pneumothorax. A needle is passed at a point just lateral to the midclavicular line and inferior to a line passing transversely through the sternal notch toward the third portion of the subclavian artery (AMPLATZ and HARNER, 1962). The subclavian artery is palpated at the supraclavicular fossa and the needle is advanced in the medial, superior and posterior direction.

A Rochester needle with a Teflon sleeve is recommended for the subclavian angiography.

OTHER TECHNIQUES OF VERTEBRAL ANGIOGRAPHY

There have been various methods proposed in the literature, but these techniques are usually utilized when the previously described techniques are unsuccessful.

RADNER's technique (1947) of the transradial catheterization has the disadvantage of sacrificing the radial artery. The vertebral angiography can be performed by puncturing the vertebral artery between the atlas and occipital bone (MASLOWSKI, 1955). This technique harbors similar advantages and disadvantages of the direct vertebral puncture technique previously described.

The right vertebral angiogram may be performed by the right common carotid injection with a needle pointing proximally and compression of the distal carotid artery. Definition of vascular beds is usually poor with this technique.

Intravenous angiography reveals vascular lesions in the origin of the vertebral arteries (STEINBERG and EVANS, 1961), but is not satisfactory for demonstration of the cervical and intracranial lesions.

CONTRAST MEDIA

Water soluble contrast media are used for angiography. The most commonly used contrast media are diatrizoate (Urografin, Renografin, Urovison, Angiografin, Hypaque), iothalamate (Conray, Angioconray), metrizoate (Isopaque), and iodamide (Conraxin, Uromiro) salts. Methylglucamine and sodium salts of these acids are usually used singly or in various combinations of the two salts.

Clinical and experimental studies have shown that methylglucamine salts of the above-mentioned salts have less effects on the circulatory and central nervous system than the sodium salts, while the methylglucamine salts are more viscous than the sodium salts. Since viscosity is not a matter of great concern in cerebral angiography in contradiction to the angiography of other parts of the body, methylglucamine salts are commonly used for cerebral angiography with or without addition of sodium salts.

In order to reduce cerebral complications, the contrast media should have proper concentration. Concentration of iodine should be in the vicinity of 300 mg/cc and not greater than 350 mg/cc for cerebral angiography. Therefore, contrast media with mollecular concentration of 60% to 65% are ideal for carotid and vertebral angiography. We have used Isopaque 280 (59%, Iodine conc.: 280 mg/cc), Urografin 60 (60%, Iodine conc.: 292 mg/cc), Angiografin (65%, Iodine conc.: 306 mg/cc), and Conray (60%, Iodine conc.: 282 mg/cc). There does not appear to be any significant difference in the rate of cerebral complications among these contrast media.

The amount of contrast media per injection depends upon the size of the artery and body weight of the patients. Approximately 6 to 8 cc are injected for selective injection of the vertebral artery in adults. In infants and children 5 to 7 cc may be employed for selective study. For non-selective angiograms such as subclavian and retrograde brachial angiograms 20 to 40 cc may be required.

There should be an interval of 5 to 7 minutes between injections into the same vertebral artery. When 5 to 8 cc are used for each injection, it is permissible to do up to 10 injections in the same vessel in any one session.

RADIOGRAPHIC TECHNIQUE

Layout of a room for biplane cerebral angiography is shown (Fig. 7).

Routinely, lateral and half-axial (Towne) projections are obtained. An additional view in the straight anteroposterior projection may be obtained in patients with posterior fossa tumors and in the presence of superimposition of the cerebellar arteries. This projection enables one to evaluate the anterior and posterior inferior cerebellar arteries to good advantage.

Following a preliminary exposure for subtraction base, the contrast media is injected by hand as rapidly as possible or by a pressure injector (Fig. 8). With selective vertebral injections, the exposures are started at the beginning of the injection. There should be 1 to 2 seconds lag between the start of injection and the initial exposure for serial films with non-selective subclavian and brachial injections. In infants and children as well as in adults with arteriovenous malforma-

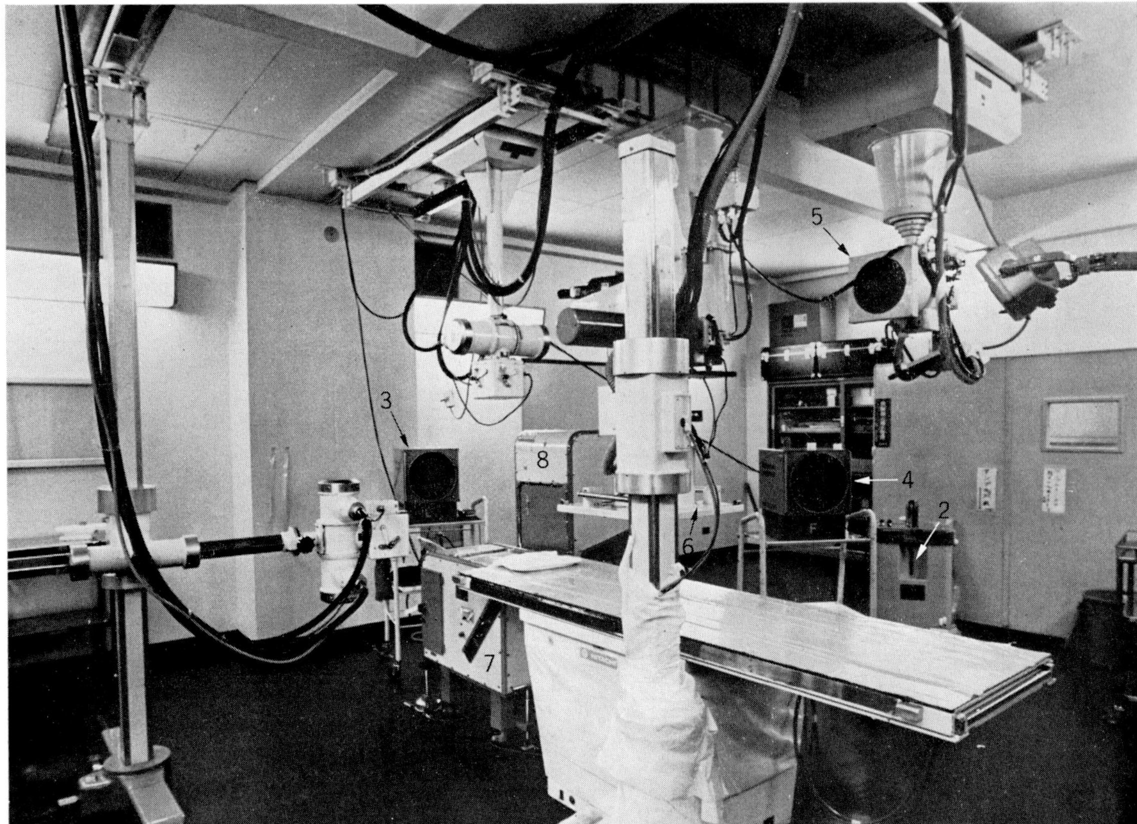

A

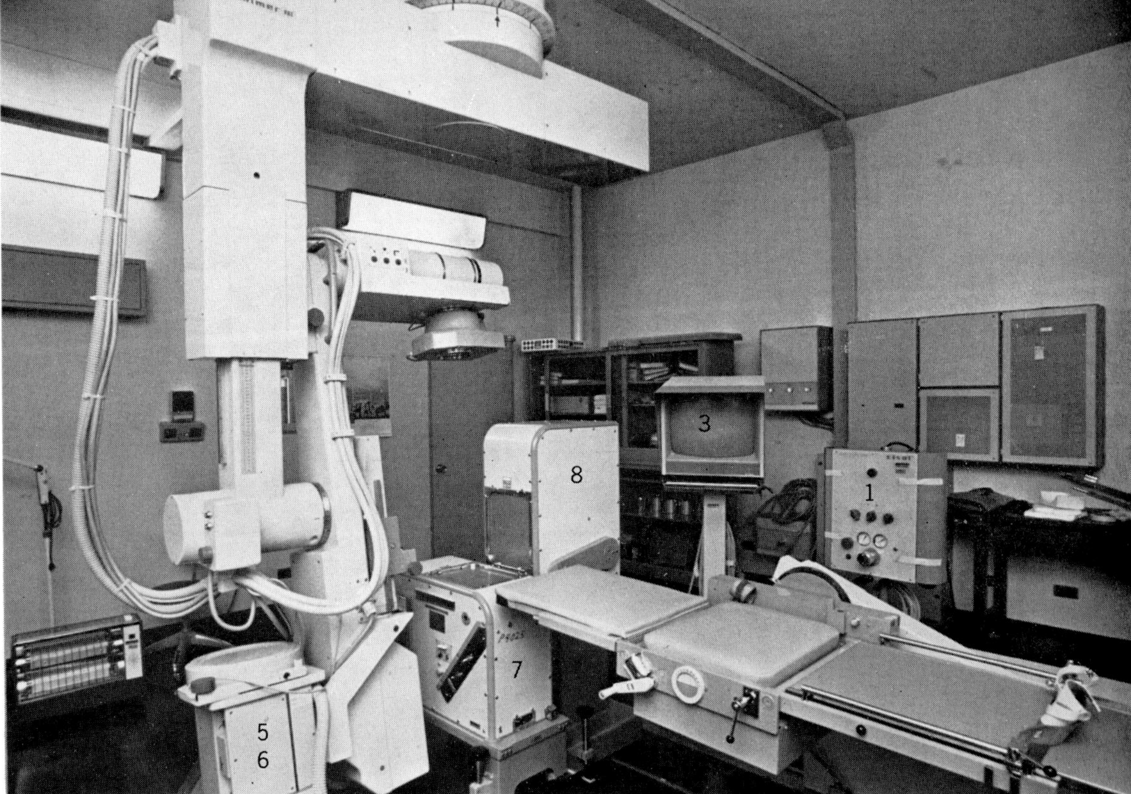

B

Fig. 7 Layout of an angiographic room. A: Biplane cerebral angiography. B: Monoplane cerebral angiography by Mimer III.
1 = Pressure injector (Cisal I). 2 = Pressure injector (Gidlund). 3 = Television for lateral fluoroscopy. 4 = Television for frontal fluoroscopy. 5 = Image intensifier for lateral fluoposcopy. 6 = Image intensifier for frontal fluoroscopy. 7 = Rapid serial film changer for frontal projection (AOT). 8 = Rapid serial film changer for lateral projection (AOT).

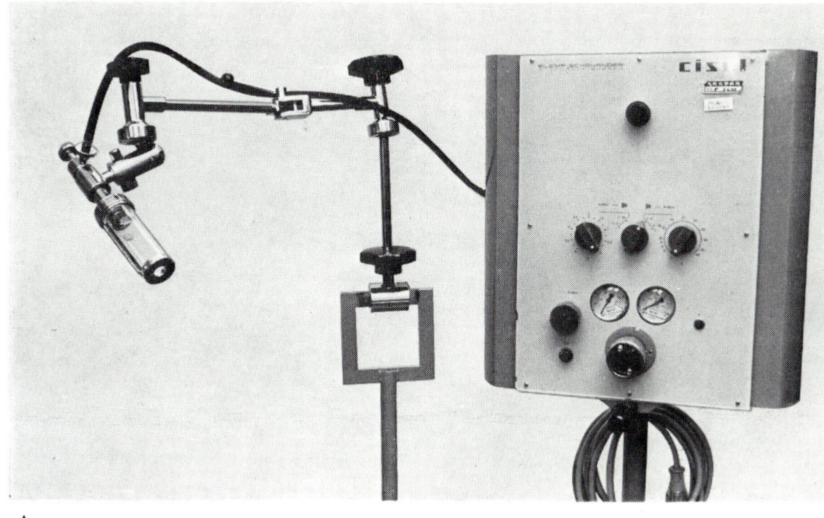

A

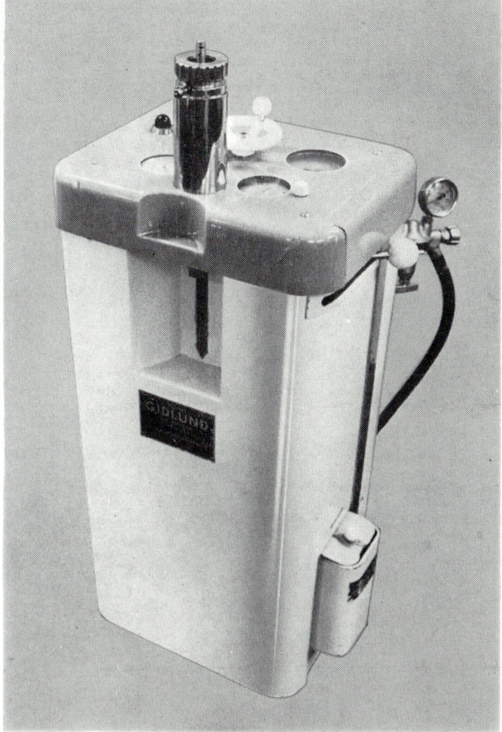

B

Fig. 8 Pressure injectors used for cerebral angiography.
A: Cisal I B: Gidlund.

tions, serial films are exposed at a rate of 3 per second for 2 seconds followed by one per second for 6 seconds. In adults, the rate of 2 per second for 3 seconds followed by one per second for 6 seconds usually provides satisfactory informations.

COMPLICATIONS

Types of complications

The complications of vertebral angiography can be divided into local, general and neurologic complications. The local complications are those closely associated with the traumatic effects at the puncture site. With the direct vertebral puncture technique, subintimal injections, hematomas and postoperative bleeding are the main complications. Brachial neuritis can occur. Arteriovenous fistulae have been reported at the puncture site following direct puncture vertebral angiography (Lester, 1966; Newton and Darroch, 1966). Following catheter techniques or retrograde brachial techniques, there may be thrombosis, formation of hematomas or postoperative bleeding at the puncture site of the femoral, axillary and brachial arteries. Pneumothorax has been reported after performing subclavian puncture angiography (Amplatz and Harner, 1962). Local complications following direct pucture techniques are prone to be associated with neurologic complications, since there is usually a compromise in vertebral blood flow.

General complications are usually due to allergic reactions to contrast media or local anesthetics. Hypotensive reactions are the most common general complications. Instances of fatal complications are observed although the exact cause of deaths is difficult to evaluate.

Neurologic complications are usually secondary to effects of contrast media on the central nervous system and compromise in cerebral blood flow by a local trauma or embolization. Complications such as amblyopia, hemianopsia, visual agnosia, cortical blindness, visual hallucination, convulsive seizures and bulbar syndromes have been reported following vertebral angiography. Quadriplegia has also been reported. These complications are usually transient, but may be permanent.

Incidence of neurologic complications

The incidence of the neurologic complications with modern contrast media have been reported by various authors (Table 9). Retrograde brachial technique appears to be associated with lower incidence of neurologic complications. It is noted that fatal complications have not followed the transfemoral or transaxillary catheter techniques.

Vertebral angiography usually has a higher complication rate than carotid angiography.

Table 9 Neurologic Complications of Vertebral Angiography in the Literature.

	Technique	No. Exams.	No. Neurologic Complications	(Transient)	(Permanent)	(Death)
Lester and Klee (1965)	Direct puncture	337	7	(5)	(0)	(2)
Ruggiero et al. (1958)	Direct puncture	277	9			(2)
Mones (1961)	Direct puncture	128	14	(13)	(1)	(0)
Scott et al. (1963)	Retrograde brachial	98	2	(0)	(1)	(1)
Tatelman and Sheehan	Transbrachial catheter with subclavian injection	220	5	(4)	(1)	(0)
Pribrum (1964)	Subclavian puncture	140	4	(4)	(0)	(0)
Takahashi et al. (1969)	Transfemoral and axillary	250	8	(7)	(1)	(0)
Newton (1966)	Transfemoral and axillary	170	9	(9)	(0)	(0)
Takahashi and Kawanami (1972)	Transfemoral and axillary	346	9	(6)	(3)	(0)

Factors causing neurologic complications

There is definitely higher incidence of neurologic complications in patients with cerebrovascular diseases (Takahashi and Kawanami, 1972). In addition, the complications are incurred when the diseased vessels are punctured (Pribrum, 1965). Therefore, a meticulous technique should be exercised in performance of vertebral angiography and the direct vertebral puncture technique is even avoided in the patients with marked atherosclerosis in the vertebral artery.

There have been reports that more complications are associated with patients in older age group, while some authors report that there is no relationship between the age of patients and incidence of complications.

According to Takahashi and Kawanami (1972) higher complication rate is encountered when a vertebrobasilar system is quite small and the posterior cerebral arteries receive their blood supply mainly from the carotid system. In addition, complications are apt to occur in cases with better reflux into the contralateral vertebral artery, suggesting the size of the catheters and the speed of injection might be another important factor (Table 10).

Prevention of complications

Sensitivity test to contrast media should be performed on the previous day or on the same day on the angiographic table to avoid allergic reactions. The use of antihistamine to prevent reactions may be advisable in patients with a positive sensitivity test.

Local complications may be reduced when angiography is performed with meticulous techniques by the experienced examiner.

When selective catheterization is performed in small arteries, use of smaller catheters and adjustment of injection pressure must be required, since the incidence of neurologic complications increases in proportion to the speed of contrast media within the vessels. It should also be emphasized that patients with cerebrovascular diseases are subjected to angiography under absolute indications.

Table 10 Complications Observed in 540 Catheter Vertebral Angiograms.

Neurologic	
1) Vertebrobasilar insufficiency clearing over 5 month period (34, M., Vertebral)	1
2) Basilar artery thrombosis (34, F., Vertebral)	1
3) Tonsillar herniation (5, F., Vertebral)	1
4) Transient nystagmus lasting 5 minutes (35, M., Vertebral)	1
5) Transient disorientation lasting 60 minutes (41, F., Vertebral and bilat. carotid; 54, M., Subclavian vertebral)	2
6) Hemiparesis clearing over 5 hours (47, F., Vertebral)	1
7) Transient disorientation lasting 5 hours (43, M., Vertebral and bilat. carotid)	1
Total	8
General and Local	
1) Thrombosis at the puncture site requiring thrombectomy (23, F., Bilat. carotid and vertebral)	1
2) Hypotensive reaction (44, M., Vertebral)	1
3) Hypotensive reaction (60, F., Vertebral and carotid)	1
Total	3

ANGIOGRAPHIC DEMONSTRATION OF COMPLICATIONS

Subintimal Injection and Dissection of the Left Vertebral Artery

A 20-year-old female: Figs. 9 and 10 (Through the courtesy of Dr. YAMAGUCHI, Research Institute of Brain & Blood Vessels, Akita)

Fig. 9 Anteroposterior projection of the neck. The catheter tip was placed in the left vertebral artery and contrast media was injected. The blood flow in the vertebral artery is slowed with reflux of contrast media into the subclavian artery. There is irregular filling of the vertebral artery. The proximal portion is densely opacified, while the distal segment is visualized faintly.

Fig. 10 Capillary phase in the anteroposterior projection. There is continued opacification of the left vertebral artery with no filling of the intracranial segments. There is irregular, interrupted filling of the vertebral artery, indicating dissection.

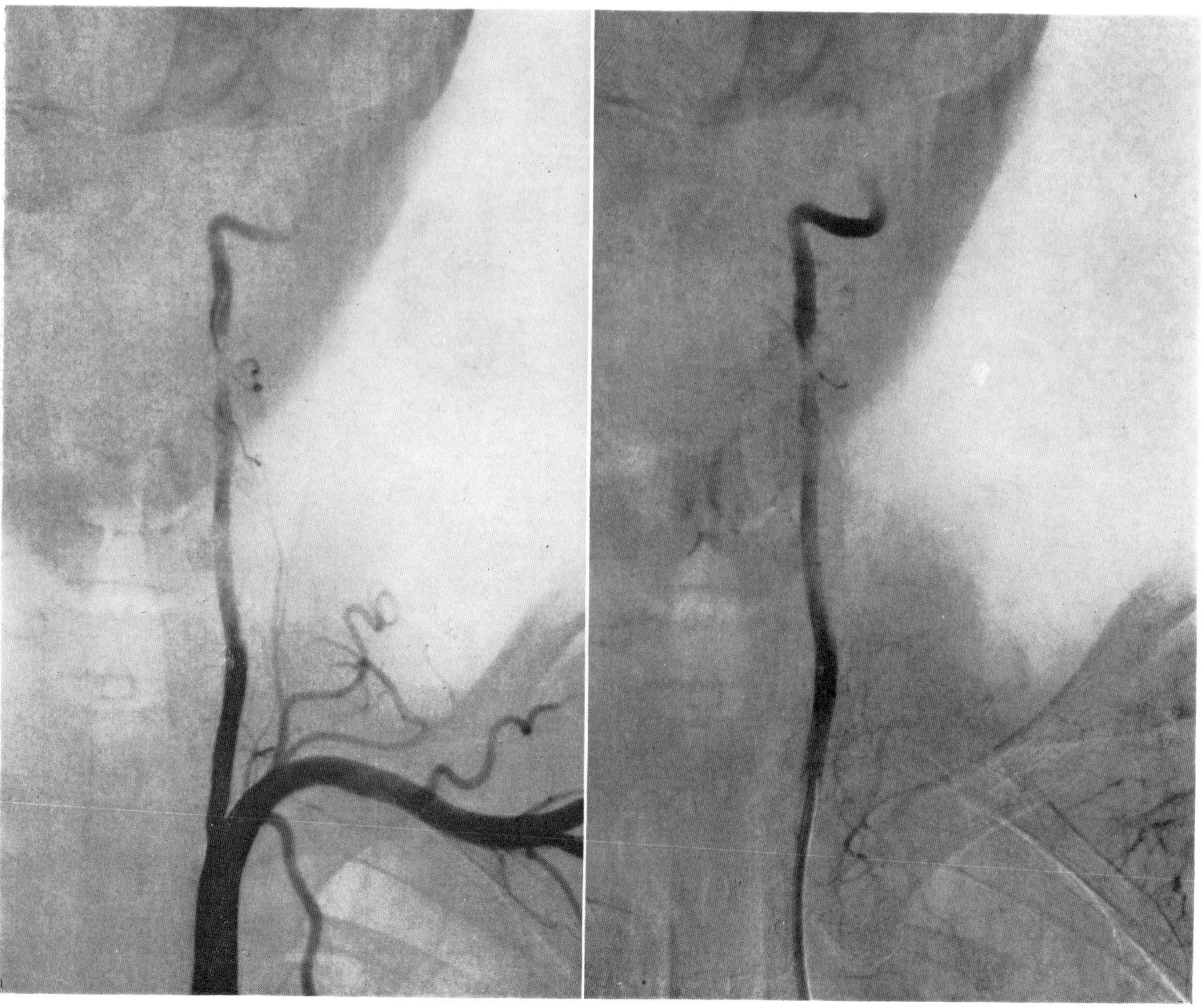

Fig. 9 **Fig. 10**

Occlusion of the Distal Vertebral Artery during Catheter Vertebral Angiography

A 34-year-old male: Fig. 11

Fig. 11 Arterial phase in the Towne projection. There developed occlusion of the distal vertebral or proximal basilar artery on the third injection (an arrow). The first and second injections were uneventful. This is probably due to spasm or embolism. The patient soon developed vertigo, dysphagia, left ptosis and left facial palsy, which cleared over a period of 5 months. There was moderate atherosclerotic disease in the carotid system.

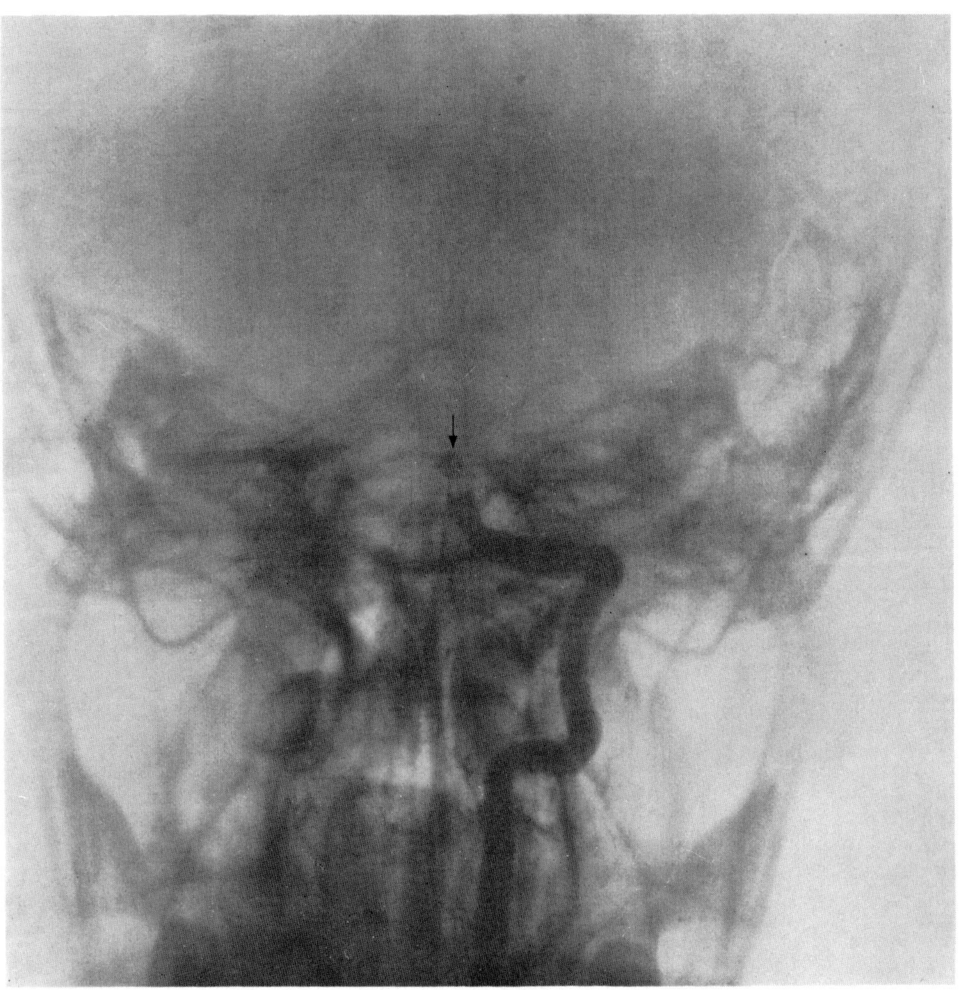

Fig. 11

Occlusion of the Basilar Artery Following Catheter Vertebral Angiography

A 29-year-old female: Figs. 12 and 13

The initial vertebral angiogram was entirely normal. The patient slowly developed drowsiness, slurring of speech and slow response to verbal stimuli approximately 8 hours after the examination. Within the next 5 hours, she developed decerebrate rigidity, soon followed by quadriplegia. She was studied for frontal astrocytoma.

Fig. 12 Arterial phase in the anteroposterior projection. This is the second vertebral angiogram 30 hours after the initial study. The anteroposterior projection shows occlusion of the basilar artery just distal to the origin of the arterior inferior cerebellar artery (an arrow). The latter artery is well shown.

Fig. 13 Arterial phase in the lateral projection. There is occlusion of the basilar artery (an arrow). The anterior inferior cerebellar artery is well opacified. There is collateral supply to the superior cerebellar artery via the posterior and anterior inferior cerebellar arteries. The posterior meningeal artery is enlarged and probably contributing to the collaterals.

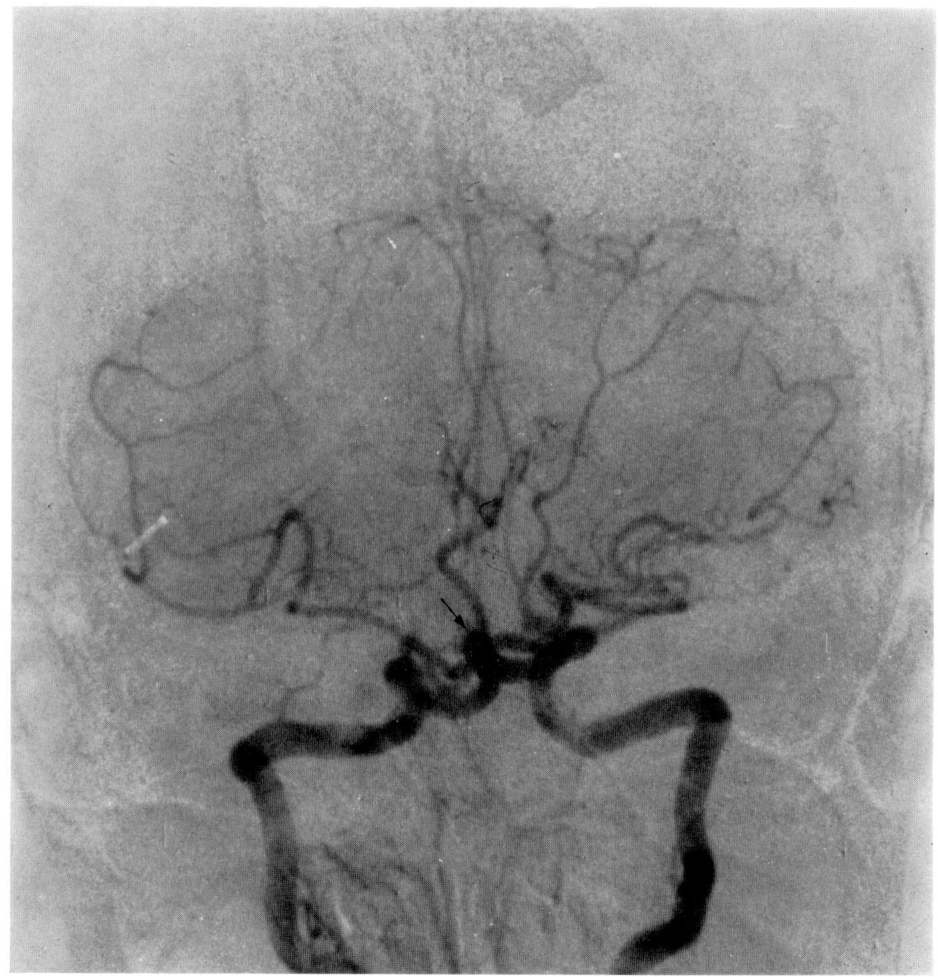

Fig. 12

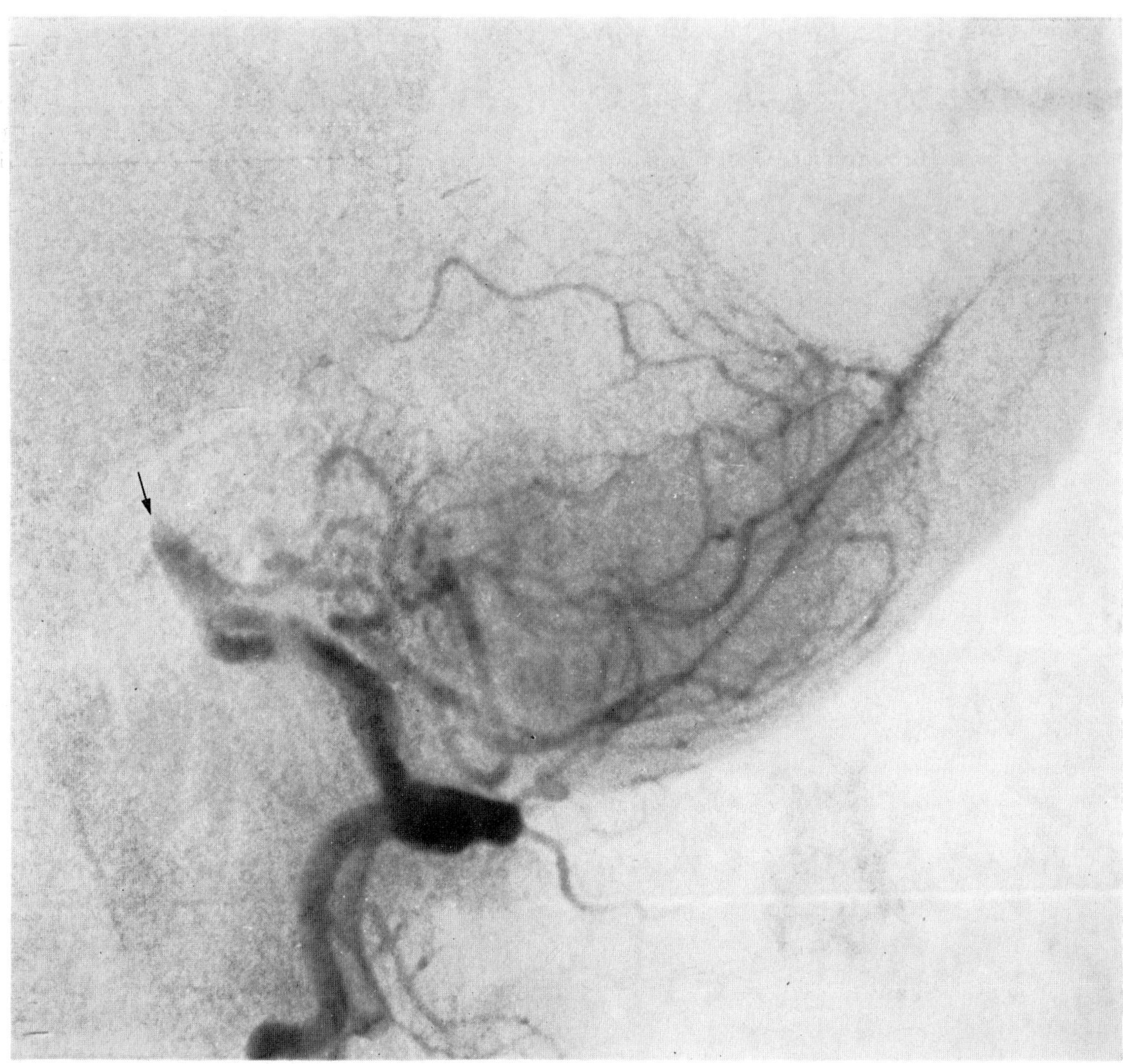

Fig. 13

4

Anatomy of the Vertebrobasilar Vascular System

Arterial System

VERTEBRAL ARTERY

Normal anatomy of the vertebrobasilar system is illustrated in a schematic diagram (Fig. 14).

The vertebral artery arises from the subclavian artery as the first branch and courses through the costotransversal foramen. The origin of the left vertebral artery may be from the thoracic aorta. There may also be other anomalies in the origin of the artery. It enters the skull by way of the foramen magnum and ends by uniting with the vertebral artery on the opposite side. Four segments can be distinguished in the course of the vertebral artery.

First segment

This is the initial part of the vertebral artery from its origin to the entry into the costotransversal foramen of the sixth cervical vertebra. The artery may enter the costotransversal foramen of the fifth vertebra.

Second segment

The second segment courses within the costotransversal foramen of the sixth cervical vertebra to the second cervical vertebra. The posterior surface of the artery is crossed by the cervical nerve roots.

Third segment

This segment lies within the transverse process of the axis and the atlas. After passing through the costotransversal foramen of the second cervical vertebra, the vertebral artery swings laterally towards the costotransversal foramen of the atlas. The artery passes through the costotransversal foramen of the atlas and then runs posteriorly within the vertebral groove.

This segment is curved with considerable redundancy.

Fourth segment

This segment begins at the exit from the transverse process of the atlas and ends at the unification with the vertebral artery from the opposite side. As soon as it comes out from the transverse process of the atlas, the artery courses horizontally backwards in the vertebral groove of the atlas, and then extends supero-anteriorly into the skull by the lateral aspect of the foramen magnum.

After penetrating the dura at the level of the foramen magnum the artery courses superiorly and medially, uniting with the vertebral artery on the opposite side at the level of the pontomedullary sulcus of the brain stem.

BRANCHES OF THE VERTEBRAL ARTERY

Many branches arise from the vertebral artery and supply the intracranial and extracranial structures. The posterior inferior cerebellar artery will be discussed in a separate section.

Muscular branches

The muscular branches of the vertebral artery arise from its first, second and third segments. They are small arterial branches. They not only supply the

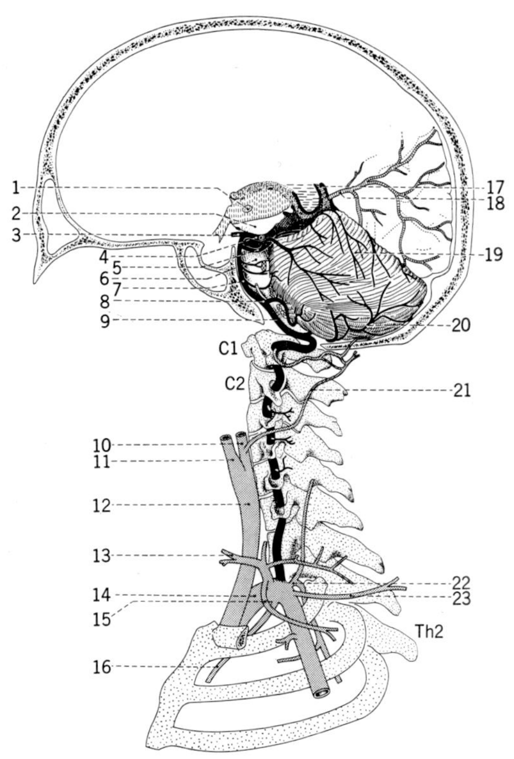

Fig. 14 Extracranial and intracranial course of the vertebral artery and its branches.
1 = Massa intermedia
2 = Cerebral peduncle
3 = Posterior communicating artery
4 = Posterior cerebral artery
5 = Superior cerebellar artery
6 = Pons
7 = Basilar artery
8 = Anterior inferior cerebellar artery
9 = Left vertebral artery
10 = External carotid artery
11 = Internal carotid artery
12 = Common carotid artery
13 = Thyrocervical arteries
14 = Subclavian artery
15 = Suprascapular artery
16 = Internal mammillary artery
17 = Splenium
18 = Right posterior cerebral artery
19 = Superior cerebellar artery
20 = Posterior inferior cerebellar artery
21 = Occipital artery
22 = Costocervical artery
23 = Transverse artery of the neck
(Through the courtesy of Butterworth & Co., Ltd. From KRAYENBÜHL and YASARGIL: Cerebral Angiography. Butterworth & Co., Ltd., 1968)

muscles in the neck, but also supply the dura and meninges in the spinal canal. There are abundant anastomoses with the spinal arteries as well as muscular branches of the occipital artery, thyrocervical trunk and costocervical trunk. The occipital artery may be visualized by injection into the vertebral artery via anastomotic branches.

Posterior spinal arteries

These arteries arise from the intracranial segment of the vertebral artery or from the posterior inferior cerebellar artery. The right and left arteries converge with each other on the posterior surface of the medulla and course downwards on the posterior aspect of the medulla and spinal cord.

These arteries are infrequently seen on vertebral angiograms.

Anterior spinal artery

The anterior spinal artery arises from the intracranial segment of the vertebral artery. The artery converges with the artery from the opposite side forming a single vessel. The artery runs inferiorly over the anterior surface of the medulla and the spinal cord.

This artery is quite frequently visualized on vertebral angiograms of good quality.

Anterior meningeal artery

This artery originates from the second segment of the extracranial vertebral artery below its first bend at the level of the axis. It enters the spinal canal and courses superiorly and medially in the anterior aspect of the canal. This artery supplies the dura at the foramen magnum.

Incidence of angiographic visualization of this artery is approximately 48 per cent (NEWTON, 1968). In the frontal projection, the artery courses superiorly and medially towards the foramen magnum, while it lies parallel to the posterior surface of the vertebral bodies.

Posterior meningeal artery

This artery arises from the extracranial vertebral artery between the arch of the atlas and the foramen magnum. The artery courses superiorly and medially towards the posterior rim of the foramen magnum, where the artery enters the skull and courses within the falx cerebelli near the midline. There are two branches of this artery which ramify within the dura. The medial branch courses superiorly in the falx cerebelli parallel to the occipital bone and frequently enters the posterior portion of the falx cerebri. The lateral branch supplies the medial aspect of the dura in the posterior fossa.

The extracranial course of this artery is slightly tortuous, but the artery shows straighter course within the skull. Incidence of angiographic visualization is approximately 35 per cent (NEWTON, 1968).

The vermian segment of the posterior inferior cerebellar artery may be confused with this artery, but differentiation is not difficult when the origin and course of this artery is taken into consideration.

POSTERIOR INFERIOR CEREBELLAR ARTERY

The posterior inferior cerebellar artery is divided into various segments and branches. Terminology proposed by HUANG and WOLF (1969) will be used in this section (Fig. 15).

Anterior medullary segment

The posterior inferior cerebellar artery originates from the distal vertebral artery and courses posteriorly and inferiorly around the medulla oblongata. This initial segment is referred to as the anterior medullary segment.

Lateral medullary segment

The artery continues backwards towards the inferior pole of the tonsil encircling the lateral aspect of the medulla. This portion of the artery is called the lateral medullary segment.

Posterior medullary segment

On reaching the inferior pole of the tonsil the vessel turns upward and courses superiorly on the posterior surface of the medulla. The inferiorly convex curve of the artery is designated as the caudal loop and this segment along the posterior surface of the medulla as the posterior medullary segment. The caudal loop usually courses down to the inferior aspect of the tonsil, but may extend below the level of the inferior tonsil or courses in the upper part of the cerebellomedullary fissure.

Supratonsillar segment

As soon as the posterior medullary segment reaches the anterior and superior aspect of the tonsil, the artery courses posteriorly over the superior pole of the tonsil. This segment is called the supratonsillar segment, the cranial loop or the choroid arc. This segment runs over the roof of the fourth ventricle. The supratonsillar segment may run transversely below the superior pole of the tonsil. In some cases the supratonsillar and the posterior medullary segment may be absent and the artery continues under the inferior pole of the tonsil, reaching the cerebellar hemisphere and paravermian sulcus. According to HUANG (1969), the choroidal point, the beginning of the supratonsillar segment, is 0.4 mm behind the anterior one-third point of a line connecting the anterior margin of the foramen magnum and the torcular (TAKAHASHI et al., 1973).

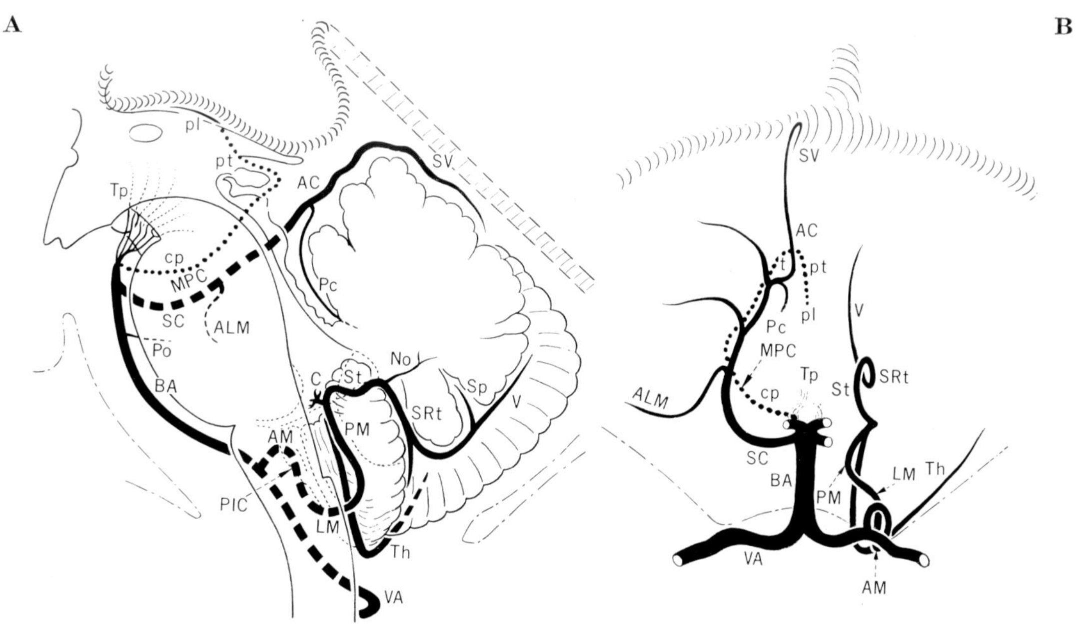

Fig. 15 Schematic diagram of the major arteries in the posterior fossa. A: Lateral projection, B: Towne projection. AC = Anterior culminate segment. ALM = Anterior lateral marginal branch. AM = Anterior medullary segment. BA = Basilar artery. C = Choroidal arteries. cp = Circumpeduncular segment. LM = Lateral medullary segment. MPC = Medial posterior choroidal artery. No = Nodular branch. Pc = Precentral cerebellar artery. PIC = Posterior inferior cerebellar artery. pl = Plexal segment. PM = Posterior medullary segment. Po = Pontine artery. pt = Pretectal segment. SC = Superior cerebellar artery. Sp = Suprapyramidal branch of the posterior inferior cerebellar artery. SRt = Superior retrotonsillar segment of the posterior inferior cerebellar artery. St = Supratonsillar segment of the posterior inferior cerebellar artery. SV = Vermian segment. Th = Tonsillohemispheric branch. Tp = Thalamoperforate arteries. V = Vermian segment. VA = Vertebral artery. t = Tectal segment. (Through the courtesy of HUANG and WOLF, Neuroradiology, 1:4, 1970)

Superior retrotonsillar segment

The supratonsillar segment continues backwards and downwards along the posterior aspect of the tonsil in the retrotonsillar fissure. This portion is the superior retrotonsillar segment.

Vermian branch

The superior retrotonsillar segment courses further downwards and then form a downward loop around the copula pyramidis. Then, the artery continues upwards and backwards in the paravermian sulcus as the vermian branch. This branch supplies the inferior vermis and its adjacent cerebellum.

Tonsillohemispheric branch

This branch originates from the distal end of the posterior medullary segment and courses over the medial surface of the tonsil. This branch sends several arterial branches to the inferior surface of the cerebellar hemisphere as well as to the tonsil.

Nodular and choroidal branches

Small arterial branches arise from the supratonsillar segment and run superiorly, supplying the choroid plexus of the fourth ventricle and the nodulus. They are infrequently seen in normal cases, but may be enlarged in tumors of the fourth ventricle and the nodulus (TAKAHASHI et al., 1973).

Variation of the posterior inferior cerebellar artery

Many variations in the origin and course of the posterior inferior cerebellar artery have been observed in association with the anomalies of the anterior inferior cerebellar artery. The size of the posterior inferior cerebellar artery is frequently inversely related to the size of the anterior inferior cerebellar artery. When the posterior inferior cerebellar artery is hypoplastic or absent, the medial branch of the anterior inferior cerebellar artery may supply the areas which would normally receive blood from the posterior inferior cerebellar artery. Conversely, the posterior inferior cerebellar artery may supply the areas normally supplied by the anterior inferior cerebellar artery. The posterior inferior cerebellar artery may arise as a common trunk with the anterior inferior cerebellar artery. Various anomalies in the origin and course of the anterior and posterior inferior cerebellar arteries have been observed (Figs. 16 and 17).

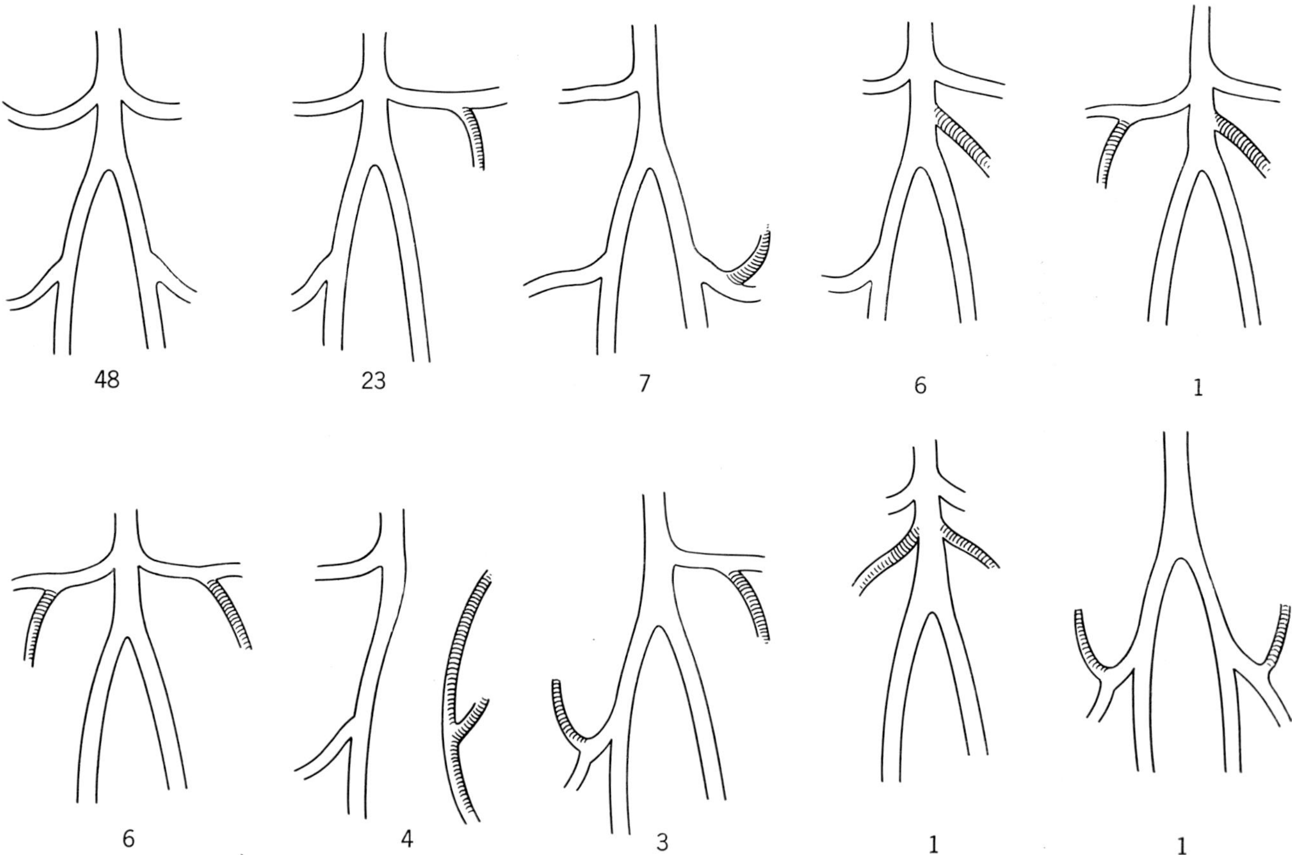

Fig. 16 Schematic diagram showing variations of the posterior inferior and anterior inferior cerebellar arteries in 100 normal patients. Statistics were obtained on the subjects with excellent visualization of both arteries. The diagram is shown with a disregard of the side.
(Through the courtesy of Radiology. From TAKAHASHI et al.: Radiology, 90: 281, 1968)

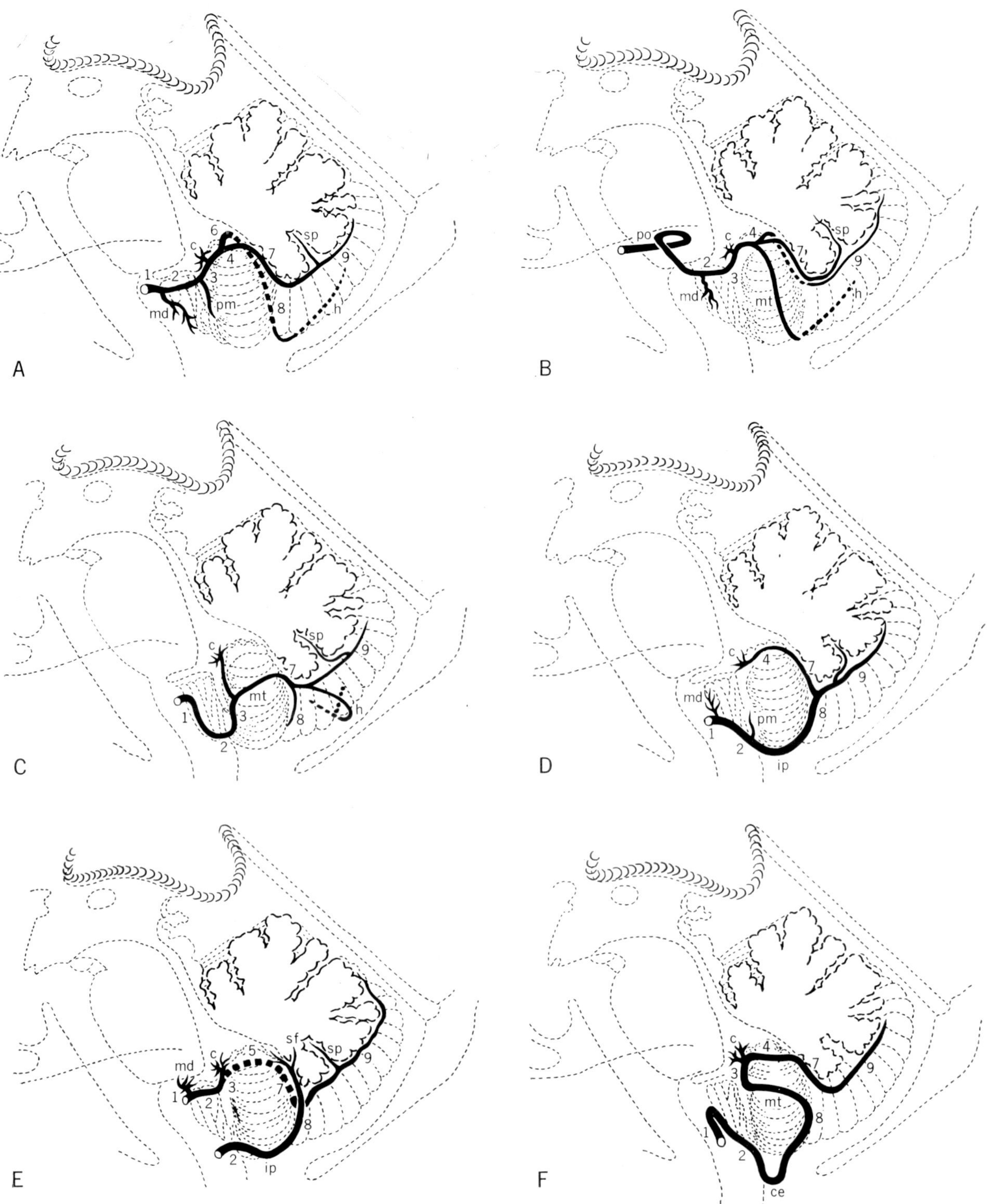

Fig. 17 Variations in the course of the posterior inferior cerebellar artery and its branches. 1 = The anterior medullary segment. 2 = Lateral medullary segment. 3 = Posterior medullary segment. 4 = Medial supratonsillar segment. 5 = Lateral supratonsillar segment. 6= Transverse supratonsillar segment. 7 = Superior retrotonsillar segment. 8 = Inferior retrotonsillar segment. 9 = Vermian segment. c = Choroidal branch. ce = Cervical segment. h = Hemispheric segment. ip = Inferior polar segment. md = Medullary branch. mt = Medial tonsillar segment. pm = Posterior medullary branch. po = Pontine segment. sf = Arterial twig in the secondary fissure behind the uvula. sp = The suprapyramidal branch. (Through the courtesy of Huang and Wolf: Am. J. Roentgenol., 107: 543, 1969)

BASILAR ARTERY AND ITS PONTINE BRANCHES

The basilar artery is formed by the junction of the two vertebral arteries at about the level of the pontomedullary sulcus. It courses superiorly in a median shallow groove of the anterior surface of the pons. Within the interpeduncular cistern the artery divides into two posterior cerebral arteries just after passing between the two abducent nerves.

The course and size of the artery

The course of the basilar artery is straight or slightly curved without deviation from the midline in young individuals. In older age group, the basilar artery is curved and dislocated from the midline, showing "S"-shaped curve. This latter configuration is usually due to marked atherosclerosis or unequal vertebral arteries. When one vertebral artery is hypoplastic, the basilar artery usually shows first convexity towards the ipsilateral side and then swings back with the second convexity towards the contralateral side.

Level of bifurcation

The basilar artery is bifurcated into the posterior cerebral arteries within the interpeduncular cistern and the level of the bifurcation is usually close to the midline and located above, below or at the level of the dorsum sellae. The terminal segment of the artery may indent the floor of the third ventricle.

Variations and anomalies

The lumen of the basilar artery may be divided by a complete septum. This anomaly is quite uncommon. A portion of this artery may be duplicated, forming a window in the center. This is called "fenestration". This is also an infrequent anomaly and is usually observed in the lower half of the basilar artery. Complete duplication of the basilar artery has also been described. In this anomaly the vertebral artery continues as the basilar artery on each side.

Pontine branches of the basilar artery

The pontine branches can be classified into 2 groups: median and transverse pontine arteries. The median pontine branches are numerous minute twigs which run posteriorly and perforate the pons perpendicularly. The transverse pontine branches originate from the posterolateral aspects of the basilar artery and course laterally and then posteriorly encircling the pons. They are variable in size and number. They give perforating branches along their course.

These pontine branches are faintly visualized in lateral projections, but infrequently seen in the Towne projections. Gabrielsen and Amundsen (1969) identified these branches in 84 per cent of the vertebral angiographies in the lateral projection and 41 per cent in the anteroposterior projection. These arterial branches are useful in locating the anterior border of the pons.

ANTERIOR INFERIOR CEREBELLAR ARTERY

The anterior inferior cerebellar artery originates from the proximal portion of the basilar artery and its main branch traverses the cerebellopontine angle.

Within the cerebellopontine angle, the artery runs in contact with either the dorsal or ventral aspect of the roots of the facial, intermediate and acoustic nerves. The artery gives off the internal auditory artery which passes into the internal auditory meatus. This latter artery may take origin directly from the basilar artery above the origin of the anterior inferior cerebellar artery.

The anterior inferior cerebellar artery ramifies into two branches within the cerebellopontine angle. The main branch comes out from the cerebellopontine angle and then courses laterally in the horizontal fissure between the superior and inferior semilunar lobules of the cerebellum. This branch sends abundant anastomoses to the branches of the superior cerebellar and posterior inferior cerebellar arteries. The medial branch courses downwards towards the biventral lobule, forming abundant anastomoses with the branches of the posterior inferior cerebellar artery.

There have been many variations in association with the anomalies of the posterior inferior cerebellar artery. This has been described previously (Fig. 16).

In order to visualize the anterior inferior cerebellar artery to good advantage, straight anteroposterior projections with subtraction technique may preferably be obtained.

SUPERIOR CEREBELLAR ARTERY

The superior cerebellar artery arises from the distal portion of the basilar artery. The main segment of this artery courses laterally and then posteriorly, encircling the midbrain. The main trunk of this artery can be divided into 3 main segments: Interpeduncular-crural, ambient and quadrigeminal (MANI and NEWTON, 1968). The artery supplies the tectum, the superior cerebellar hemisphere, and the superior vermis by sending small hemispheric branches: The marginal branch, the hemispheric branches and the superior vermis branches.

Interpeduncular-crural segment

This segment is the initial part which courses laterally within the interpeduncular and crural cisterns and surrounds the cerebral peduncle. The oculomotor nerve lies between this segment and the proximal portion of the posterior cerebral artery.

Ambient segment

The ambient segment courses posteriorly over the lateral surface of the midbrain within the ambient cistern. This segment is closely related to the tentorium, which separates this artery from the posterior cerebral artery and the basal vein of Rosenthal. Laterally, the artery is surrounded by an overlapping lip of the cerebellum.

Quadrigeminal segment

This segment lies within the quadrigeminal cistern which envelopes the quadrigeminal plate. The right and left superior cerebellar arteries approximate closely with rich anastomoses within this cistern.

Marginal branch

The marginal branch originates from the anterior portion of the ambient segment and courses anterolaterally along the anterior superior margin of the cerebellum, finally coursing within the horizontal fissure. This branch approaches the superior aspect of the cerebellopontine angle just before it enters the horizontal fissure. Within the horizontal fissure this branch anastomoses with the branches of the anterior and posterior inferior cerebellar arteries. According to MANI and NEWTON (1968), the size of this artery is inversely related to the size of the anterior inferior cerebellar artery.

The marginal branch is usually the direct continuation of the inferior trunk in the presence of duplication of the superior cerebellar arteries, while the superior trunk continues around the brain stem as the ambient segment. This branch may be called anterior lateral marginal branch.

Hemispheric branches

These branches arise from the ambient segment of the superior cerebellar artery. There are usually 2 to 4 branches on each side. At first, they ascend for a short distance and then course inferiorly, supplying the superior cerebellar hemisphere in a radial fasion. The initial hair-pin curve is produced by coursing over the overlapping lip of the superior cerebellum.

Superior vermis branch

This branch is the terminal branch of the superior cerebellar artery and direct continuation of the quadrigeminal segment. It courses posteriorly and inferiorly in the paravermian sulcus close to the midline. There are abundant anastomoses with the vermian branches of the posterior inferior cerebellar artery.

The superior vermis branch may be projected above the posterior cerebral arteries in the lateral projection, since the branches of the posterior cerebral artery may be below the level of the tentorial incisura.

The proximal portion of this branch, located anterior to the culmen, may be called anterior culminate segment.

POSTERIOR CEREBRAL ARTERY

The posterior cerebral artery arises from the distal end of the basilar artery within the interpeduncular cistern. At first the artery courses laterally and then posteriorly, encircling the midbrain within the crural and ambient cisterns. Upon reaching the quadrigeminal cistern the artery courses within the lateral portion of the quadrigeminal cistern and then terminates as the cortical branches. There are many branches which arise from each segment of this artery. This artery and its branches lie close above the edge of the tentorium, and are separated from the superior cerebellar artery by the oculomotor nerve. Normal anatomy of the artery and its branches are illustrated in a schematic diagram (Fig. 18).

The artery may be divided into 4 main segments and their cortical branches as follows. The branches to the mesencephalon will be discussed in a separate chapter.

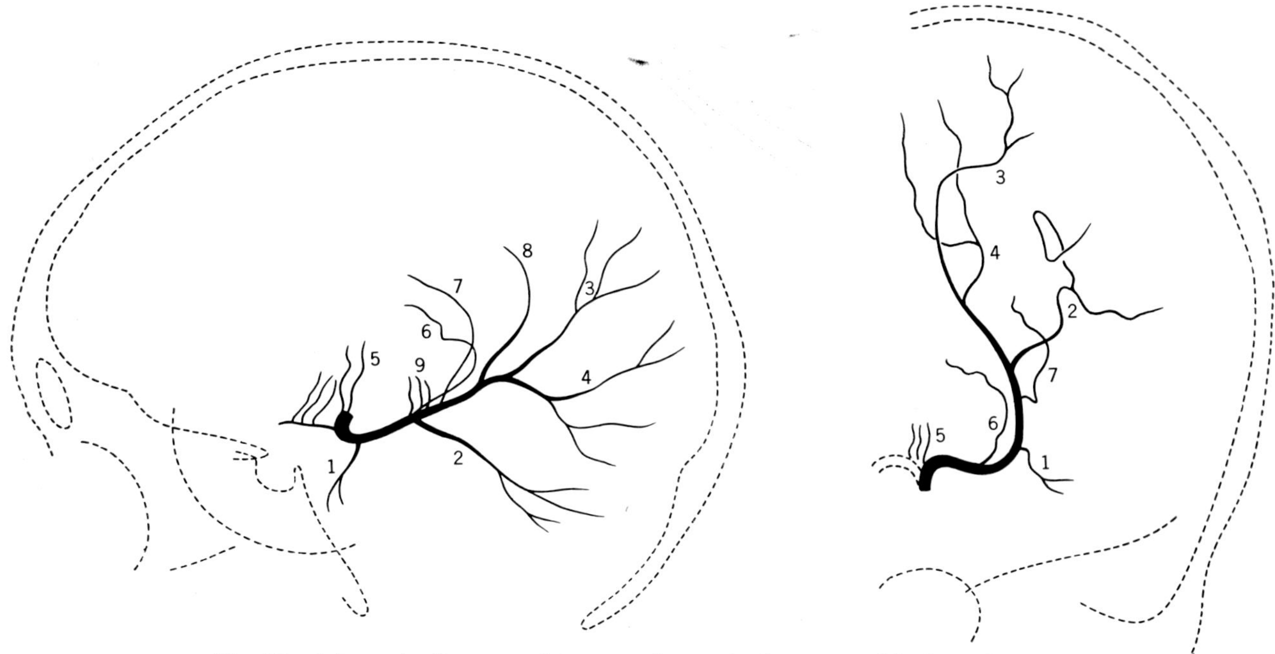

Fig. 18 Schematic diagrams of the posterior cerebral artery and its branches.
1 = Anterior temporal artery. 2 = Posterior temporal artery. 3 = Parieto-occipital artery. 4 = Calcarine artery. 5 = Thalamoperforate arteries. 6 = Medial posterior choroidal artery. 7 = Lateral posterior choroidal artery. 8 = Posterior pericallosal artery. 9 = Colliculi quadrigemini and corpori geniculati arteries.

Interpeduncular segment

This segment is the short initial part to the origin of the posterior communicating artery. This segment measures 0.5 to 1.0 cm in length.

On the half-axial views this segment extends anterolaterally, while it cannot be identified on the lateral views.

Crural segment

This segment is the portion encircling the anterolateral aspect of the peduncle.

Ambient segment

This segment courses around the upper brain stem within the ambient cistern, and usually describes a concave curve superiorly.

According to Wackenheim and Braun (1970), the maximum distance between the two segments is 3.5 to 5.5 cm.

Quadrigeminal segment

This segment is the portion which lies in the quadrigeminal cistern and corresponds to the free posterior edge of the tentorium. The segment on each side converges and shows the minimal distance between the two arteries. This distance varies from 1 to 3 cm at the level of the free margin of the tentorium (Wackenheim and Braun, 1970).

Branches to the cortex

There are 4 main cortical branches of the posterior cerebral artery: the anterior temporal, posterior temporal, parieto-occipital, and calcarine arterie (branches).

Anterior temporal artery

This artery originates from the crural segment or the proximal ambient segment of the posterior cerebral artery. It may arise from the posterior temporal artery. This artery supplies the anterior, inferior portion of the temporal lobe. Not infrequently, multiple branches arise from the same segment to supply the anterior temporal lobe.

In the lateral view the artery is projected anterior to the basilar artery, while differentiation of this artery from the marginal branch of the superior cerebellar artery may be difficult in the half-axial projection.

Posterior temporal artery

This artery arises from the middle portion of the ambient segment of the posterior cerebral artery and supplies the posterior, inferior portions of the temporal lobe and the anterior aspect of the occipital lobe. Infrequently it arises from the quadrigeminal segment of the posterior cerebral artery. In stead of one main trunk, there may be 2 or more branches directly arising from the posterior cerebral artery.

In the lateral projection this artery is located below the calcarine and parieto-occipital arteries, being superimposed upon the superior cerebellar artery. In the half-axial projection the artery extends laterally from its origin and then posteriorly.

Parieto-occipital artery

This artery is the direct continuation of the quadrigeminal segment of the posterior cerebral artery. The artery courses in the parieto-occipital fissure, supplying primarily the medial surface of the parietal and occipital lobes.

The parieto-occipital artery is the upper most cortical branch in the lateral projection. In the half-axial projection, the proximal parieto-occipital artery is the most medial of the cortical branches, while the distal branches extends lateral to the calcarine artery.

Calcarine artery

This artery arises from the parieto-occipital artery within the rostral third of the calcarine fissure and courses posteriorly deep in the calcarine fissure. There may be more than two branches.

In the lateral projection this artery is projected between the parieto-occipital and the posterior temporal arteries. In the half-axial projection the proximal calcarine artery is projected between the parieto-occipital and posterior temporal arteries. The distal segment of this artery is the most medial of the 3 posterior cortical branches.

Posterior communicating artery

This artery is frequently visualized with its anterior thalamoperforate arteries.

BRANCHES OF THE POSTERIOR CEREBRAL ARTERY SUPPLYING THE MESENCEPHALON AND ITS ADJACENT STRUCTURES

Thalamoperforate arteries

The thalamoperforate arteries arise from the interpeduncular segment of the posterior cerebral artery as well as the terminal part of the basilar artery. There are usually 2 to 6 arteries which measure less than 1 mm in diameter. The arteries course superiorly and posteriorly through the interpeduncular fossa and then penetrate the posterior perforated substance into the parenchyma. Within the parenchyma the arteries usually run along the lateral wall of the third ventricle forming anteriorly convex curves.

There are arterial branches which arise from the posterior communicating artery and take similar courses. For angiographic purposes these arteries may be called the anterior thalamoperforate arteries, while the former arteries are designated as the posterior thalamoperforate arteries.

Angiographically, the thalamoperforate arteries may be divided into cisternal and parenchymal portions. The cisternal portion courses superiorly and anteriorly and enters the parenchyma by forming a gentle curve posteriorly. The parenchymal portion runs superiorly adjacent to the midline.

Medial posterior choroidal artery

The medial posterior choroidal artery originates from the interpeduncular or crural segment of the posterior cerebral artery. The artery runs parallel to the posterior cerebral artery around the brain stem within the ambient cistern and enters the quadrigeminal cistern. Within this cistern the artery courses superiorly and anteriorly, passing lateral to the pineal gland. This arterial segment forms a figure "3". The final course of this artery is towards the foramen of Monro within the velum interpositum alongside the internal cerebral vein. During the latter course the artery supplies the choroid plexus of the third ventricle.

It is quite difficult to identify the medial posterior choroidal artery in the anteroposterior projection, unless the technique is of supreme quality. In the lateral projection, the segment encircling the brain stem is superimposed over the posterior cerebral artery. Therefore, the segment beyond the quaridgeminal cistern is identifiable on angiograms. As previously stated, this segment shows a figure "3" in close association with the pineal body and is usually localized anterior to the lateral posterior choroidal artery.

Lateral posterior choroidal arteries

These arteries arise from the crural or ambient segments of the posterior cerebral artery. There are usually 2 to 6 arteries on each side. They immediately enter the choroid fissure and supply the choroid plexus of the lateral ventricle. The anterior branch of these arteries supplies the choroid plexus of the anterior portion of the temporal horn together with the anterior choroidal artery from the internal carotid artery. The posterior branches enter the choroid fissure, course over the thalamus and enter the lateral ventricle. They terminate in the choroid plexus of the lateral ventricle, the trigone and the tela choroidea over the thalamus.

Angiographically, the posterior branches of the lateral posterior choroidal arteries describe a large anteriorly convex curve over the pulvinar. They may be projected posterior to the medial posterior choroidal arteries or superimposed over this latter artery. They do not form a figure "3" appearance unlike the medial posterior choroidal artery.

Posterior pericallosal artery

This artery usually arises from the parieto-occipital branch of the posterior cerebral artery within the quadrigeminal cistern. It courses posteriorly and superiorly around the posteroinferior margin of the splenium, forming a smooth curve. The artery then enters the pericallosal cistern and courses anteriorly over the corpus callosum. There are rich anastomoses between the posterior and anterior pericallosal arteries. The artery may extend beyond the cingulate gyrus and supply the callosomarginal sulcus.

The artery may arise from a trunk common with the medial posterior choroidal artery or from the calcarine branch of the posterior cerebral artery.

Angiographically, this artery is located about 1.0 cm behind the curve of the lateral posterior choroidal arteries, and usually shows backward bends at the posteroinferior margin of the splenium. The artery cannot be localized in the frontal projections.

The distance between the most posterior point of the lateral posterior choroidal artery and the posterior pericallosal artery is less than 21 mm in normal subjects when the mesurement is made on a line from the tuberculum sellae to the most posterior curve of the lateral posterior choroidal arteries (GALLOWAY et al., 1964).

Colliculi quadrigemini and corpori geniculati arteries

These arteries arise from the ambient and quadrigeminal segments of the posterior cerebral artery and supply the quadrigeminal colliculi and the geniculate bodies. They are rarely opacified in routine angiograms.

NORMAL ARTERIAL PHASES OF VERTEBRAL ANGIOGRAMS

Normal Arterial Phase of a Vertebral Angiogram

A 35-year-old female: Figs. 19 and 20

Fig. 19 Arterial phase in the lateral projection. The arteries show normal course and branching. The posterior inferior cerebellar artery shows normal course except for the small caudal loop (an arrow) and anomalous origin of the tonsillohemispheric branch (a crossed arrow). The latter artery originates from the distal portion of the cranial loop. The anterior temporal arteries are superimposed over the ambient segment of the superior cerebellar arteries (3 arrowheads). The arterial branches to the mesencephalon are well visualized.

Fig. 20 Arterial phase in the Towne projection. There is good visualization of normal anterior inferior cerebellar artery on the right. The parieto-occipital branch is prominent, while the calcarine branch is somewhat hypoplastic.

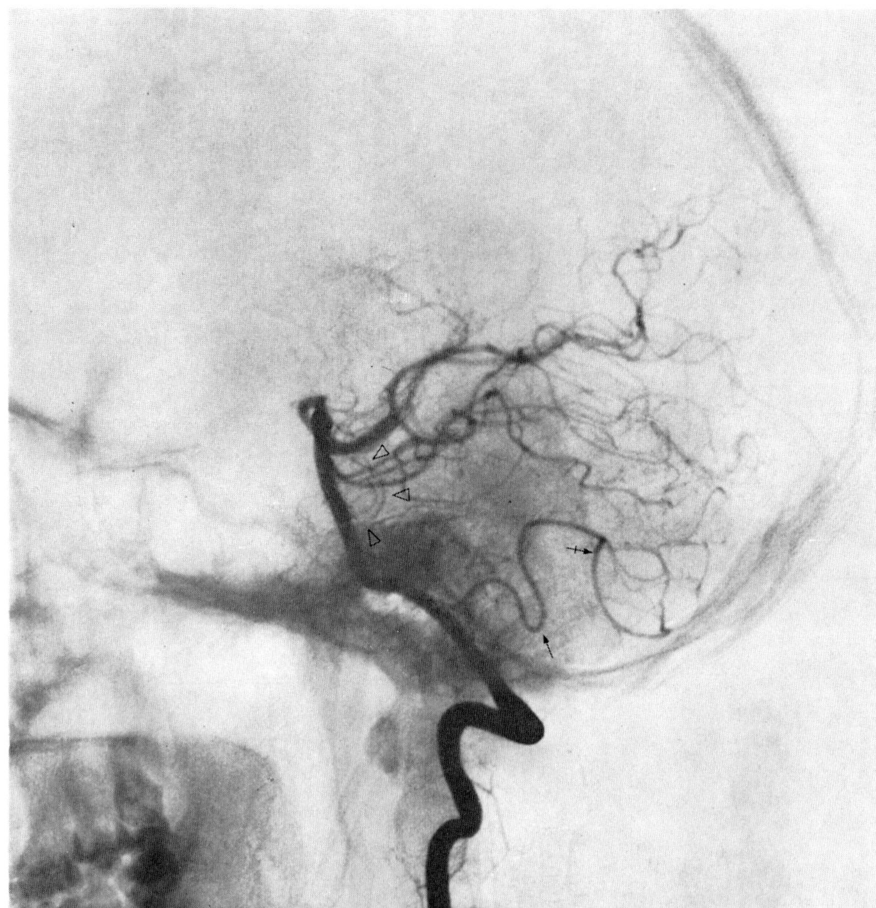

Fig. 19

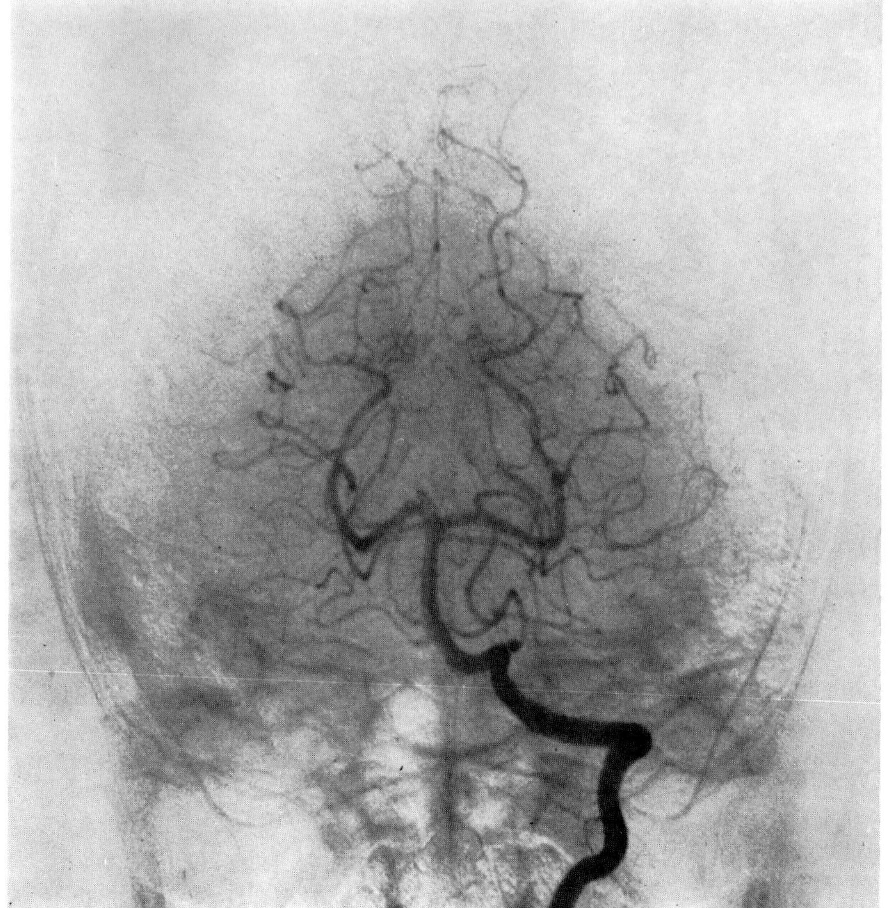

Fig. 20

Normal Arterial Phase of a Vertebral Angiogram

A 61-year-old male: Figs. 21–23

Fig. 21 Arterial phase in the lateral projection. The arteries are slightly tortuous. The right vertebral artery is hypoplastic with good reflux of contrast media (2 arrows). Four superior cerebellar arteries are superimposed at the proximal segments (2 opposing arrowheads). The arterial branches to the mesencephalon are well shown.

Fig. 22 Arterial phase in the Towne projection. The anterior and posterior inferior cerebellar arteries are superimposed and cannot be separated.

Fig. 23 Straight anteroposterior projection. There is common origin of the anterior inferior and posterior inferior cerebellar arteries on both sides. The right common trunk arises from the basilar artery and the left trunk from the vertebral artery. There are two superior cerebellar arteries on each side.

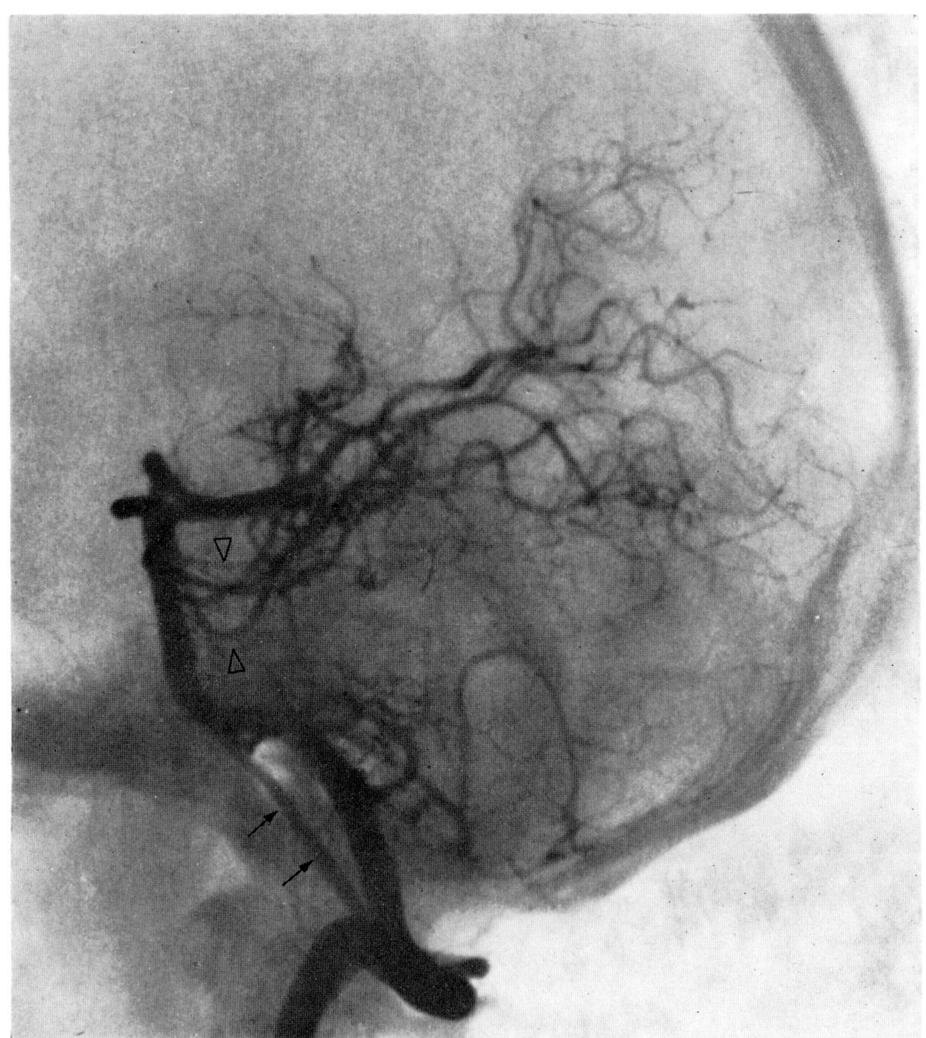

Fig. 21

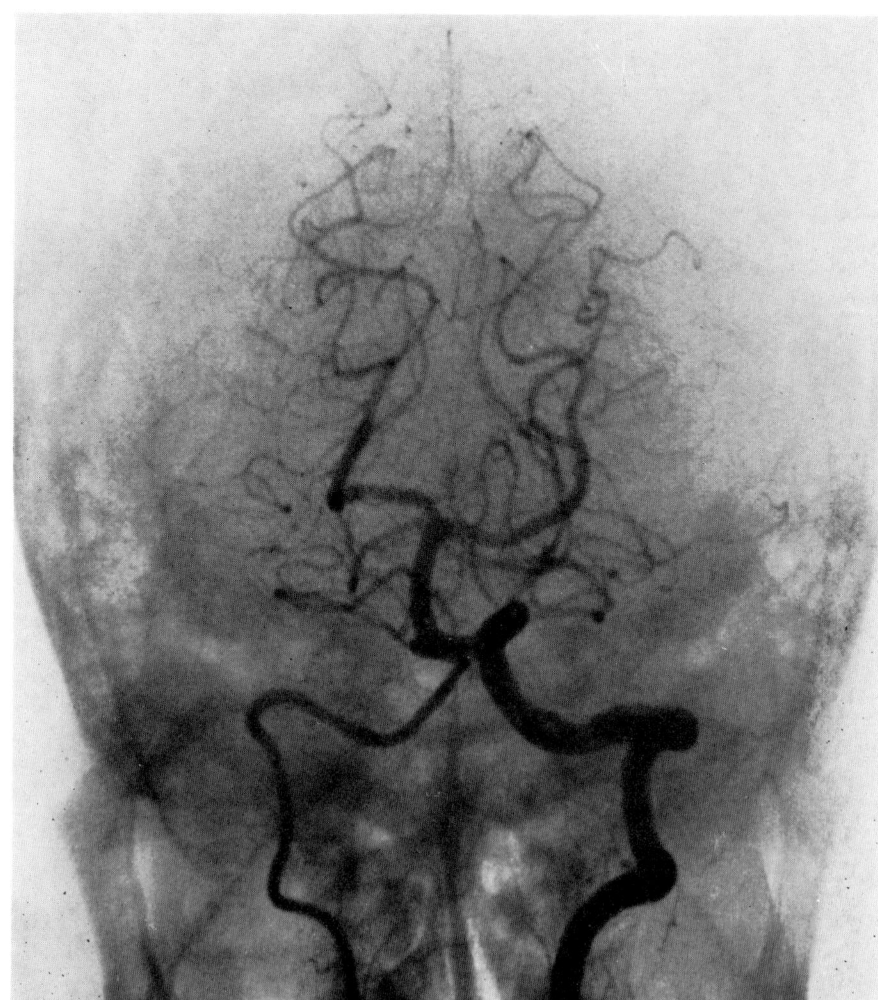

Fig. 22

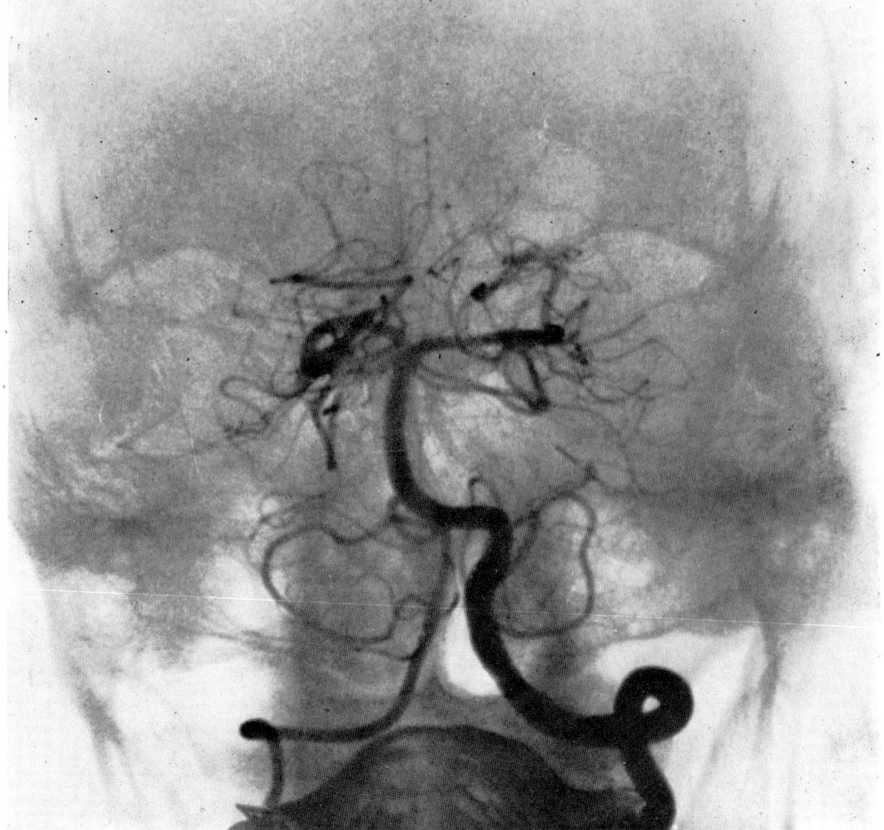

Fig. 23

Normal Arterial Phase of a Vertebral Angiogram

A 37-year-old female: Figs. 24 and 25

Fig. 24 Arterial phase in the lateral projection. The posterior inferior cerebellar arteries appear to have a high origin. The quadrigeminal and anterior culminate segments of the superior cerebellar arteries are projected above the posterior cerebral artery (3 arrows). The course of the posterior temporal artery is well shown (3 arrowheads). The remaining arterial branches show normal course and branching.

Fig. 25 Arterial phase in the Towne projection. The anterior inferior and posterior inferior cerebellar arteries on the left arise as a common trunk from the basilar artery. There are normal origins on the right. Good reflux into the right vertebral artery is seen.

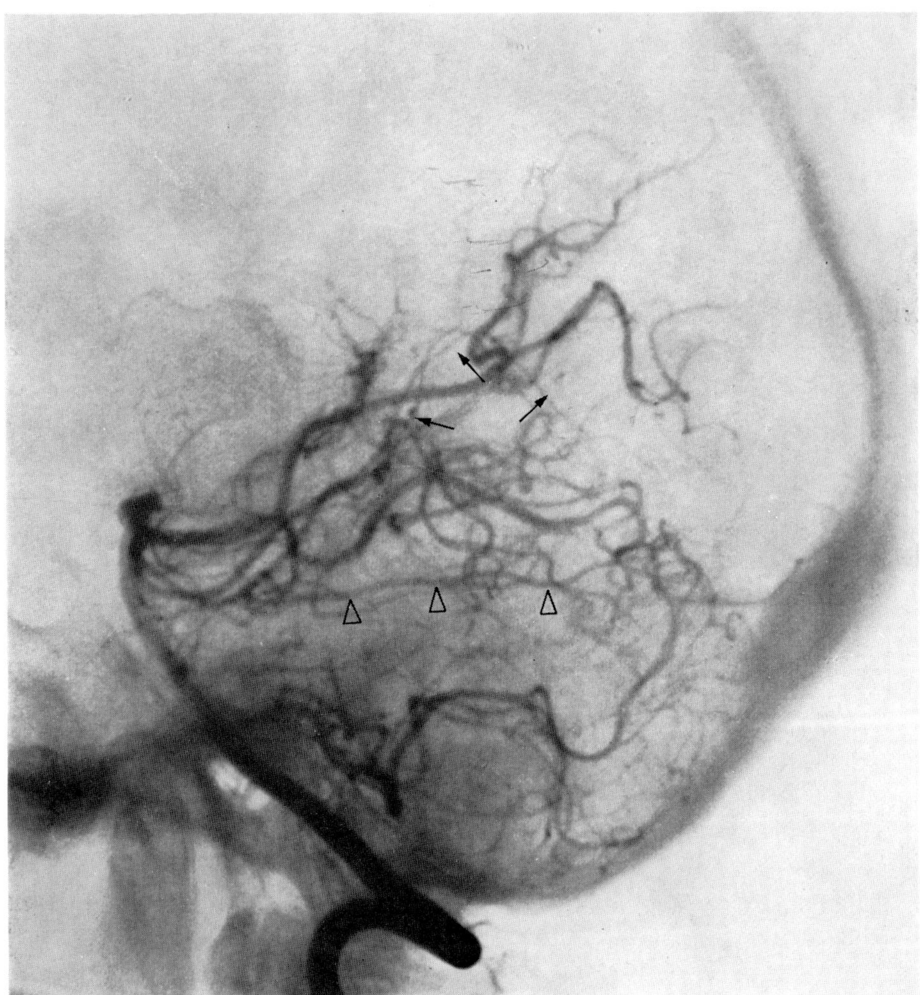

Fig. 24

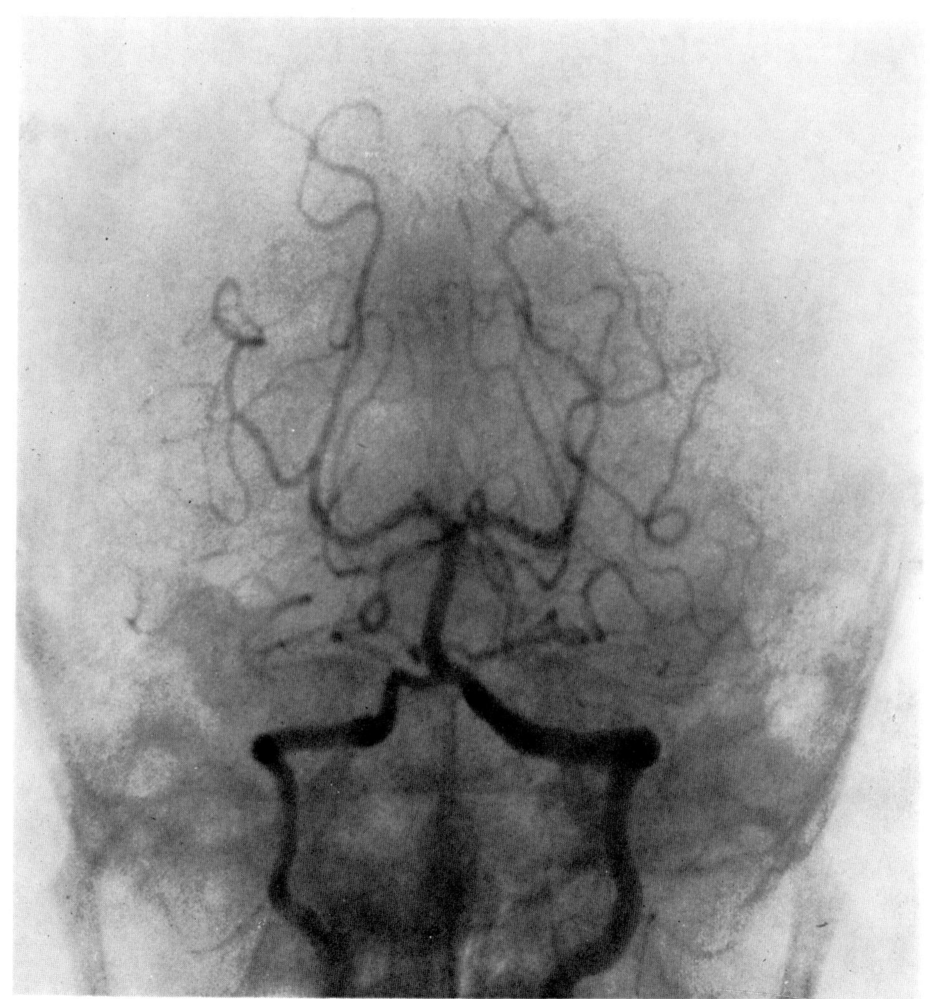

Fig. 25

Normal Posterior Inferior Cerebellar Artery

A 2-year-old female: Fig. 26

Fig. 26 Arterial phase in the Towne projection. There is spasm of the basilar artery at the time of injection with good reflux into the right vertebral artery. The normal branching of the tonsillohemispheric and vermian branches is shown to good advantage. There is an accessory hemispheric branch on the right which arises from the vermian branch (2 arrows).

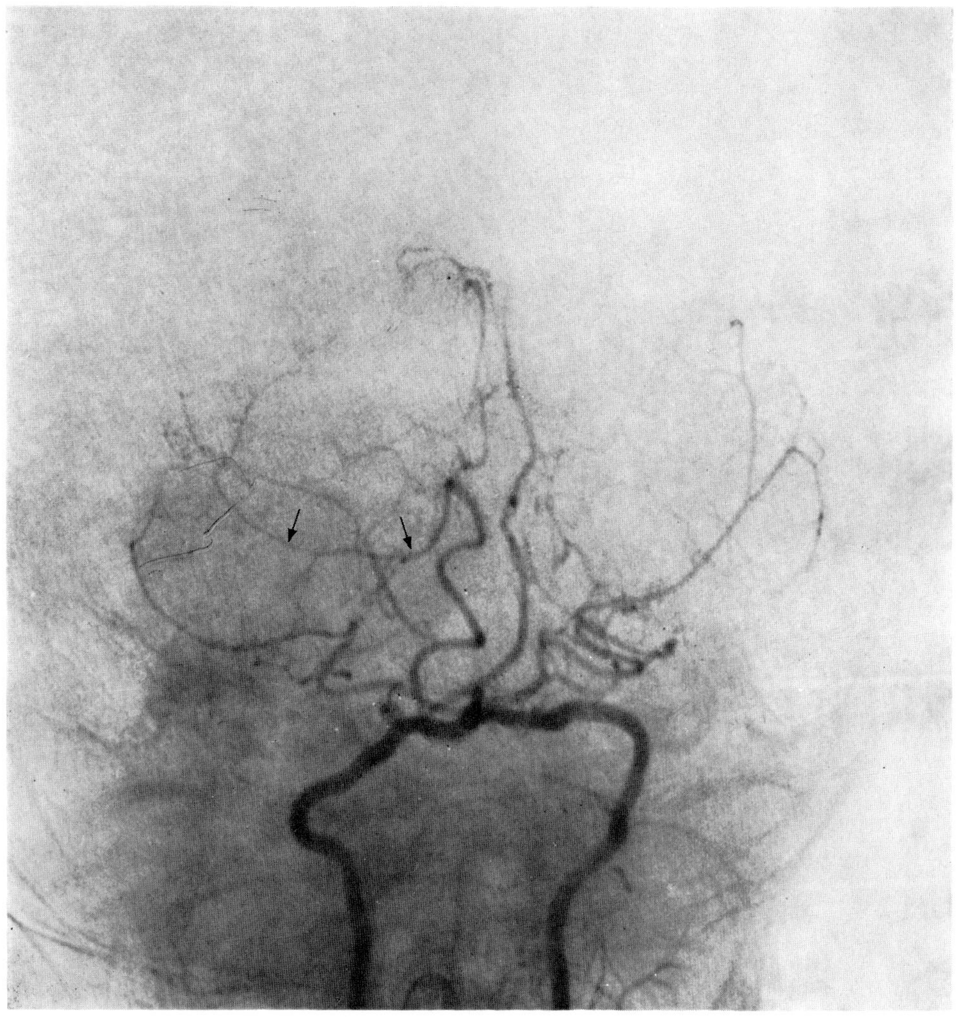

Fig. 26

Anomalous Course of the Posterior Inferior Cerebellar Artery

A 35-year-old male: Fig. 27

Fig. 27 Arterial phase in the lateral projection. The caudal loop of the left posterior inferior cerebellar artery is below the level of the foramen magnum (5 arrows). The right posterior inferior cerebellar artery takes normal course and branching (4 arrowheads). The right vertebral artery is somewhat hypoplastic.

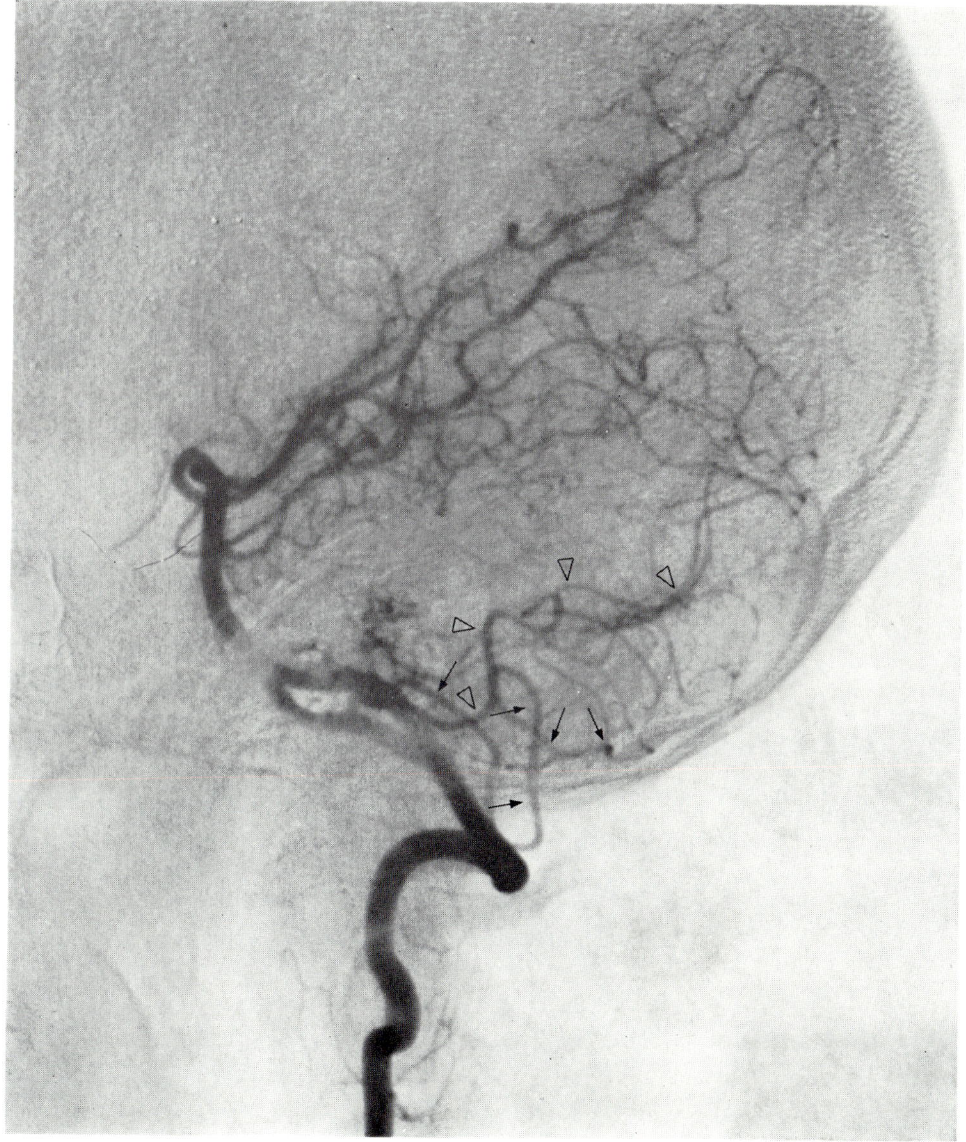

Fig. 27

Anomalous Origin and Course of the Posterior Inferior Cerebellar Artery in a Patient with a Clivus Tumor

A 53-year-old male: Figs. 28–30

Fig. 28 Arterial phase in the lateral projection. The left posterior inferior cerebellar artery originates from the third segment of the vertebral artery just above the transverse foramen of the axis (an arrow). The artery enters the spinal canal at this level and ascends toward the posterior aspect of the foramen magnum. The proximal intracranial segment of the vertebral artery, and the basilar artery are displaced posteriorly by a clivus tumor (2 open arrowheads). The posterior medullary segments of the posterior inferior cerebellar artery are also displaced backwards (2 closed arrowheads).

Fig. 29 Arterial phase in the Towne projection. The left posterior inferior cerebellar artery arises from the third segment of the vertebral artery. The course of this artery is well shown (4 arrows).

Fig. 30 Capillary phase in the Towne projection. The origin and course of the left posterior inferior cerebellar artery is demonstrated to good advantage.

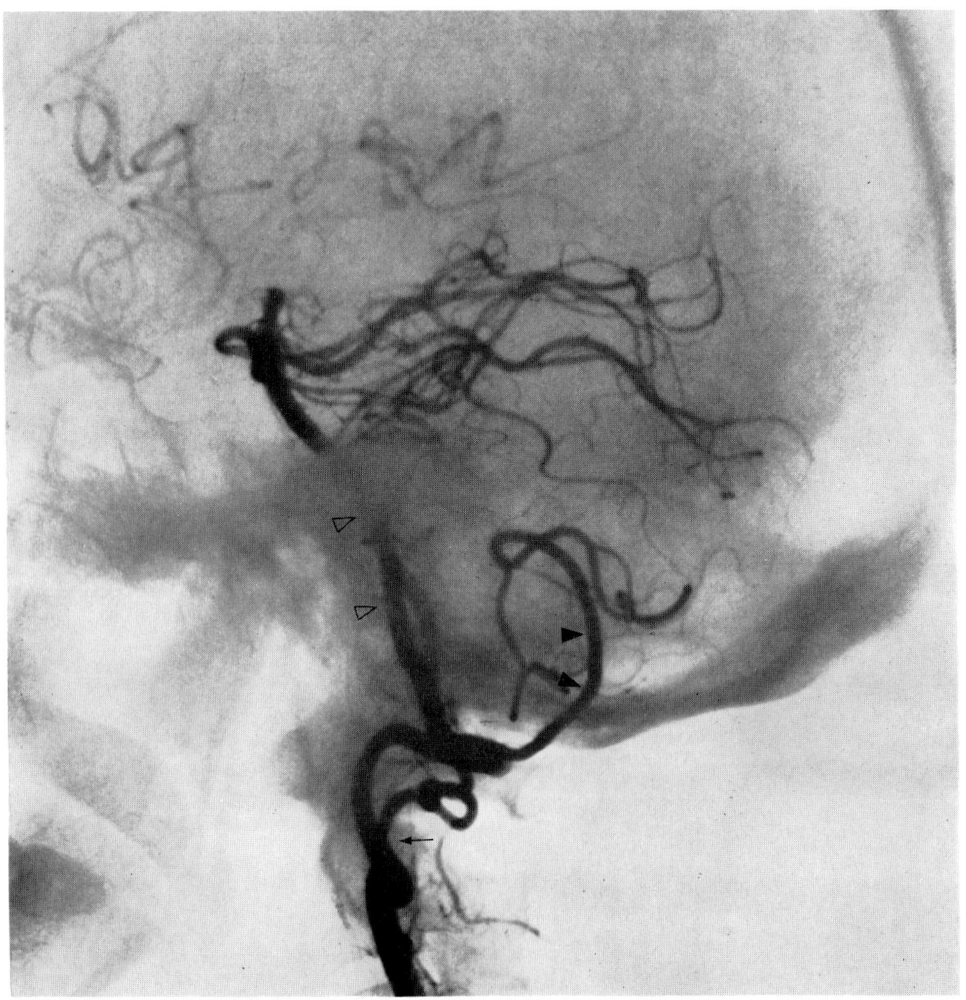

Fig. 28

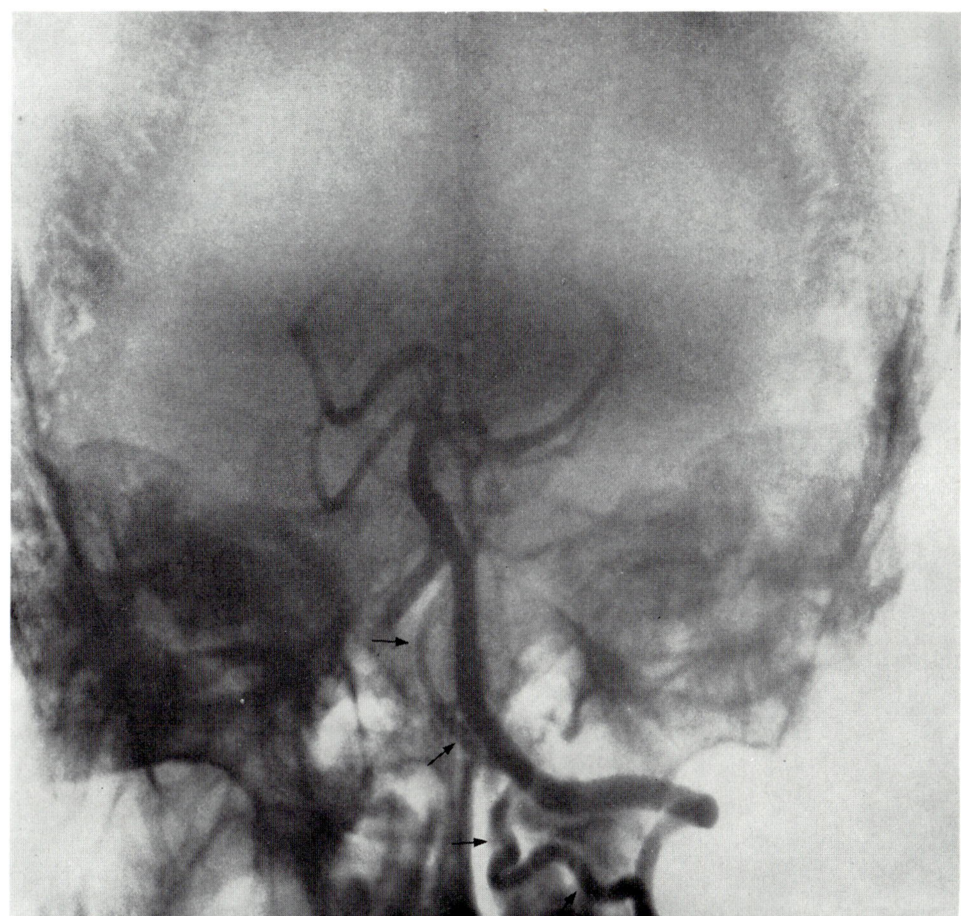

Fig. 29

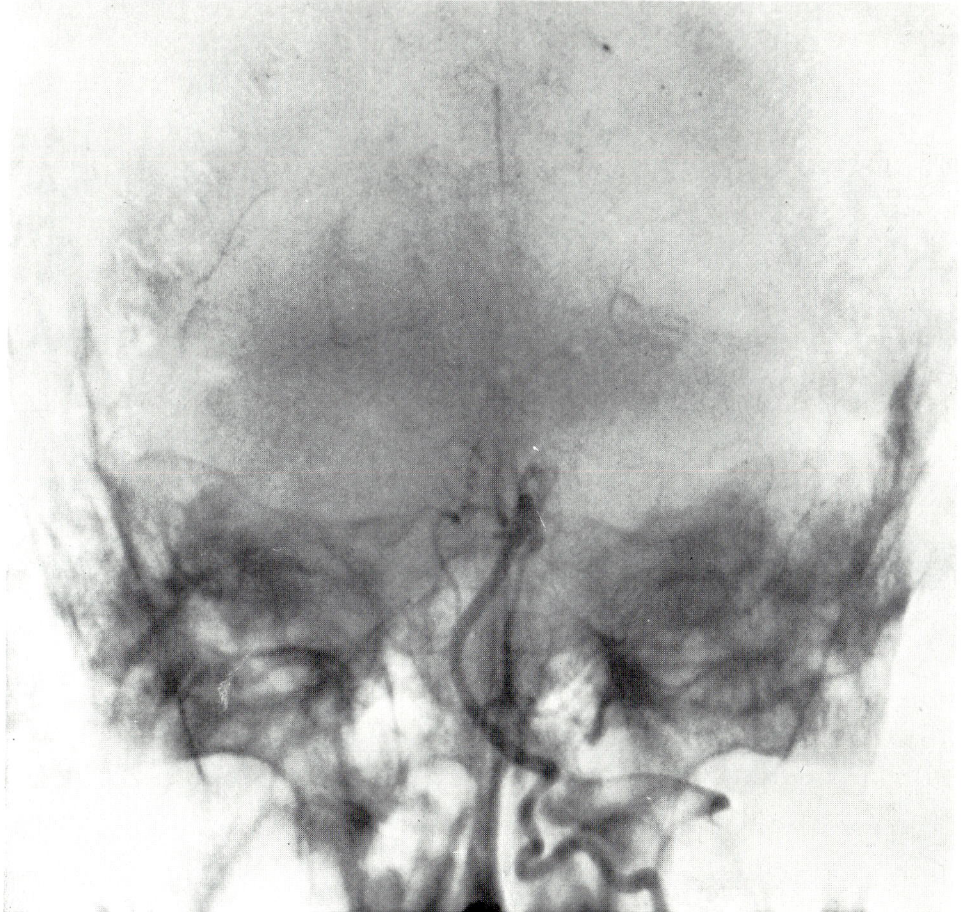

Fig. 30

Variations of the Anterior Inferior Cerebellar Arteries and Posterior Inferior Cerebellar Arteries in 5 Patients

Figs. 31–35 (Through the courtesy of Radiology. From TAKAHASHI et al.: Radiology, 90: 281, 1968)

Fig. 31 The usual pattern: both anterior inferior cerebellar arteries arise from the basilar artery and the posterior inferior cerebellar arteries from the vertebral arteries.

Fig. 32 The right anterior inferior cerebellar artery supplies the area which is ordinarily supplied by the posterior inferior cerebellar artery. Note the hypoplastic right vertebral artery and absence of the right posterior inferior cerebellar artery. There is the usual pattern on the left.

Fig. 33 The right posterior inferior cerebellar artery arises from the basilar artery just below the origin of the right anterior inferior cerebellar artery. The usual pattern on the left.

Fig. 34 The left posterior inferior cerebellar artery arises from the basilar artery. The usual pattern on the right.

Fig. 35 The anterior inferior and posterior inferior cerebellar arteries arise as a common trunk from the basilar artery on both sides. Two superior cerebellar arteries are noted bilaterally.

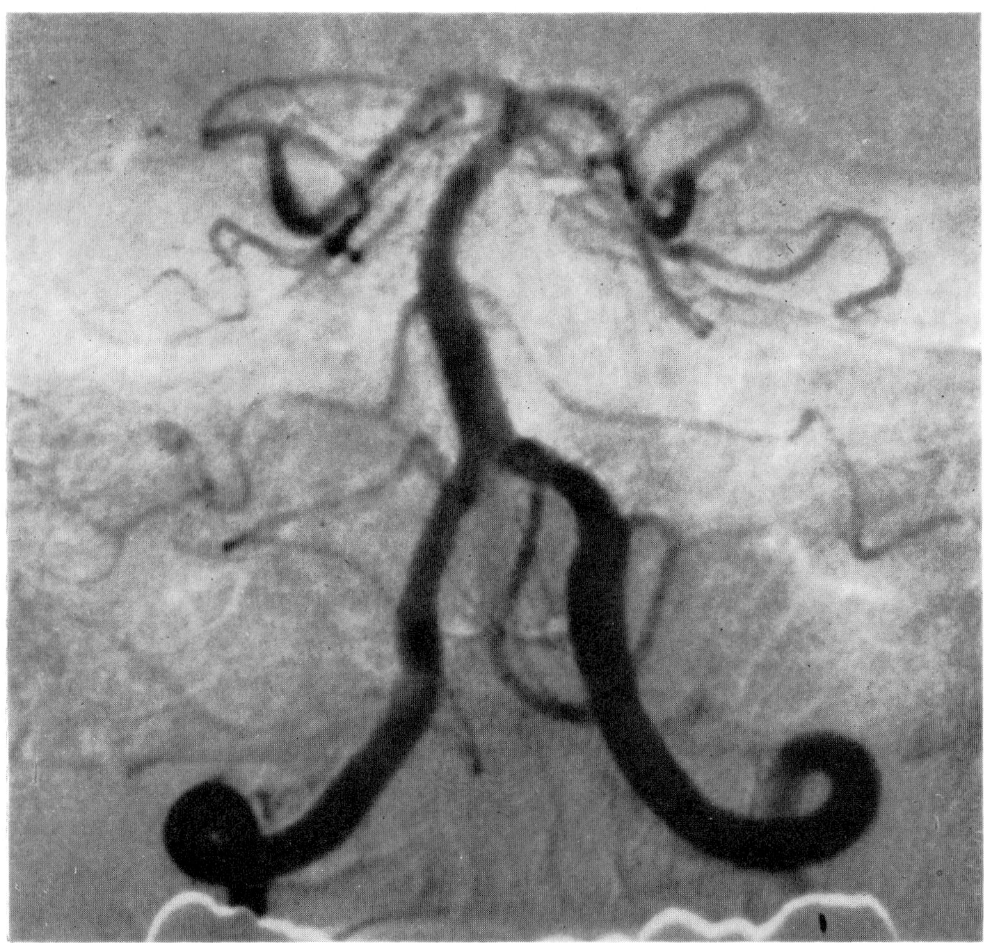

Fig. 31

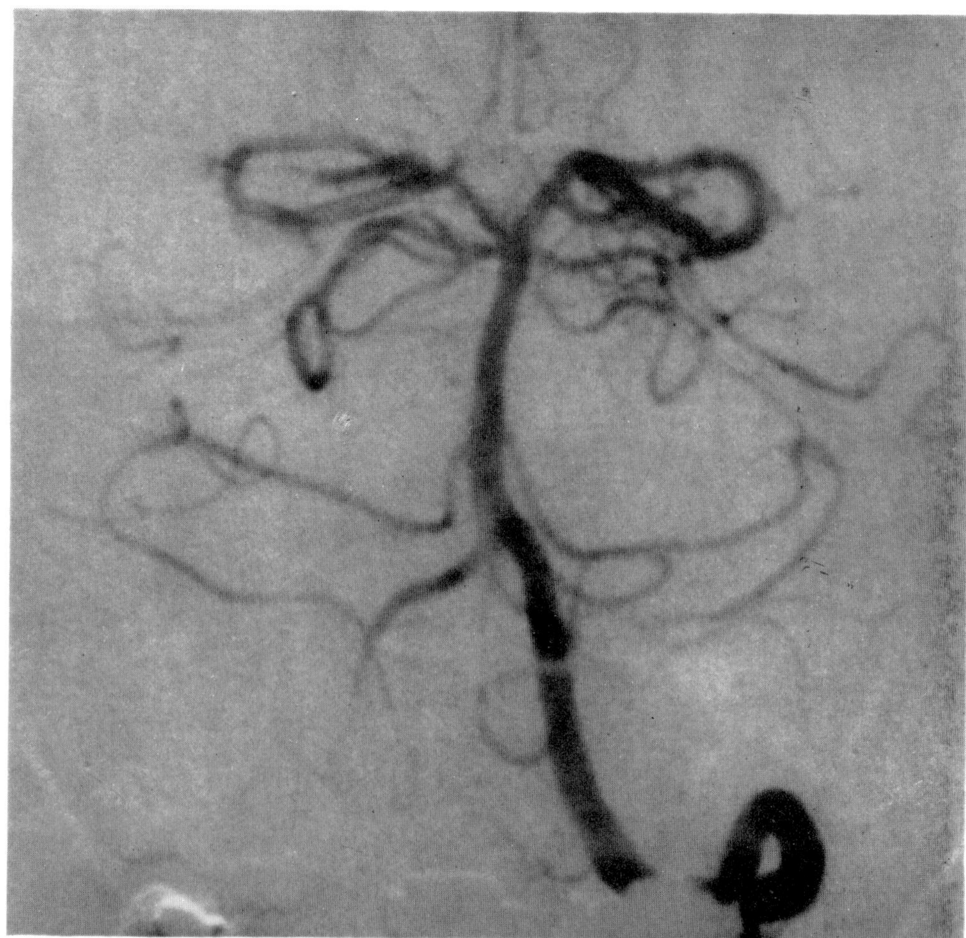

Fig. 32

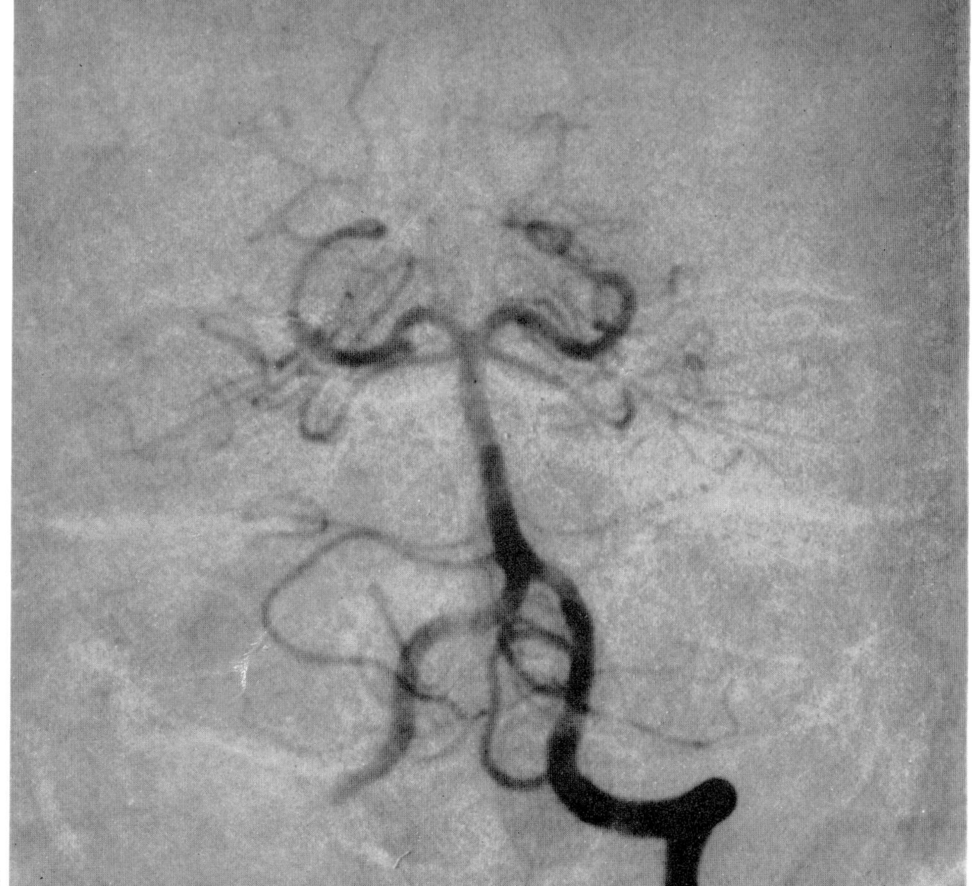

Fig. 33

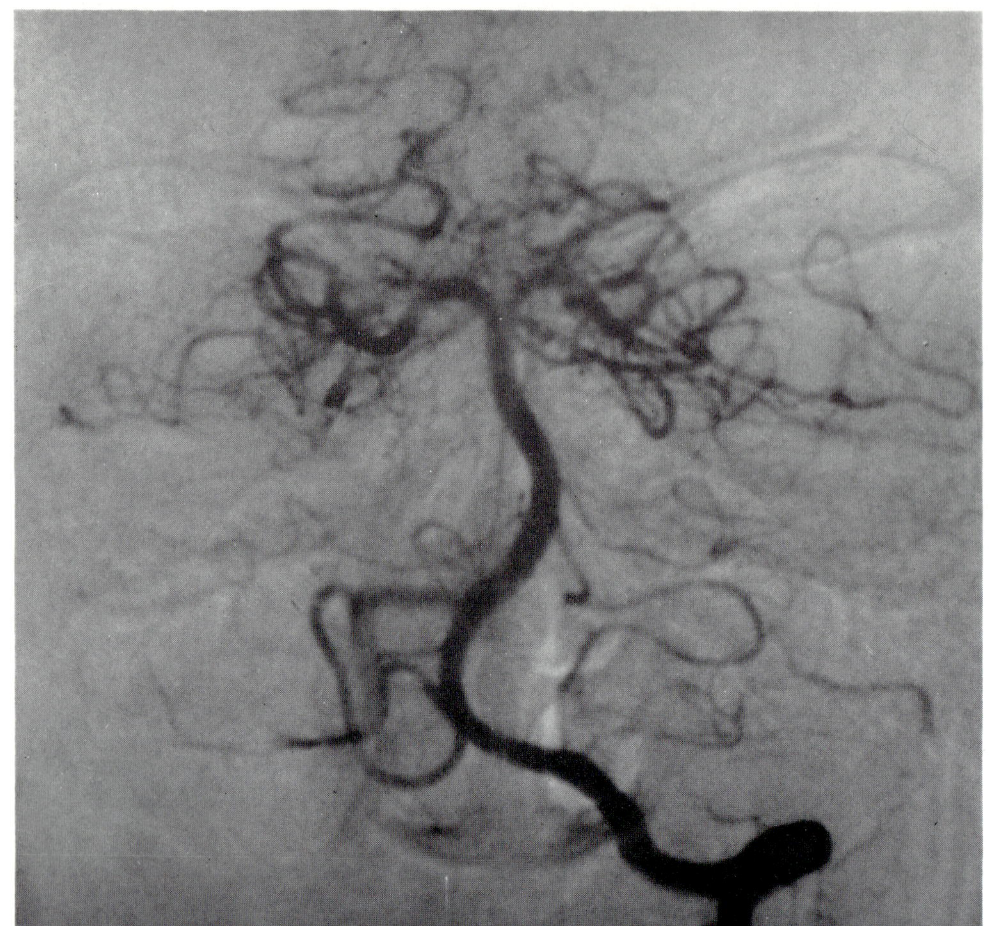

Fig. 34

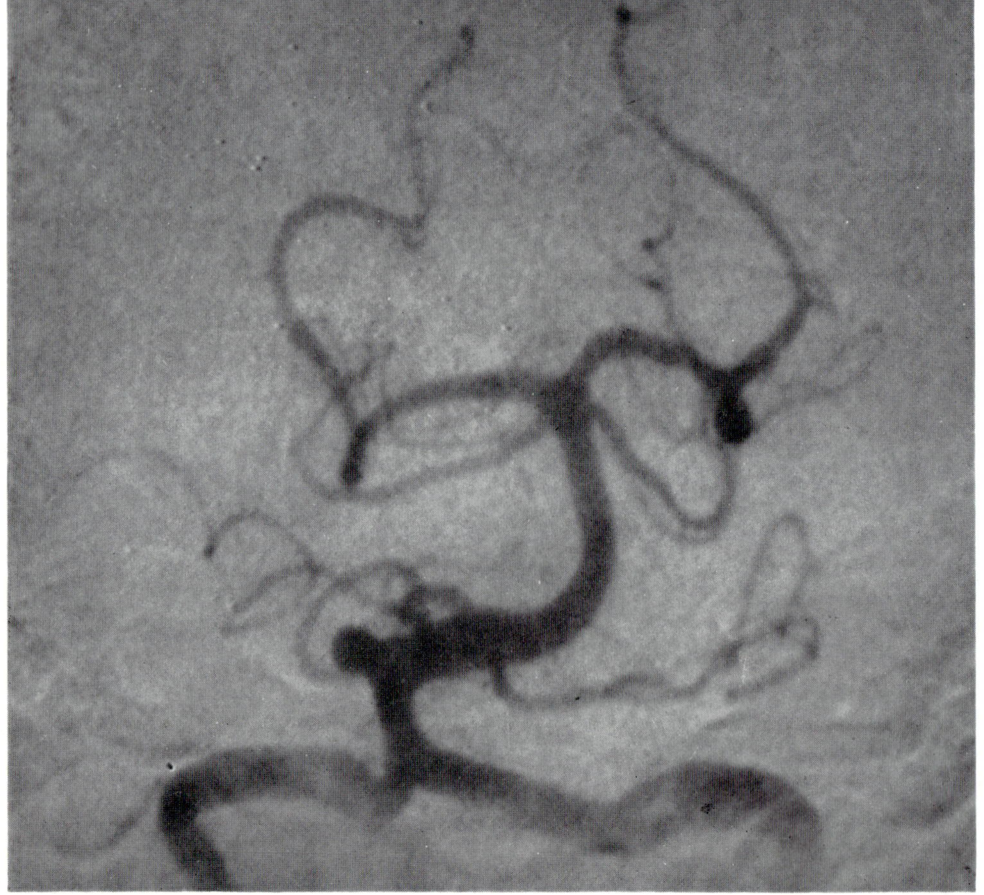

Fig. 35

Anomalous Origin and Course of the Vertebral and Posterior Inferior Cerebellar Arteries

A 37-year-old male: Figs. 36 and 37

Fig. 36 Arterial phase in the lateral projection. The left vertebral artery swings posteriorly between C_1 and C_2, entering the spinal canal below the atlas (an arrow). The posterior inferior cerebellar artery originates below the foramen magnum (a crossed arrow).

Fig. 37 Arterial phase in the Towne projection. The vertebral artery enters the spinal canal below the atlas (an arrow). There is considerably low origin of the posterior inferior cerebellar artery (a crossed arrow).

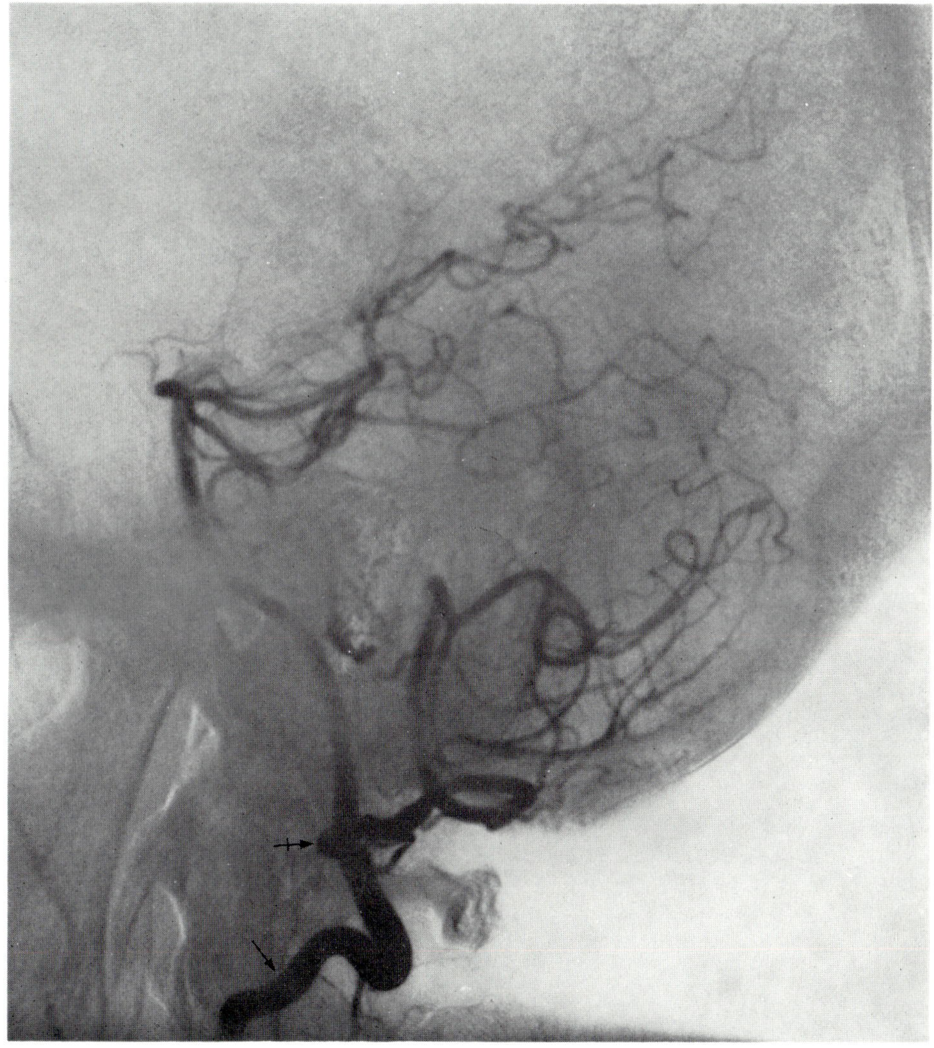

Fig. 36

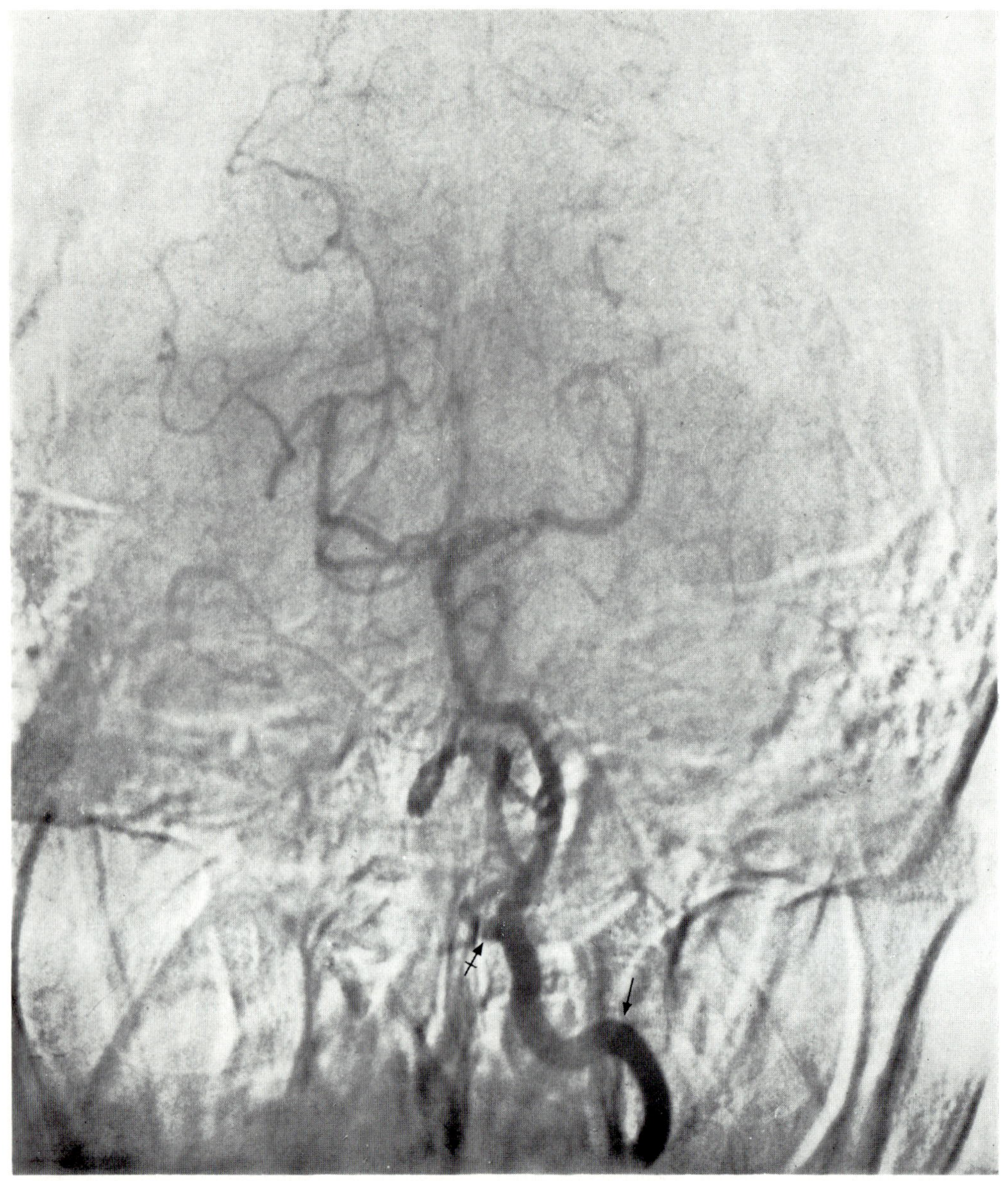

Fig. 37

Hyperplasia of the Superior Cerebellar Artery with Hypoplastic Posterior Inferior Cerebellar Artery in a Patient with Membranous Occlusion of the Foramen of Magendie

A 42-year-old male: Figs. 38 and 39

Fig. 38 Arterial phase in the lateral projection. The right superior cerebellar artery is considerably large and, in addition to the superior vermis, supplies the inferior vermis and its adjacent cerebellum which are normally vascularized by the vermian branch of the posterior inferior cerebellar artery (4 arrows). The vermian branches of the posterior inferior cerebellar artery are hypoplastic.

Fig. 39 Arterial phase in the Towne projection. Hyperplasia of the right superior cerebellar artery is well shown (5 arrows). There is filling of the hemispheric branches over the inferior cerebellar hemisphere, which are usually supplied by the posterior inferior cerebellar artery.

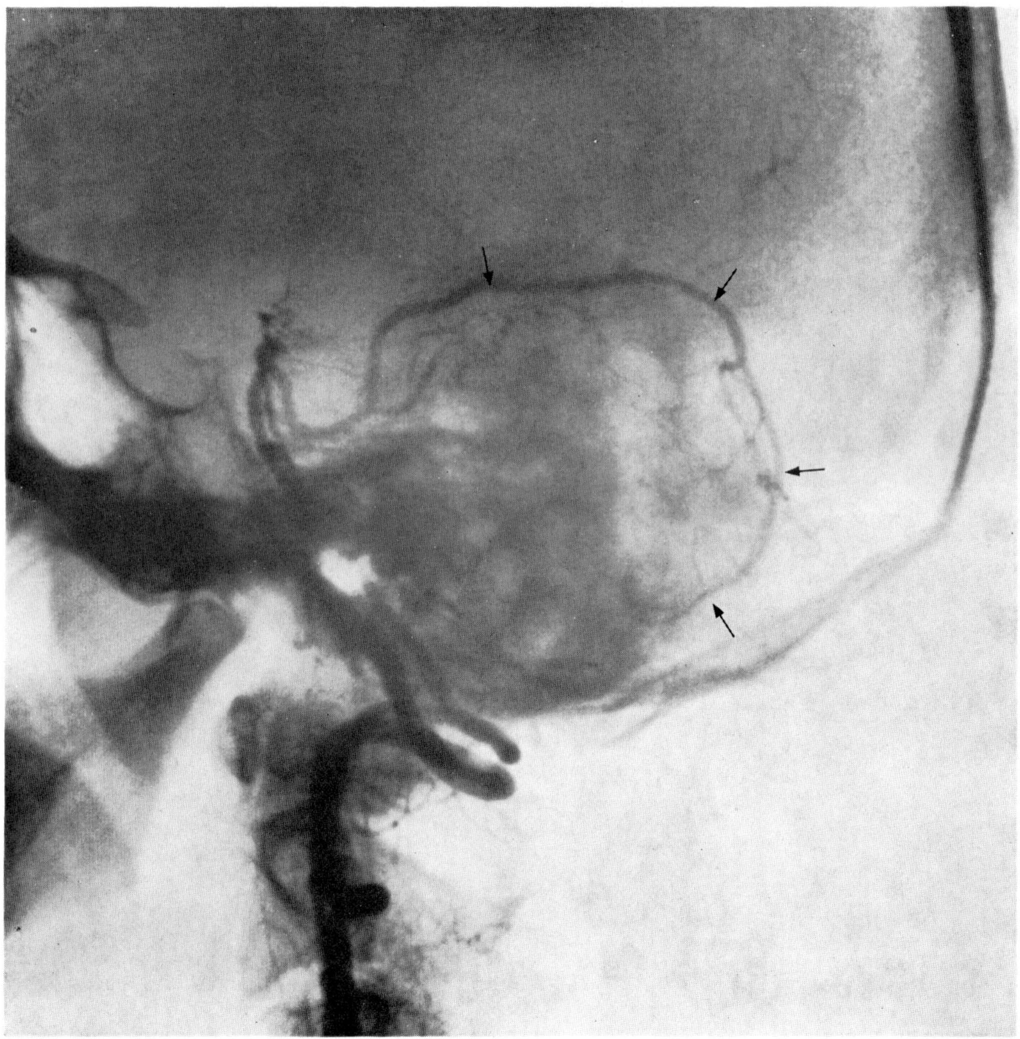

Fig. 38

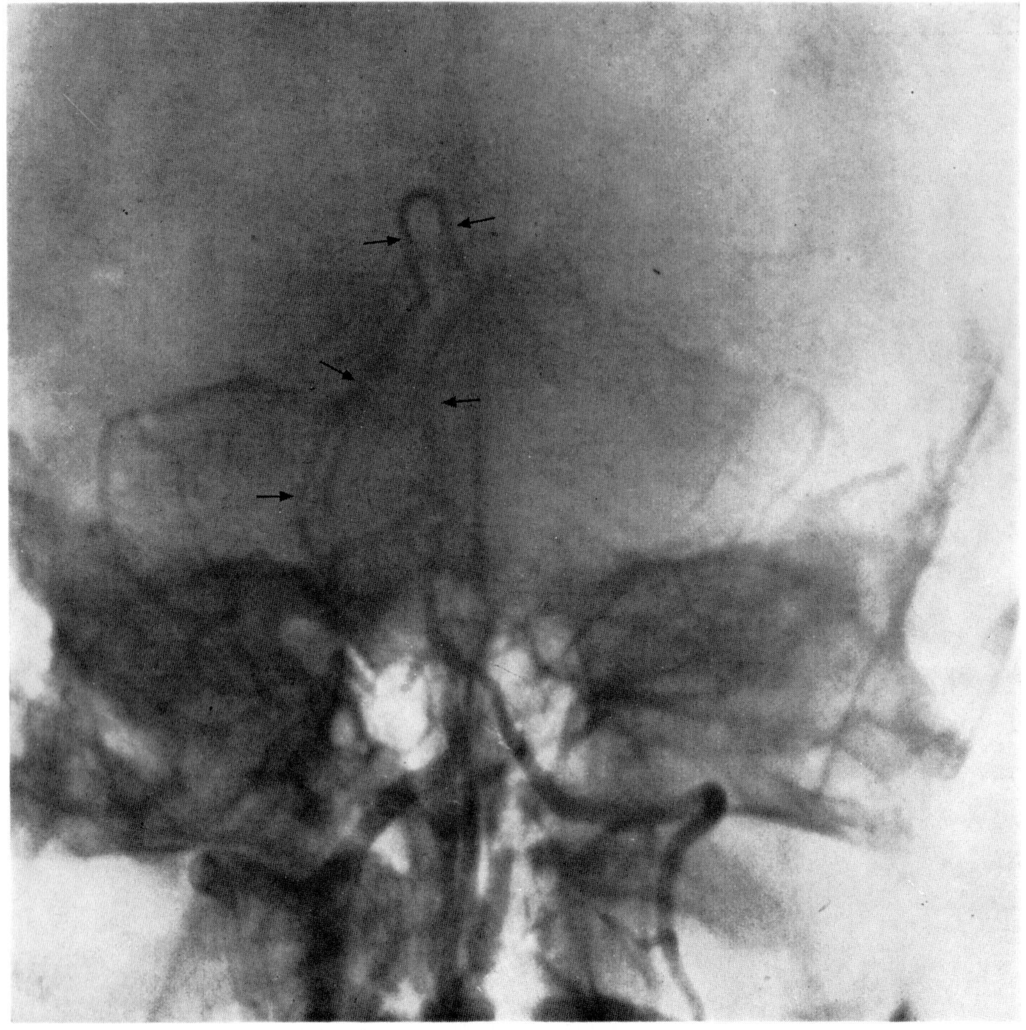

Fig. 39

Venous System

Three major drainage systems are distinguished in the posterior fossa on the basis of direction of drainage and venous terminations: (1) a superior group or Galenic draining group; (2) an anterior group or petrosal draining group; and (3) a posterior group or torcular draining group (Fig. 40). In addition, a part of the supratentorial venous system is also visualized since the vertebrobasilar arterial system supplies the supratentorial cerebral structures (Fig. 41).

Brief descriptions will be given on these venous systems. Terminology used is that of HUANG and his associates since their extensive work in this field seems to have been standardized and accepted widely.

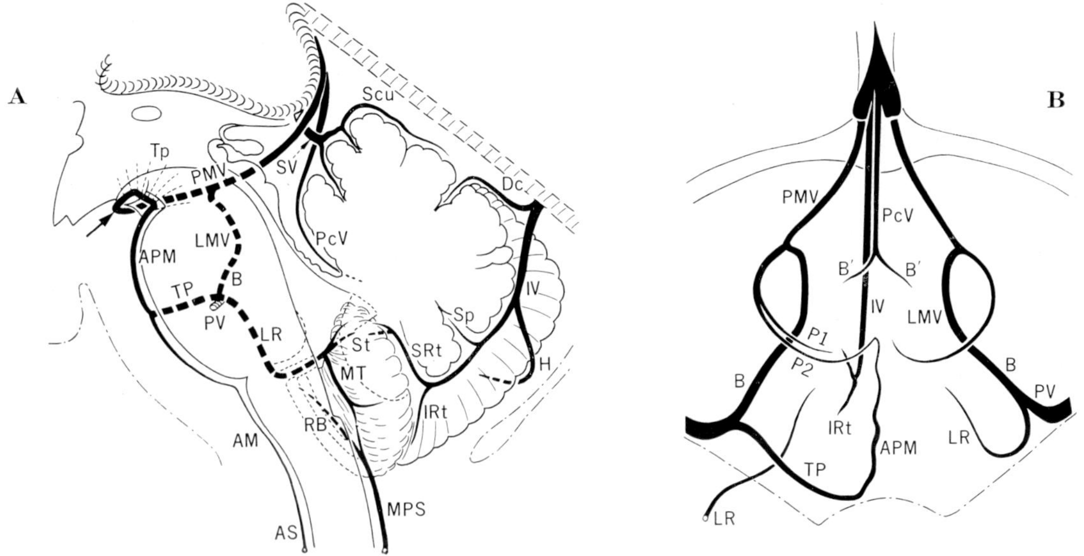

Fig. 40 Schematic diagrams of the major veins in the posterior fossa. A: Lateral projection. B: Towne projection. AM = Anterior medullary vein. APM = Anterior pontomesencephalic vein. AS = Anterior spinal vein. B = Brachial tributary of the petrosal vein. B′ = Brachial tributary of the precentral cerebellar vein. Dc = Declival vein. H = Hemispheric vein. IRt = Inferior retrotonsillar vein. IV = Inferior vermian vein. LMV = Lateral mesencephalic vein. LR = Vein of the lateral recess of the fourth ventricle. MPS = Median posterior spinal vein. MT = Medial tonsillar vein. PcV = Precentral cerebellar vein. P1, P2 = Peduncular vein. PMV = Posterior mesencephalic vein. PV = Petrosal vein. RB = Vein of the restiform body. Scu = Supraculminate vein. Sp = Suprapyramidal vein. SRt = Superior retrotonsillar vein. St = Supratonsillar vein. SV = Superior vermian vein. Tp = Thalamoperforating vein. TP = Transverse pontine vein. (Through courtesy of HUANG and WOLF: Neuroradiology, 1: 4, 1970)

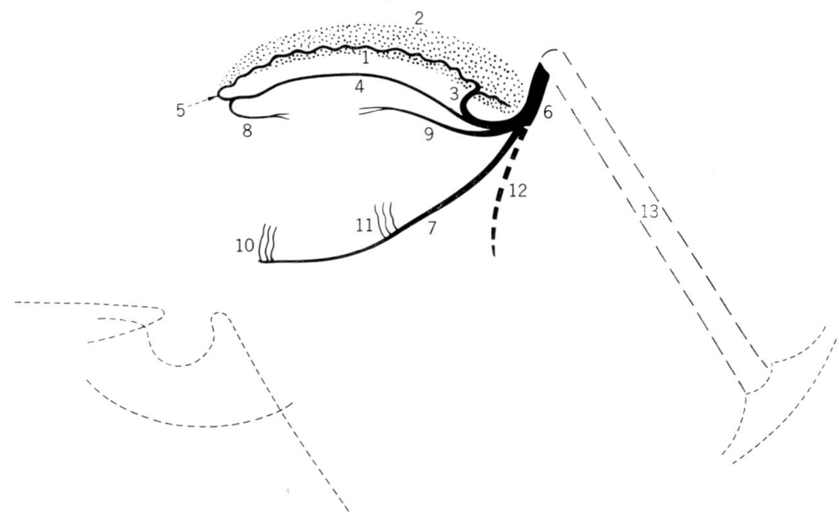

Fig. 41 Schematic illustration of the supratentorial venous system by vertebral artery injection. The numbers indicate the following veins and their percentage visualization.
1 = Superior choroid vein (97%). 2 = Choroid plexus (Lateral, 84%; Towne, 29%). 3 = Connecting vein (63%). 4 = Internal cerebral vein (97%). 5 = Venous angle. 6 = Great vein of Galen (100%). 7 = Basal vein of Rosenthal (67%). 8 = Anterior thalamic vein (78%). 9 = Superior thalamic vein (95%). 10 = Inferior thalamic vein (13%). 11 = Posterior thalamic vein (19%). 12 = Precentral cerebellar vein. 13 = Straight sinus. (Through courtesy of Radiology. From TAKAHASHI and OKUDERA: Radiology 103: 113, 1972)

SUPERIOR GROUP

The superior group are those veins draining superiorly into the Galenic system. This group primarily drain the superior and anterior surface of the cerebellum via the precentral cerebellar vein and the superior vermian vein as well as the brain stem via the posterior mesencephalic vein and anterior pontomesencephalic vein.

Precentral cerebellar vein

This vein originates in the precentral cerebellar fissure between the central lobule of the cerebellum and the lingula. This vein is formed by the union of two small lateral tributaries originating from the lateral extensions of the precentral cerebellar fissure. After forming a single trunk, the vein courses upwards and forwards parallel and posterior to the superior roof of the fourth ventricle. This portion of the vein within the precentral fissure is called the first portion.

The precentral cerebellar vein reaches the surface of the cerebellum on emerging from the precentral fissure and then courses superiorly over the culmen of the cerebellum within the quadrigeminal cistern. This portion is called the second portion. At the point of exit from the fissure the vein changes its course posteriorly and upwards, forming an obtuse angle between the inferior colliculi and the central lobule of the cerebellum. The point of this angle is called the "colliculocentral point" and the angle is referred to as the "colliculocentral angle".

The third portion of the precentral cerebellar vein is the direct continuation of the second portion above the cerebellum and terminates in the distal portion of the vein of Galen. There is usually a slight anteriorly convex curve to the second and third portions or the precentral cerebellar vein.

Variations of the precentral cerebellar vein are not uncommon. The two brachial tributaries may not unite and continue as separate veins for variable distance before they unite. The precentral cerebellar vein may join the superior vermian vein and drain into the vein of Galen as a common trunk.

According to HUANG et al. (1966), the minimal distance of the colliculocentral point to the clivus averages 3.9 cm in adults and the perpendicular line drawn from this point to Twining's line bisects the latter line in normal cases.

Superior vermian vein

The main trunk of this vein courses in the midline superiorly and anteriorly on the posterior aspect of the culmen. This segment may be referred to as "supraculminate vein". The vein enters the quadrigeminal cistern above the apex of the culmen, turning posteriorly and upwards and draining into the vein of Galen. The point of drainage is located more anteriorly than the precentral cerebellar vein. There are usually small tributaries of this vein arising from the lateral, superior aspect of the cerebellum as well as from the fissures of the culmen. These tributaries unite and drain into the supraculminate vein. As previously mentioned, the superior vermian vein and the precentral cerebellar vein may form a single trunk which enters the vein of Galen.

The distance of the supraculminate vein to the straight sinus represents the width of the supracerebellar cistern and the distance to the colliculocentral point the width of the culmen.

Posterior mesencephalic vein

This vein arises from the lateral aspect of the cerebral peduncle and courses backwards within the ambient cistern encircling the brain stem. The basal vein of Rosenthal usually runs parallel to this vein. The vein drains into the vein of Galen or one of its tributaries within the quadrigeminal cistern.

In the absence of the basal vein of Rosenthal, this vein enlarges and drains the tributaries of the former vessel. The posterior mesencephalic vein is frequently connected with the lateral mesencephalic vein and the interpeduncular segment of the anterior pontomesencephalic vein.

In the Towne projection the posterior mesencephalic vein form an inverted "V" appearance and the distance of the two veins represents the width of the brain stem.

Lateral mesencephalic vein

This vein runs superiorly within the lateral mesencephalic sulcus and drains into the basal vein of Rosenthal. However, there is frequent connection with the posterior mesencephalic vein and the petrosal vein at the same time. This vein may become a prominent anastomotic channel between the basal vein or the posterior mesencephalic vein and the petrosal vein.

The position of the vein represents the junction of the tegmen of the brain stem and the cerebral peduncle (HUANG and WOLF, 1965).

Anterior pontomesencephalic vein

This vein courses upwards in the midline along the basilar sulcus of the pons and extends into the interpeduncular fossa. It then emerges from the interpeduncular fossa, encircling the upper margin of the cerebral peduncle, and unites with the basal vein of Rosenthal or the posterior mesencephalic vein. The inferior portion of this vein drains into the petrosal vein via the transverse pontine vein. The segment related to the interpeduncular fossa is called the interpeduncular segment, while the segment related to the anterior aspect of the pons may be referred to as the pontine segment.

This vein is considerably important angiographically since it outlines the anterior aspect of the pons and the roof of the interpeduncular fossa.

ANTERIOR GROUP

The anterior group consist of the multiple venous tributaries which drain a major part of the anterior portions of the cerebellar hemispheres as well as antero-lateral aspect of the pons and medulla. These tributaries form a single trunk, the petrosal vein, within the cerebellopontine angle, which in turn joins the superior petrosal sinus.

Petrosal vein

The petrosal vein originates at the anterior angle of the cerebellum by receiving many tributaries from the cerebellum and brain stem. It courses anteriorly and laterally as a short trunk within the cerebellopontine angle cistern below the course of the fifth nerve and drains into the superior petrosal sinus just above the internal auditory meatus.

The major tributaries can be classified as follows:

(a) The transverse pontine vein
(b) The brachial vein
(c) The superior hemispheric vein
(d) The vein of the great horizontal fissure and other inferior hemispheric veins
(e) The vein from the cerebello-medullary fissure
(f) The vein of the lateral recess of the fourth ventricle

Transverse pontine vein

This vein arises from the venous plexuses of the anterior aspect of the pons as well as from the pontine segment of the anterior pontomesencephalic vein and courses laterally over the anterior surface of the pons to drain into the petrosal vein.

The distance of this vein to the clivus represents the width of the prepontine cistern.

Brachial vein

The brachial vein originates in the lateral extensions of the precentral cerebellar fissure, runs along the anterior superior margin of the cerebellum and drains into the petrosal vein at the anterior angle. This vein is frequently connected with the posterior mesencephalic vein or the basal vein of Rosenthal via the lateral mesencephalic vein.

Superior hemispheric veins

These veins are usually paired and originate from the fissures over the anterior, superior surface of the cerebellum. These veins usually drain into the petrosal vein at the anterior angle directly or indirectly via a small venous channel. They may join the vein of the great horizontal fissure.

Vein of the great horizontal fissure and other inferior hemispheric veins

As the greatest vein of the inferior hemispheric veins, the vein of the great horizontal fissure drains the anterior inferior aspect of the cerebellum. The vein originates in the posterior portion of the fissure, runs within the fissure towards the cerebellopontine angle and then drains into the petrosal vein at the anterior angle.

There are several other inferior hemispheric veins running in the various fissures of the inferior cerebellar hemisphere. They usually form a single trunk and enters the petrosal vein.

The veins from the cerebellomedullary fissure

These veins include the retro-olivary vein, the vein of the restiform body and the medial tonsillar vein (Huang and Wolf, 1968). They all drain into the petrosal vein.

The vein of the lateral recess of the fourth ventricle

This vein originates from the medial surface of the tonsil as the supratonsillar and medial tonsillar veins, runs forwards and laterally and then enters the cerebellopontine angle by way of the lateral recess of the fourth ventricle. This segment is relatively constant in position and referred to as the first segment. The second segment is the portion below the flocculus within the cerebellopontine angle. The third segment courses superiorly and anteriorly over the brachium pontis to enter the petrosal vein at the anterior angle (Huang and Wolf, 1967).

POSTERIOR GROUP

The posterior group consist of those vessels draining posteriorly or laterally into the torcular and adjacent straight or lateral sinuses. This group primarily drain the posterior inferior surface of the cerebellum and the tonsils.

Inferior vermian vein

The inferior vermian vein is formed below the copula pyramidis by the union of the superior and inferior retrotonsillar tributaries and the medial tonsillar tributary. The inferior vermian vein then courses superiorly and posteriorly alongside the inferior vermis within the paravermian sulcus. This vein enters the lateral sinus or the straight sinus near the confluence with an angle opposing their flows.

There are additional tributaries: The suprapyramidal vein running in the suprapyramidal fissure between the pyramid and the tuber and the declival vein arising from the primary fissure. These veins usually drain into the main trunk of the inferior vermian vein.

Angiographically the inferior vermian vein shows an arcuate course with medial and posterior convexity. The vein is usually located 2 to 5 mm lateral to the midline and 5 to 10 mm anterior to the inner table of the occipital bone.

The copular point, designated by HUANG et al. (1969) as the most anterior point of the curve formed by the superior retrotonsillar tributary and the inferior vermian vein, falls within a circle of 6 mm radius with its center located 4 mm behind and below the midpoint of a line connecting the anterior margin of the foramen magnum and the torcular.

Inferior hemispheric veins

The hemispheric veins, draining the inferior posterior aspect of the cerebellum, usually enter the inferior vermian vein and the petrosal vein. However, several inferior hemispheric veins usually located laterally, course upwards over the posterior inferior aspect of the cerebellum and drains directly into the lateral portion of the lateral sinus. These veins should not be confused with the inferior vermian vein in the lateral projection.

SUPRATENTORIAL GROUP

The supratentorial veins, draining the areas supplied by the posterior cerebral artery and its branches, are visualized on vertebral angiograms. These veins drain the mesencephalon, the posterior portion of the diencephalon, the lateral ventricle, the occipital lobe, the posterior temporal lobe and the posterior parietal lobe. They join the vein of Galen, the superior sagittal sinus, the straight sinus or the lateral sinus.

Basal vein of Rosenthal

This vein is formed by junction of small veins from the olfactory, insular, orbital and lenticulostriate regions. One of the main contributing veins comes from the deep middle cerebral vein originating from the insular regions. This vein courses posteriorly and passes through the lateral portion of the interpeduncular fossa, where there are abundant anastomoses with the opposite side and with the tributaries of the posterior mesencephalic and anterior pontomesencephalic veins. Then, the vein runs within the crural and ambient cisterns in the posterior and superior direction, encircling the brain stem and terminating in the great vein of Galen. The portion of the vein anterior to the interpeduncular fossa is referred to as the anterior segment, while the posterior portion is called the posterior segment. In selective vertebral angiography, only the posterior segment of the basal vein is visualized. The vein begins in the interpeduncular fossa by junction of the interpeduncular segment of the anterior pontomesencephalic vein, the interpeduncular venous plexus and the proximal portion of the posterior mesencephalic vein.

There are numerous anomalies of the basal vein of Rosenthal. The basal vein may drain into the straight sinus or lateral sinus instead of flowing into the vein of Galen. There may be absence of the entire vein, the anterior segment or the posterior segment. In the absence of the posterior segment, the basal vein drains into the petrosal vein via the anastomotic lateral mesencephalic vein.

The choroid plexus and the superior choroid vein

The choroid plexus begins at the foramen of Monro, extends posteriorly on the floor of the lateral ventricle to the atrium, where it enlarges and forms the glomus, and then courses anteriorly and inferiorly along the roof of the temporal horn. The choroid plexus is drained by the superior choroid vein and choroid branches of the veins of the posterior and inferior horns. These veins are embedded in the choroid plexus and have abundant anastomoses.

The superior choroid vein is located in the floor of the body and trigone of the lateral ventricle, embedded in the choroid plexus. This vein flows into the thalamostriate vein near the foramen of Monro or occasionally directly into the internal cerebral vein near this foramen. Drainage of the choroid plexus of the trigone is supplemented by a small choroid vein, which enters the choroid fissure under the edge of the crus fornices. This latter vein drains directly into the internal cerebral vein or the great vein of Galen or indirectly into these veins via the vein of the posterior horn or the medial atrial vein. This vein is referred to as "the connecting vein" (TAKAHASHI and OKUDERA, 1972).

The choroid plexus of the inferior horn is drained by a small choroid vein, which drains into the basal vein via the veins of the inferior horns.

Angiographically, the lateral projections show the choroid plexus to be a faint blush on the floor of the body and trigone of the lateral ventricle, which are closely associated with the lateral posterior choroidal arteries and contiguous with the internal cerebral vein at the foramen of Monro. This appears at the late arterial phase and remains to the venous phase. The superior choroid vein is visualized as the interrupted lines or band-like densities within the choroid blush. The internal cerebral vein is seen just below the choroid plexus, draining into the great vein of Galen. The connecting vein originates from the choroid plexus in the form of a "Y" and drains into the internal cerebral vein or the great vein of Galen.

In the Towne projection the blush of the choroid plexus appears as an arcuate band-like density extending laterally from the area of the sinus confluence with its convexity postero-superiorly.

The choroid plexus and the choroidal branches of the vein of the inferior horn are not visualized on vertebral angiograms, since the anterior choroidal artery participates in the blood supply of this area.

The widest distance between the choroid vein and the internal cerebral vein is 0.81 cm with a standard deviation of 0.21 cm. There is no significant difference between the values of adults and children (TAKAHASHI and OKUDERA, 1972).

Internal cerebral vein

The internal cerebral vein is opacified below the superior choroid vein and is intimately associated with the medial posterior choroidal artery. This vein begins at the foramen of Monro by drainage of the superior choroid vein, and courses posteriorly to drain into the great vein of Galen. The margin of the internal cerebral vein is not outlined sharply because this vein is embedded in the choroid plexus of the roof of the third ventricle.

Thalamic veins

There are four thalamic veins on each side: The superior, anterior, inferior and posterior thalamic veins (GIUDICELLI and SALAMON, 1970).

The superior thalamic vein drains the posteromedial aspect of the thalmus. This vein runs below the internal cerebral vein for a short distance and drains into the terminal portion of the internal cerebral vein or the basal vein of Rosenthal. The anteromedial portion of the thalamus is drained by the anterior thalamic vein, which courses anteriorly and superiorly and flows into the internal cerebral vein at the foramen of Monro. A small vein may connect the anterior and superior thalamic veins.

The inferior thalamic vein drains the anterolateral aspect of the thalamus and unites with the interpeduncular portion of the posterior mesencephalic vein or the basal vein. The posterolateral portion of the thalamus is drained by the posterior thalamic vein which empties into the posterior part of the basal vein or the posterior mesencephalic vein. The last two veins are infrequently visualized.

Other supratentorialveins

(KRAYENBÜHL and YASARGIL, 1968)

The ascending occipital cerebral vein is formed by the junction of the veins of the dorsal surface of the occipital lobe, courses superiorly and anteriorly along the superior sagittal sinus and drains into this sinus near the parieto-occipital sulcus. The veins of the posterior and lateral surface of the occipital lobe flow into the lateral sinus after they form one or more main vessels. They are referred to as the descending dorsal occipital veins.

The veins over the cuneus and precuneus drain singly or jointly into the straight sinus or into the posterior portion of the vein of Galen. They are called the descending medial occipital veins.

The posterior cerebral vein or the dorsal pericallosal vein drains the dorsal aspect of the splenium and medial aspect of the longitudinal cerebral fissure, courses over the splenium and finally unites with the middle portion of the vein of Galen.

NORMAL VENOUS PHASES OF VERTEBRAL ANGIOGRAMS

Normal Venous Phase of a Vertebral Angiogram

A 27-year-old male: Figs. 42 and 43

Fig. 42 Lateral projection. The precentral cerebellar vein and the superior vermian vein form a single trunk which drains superiorly into the vein of Galen (2 arrows). There is good visualization of the superior petrosal sinus, but the petrosal vein is obscured by the mastoid. One of the inferior vermian veins runs posterior to the usual course (2 arrowheads).

Fig. 43 Towne projection. The petrosal vein (an arrow) and the vein of the lateral recess of the fourth ventricle (2 arrowheads) are well shown bilaterally. The right hemispheric vein drains into the inferior vermian vein, which shows an anomalous course in the lateral projection.

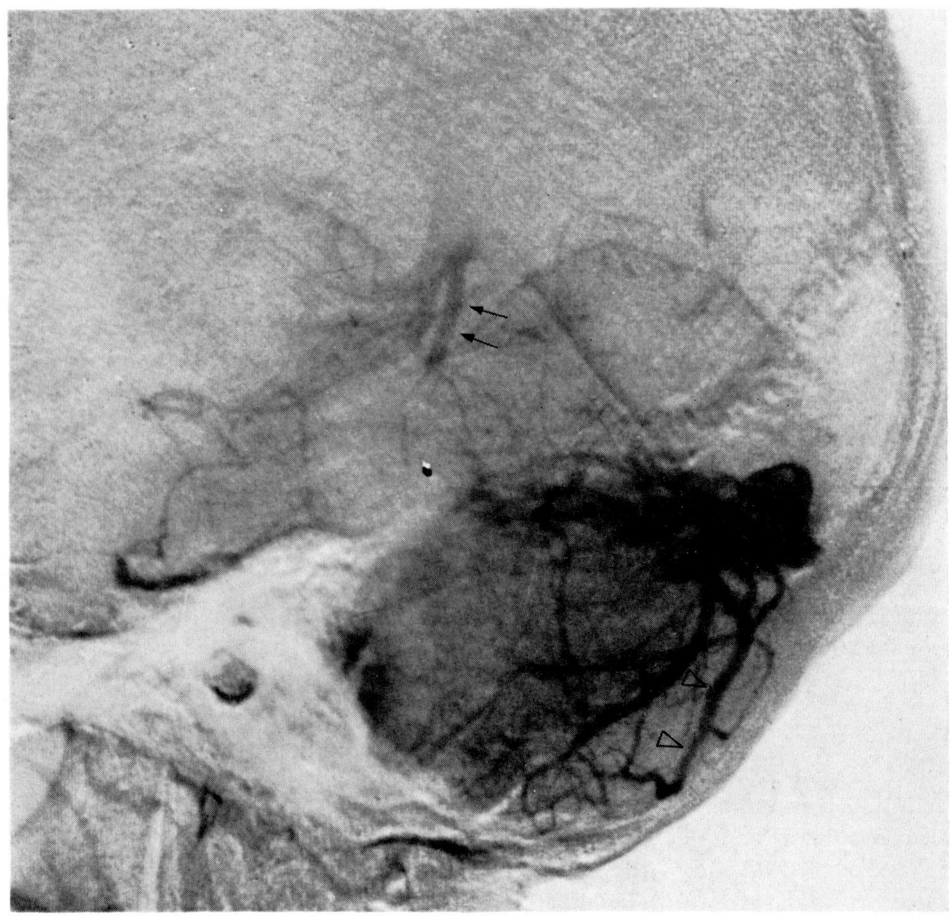

Fig. 42

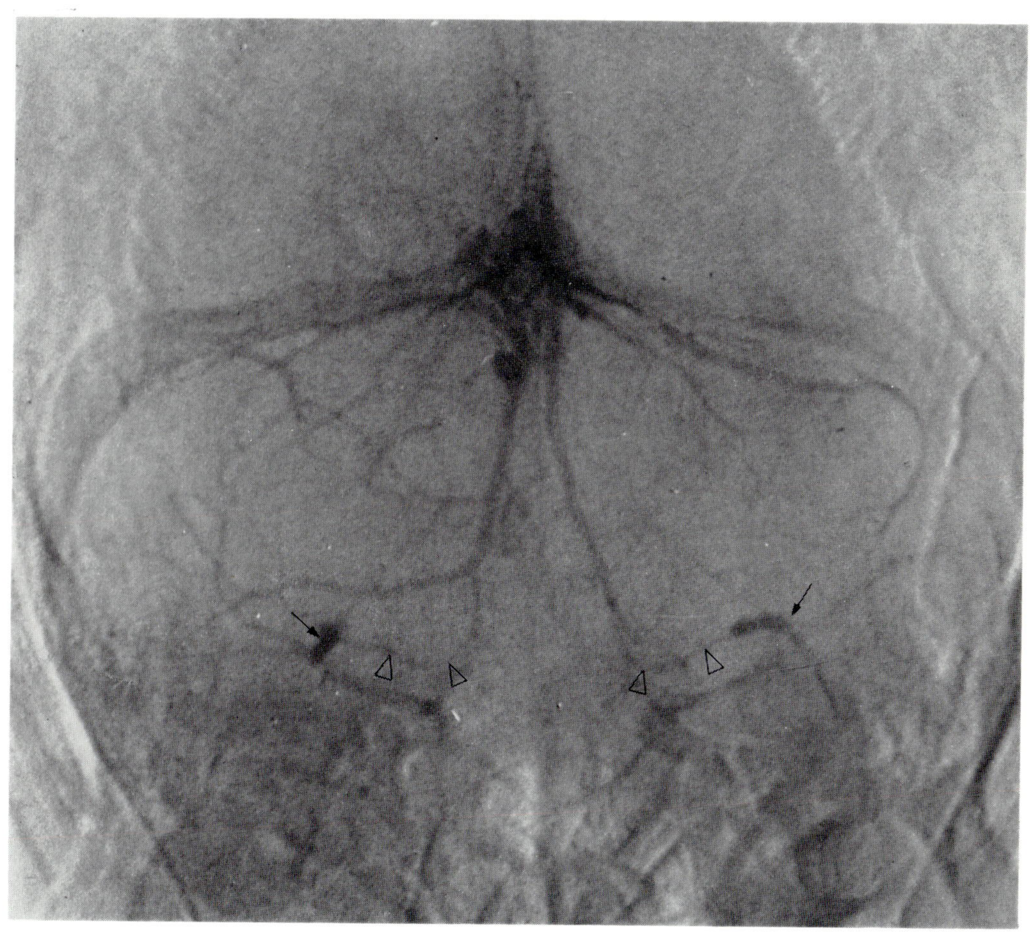

Fig. 43

Normal Venous Phase of a Vertebral Angiogram

A 15-year-old female: Figs. 44 and 45

Fig. 44 Lateral projection. The superior vermian vein anomalously drains into the sinus confluence (2 arrows). The petrosal vein and its tributaries are shown to good advantage (an arrowhead). The vein of the lateral recess of the fourth ventricle is opacified faintly (2 crossed arrows).

Fig. 45 Towne projection. The petrosal vein and its tributaries are well shown (an arrowhead) with the lateral segment of the superior petrosal sinus. The inferior vermian veins and the precentral cerebellar vein take a parallel course (2 opposing arrows).

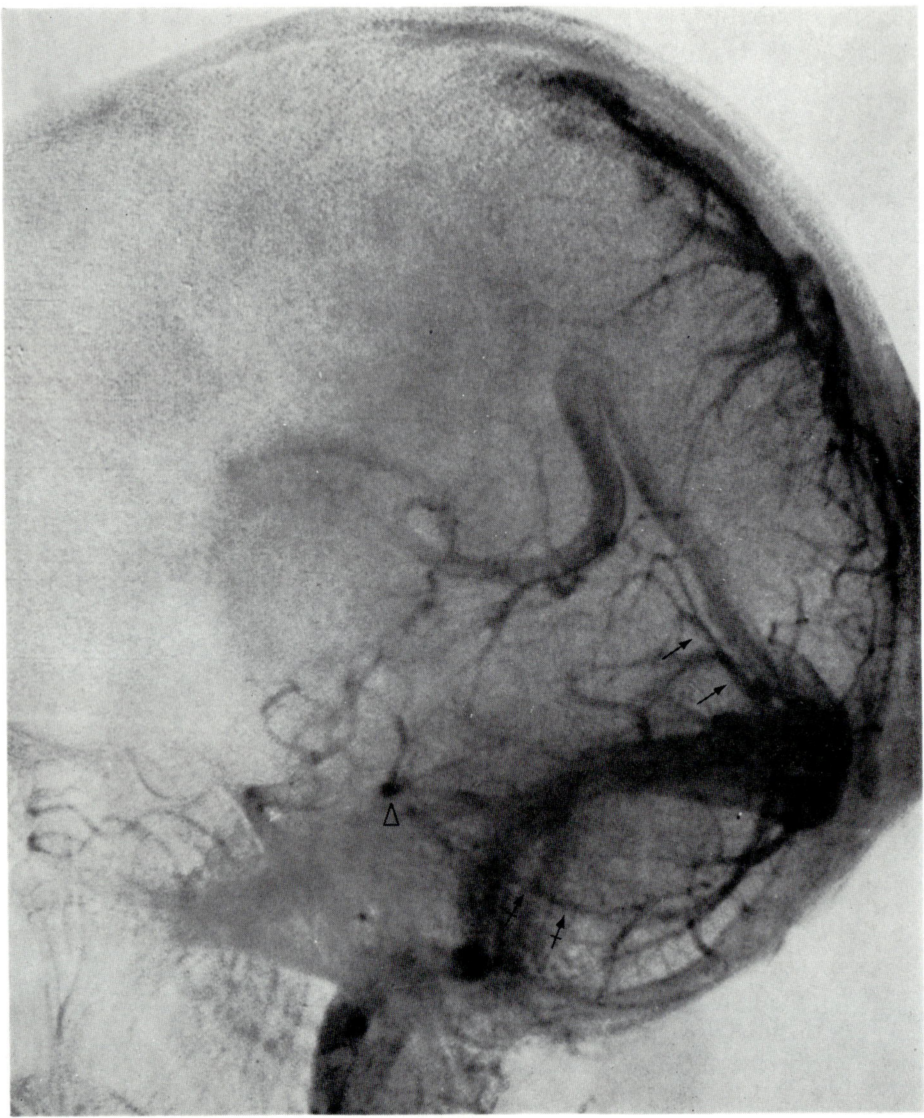

Fig. 44

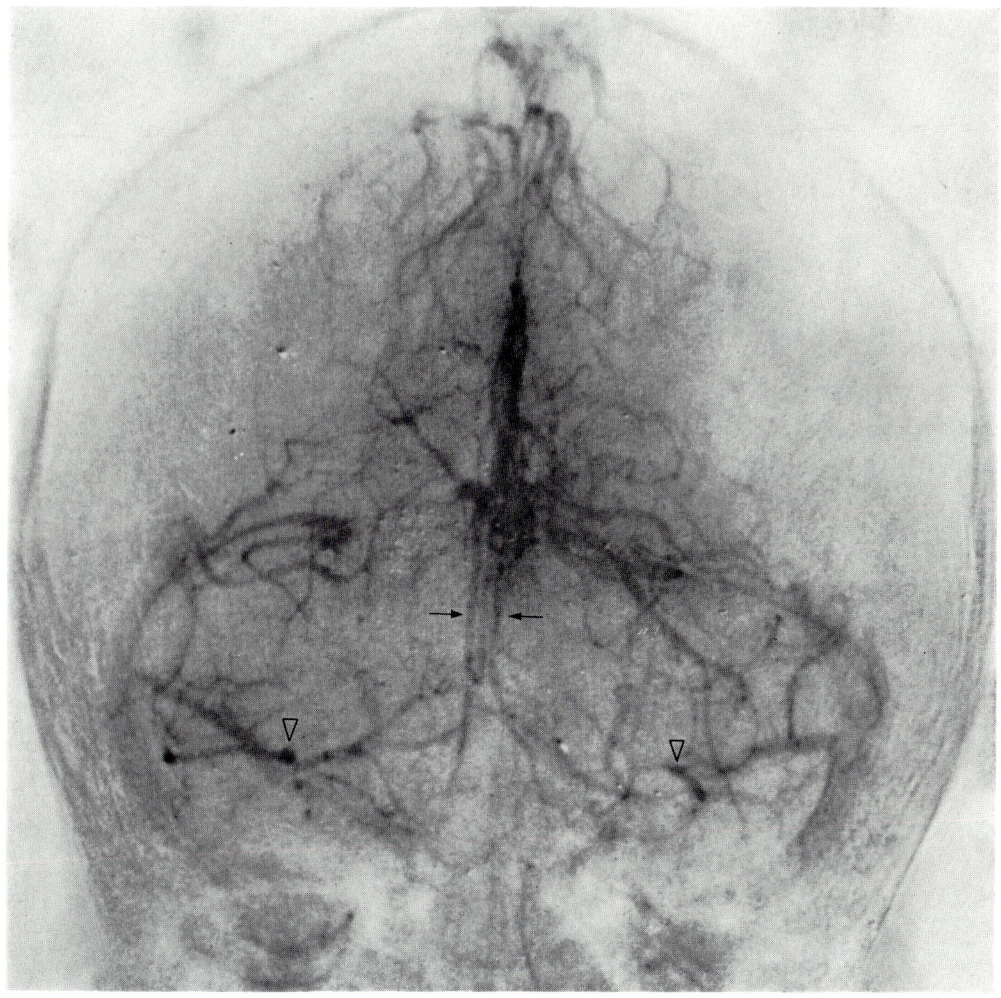

Fig. 45

Normal Petrosal Vein and its Tributaries in 2 Patients

Figs. 46 and 47

Figs. 46, 47 Towne projection. 1. Petrosal vein, 2. Transverse pontine vein, 3. Anterior pontomesencephalic vein, 4. Brachial vein, 5. Superior hemispheric vein, 6. Inferior hemispheric vein, 7. Superior petrosal sinus. The vein of the lateral recess of the fourth vertricle is also shown (2 arrows).

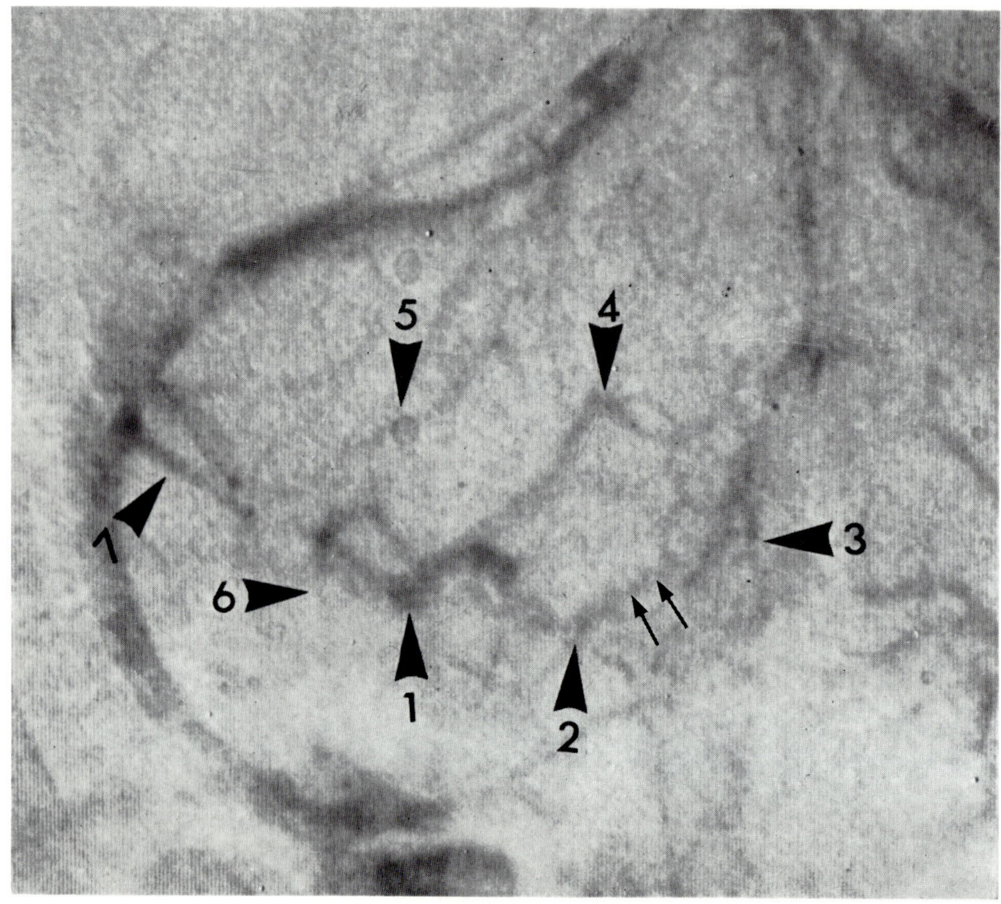

Fig. 46

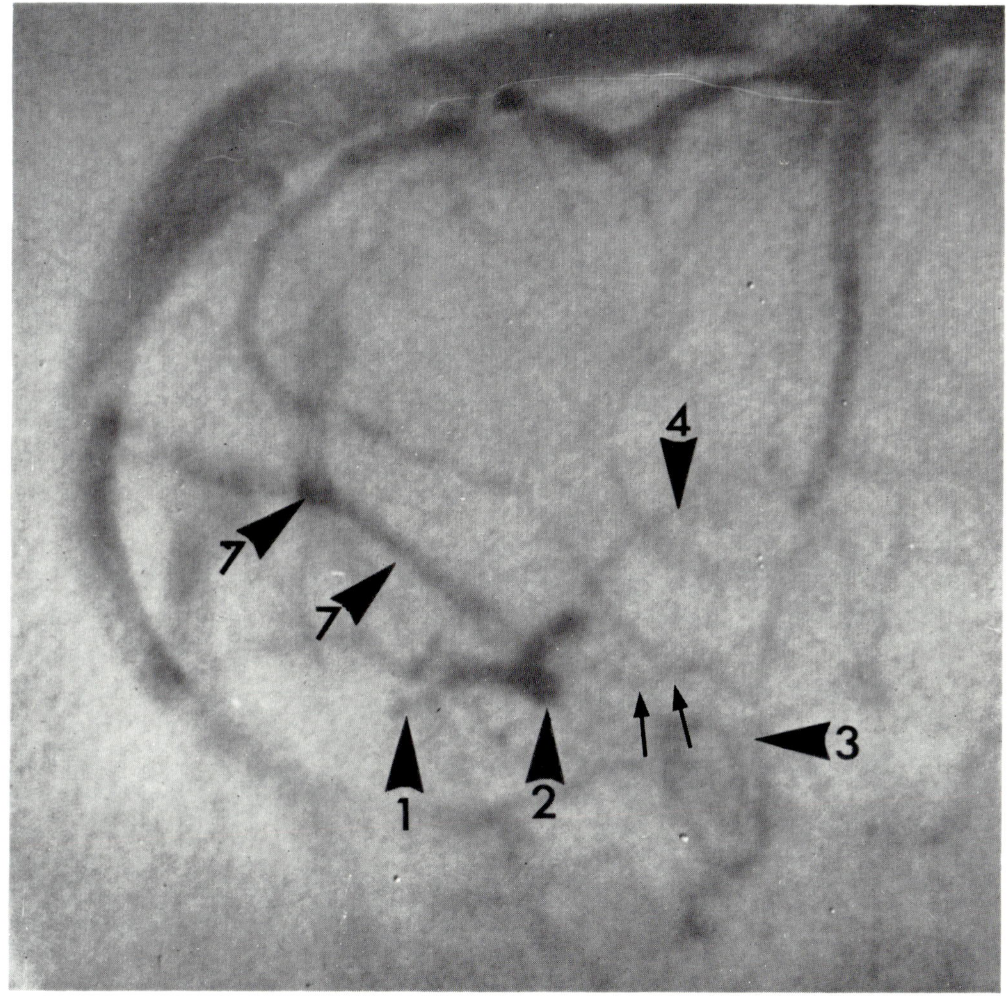

Fig. 47

Anomalous Inferior Vermian Vein Draining into the Superior Vermian Vein

A 56-year-old male: Fig. 48

Fig. 48 Lateral projection. The inferior vermian vein continues as the superior vermian vein and drains into the vein of Galen. The superior and inferior vermis is outlined by this anomalous vein (4 arrows).

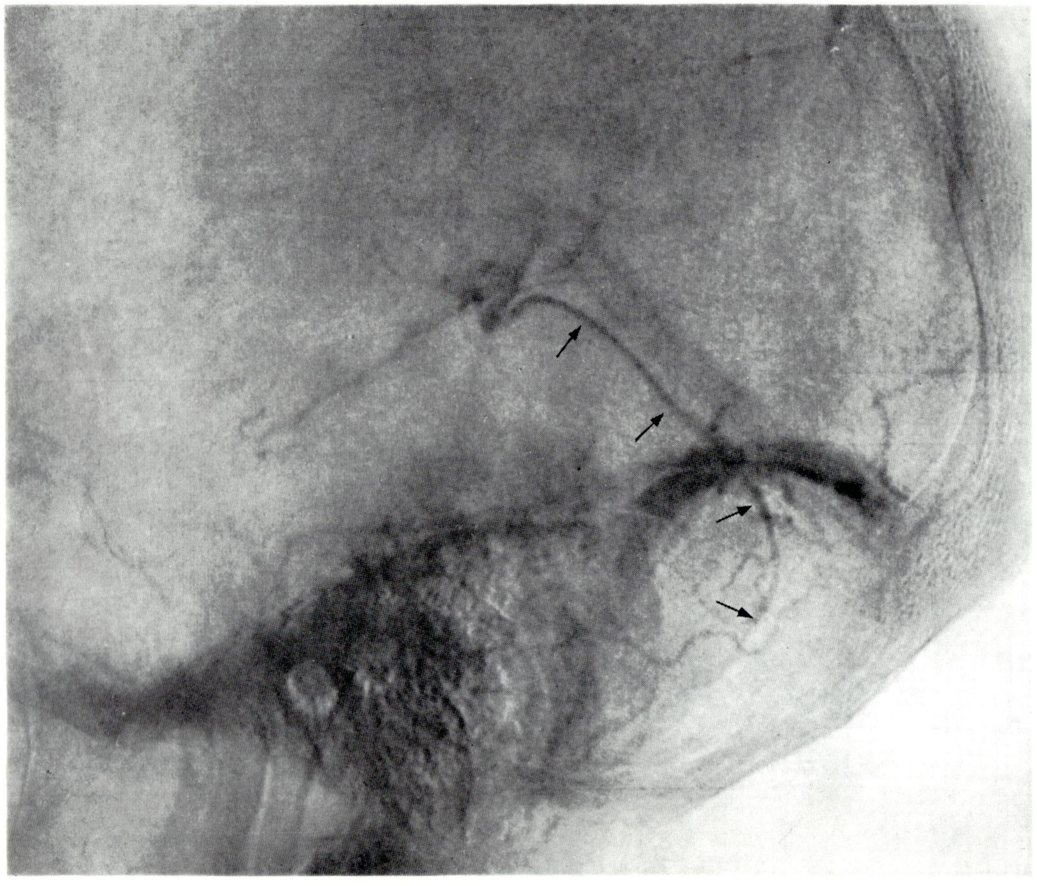

Fig. 48

Normal Supratentorial Venous System by Vertebral Artery Injection

A 48-year-old male: Figs. 49–54

Fig. 49 Capillary phase in the lateral projection.
Fig. 50 Venous phase in the lateral projection.
Fig. 51 Schematic illustration of Fig. 50
Fig. 52 Capillary phase in the Towne projection.
Fig. 53 Venous phase in the Towne projection.
Fig. 54 Schematic illustration of Fig. 53.

The numbers indicate the following veins: 1. Superior choroid vein, 2. Choroid plexus, 3. Connecting vein, 4. Internal cerebral vein, 5. Venous angle, 6. Great vein of Galen, 7. Basal vein of Rosenthal or posterior mesencephalic vein, 8. Anterior thalamic vein, 9. Superior thalamic vein.

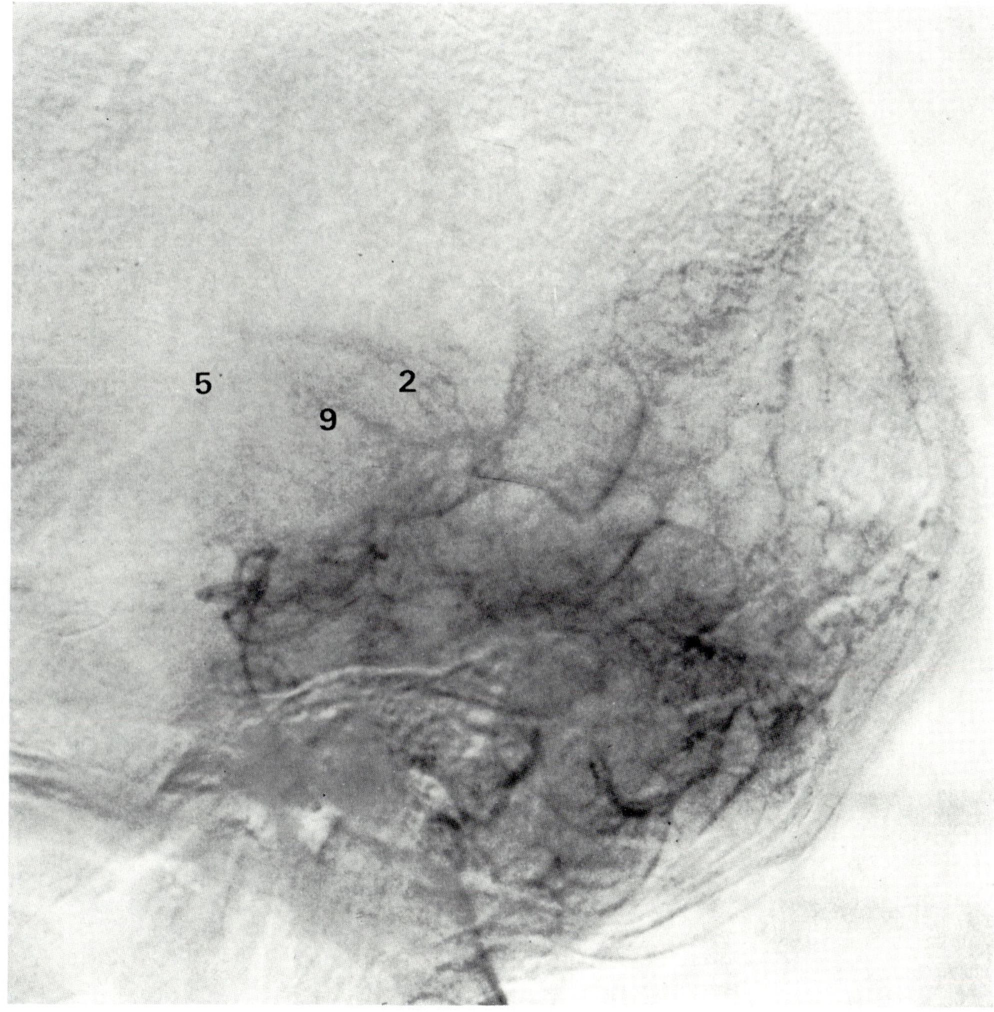

Fig. 49

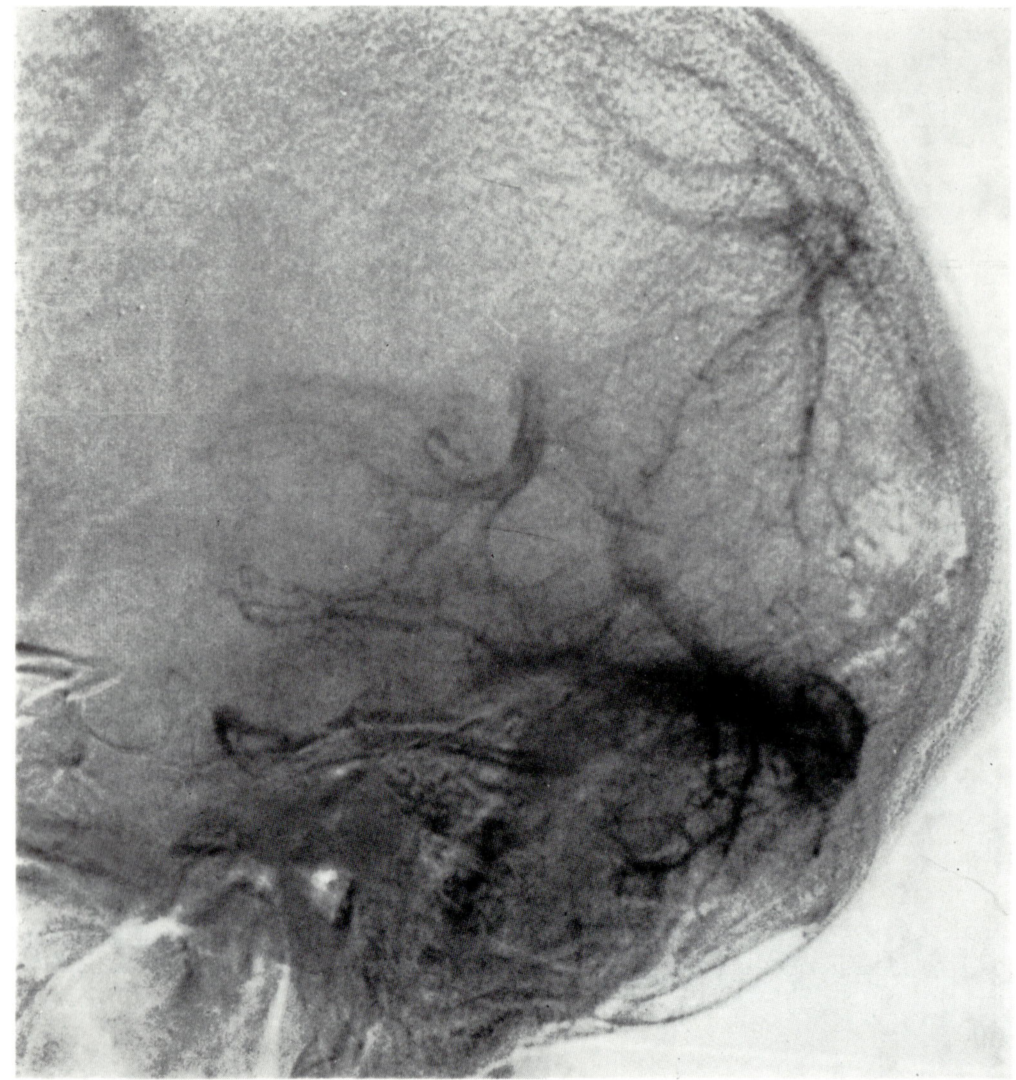

Fig. 50

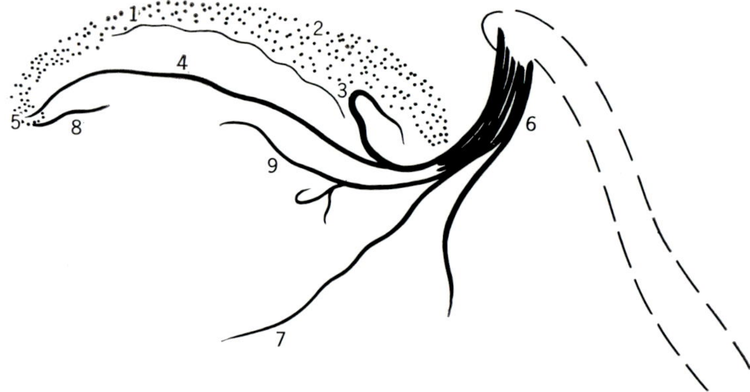

Fig. 51

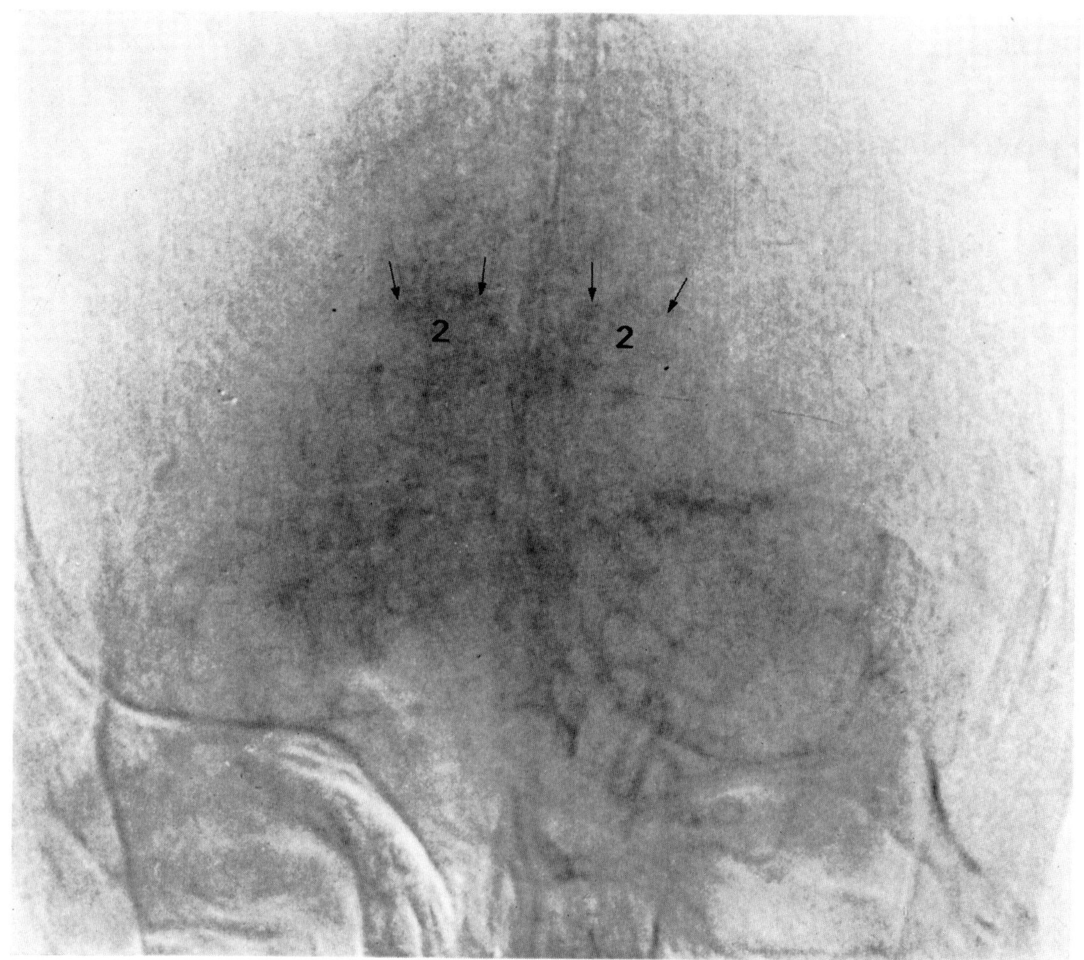

Fig. 52

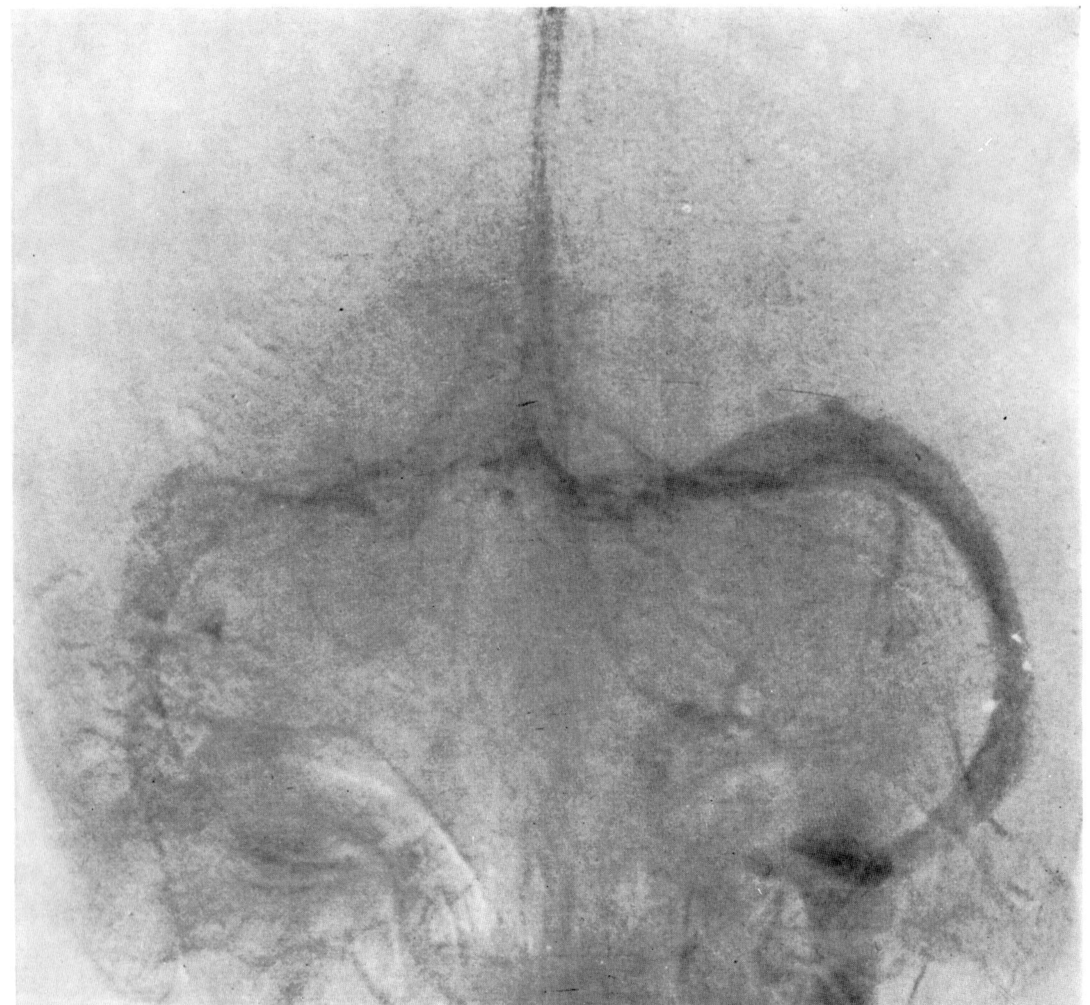

Fig. 53

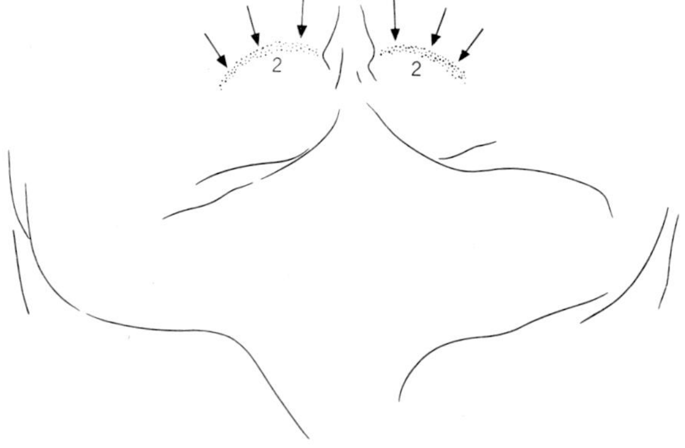

Fig. 54

5

Statistics and General Angiographic Manifestations of Intracranial Tumors

STATISTICAL DATA OF INTRACRANIAL TUMORS

Incidence of histologic type of brain tumors is listed in a table (Table 11) as reported by Cushing (1932), Olivecrona (1955) and Zülch (1965). The figures come close to each other.

The knowledge of relative frequency of brain tumors at various locations is very important in arriving at a correct angiographic diagnosis. Since various authors report similar figures, Zülch's data (1965) are quoted (Table 12).

In childhood incidence of histologic type of brain tumors is considerably different from the data for the entire age group (Fig. 55). Proportion of gliomas is 70 to 80%, while meningioma is quite rare and neurinoma is practically absent in childhood. Furthermore, 50 to 60% of all intracranial tumors occur in the posterior fossa in childhood. The relative frequency at various locations is also slightly different, especially, in the posterior fossa (Fig. 56).

The relative frequency of tumor types in different locations can be summarised according to Zülch (1965). The less commonly occurring types are shown in brackets.

Temporal lobes
Temporolateral: Oligodendrogliomas—glioblastomas—meningiomas (sylvian fissure)—astrocytomas
Temporobasal: Gangliocytomas—meningiomas—chordomas
Temporomedial: Glioblastomas—oligodendrogliomas
Parietal lobes
Parietolateral: Astrocytomas—oligodendrogliomas—glioblastomas—ependymomas and spongioblastomas (in adolescence)—meningiomas (of the convexity)
Parietodorsal: Glioblastomas—astrocytomas—meningiomas (parasagittal)
Parietomedial: Astrocytomas
Occipital lobes
Glioblastomas spreading from the corpus callosum or its radiation—meningiomas (posterior third of the sagittal sinus—tentorium/torcular)—[astrocytomas and oligodendrogliomas spreading from the temporal or parietal region]

Table 11 Classification and Incidence of Tumor Types (Through the courtesy of Springer-Verlag. From Zülch : Brain Tumors, 1965).

	Zülch (6,000 cases)	Cuching's (2,023 cases)	Olivecrona (5,250 cases)
Medulloblastomas	3.8(%)	4.3(%)	(%)
Spongioblastomas (incl. the so-called cerebellar astrocytoma)	7.0	6.1	
Oligodendrogliomas	8.2	1.3	
Astrocytomas	6.4	9.8	
Glioblastomas	12.3	10.3	46.5
Ependymomas	4.3	1.3	
Plexus papillomas	0.5	0.6	0.3
Pinealomas	0.4	0.7	
Neurinomas	7.6	8.7	8.0
Gangliocytomas	0.4	0.2	
Meningiomas	18.0	13.4	19.2
Angioblastomas	1.3	1.2	2.4
Fibromas	0.1		
Sarcomas	2.7	0.7	
Chondromas	0.3	0.1	
Lipomas	0.1		
Osteomas	0.5	0.7	
Chordomas	0.2	0.1	
Craniopharyngiomas	2.5	4.6	1.7
Pituitary adenomas	8.0	17.8	8.5
Cylindromatous epitheliomas	0.2		
Epidermoids	1.7	0.7	0.7
Dermoids	0.2		
Teratomas	0.2	0.2	0.3
Angiomas and aneurysms	2.5	1.0	7.0
Unclassified tumors	3.7	9.6	
Metastases	4.0	3.2	3.4
Parasites	0.1	0.1	
Granulomas	0.7	2.2	1.0
Arachnoiditis and ependymitis	1.5	1.1	
Miscellaneous (myelomas, Schüller-Christian's disease, etc.)	0.6		1.0
Total	100.0(%)	100.0(%)	100.0(%)

Table 12 Relative Frequency (%) of Tumor Types Found at the Various Locations (Through the courtesy of Springer-Verlag. From Zülch: Brain Tumors, 1965).

	Frontal (629 cases)	Temporal (414 cases)	Parietal (345 cases)	Occipital (130 cases)	Region of the chiasm (352 cases)	Third ventricle (28 cases)	Lateral ventricle (41 cases)	Upper brain stem (87 cases)	Quadrigeminal plate (49 cases)	Aqueduct (24 cases)	Cerebellum and fourth ventricle (482 cases)	Pontocerebellar angle (282 cases)	Lower brain stem (27 cases)	Spinal cord (96 cases)
Medulloblastoma									10.1		24.8	0.4		1.2
Spongioblastoma	0.6	1.2	0.3	3.7	6.5	39.6	7.3	2.3	6.1	29.4	28.8		7.4	9.2
Oligodendroglioma	15.7	12.4	8.7	5.1		3.6		12.6	2.1		0.2		3.7	
Astrocytoma	17.4	11.8	12.2	6.6		10.8		10.4	6.1	4.2	0.2		22.2	3.2
Glioblastoma multiforme	19.4	28.8	21.8	25.6				52.9	2.1				22.2	2.2
Ependymoma	2.4	2.6	7.5	6.6		18.0	16.9		12.1		11.1	0.4	14.8	7.2
Plexus papilloma		0.2				3.6	14.5				2.0			
Pinealoma									26.1					
Neurinoma		0.2										79.2		15.2
Gangliocytoma	0.3	1.0	0.9	1.5			4.9		2.1					2.2
Meningioma	30.6	26.2	31.3	27.0	9.9		9.7	1.1			5.3	6.7	3.7	22.2
Angioblastoma			0.3								11.6	0.4		4.2
Fibroma	0.5				0.4							0.4		
Sarcoma	1.3	1.4	1.7	1.5	0.4		2.5	2.3	2.1		0.6			6.2
Chondroma	0.2	0.5										0.7		
Lipoma														2.2
Osteoma	0.6	0.5	0.3	0.7										
Chordoma					1.2							0.4	3.7	
Craniopharyngioma					21.9									
Pituitary adenoma					52.2									
Epidermoid	0.2	1.9		1.5	0.7		9.7	2.3	4.1		0.6	4.6	7.4	2.2
Dermoid		0.2									0.6			
Teratoma		0.5							14.1		0.4			
Angioma and aneurysm	0.9	1.4	2.9	8.8	1.2			2.3			0.6	0.4	3.7	
Unclassif. tumors	3.2	4.8	6.4	2.9	4.0	10.8	14.5	4.6	6.1		2.7	2.5	7.4	11.2
Metastases	5.4	2.9	5.2	6.6	0.4			5.7			2.5	1.4	3.7	4.2
Parasites											0.2			
Granuloma	0.5	0.2	0.3	0.7			7.3	3.5			1.9			2.2
Adhesive arachnoiditis	0.3	0.5	0.3		0.7				6.1		5.3	0.7		1.2
Ependymitis										46.2				
Misc.	0.3	0.2		0.7	0.4		12.1			21.0	1.7			
Colloidal cyst						14.4								
Neurofibroma														1.2
Cyst														1.2
"Glioma"														1.2

Chiasmal region
Spongioblastomas and craniopharyngiomas (adolescence)—pituitary adenomas—meningiomas—epidermoids—adhesive arachnoiditis—chordomas—aneurysms of the anterior communicating and carotid arteries (parasellar)—parasellar teratomas

Third ventricle
Ependymal cysts (foramen of Monro)—ependymomas—spongioblastoms (of the hypothalamus)—plexus papillomas—[epidermoids]—meningiomas of the velum interpositum

Lateral ventricles
Ependymomas—meningiomas—plexus papillomas—epidermoids—[chondromas—teratomas—lipomas—the ventricular tumors of tuberous sclerosis]

Corpus callosum and septum pellucidum
Anterior: Glioblastomas—oligodendrogliomas—astrocytomas (diffuse)—[lipomas]
Posterior : Gliobrastomas—oligodendrogliomas—[lipomas]

Tumors of the septum pellucidum
Spongioblastomas (which have generally grown in from the surroundings)—astrocytomas—oligodendrogliomas—glioblastomas—cysts of the septum pellucidum

Rostral brain stem and basal ganglia
Glioblastomas—oligodendrogliomas (adolescence)—astrocytomas (often bilateral, growing across the massa intermedia)

Region of the quadrigeminal plate
Pinealomas—medulloblastomas / pineoblastomas—spongioblastomas—[glioblastomas]—ependymomas (aqueduct and posterior third ventricle)—ependymal cysts—arachnoidal cysts—teratomas—meningiomas—[capillary angioma]

Aqueduct
Spongioblastomas (adolescence)—ependymitis—malformations—[ependymomas]

Cerebellar vermis
Medulloblastomas—spongioblastomas (so-called astrocytomas)—[epidermoids—dermoids—teratomas]—meningiomas (torcular)

Cerebellar hemispheres
Medulloblastomas—spongioblastoms (so-called astrocytomas)—angioblastomas—meningiomas (tentorial)

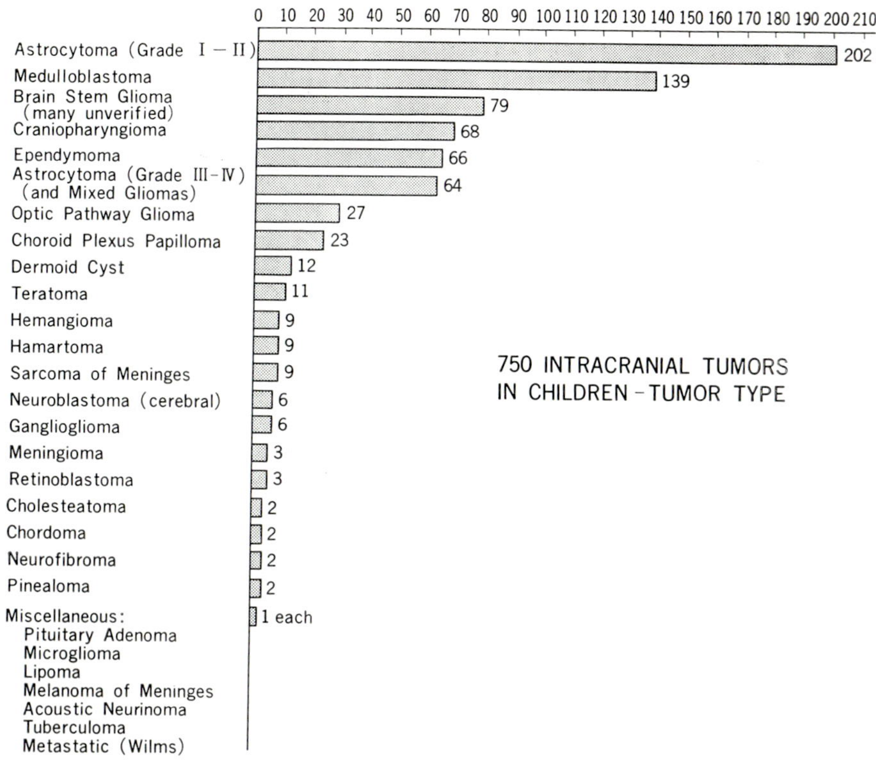

Fig. 55 Classification and incidence of tumor types based upon 750 cases in childhood (Through the courtesy of Charles C. Thomas Publisher. From MATSON: Neurosurgery of Infancy and Childhood, 1969).

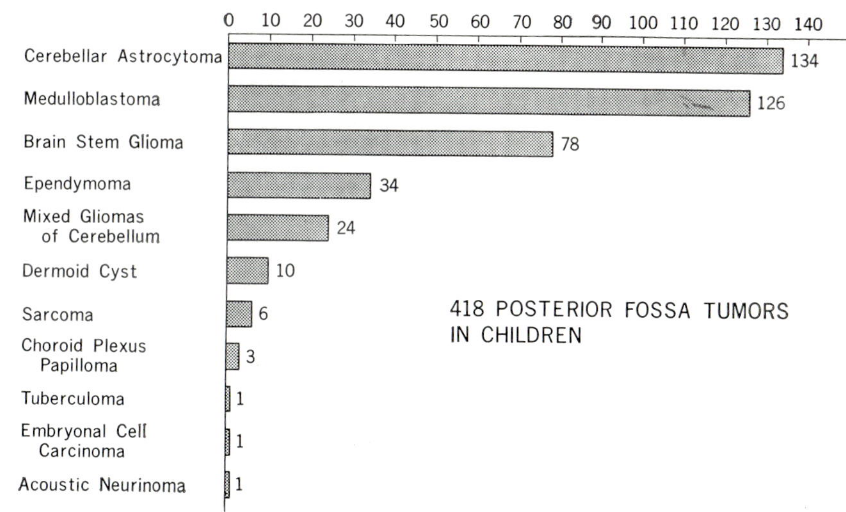

Fig. 56 Relative frequency of 418 tumor types at the various locations of the posterior fossa in childhood (Through the courtesy of Charles C. Thomas Publisher. From MATSON: Neurosurgery of Infancy and Childhood, 1969).

Fourth ventricle

Ependymomas—plexus papillomas—spongioblastomas—angioblastomas (calamus scriptorius)—adhesive arachnoiditis

Cerebello-pontine angle

Neurinomas—meningiomas—epidermoids—[plexus papillomas—ependymomas—ependymal cysts—adhesive arachnoiditis]

Caudal brain stem (pons and medulla)

Astrocytomas—spongioblastomas—glioblastomas—gangliocytomas—chordomas—meningiomas (clivus/craniospinal)

Spinal tumors

Intradural: Ependymomas—spongioblastomas—astrocytomas—oligodendrogliomas—meningiomas—neurinomas—angioblastomas—epidermoids—lipomas—[teratomas]

Extradural: Sarcomas—cavernous angiomas of the vertebral bodies and epidural space, especially in the thoracic region—metastases—[tumors of thyroid origin—dumbbell neurinomas]—gangliocytomas of the sympathetics

Base of the skull

Medial group: Chordomas—nasopharyngeal tumors (fibromas of the nasopharynx, "cylindromas," squamous cell carcinomas, lymphosarcomas, reticulum cell sarcomas)

Paramedial group: Chondromas/osteochondromas of the petrous tip—neurinomas of the Gasserian ganglion—aneurysms of the carotid (infra- and suprasellar)—meningiomas of Meckel's cave—craniospinal meningiomas and meningiomas of the clivus—parasellar teratomas—"cylindromas"

INCREASED INTRACRANIAL PRESSURE

Arteriographic features

The basilar and intracranial vertebral arteries are compressed against the clivus with decreased distance between the arteries and the clivus. In the lateral projection, the anterior culminate and vermian segments of the superior cerebellar arteries are displaced superiorly and posteriorly in an arcuate fashion, while these segments are separated laterally in the Towne projection. The latter findings are frequently associated with upward transtentorial herniation of the superior vermis. The anterior inferior cerebellar artery may be straightened and compressed against the clivus with markedly increased intracranial pressure. The supratonsillar segment of the posterior inferior cerebellar artery is stretched and slightly displaced downward. The vermian segments of this artery may show stretching and compression against the occipital bone. Such downward displacement of the posterior inferior cerebellar artery may be associated with tonsillar herniation. In addition, small arterial branches in the posterior fossa visualized during the course of the vertebral angiography are frequently stretched and diminished in caliber. While some of the above findings may be specific signs of the posterior fossa masses, they are usually indicative of increased intracranial pressure in the posterior fossa.

Small supratentorial arteries such as the thalamoperforate, posterior choroidal and posterior pericallosal arteries show sharp, increased visualization in the presence of increased intracranial pressure. The thalamoperforate arteries are stretched and lose their wavy course. In addition, arteriographic findings of dilatation of the supratentorial vertricles are demonstrated by these arteries.

Venographic features

The pontine segment of the anterior pontomesencephalic vein is compressed against the clivus and its interpeduncular segment is depressed downward with inferior displacement of the upper brain stem. With the same reasons the posterior mesencephalic and basal vein of Rosenthal is depressed downward. The supraculminate and superior vermian veins are compressed against the straight sinus and the inferior vermian vein is displaced downward. The fissural segment of the precentral cerebellar vein is displaced superiorly and posteriorly with angulation at the colliculocentral point. In addition, the veins of the posterior fossa are frequently reduced in caliber and straightened. Venographic signs of dilatation of the lateral ventricles are also present. In particular, the distance between the superior choroid vein and the internal cerebral vein is reduced due to dilatation of the lateral ventricle.

Other angiographic findings

Increased intracranial pressure lowers the speed of blood flow especially on the side of tumors. Therefore, the normal brain tissue in the posterior fossa may show diffuse stain in the capillary phase secondary to prolonged flow in the capillaries. Visualization of the posterior fossa veins is frequently slowed. This finding is apparent when normal and abnormal sides are compared.

Large Medulloblastoma Filling the Ballooned Fourth Ventricle and Producing Bilateral Tonsillar Herniation

An 8-year-old female: Figs. 57–64

At surgery the aqueduct was enlarged and the lateral recess of the fourth ventricle on the right was infiltrated. No mass was present in the vallecula.

Fig. 57 Preoperative vertebral angiogram (arterial phase in the lateral projection). The arteries in the posterior fossa are slightly diminished in caliber. The anterior culminate and vermian segments of the superior cerebellar artery are stretched in an arcuate fashion (3 arrows). The precentral cerebellar artery is displaced anteriorly (3 open arrowheads). There is stretching of the thalamoperforate arteries (closed arrowheads). The posterior inferior cerebellar artery is depressed with marked downward displacement of the supratonsillar segment (2 long arrows). The vermian segment and its branches are also stretched and depressed (3 crossed arrows).

Fig. 58 Postoperative vertebral angiogram (arterial phase in the lateral projection) for comparison. The posterior inferior cerebellar artery has been ligated. The caliber of the arteries is now normal. The anterior culminate segments (3 arrows) and thalamoperforate arteries (arrowheads) are normal in position. The precentral cerebellar artery is not visualized.

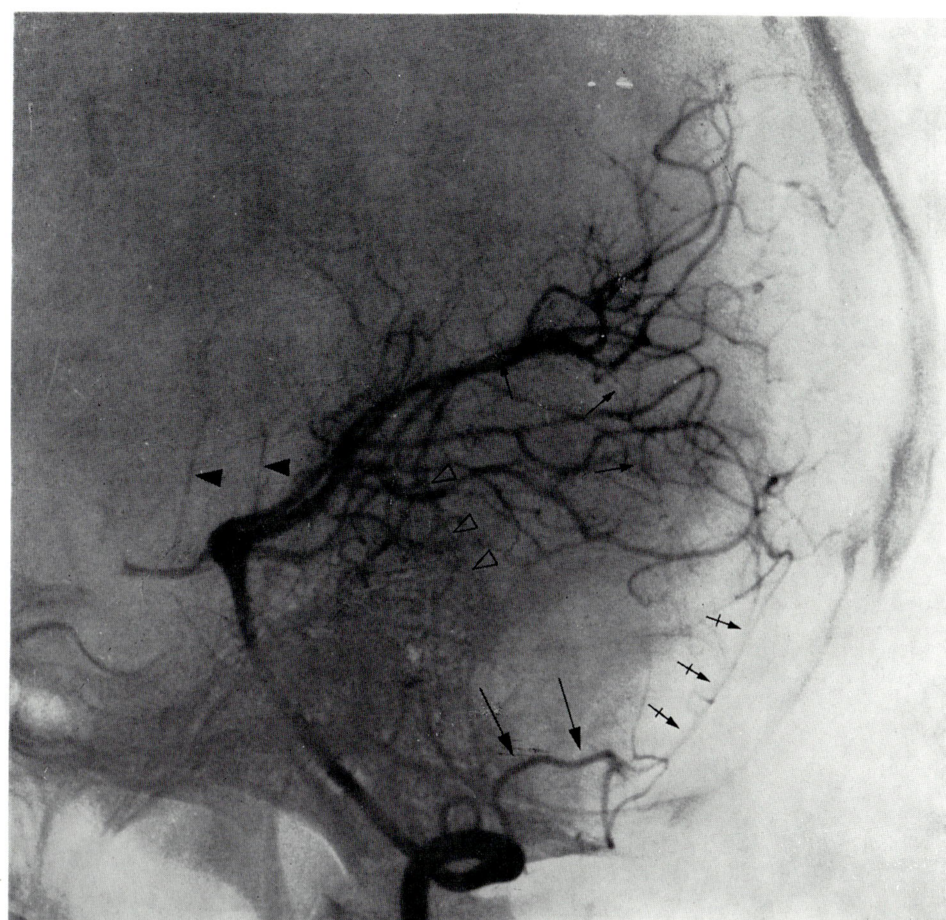

Fig. 57

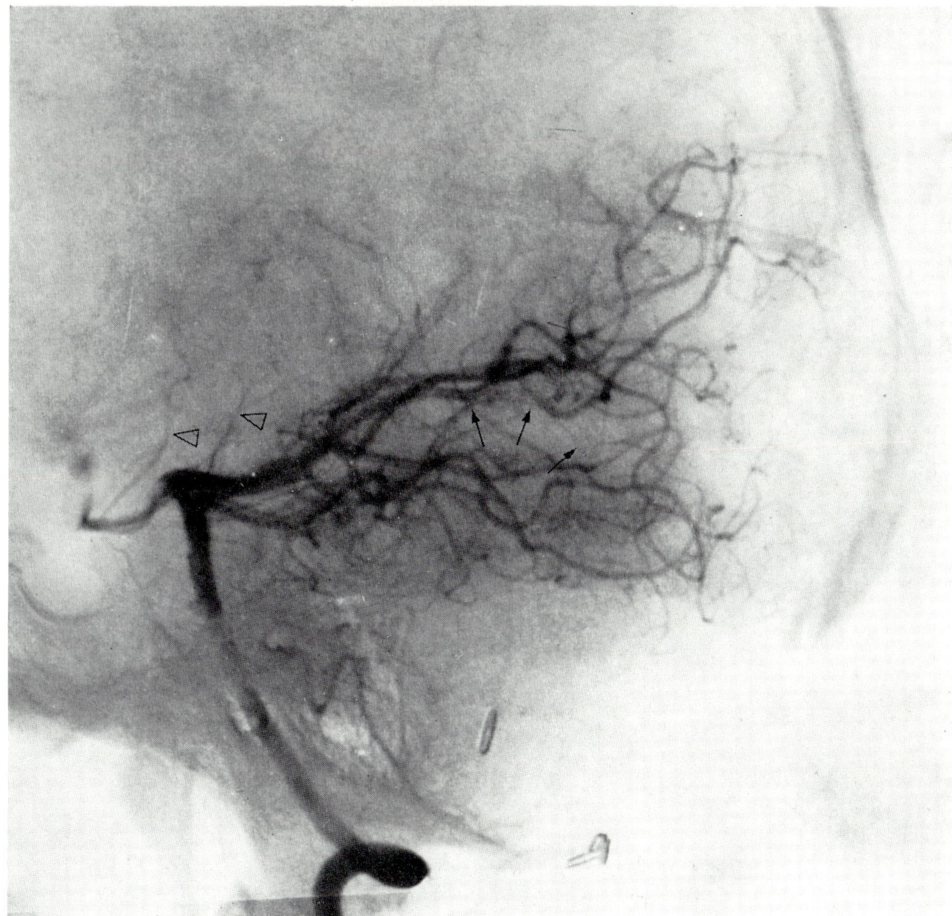

Fig. 58

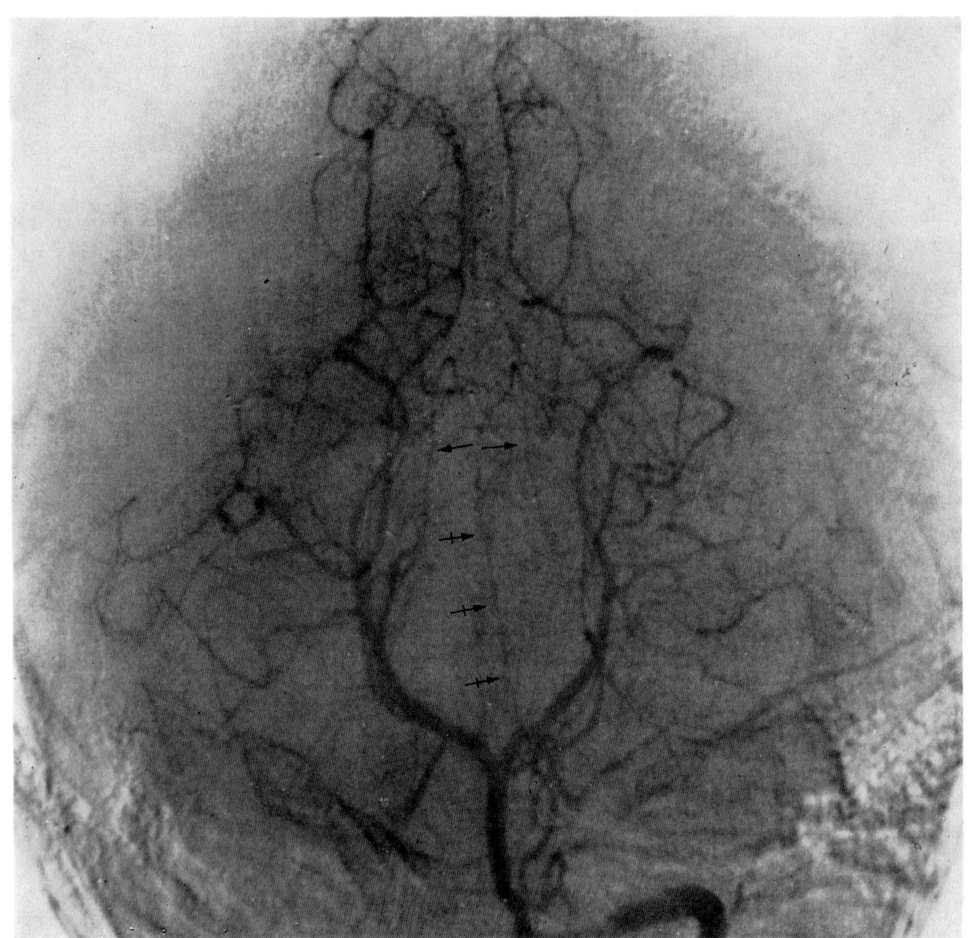

Fig. 59

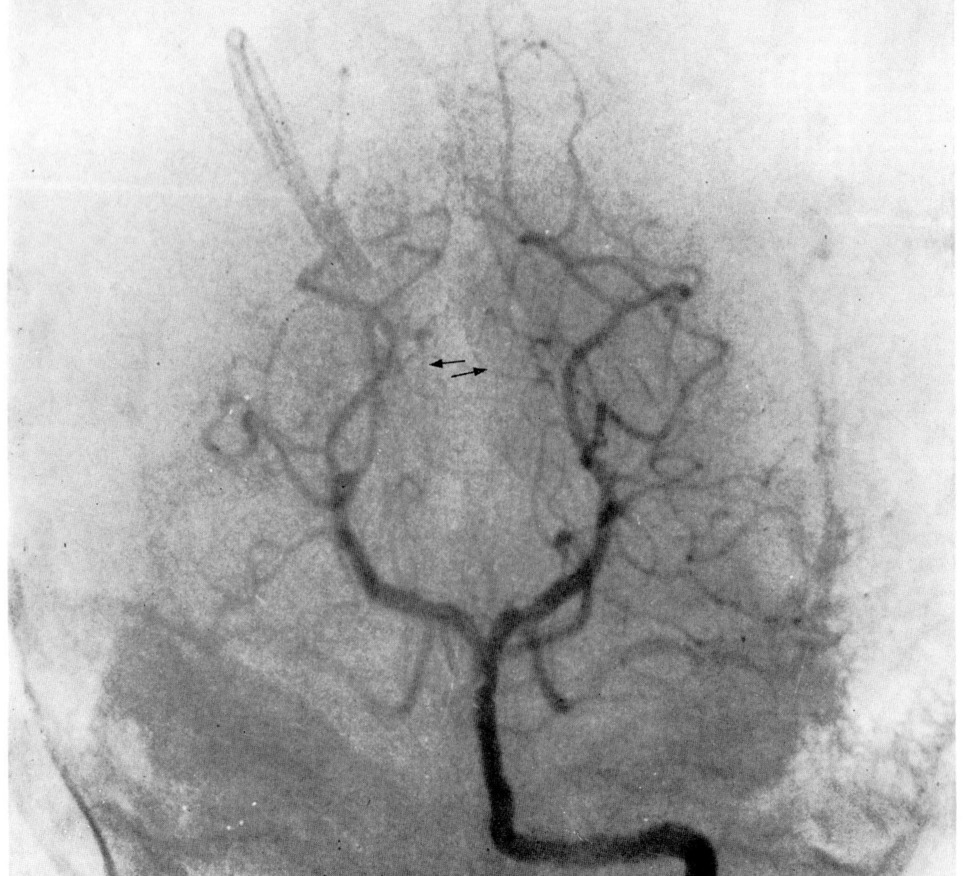

Fig· 60

Fig. 59 Preoperative vertebral angiogram (arterial phase in the Towne projection). The caliber of the arterial branches is all diminished and small branches such as marginal and anterior inferior cerebellar arteries are straightened. The quadrigeminal segments of the superior cerebellar arteries are displaced laterally, indicating upward transtentorial herniation (arrows). The vermian segment of the posterior inferior cerebellar artery is straightened and displaced slightly to the left (3 crossed arrows).

Fig. 60 Postoperative vertebral angiogram (arterial phase in the Towne projection) for comparison. The anterior culminate segments of the superior cerebellar arteries are normally located (arrows). The posterior inferior cerebellar artery has been clipped.

Fig. 61 Preoperative vertebral angiogram (venous phase in the lateral projection). The anterior pontomesencephalic vein is compressed against the clivus (a closed arrowhead) and the interpeduncular segment of this vein is depressed (an arrow). The distance between the superior choroid vein and the internal cerebral vein is diminished (2 opposing arrows). The precentral cerebellar vein is straightened and displaced anteriorly (3 arrows). The superior vermian vein and the inferior vermian vein are compressed against the straight sinus and the occipital bone, respectively (3 crossed arrows). The copular point is displaced downward (an open arrowhead).

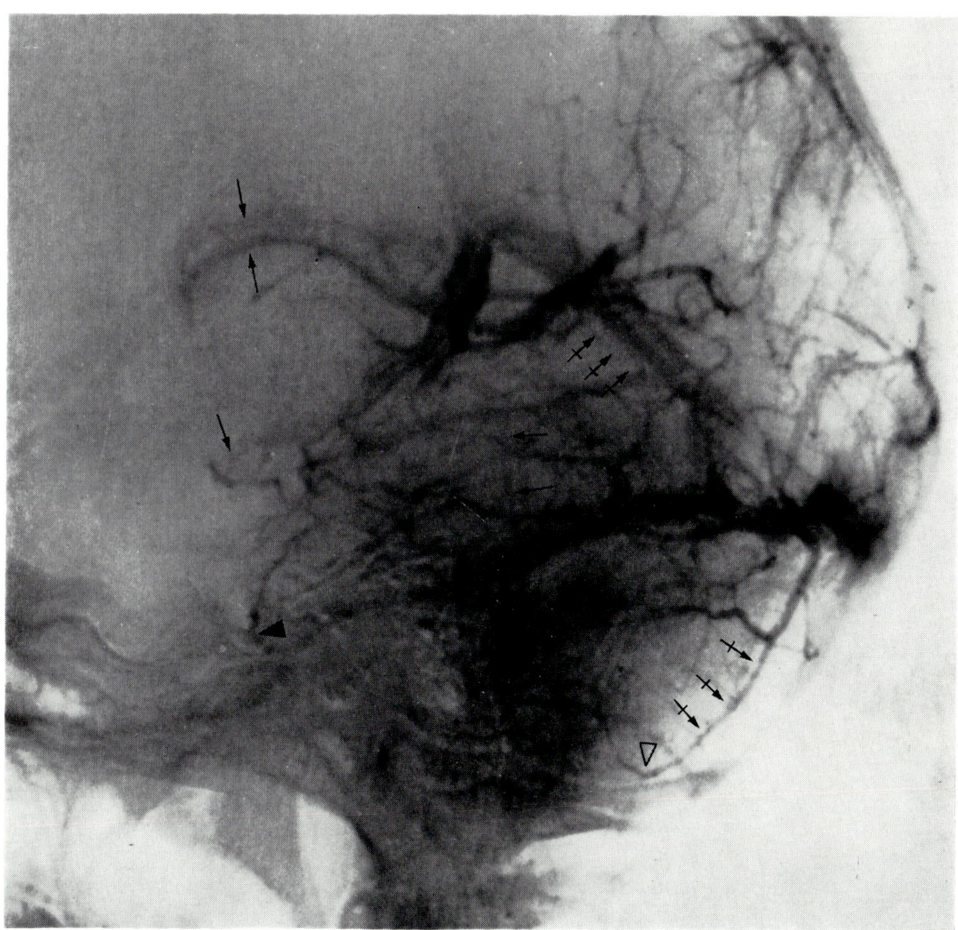

Fig. 61

Fig. 62 Postoperative vertebral angiogram (venous phase in the lateral projection) for comparison. The interpeduncular segment is now normal in position (an arrow). The distance between the superior choroid vein and internal cerebral vein is normal (2 opposing arrows). The superior vermian vein is not stretched (2 crossed arrows). The precentral cerebellar vein is not visualized in this view. The inferior vermian vein has been ligated.

Fig. 63 Preoperative vertebral angiogram (venous phase in the Towne projection). The petrosal veins and their tributaries are compressed against the petrous bone (2 arrows). The posterior mesencephalic and lateral anastomotic mesencephalic veins are slightly stretched (3 arrowheads). There is straightening of the precentral cerebellar vein, which is localized in the midline (3 crossed arrows).

Fig. 64 Postoperative vertebral angiogram (venous phase in the Towne projection) for comparison. There is no stretching of the posterior and lateral anastomotic mesencephalic vein (3 arrowheads). The petrosal veins are normal in position (an arrow). The precentral cerebellar vein is visualized with inverted "Y" at its inferior termination.

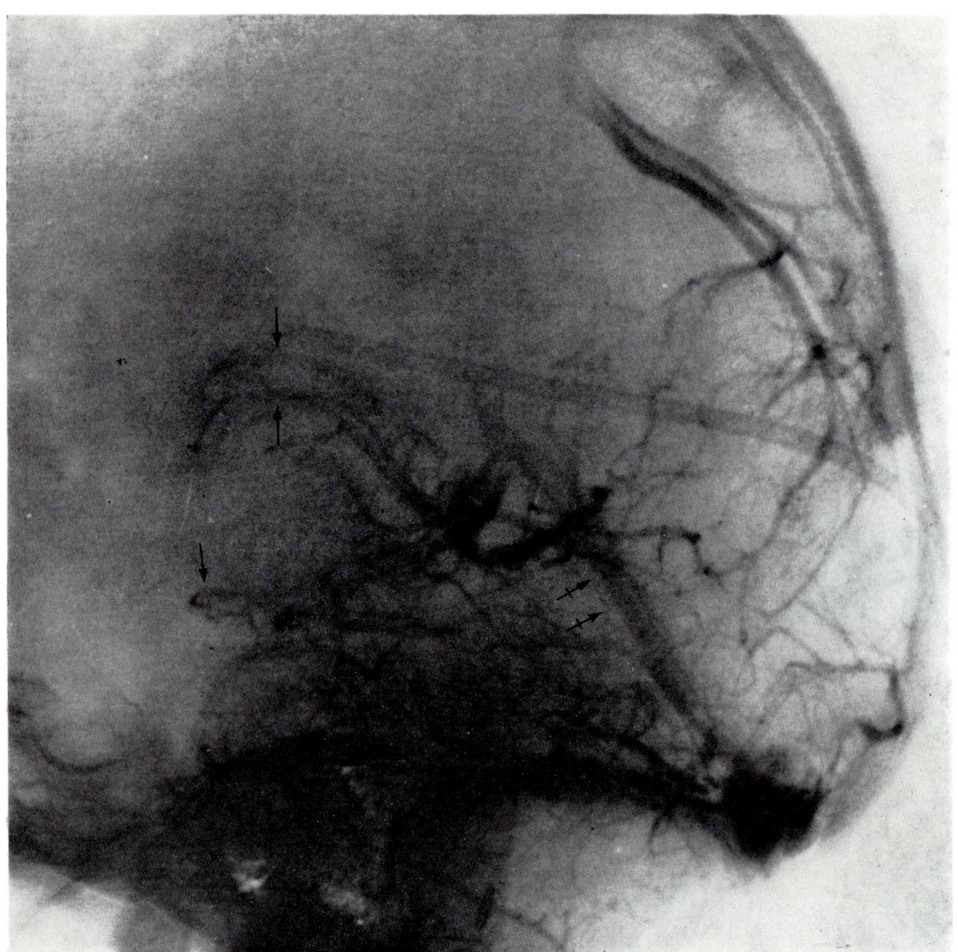

Fig. 62

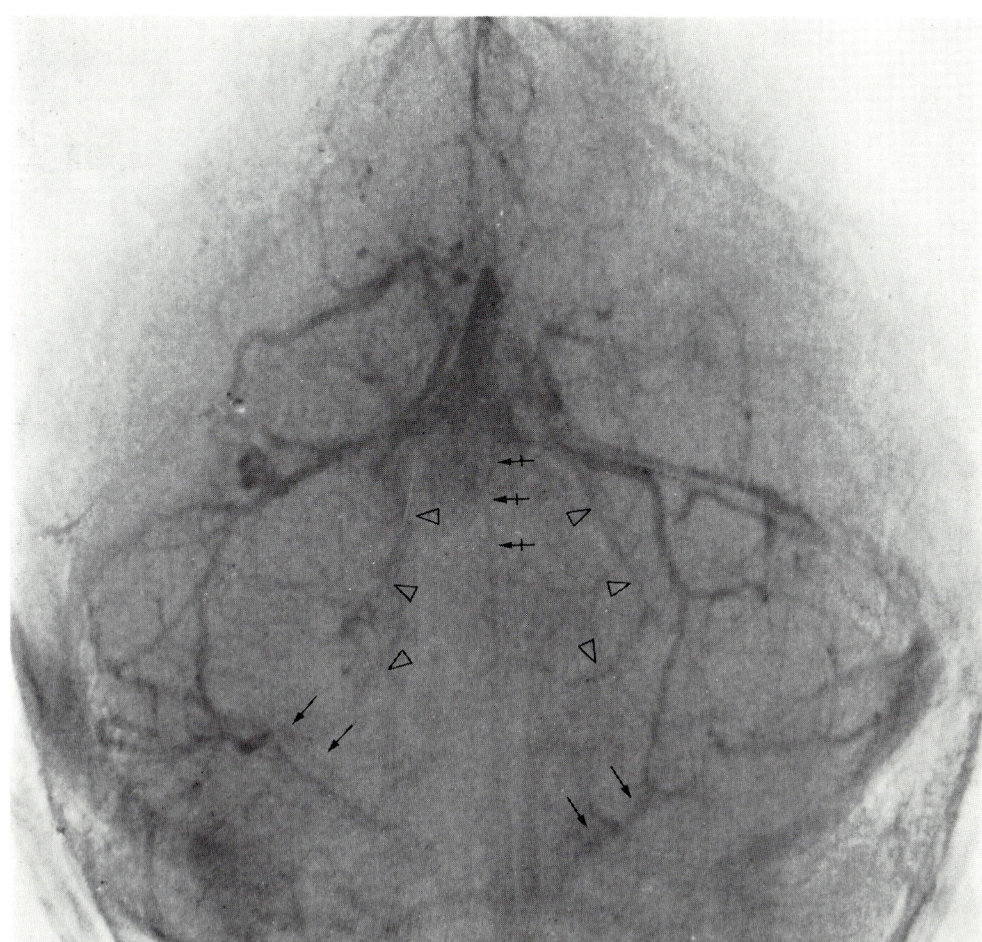
Fig. 63

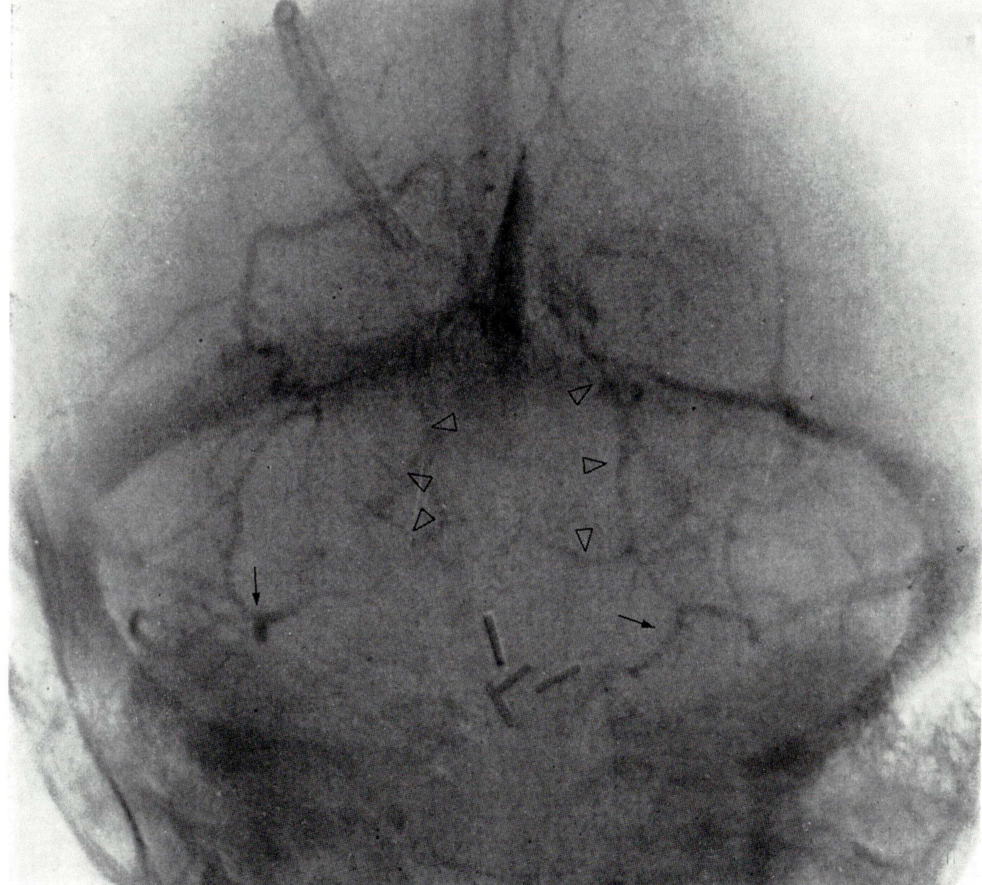
Fig. 64

PATHOLOGICAL CIRCULATION IN THE POSTERIOR FOSSA TUMORS

Demonstration of abnormal tumor circulation provides useful diagnostic information in regard to location, size and histologic nature of the tumors. Percentage visualization of pathological tumor circulation by vertebral angiography has been reported to be between 20 and 40%, primarily depending upon methods of vertebral angiographies. Direct injection technique such as transfemoral or transaxillary catheter vertebral angiography undoubtedly increases this incidence. In this section, special attention has been paid to the most common tumors of the posterior fossa.

Meningiomas

Meningiomas occur most commonly in the cerebellopontine angle, over the clivus and at the tentorial margin in the posterior fossa. However, a small number of meningiomas still develop over the cerebellar hemisphere, the undersurface of the tentorium and the vallecula.

The characteristic appearance of meningiomas is a homogeneous tumor stain with sharp margins. The tumor stain persists for a considerable period of time, usually into the capillary phase or the early venous phase. Tumor vessels are not usually demonstrated. As for the blood supply, the majority of meningiomas in the posterior fossa are supplied by the meningeal branches of the vertebral arteries as well as external and internal carotid arteries. The anterior and posterior meningeal branches of the vertebral artery may supply the meningiomas, while the meningohypophyseal artery of the internal carotid artery may send meningeal branches to the posterior fossa and to the tentorium. Posterior fossa meningiomas may also be supplied by the meningeal branches of the occipital artery or the accessory meningeal arteries entering the intracranium by way of the condyloid foramen and through the foramen lacerum. In addition, the anterior inferior and posterior inferior cerebellar arteries frequently send small arterial branches to the meningiomas in the posterior fossa.

Meningiomas do not usually show draining veins, but some meningiomas such as angioblastic meningiomas may show prominent draining veins with an increase in the speed of circulation. Such meningiomas are frequently associated with irregular tumor vessels and tumor stains.

Hemangioblastomas

These tumors are extremely vascular and frequently associated with cyst formation. Taveras and Wood (1964) described three different types of vascular patterns angiographically: 1) a mural nodule with a cyst associated with one or more draining veins; 2) a circular arrangement of abnormal vessels surrounding a clear cystic space; and 3) a large mass with many abnormal vessels and distinct abnormal veins. In our experience mural nodules usually present small, homogeneous stains and may be missed without use of subtraction technique.

Gliomas and other tumors

Glioblastoma multiforme may present irregular tumor vessels with arteriovenous communication. Enlarged feeding arteries and draining veins may be demonstrated. Glioblastomas, however, are infrequently found in the posterior fossa. Cerebellar astrocytomas are avascular tumors with frequent formation of cysts; only rarely a capillary blush may be demonstrated within a tumor. Since cerebellar astrocytomas frequently occur in the young patients, astrocytomas should be suspected in the presence of avascular hemispheric lesions in the younger age group.

Some ependymomas and medulloblastomas show enlargement of the choroidal and nodular branches of the posterior inferior cerebellar artery, which are rarely visualized in normal cases. In addition, medulloblastomas present enlargement and posterior displacement of the posterior inferior cerebellar artery. Very minimal tumor stain may be demonstrated. Other fourth ventricle tumors and cerebellar tumors with invasion of the fourth ventricle and nodulus also produce similar angiographic findings.

Metastatic tumors

These tumors in the posterior fossa show variety of abnormal pathological circulations similar to supratentorial metastatic lesions. Metastatic tumors from the kidney may show markedly irregular tumor vessels with arteriovenous communication, while a homogeneous stain may be seen in a metastatic tumor from the thyroid, breast and lung. Tumor stains may contain central radiolucency.

It has been suggested that a metastatic tumor is supplied by a single artery, but this is not always applicable.

In our experience, local edema is conspicuous in metastatic tumors. Therefore we consider a metastatic lesion when the local edema is marked in spite of a small area of pathological vessels.

Acoustic neurinomas

Tumor stains may be demonstrated in acoustic neurinomas. The stains are patchy or diffuse and supplied by the anterior inferior cerebellar artery. Tumor vessels are not demonstrated in most cases.

Networks of small arterial branches over the tumor sometimes simulate a single arterial branch displaced by the tumor; this is probably due to the tangential effects of the networks to the central X-ray. There is frequently development of abnormal veins which drain into the petrosal vein and usually measures 2 to 3 mm in the greatest diameter. The abnormal vein originates from the posterior and inferior aspect of the tumor, takes a course over the tumor and then drains into the petrosal vein. Therefore, this abnormal vein shows arched configuration with superior and posterior convexity.

Meningioma in the Right Cerebellopontine Angle

A 44-year-old male: Figs. 65 and 66

Fig. 65 Arterial phase in the anteroposterior projection. The right anterior inferior cerebellar artery is enlarged and elevated (2 arrows). Its distal branches are stretched. There is minimal displacement of the basilar artery to the left.

Fig. 66 Capillary phase in the Towne projection. There is a 3.0 cm round, homogeneous tumor stain in the right cerebellopontine angle (3 arrows). Homogeneity of the tumor stain and its persistence into the early venous phase are strongly suggestive of a meningioma. The main blood supply was from the anterior inferior cerebellar artery at surgery.

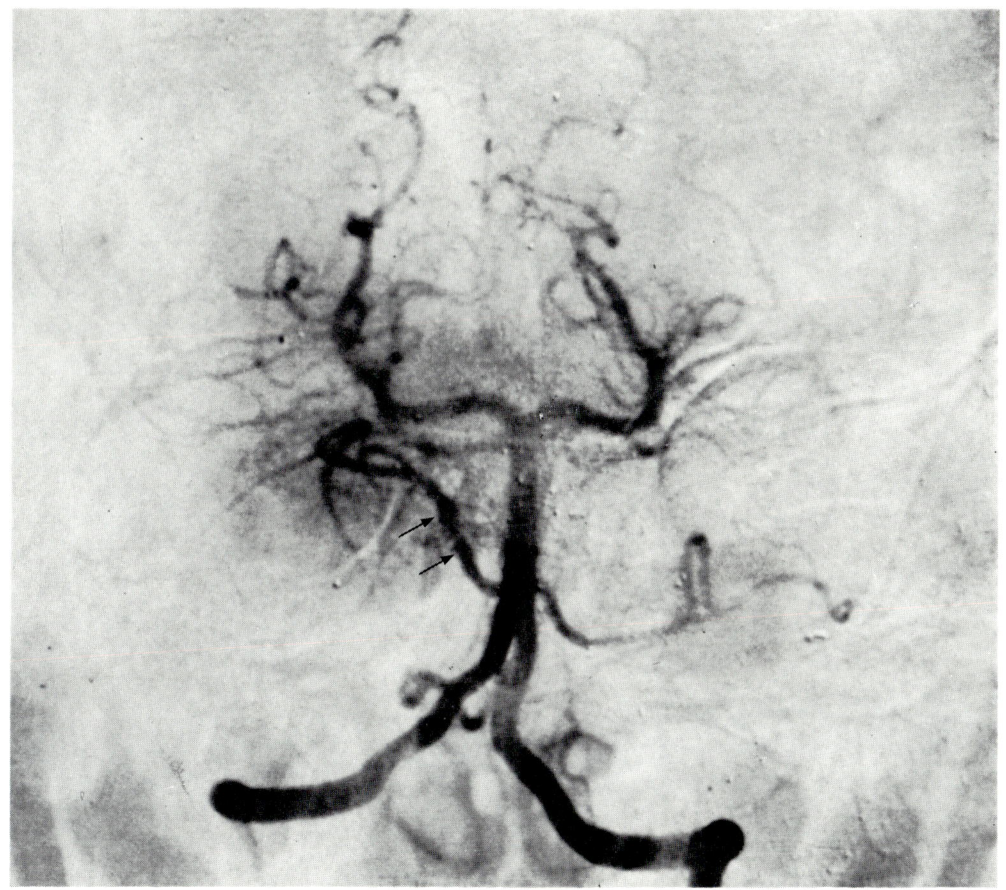

Fig. 65

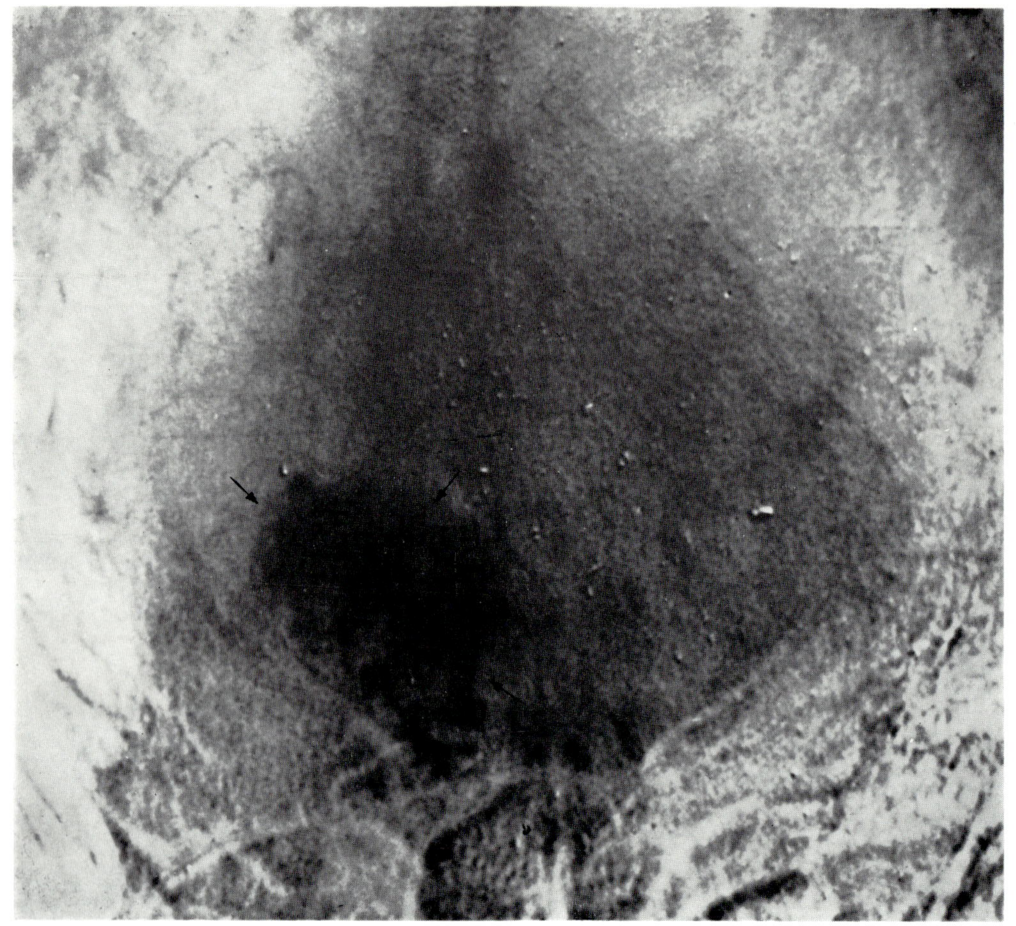

Fig. 66

Huge Hemangioblastoma Involving the Inferior Vermis, both Inferior Cerebellar Hemispheres, Vallecula and Fourth Ventricle

A 20-year-old male: Figs. 67–71

Fig. 67 Arterial phase of the left vertebral angiogram in the Towne projection. There are extensive, irregular tumor vessels in the midline extending laterally on both sides. The major blood supply is from the posterior inferior cerebellar artery with minimal supply from the superior cerebellar artery. There is separation of the superior cerebellar arteries, suggesting upward transtentorial herniation.

Fig. 68 Arterial phase of the left vertebral angiogram in the lateral projection. There is a large tumor with irregular tumor vessels in the fourth ventricle, vallecula and inferior cerebellum. The blood supply is from the enlarged posterior inferior cerebellar artery (an arrow) and the superior cerebellar artery (2 crossed arrows). The basilar artery is compressed against the clivus and the anterior culminate and vermian segments of the superior cerebellar artery are stretched superiorly.

Fig. 69 Venous phase of the left vertebral angiogram. There is a 5×5 cm area of dense tumor stains in the inferior posterior fossa, which are drained by the enlarged inferior vermian vein (2 arrows). The precentral cerebellar vein is elevated (2 crossed arrows).

Fig. 70 Arterial phase of the right vertebral angiogram in the lateral projection. There are arteriographic changes similar to the left sided study. The feeding arteries are the posterior inferior (an arrow) and superior (2 crossed arrows) cerebellar arteries.

Fig. 71 Venous phase of the right vertebral angiogram. There are similar venous changes as on venous phase of the left vertebral angiogram. The inferior vermian vein is enlarged and drains the tumor (2 arrows). The precentral cerebellar vein is elevated (a crossed arrow).

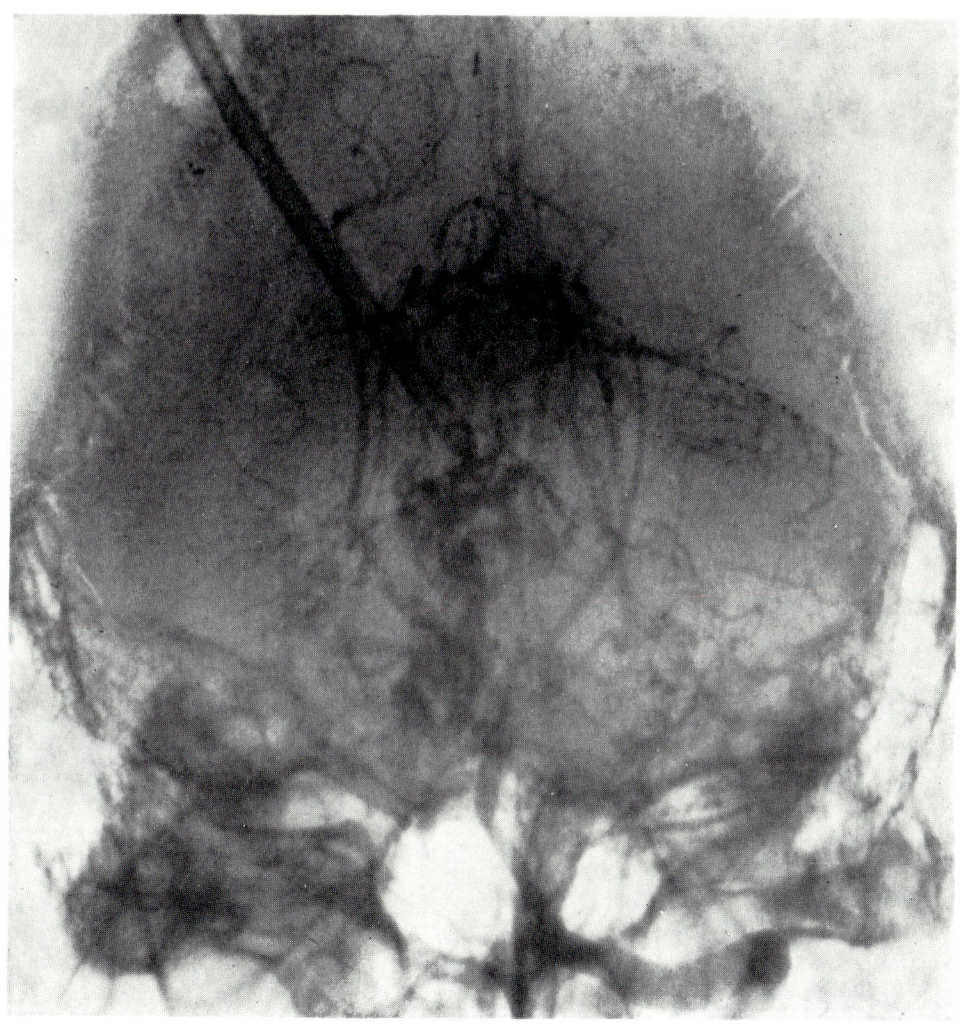

Fig. 67

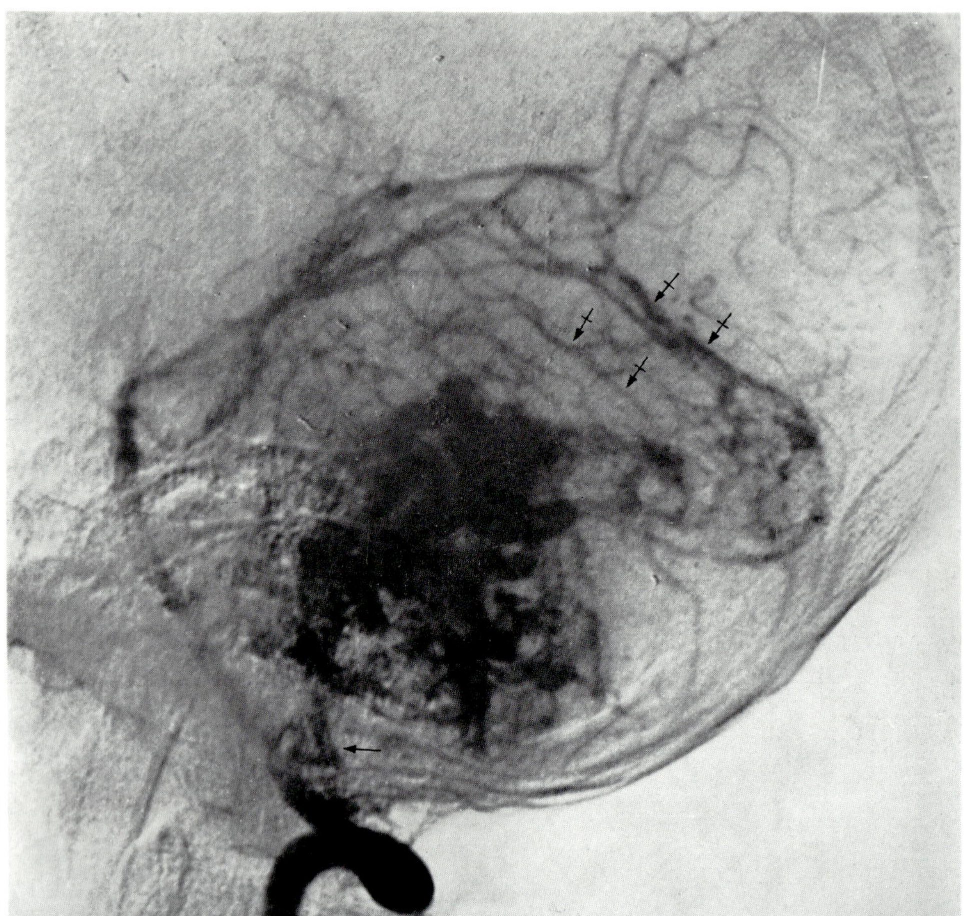

Fig. 68

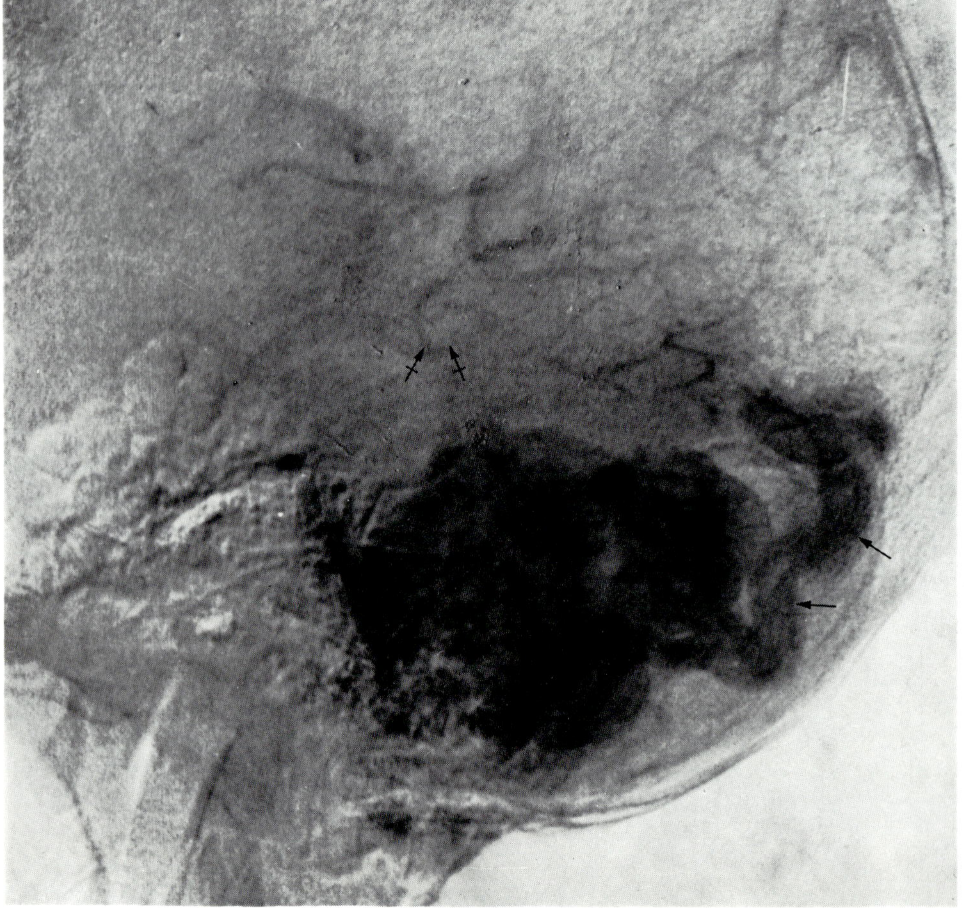

Fig. 69

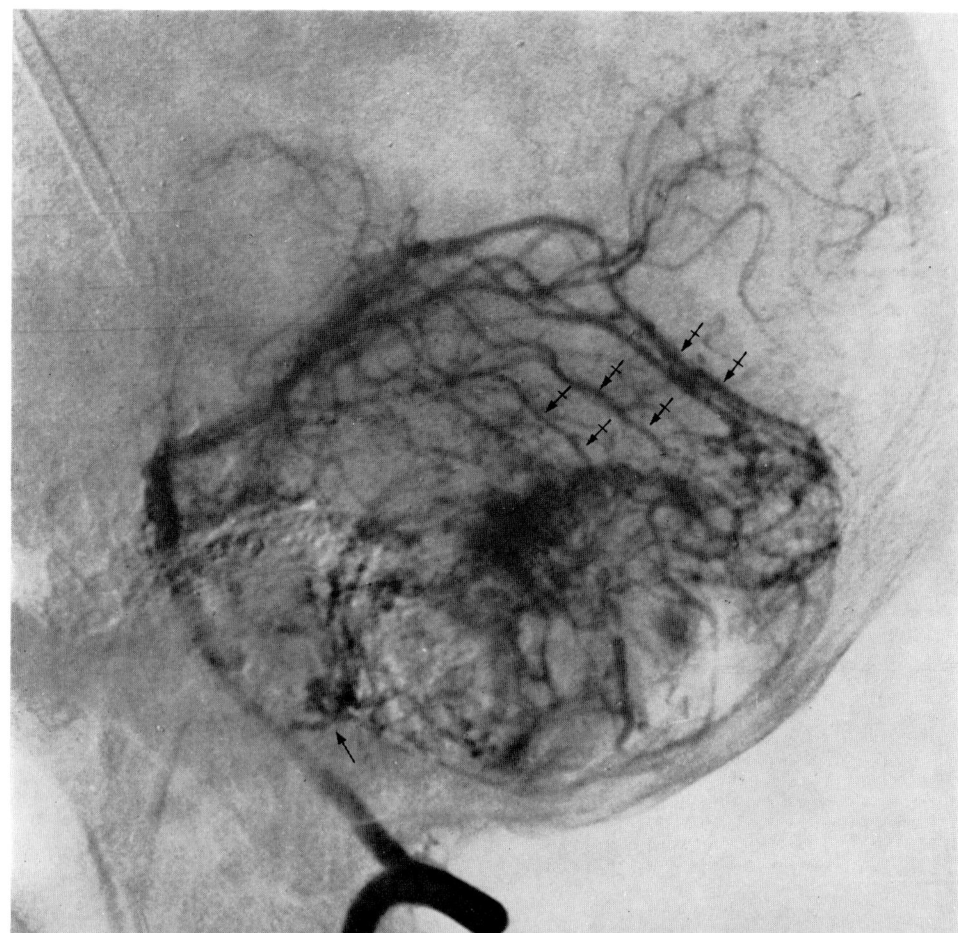

Fig. 70

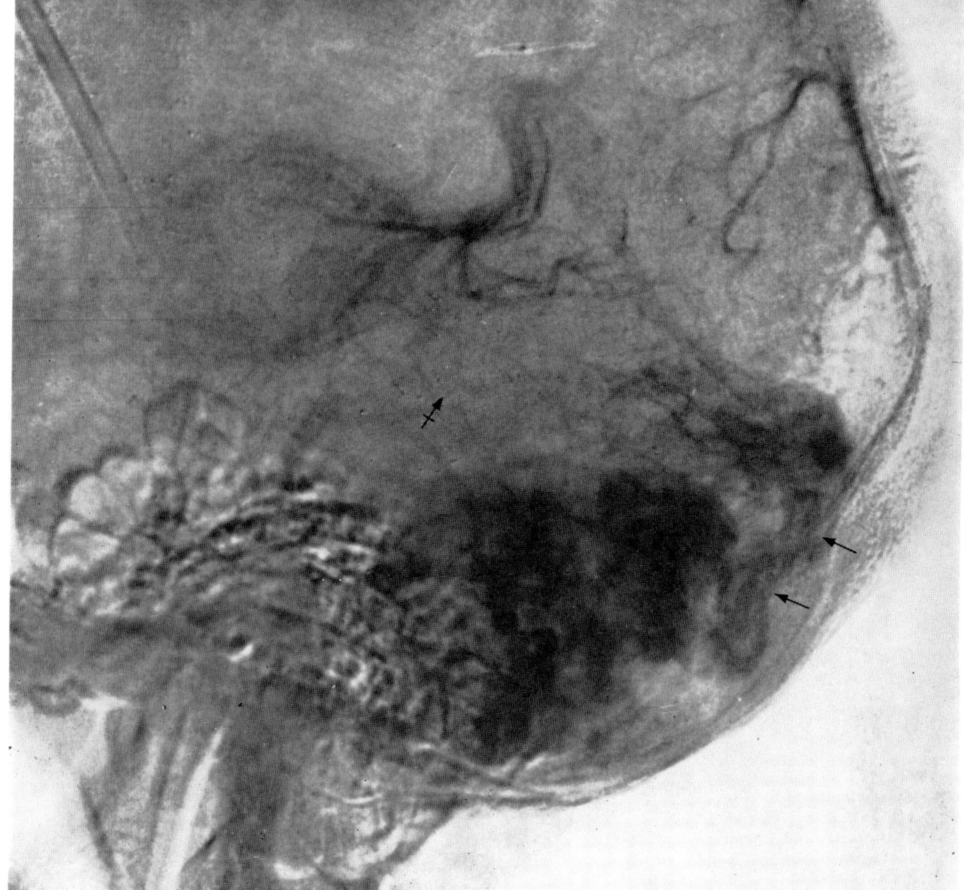

Fig. 71

Large Cystic Hemangioblastoma in the Left Cerebellar Hemisphere with a Mural Nodule

A 49-year-old female: Figs. 72–75

Fig. 72 Arterial phase in the lateral projection. The basilar artery is compressed against the clivus. There is a 1.2 cm homogeneous tumor stain in the superior aspect of the cerebellum (4 arrowheads), which appears to be supplied by an enlarged branch from the superior cerebellar artery (2 crossed arrows). The supratonsillar segment of the posterior inferior cerebellar artery is angulated and displaced anteriorly (a crossed arrow). The hemispheric and vermian branches are stretched and displaced downward (3 arrows). These arterial displacements indicate that there is a large cystic component extending into the inferior cerebellar hemisphere.

Fig. 73 Arterial phase in the Towne projection. There is an ovoid tumor stain in the superior aspect of the left cerebellum adjacent to the brain stem (4 arrowheads). Blood supply comes from an enlarged branch of the ambient segment of the superior cerebellar artery (a crossed arrow). The marginal artery is stretched (3 arrows); but the main segment of the superior cerebellar artery is not displaced. The anterior inferior cerebellar artery is depressed on the left.

Fig. 74 Capillary phase. The tumor stain contains central radiolucency which is characteristic of a hemangioblastoma.

Fig. 75 Venous phase. The tumor stain is faintly seen (3 arrowheads). The drainage is into the posterior mesencephalic vein (2 arrows), via the anastomotic lateral mesencephalic vein (3 crossed arrows).

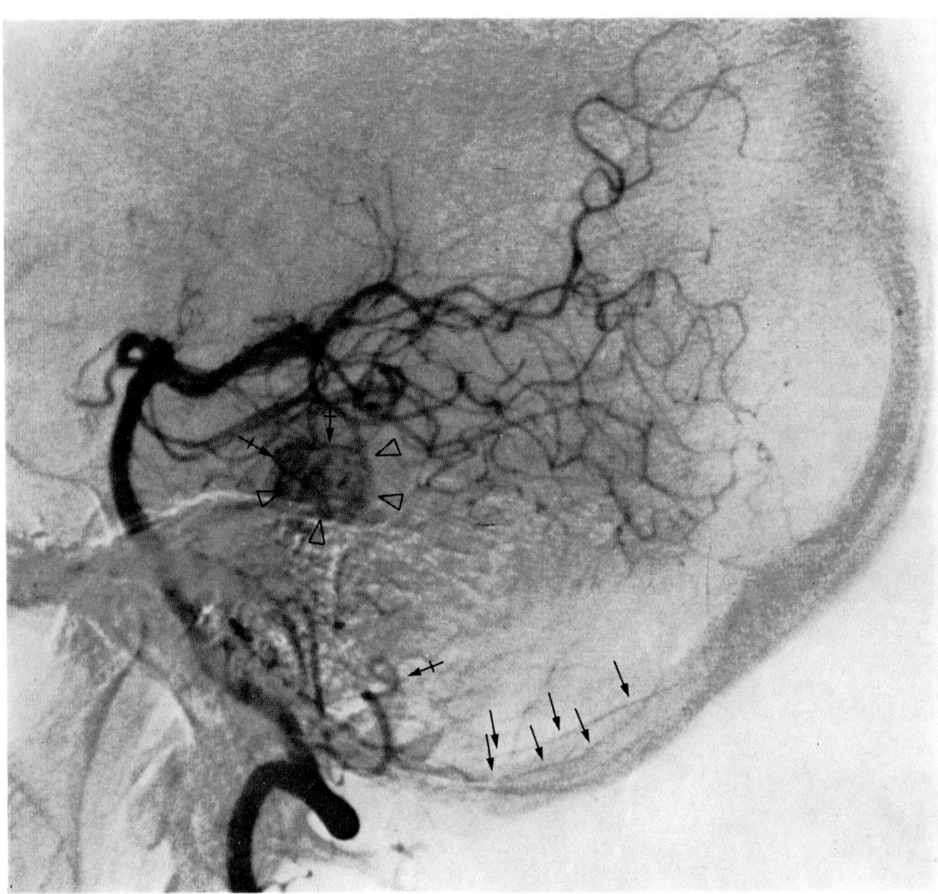

Fig. 72

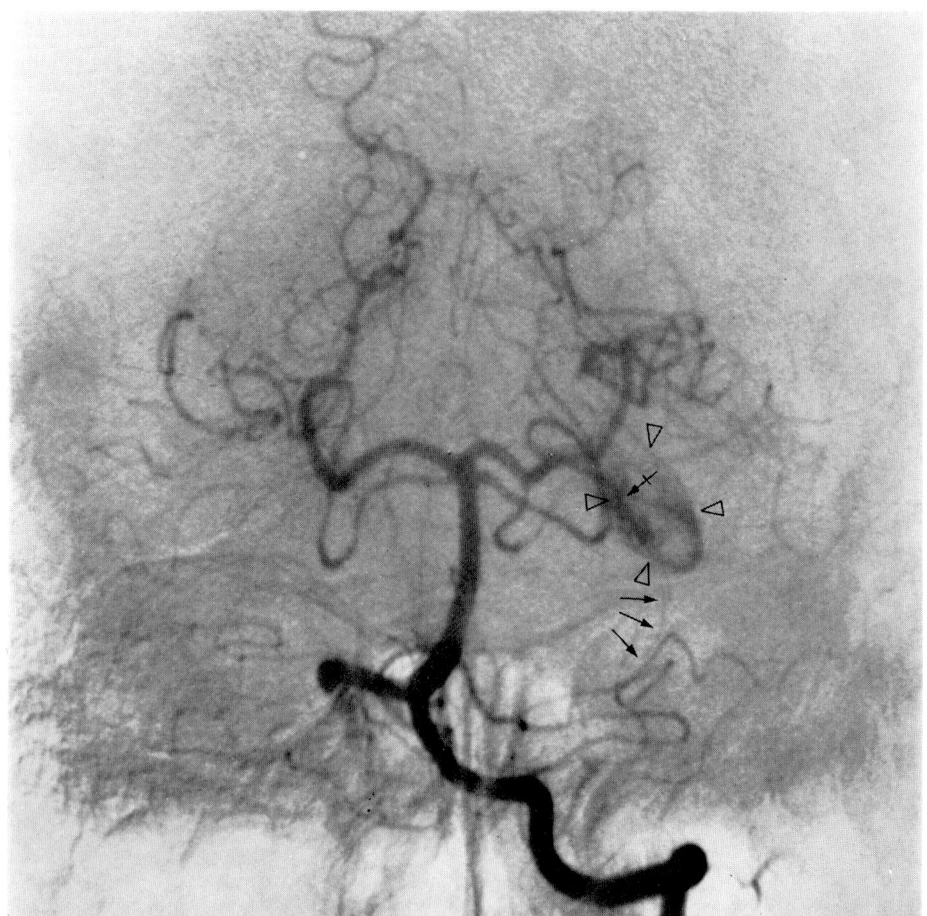

Fig. 73

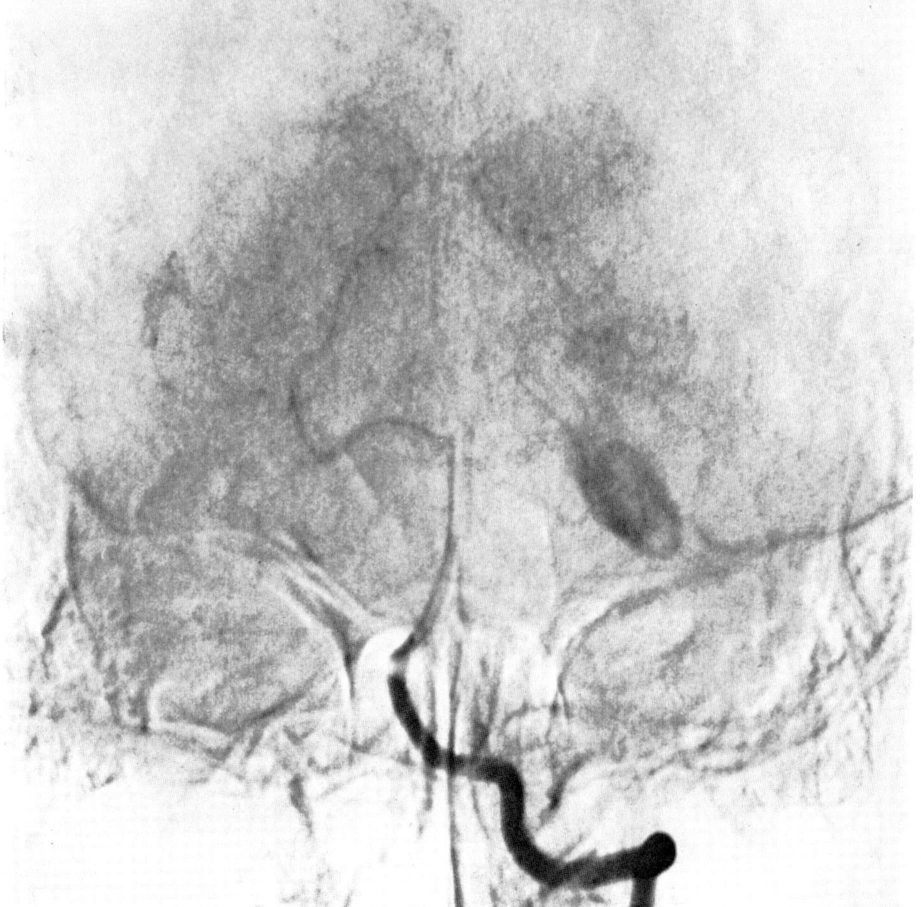

Fig. 74

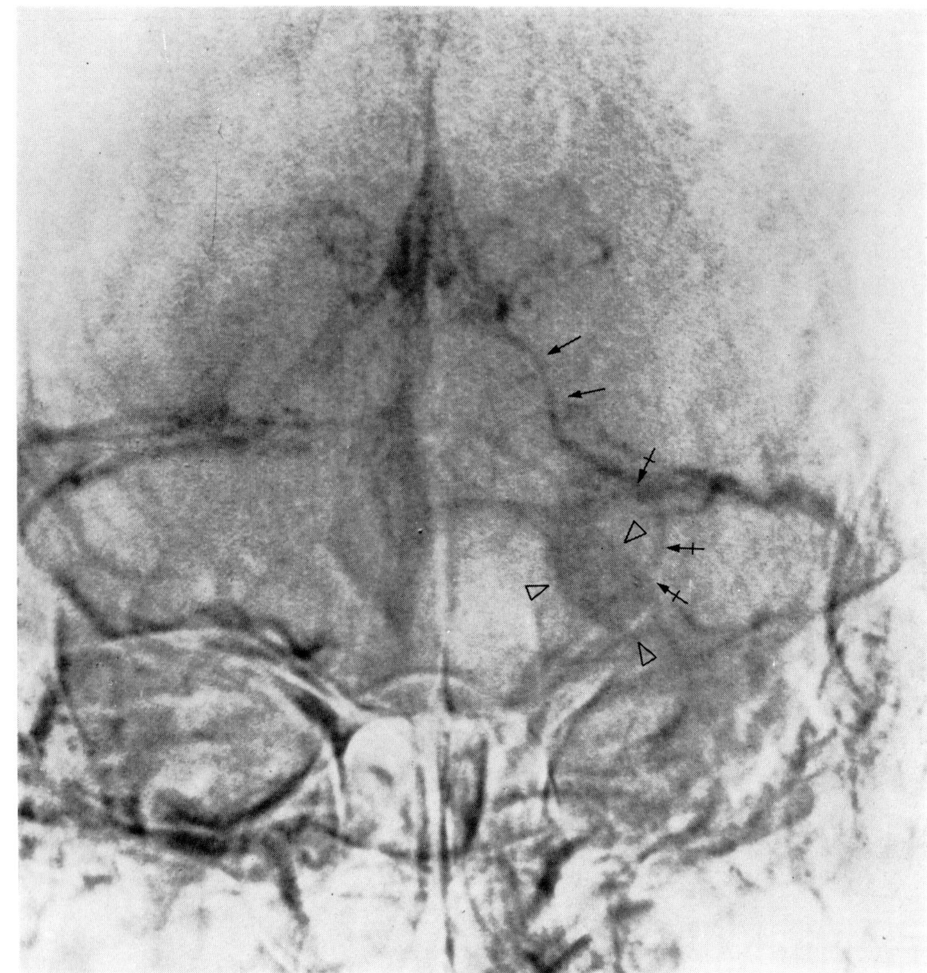

Fig. 75

Metastatic Glioblastoma in the Left Superior Cerebellar Hemisphere

A 24-year-old female: Figs. 76–81

A left occipital glioblastoma was removed 10 months previously.

Fig. 76 Arterial phase in the lateral projection. There is a 3.5 cm vascular mass in the superior cerebellum (5 arrowheads), mainly receiving blood supply from the enlarged superior cerebellar artery (a crossed arrow). The superior cerebellar artery and its branches are slightly elevated on the left. The supratonsillar segment of the posterior inferior cerebellar artery are depressed and displaced posteriorly (3 arrows). The basilar artery is compressed against the clivus and the thalamoperforate arteries are stretched, indicating increased hydrocephalus.

Fig. 77 Venous phase in the lateral projection. Enlarged abnormal veins (3 arrowheads) are noted and appear to drain into the posterior mesencephalic vein (2 arrows) and into the precentral cerebellar vein (a crossed arrow).

Fig. 78 Late venous phase in the lateral projection. The prepontine segment of the anterior pontomesencephalic vein is displaced anteriorly (2 arrows), and its interpeduncular segment has lost its normal course with marked anterior and superior displacement (2 crossed arrows). The petrosal vein is displaced downward (2 arrowheads). The precentral cerebellar vein is normal in position.

Fig. 79 Arterial phase in the Towne projection. The superior cerebellar artery on the left is enlarged, with elevation and supplies the vascular tumor (3 arrows). The vermian branches of the posterior inferior cerebellar artery are displaced to the right (4 crossed arrows).

Fig. 80 Capillary phase in the Towne projection. Abnormal veins in the tumor are well shown. Primary drainage is by the posterior mesencephalic vein (2 arrows) and the petrosal vein (2 crossed arrows). There is also drainage via the precentral cerebellar vein (an arrowhead).

Fig. 81 Venous phase in the Towne projection. The veins related to tumor circulation has disappeared. The petrosal vein on the left is markedly displaced downward (3 arrows). The inferior vermian vein is displaced to the right (3 crossed arrows).

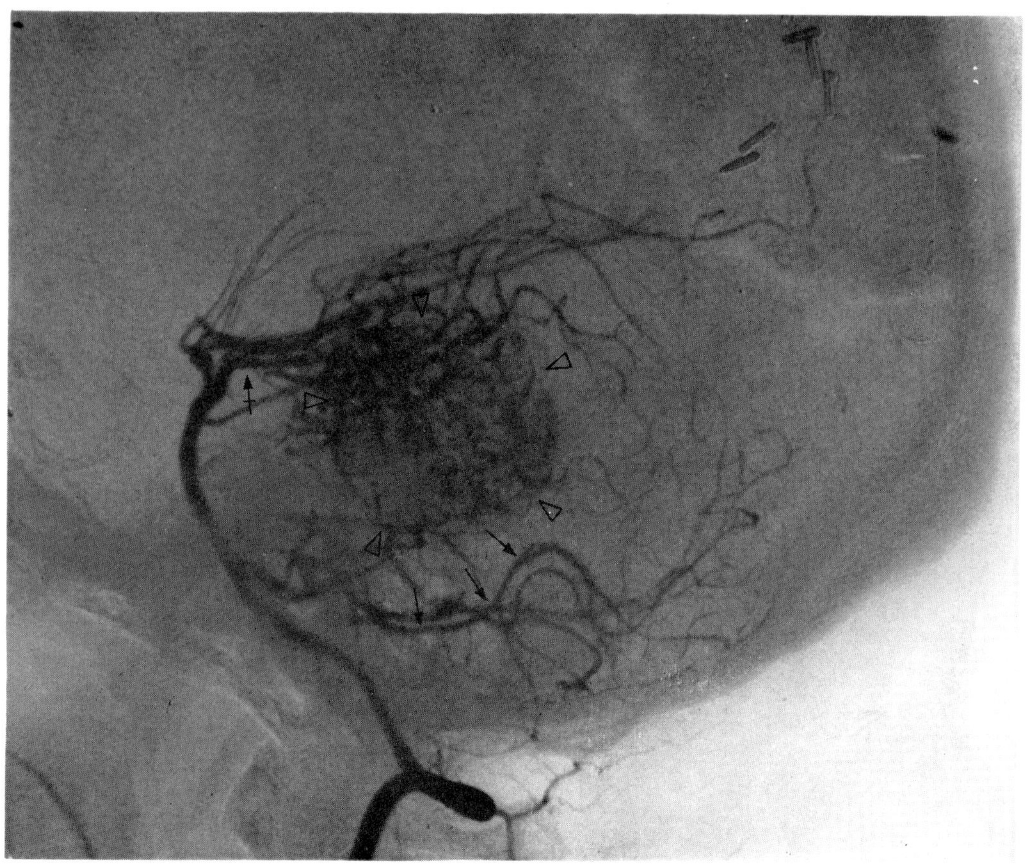

Fig. 76

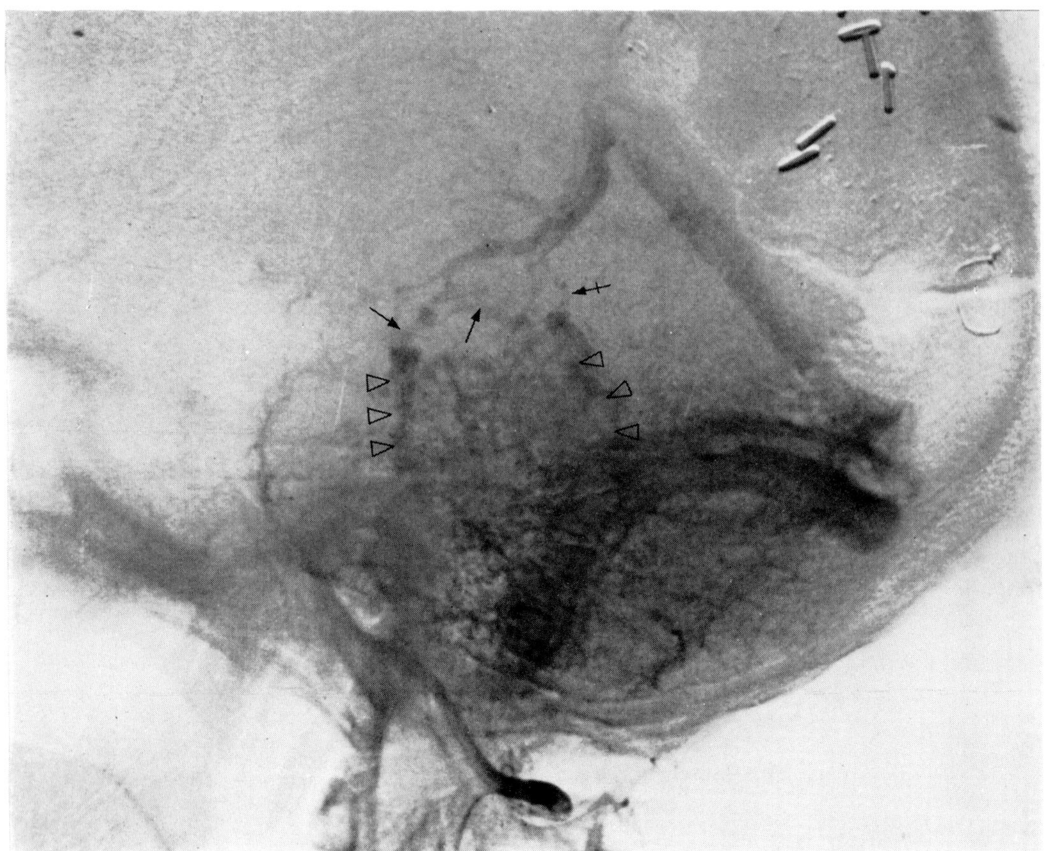

Fig. 77

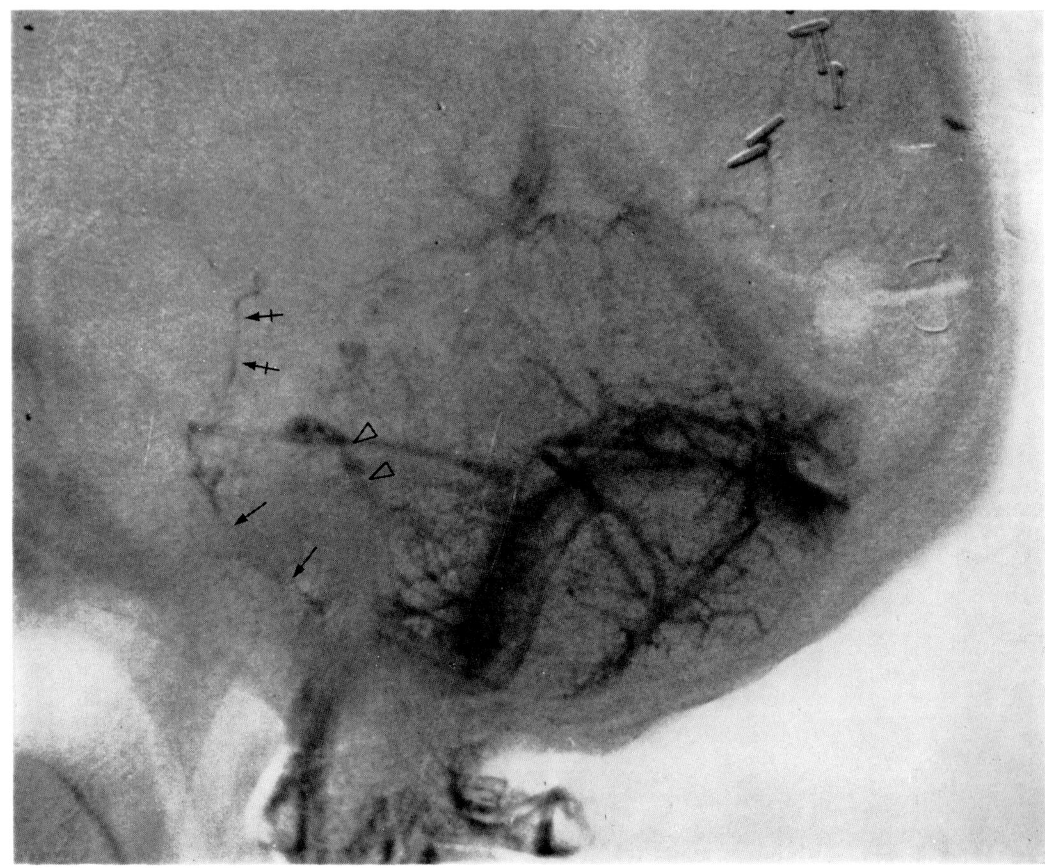

Fig. 78

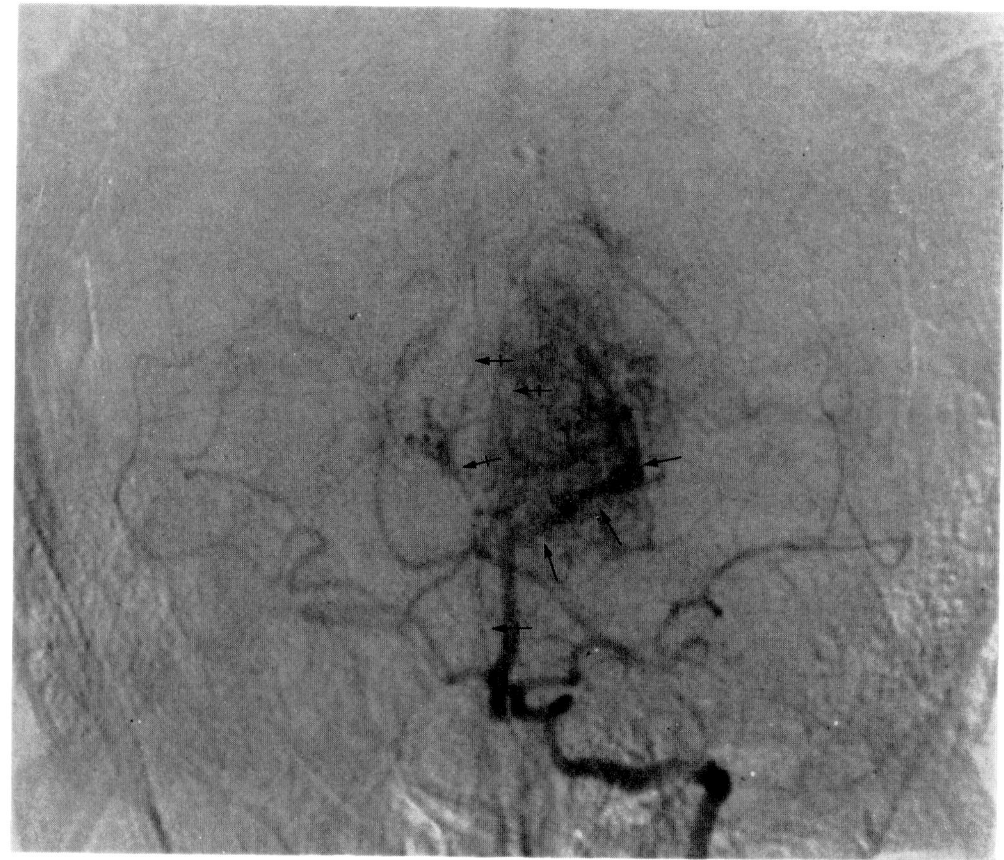

Fig. 79

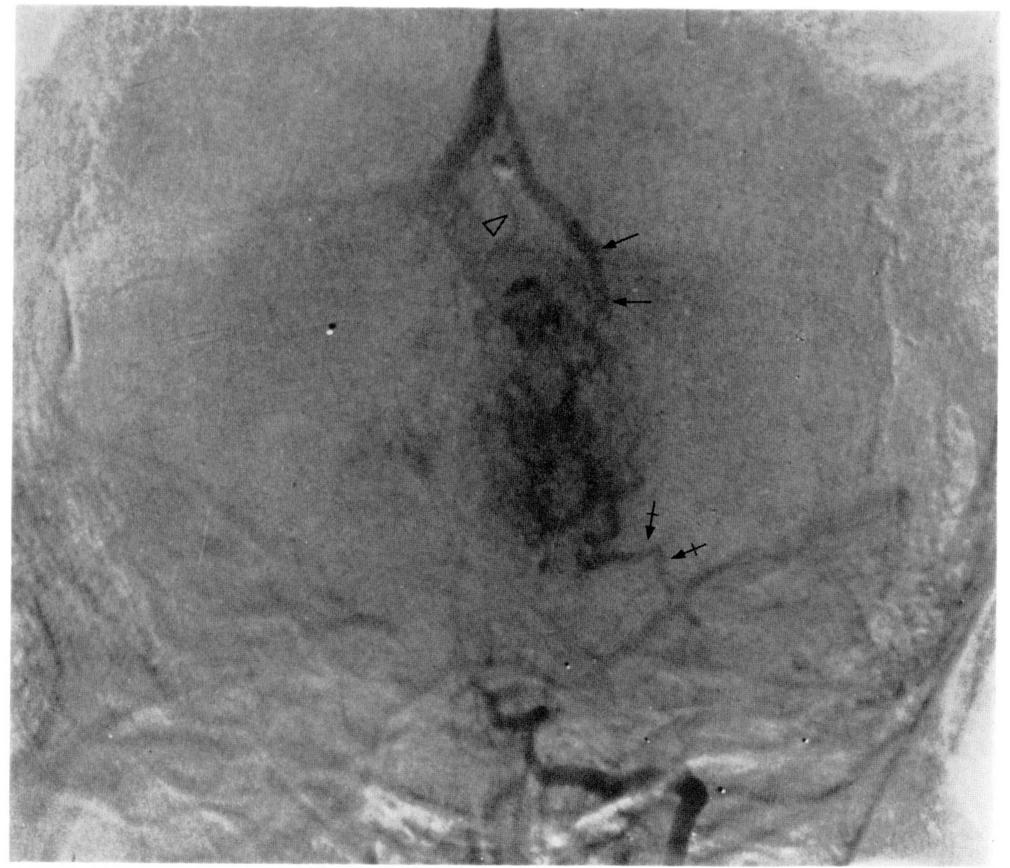

Fig. 80

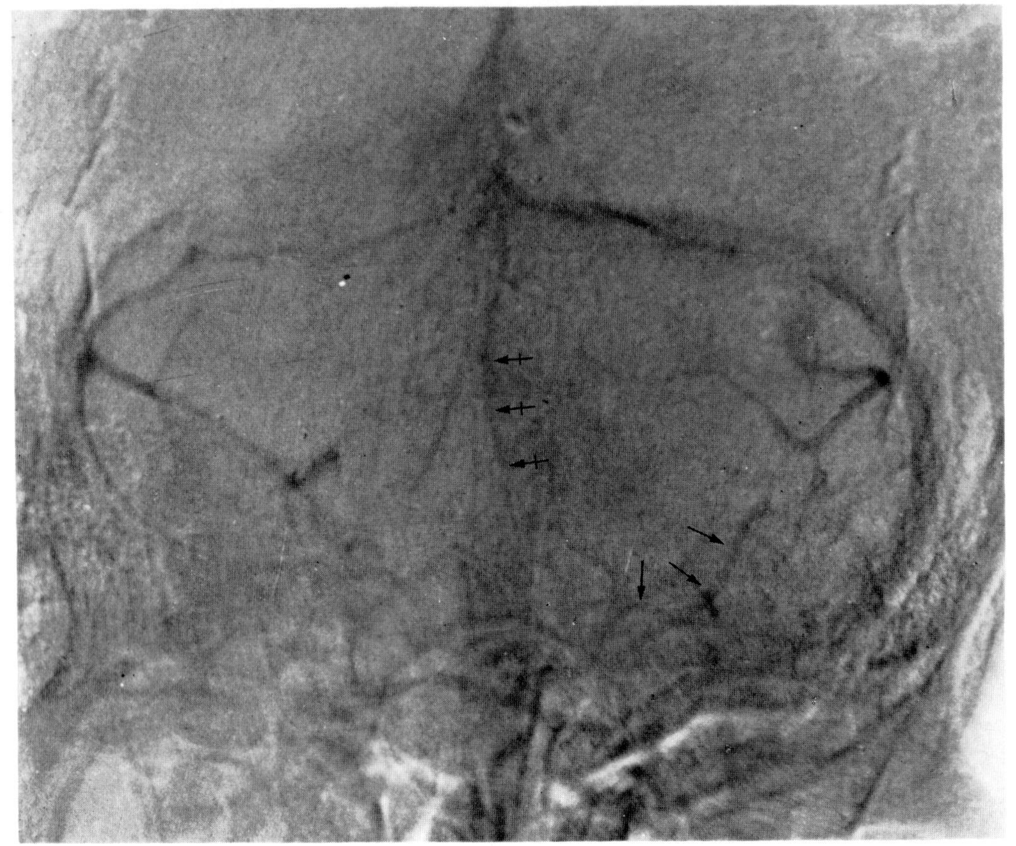

Fig. 81

Large Astrocytoma in the Left Superior Cerebellar Hemisphere with Tumor Stains and Early Venous Drainage

A 12-year-old male: Figs. 82–85

Fig. 82 Arterial phase in the Towne projection. The quadrigeminal and anterior culminate segments of the superior cerebellar artery are displaced to the right (4 crossed arrows), while the hemispheric branch is displaced laterally (4 arrows). There is early visualization of an abnormal vein in the medial aspect of the tumor (3 open arrowheads). The supratonsillar segment of the posterior inferior cerebellar artery is shifted to the right of the midline (3 closed arrowheads).

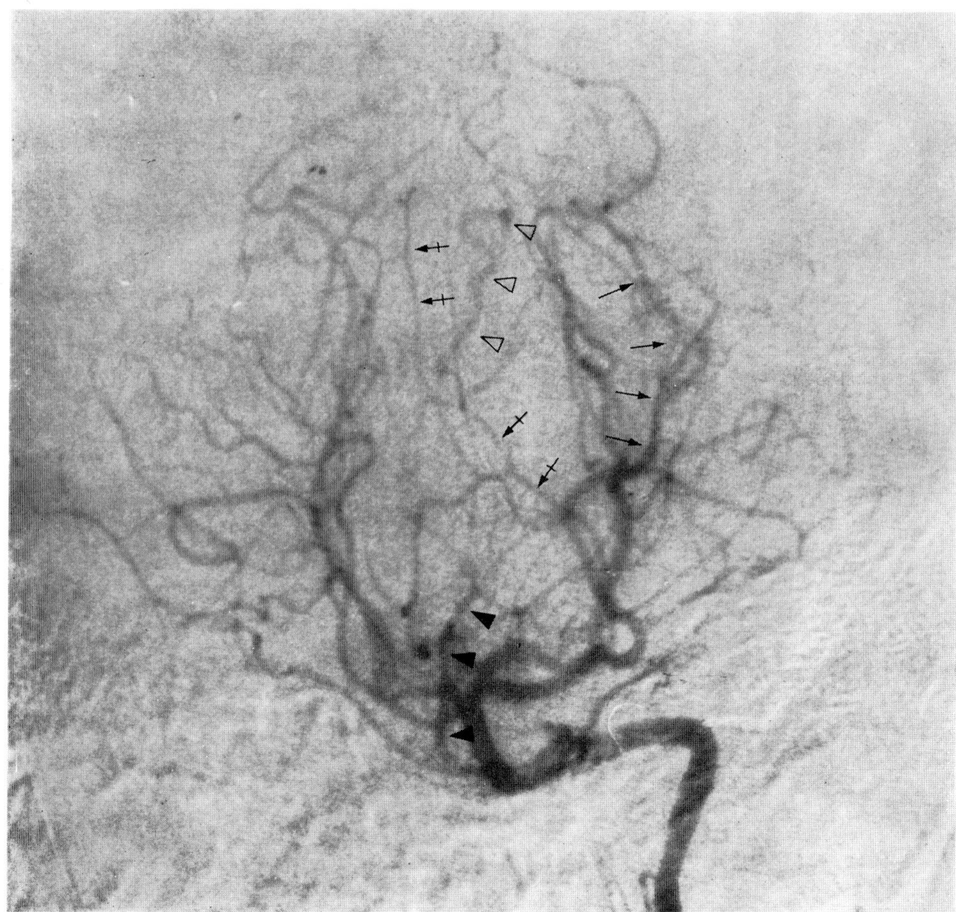

Fig. 82

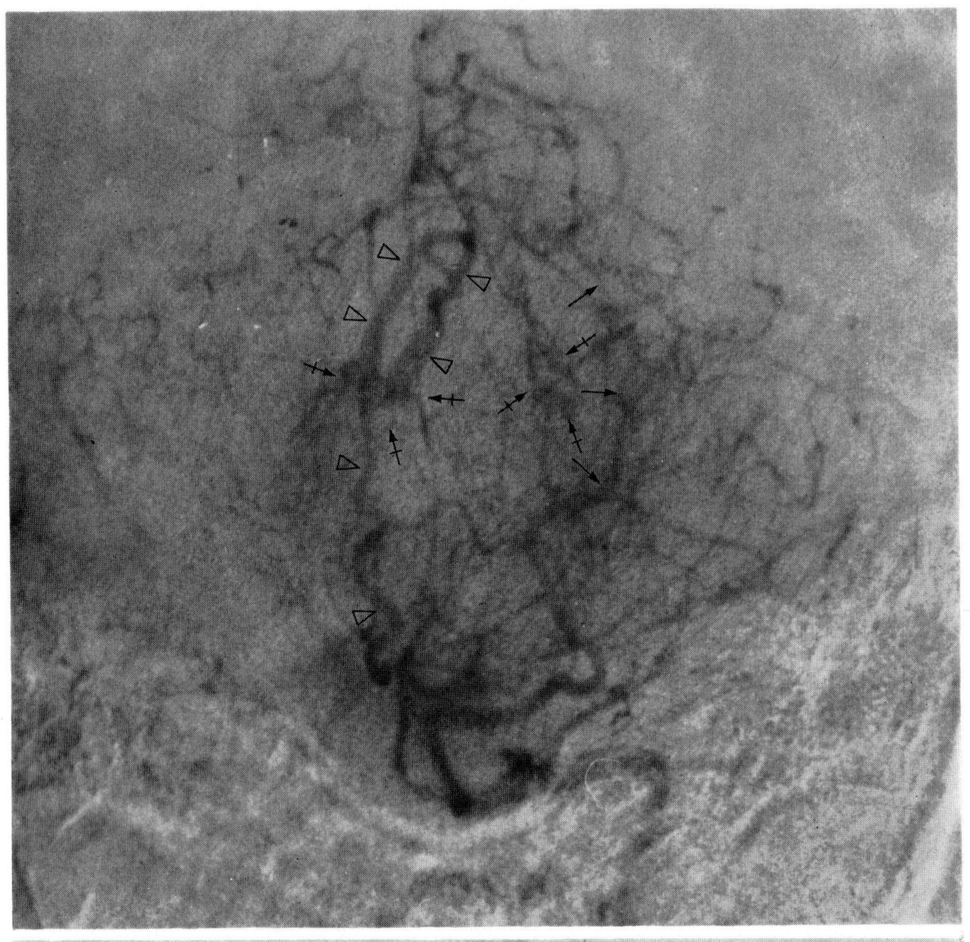

Fig. 83

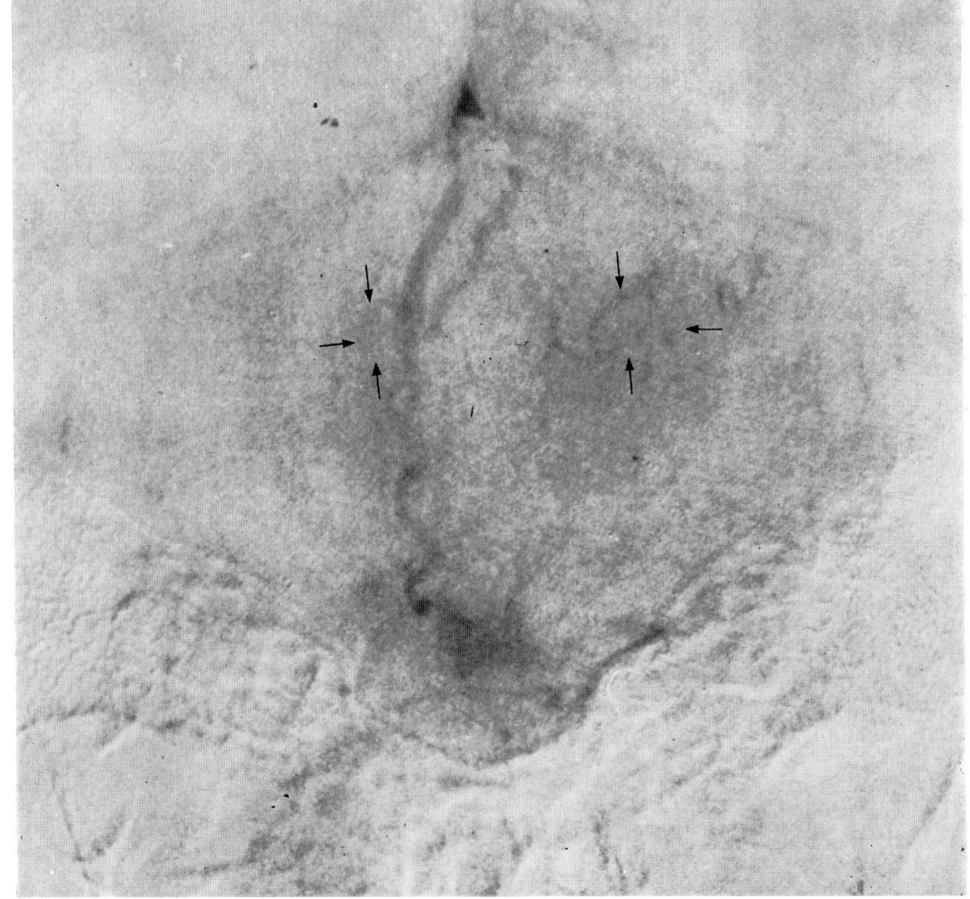

Fig. 84

Fig. 83 Late arterial phase in the Towne projection. Irregular tumor vessels are noted in two areas (3 crossed arrows). The course of the left superior cerebellar artery is well shown with its hemispheric branch displaced laterally (3 arrows). The abnormal draining vein is demonstrated (arrowheads).

Fig. 84 Capillary phase in the Towne projection. The tumor stains are noted in the two areas of the superior vermis (3 arrows). There are abnormal veins draining these areas.

Fig. 85 Capillary phase in the lateral projection. The tumor stains are again demonstrated in the superior vermis (3 crossed arrows). The abnormal draining vein appears to course over the culmen and into the lateral mesencephalic sulcus (arrowheads).

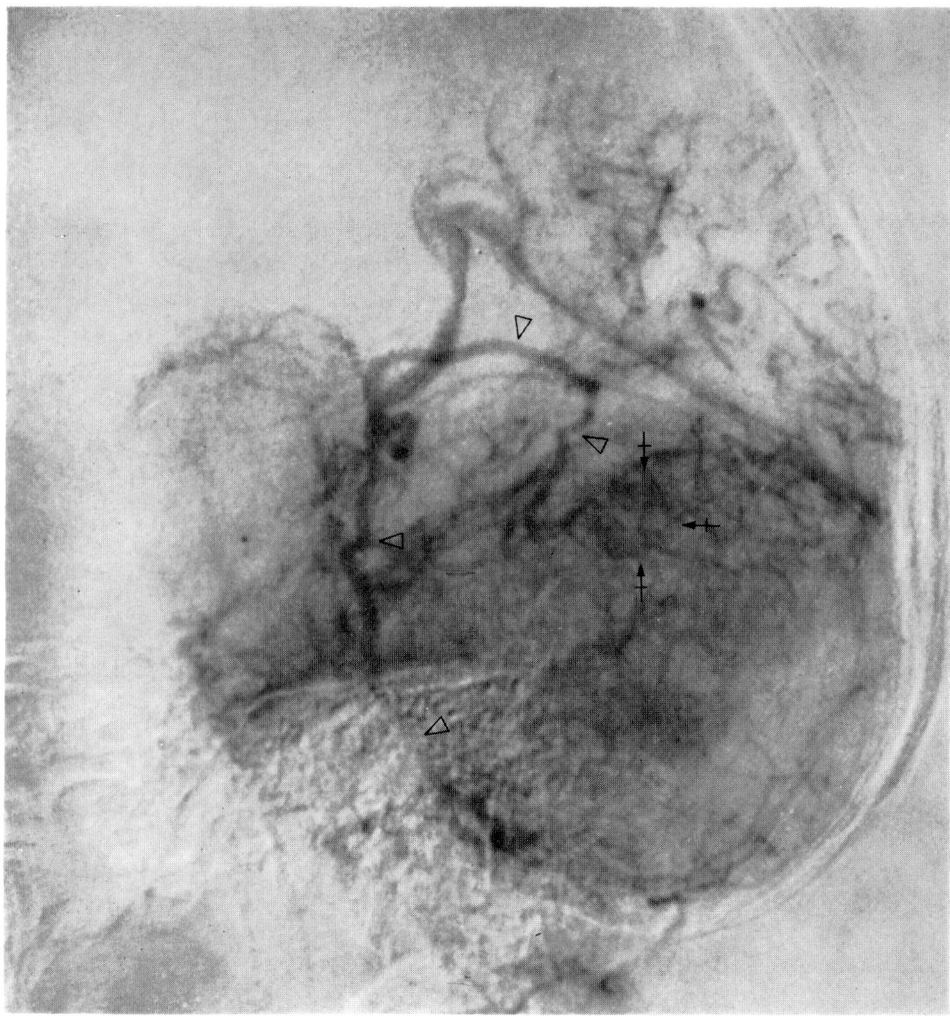

Fig. 85

TRANSTENTORIAL HERNIATION

Transtentorial herniations can be divided into descending, ascending and axial (central) herniations depending upon the structure being herniated through the tentorial slit.

Descending transtentorial herniation

The hernia may be anterior, the uncus and the anterior portion of the hippocampal gyrus forming the main portion of herniation or posterior, the hippocampal gyrus forming the main hernia. Complete descending herniation takes place when the anterior and posterior herniations occur at the same time. The herniation may be on the side of the tumor or sometimes bilateral.

Anterior descending herniation displaces the anterior portion of the posterior cerebral artery downward with a vertical orientation of the posterior communicating artery. These arteries are displaced medially in the Towne projection. The distal basilar artery may be displaced to the opposite side.

Posterior descending herniation displaces the ambient and quadrigeminal segments of the posterior cerebral artery medially and downward. The basal vein is also displaced medially and downward.

If a descending herniation is complete, there is depression and medial displacement of the posterior cerebral artery along the entire length of the tentorial notch. In bilateral herniations, the bifurcation of the basilar artery is displaced downward with a buckled appearance and there is a downward displacement of the interpeduncular segments of the anterior pontomesencephalic veins.

In addition to the above findings, the anterior choroidal artery, visualized on carotid angiograms, may be stretched and displaced in a medial and inferior direction, forming one of the most important angiographic findings in evaluation of transtentorial herniations.

Ascending transtentorial herniation

This herniation is usually posterior or posterolateral in location, the superior vermis forming the main portion of the hernia. The anterior culminate and quadrigeminal segments of the superior cerebellar arteries are stretched in an arcuate fashion and frequently projected above the posterior cerebral arteries in the lateral view. These segments of the superior cerebellar arteries are separated in the Towne projection. With the latter projection the posterior cerebral arteries may be displaced laterally. The basilar artery is usually compressed against the clivus. The vein of Galen and the basal vein may be displaced superiorly.

Axial (central) herniation

There is an inferior displacement of the brain stem along the clivus with supratentorial expanding lesions. Such displacement is called an axial or central herniation and is produced mostly by midline supratentorial tumors such as third ventricle tumors, thalamic tumors and bifrontal tumors. The basilar artery is displaced backward and downward with "accordioned" appearance or "buckled" appearance. The interpeduncular segment of the anterior pontomesencephalic vein is markedly compressed and displaced downward. The basal vein and the vein of Galen may also be displaced downward.

Downward Transtentorial Herniation Secondary to a Temporal Tumor

A 19-year-old male: Figs. 86–88

Fig. 86 Arterial phase in the Towne projection. There is marked shift of the arteries to the right. In particular, the posterior cerebral (2 arrows), superior cerebellar (2 crossed arrows) and distal basilar arteries are displaced to the right. The posterior temporal artery is stretched (3 open arrowheads). The thalamoperforate arteries are also displaced to the right (2 closed arrowheads). A branch of the middle cerebral artery is markedly displaced in the superior and medial direction (2 double-crossed arrows). These findings suggest a large expanding lesion in the left temporal region, displacing the mid-brain and the left temporal lobe to the right.

Fig. 87 Arterial phase in the lateral projection. The left posterior cerebral artery is depressed along the entire length of the tentorial edge, indicating complete downward transtentorial herniation (4 arrows). The posterior temporal artery shows sharp angulation at the tentorial edge (a crossed arrow). There are stretching of the thalamoperforate arteries (closed arrowheads) and posterior displacement of the posterior choroidal arteries (open arrowheads), probably due to displacement of the diencephalon. The posterior communicating artery is depressed (a triple-crossed arrow). The angular artery of the middle cerebral artery is elevated in an arcuate fashion (2 double-crossed arrows).

Fig. 88 Left common carotid angiogram in the anteroposterior projection. There is a large vascular tumor in the left temporal region (4 arrows) which is supplied by the enlarged middle meningeal artery (3 crossed arrows). The anterior and middle cerebral arteries are displaced to the right. The anterior choroidal artery is displaced to the right in an arcuate fashion, indicating herniation of the uncus and the hypocampal gyrus (3 arrowheads).

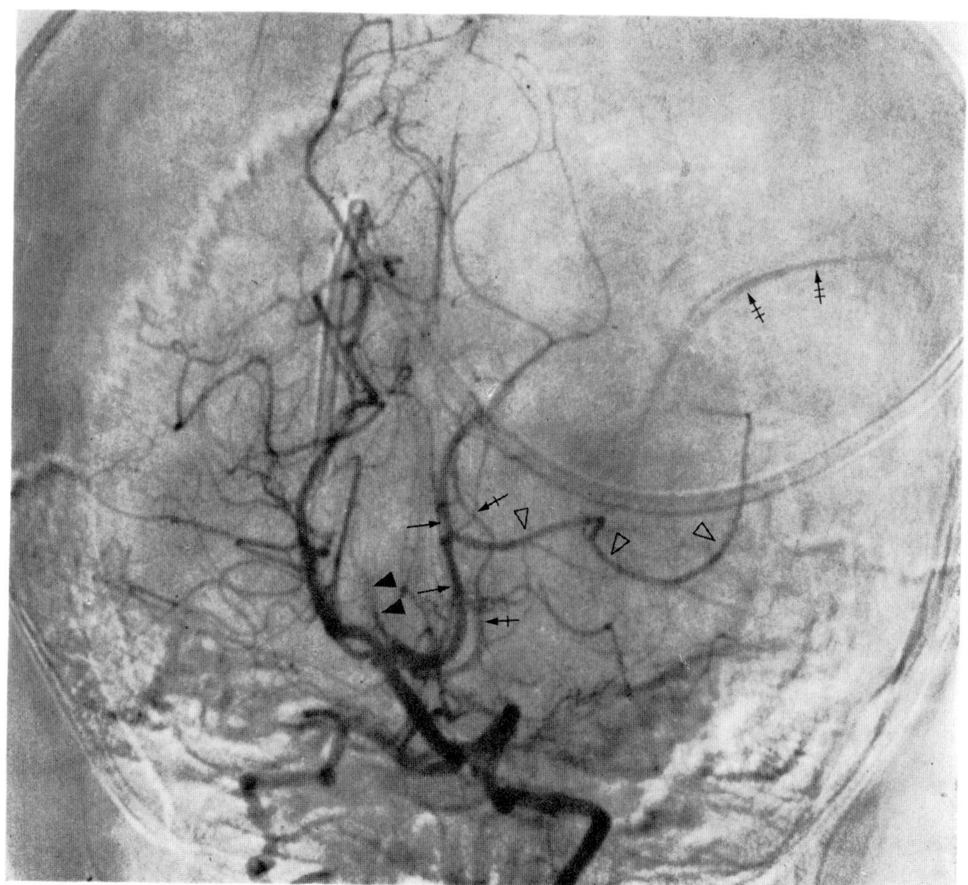

Fig. 86

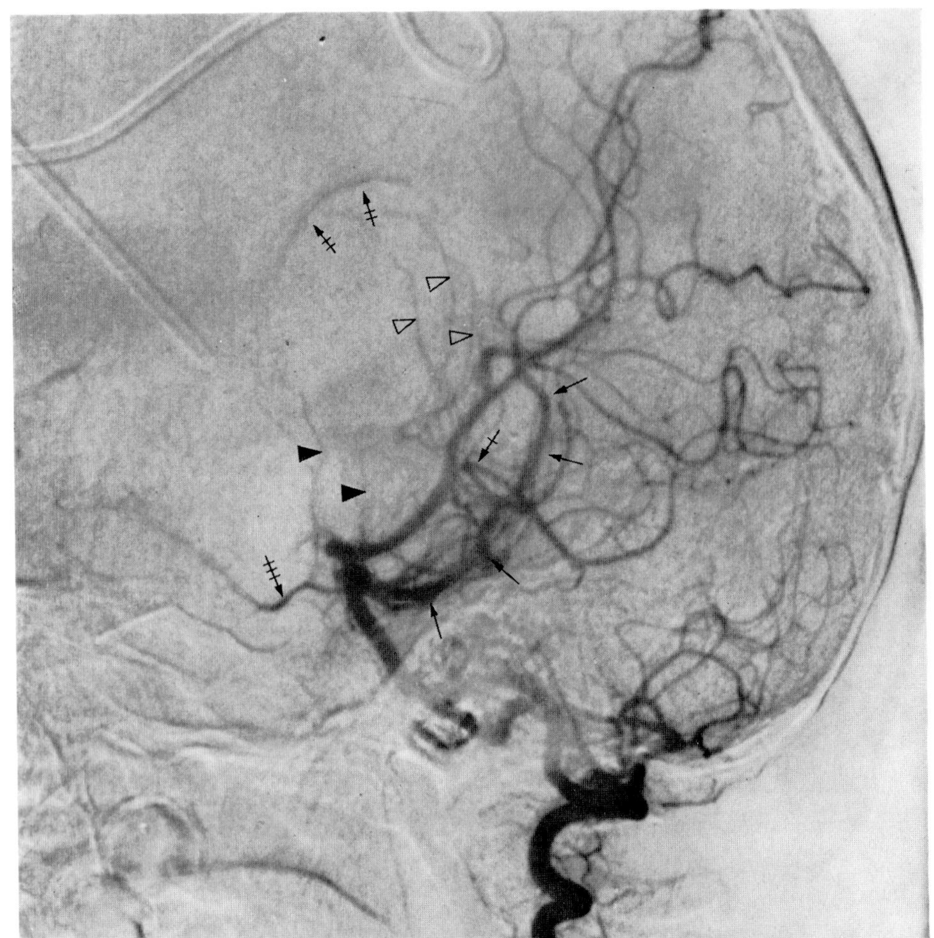

Fig. 87

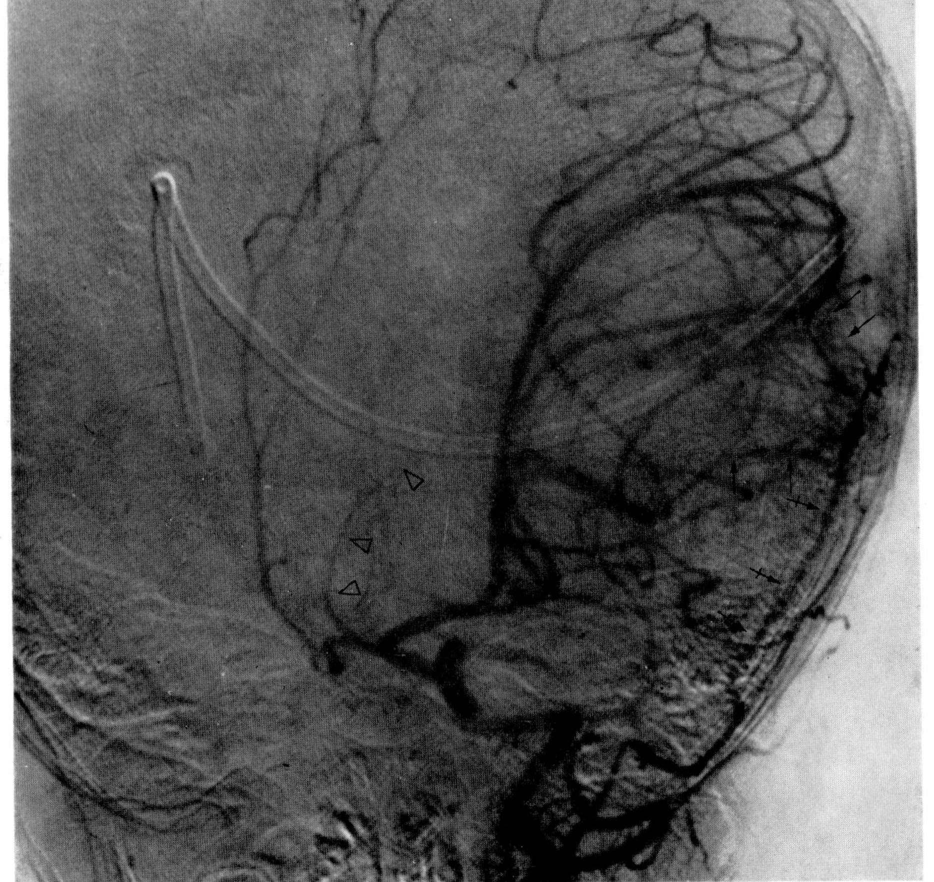

Fig. 88

Upward Transtentorial Herniation due to Hemorrhage into the Left Cerebellar Hemisphere

A 60-year-old male: Figs. 89 and 90 (Through the courtesy of Dr. YAMAGUCHI, Research Institute of Brain and Blood Vessels, Akita)

Fig. 89 Arterial phase in the lateral projection. The left posterior cerebral artery (2 crossed arrows) and superior cerebellar artery (2 arrows) are superimposed and displaced superiorly in an arcuate fashion above the tentorial incisura. The proximal segments of the superimposed arteries are marked with 2 opposing arrows. The posterior temporal artery is visualized (2 closed arrowheads). The hemispheric branch of the superior cerebellar artery is stretched and kinked at the tentorial incisura (2 open arrowheads). The basilar artery is displaced anteriorly and the posterior inferior cerebellar artery is depressed downwards.

Fig. 90 Arterial phase in the Towne projection. The main segment of the superior cerebellar artery is straightened (2 crossed arrows) with markedly stretched arterial branches (2 arrows). The posterior cerebral artery is laterally displaced (3 arrowheads). The arteries on the right are poorly visualized probably due to spasm.

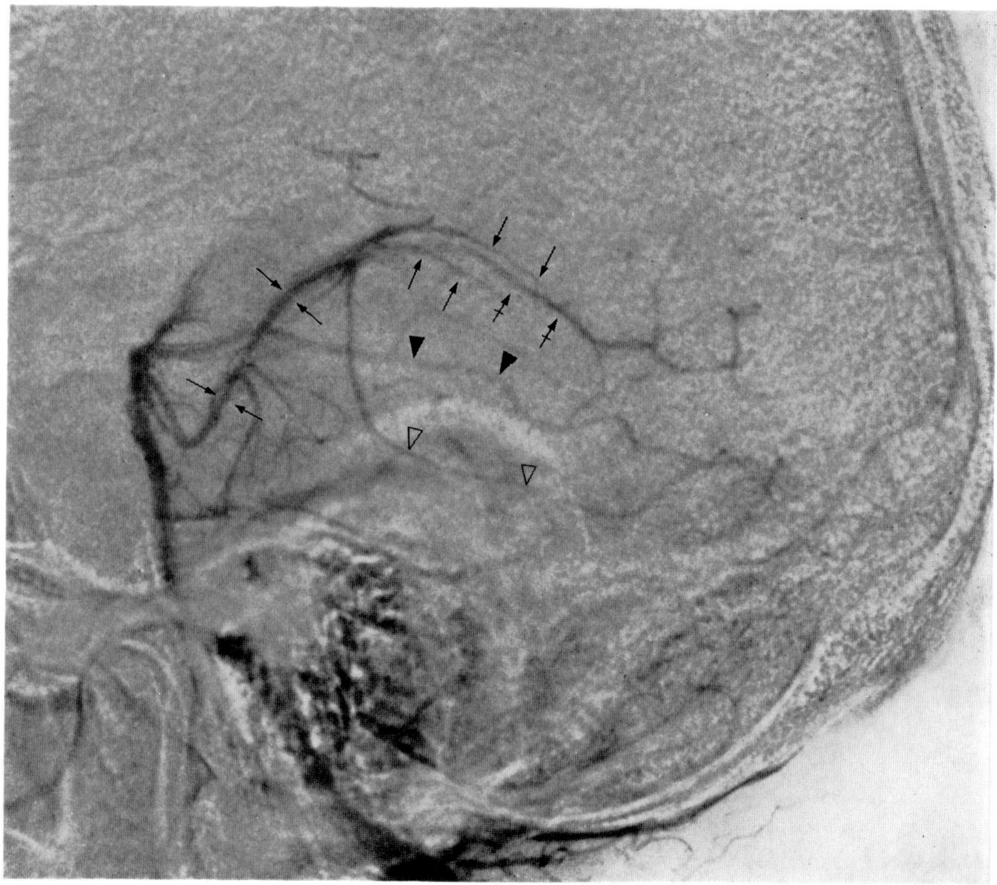

Fig. 89

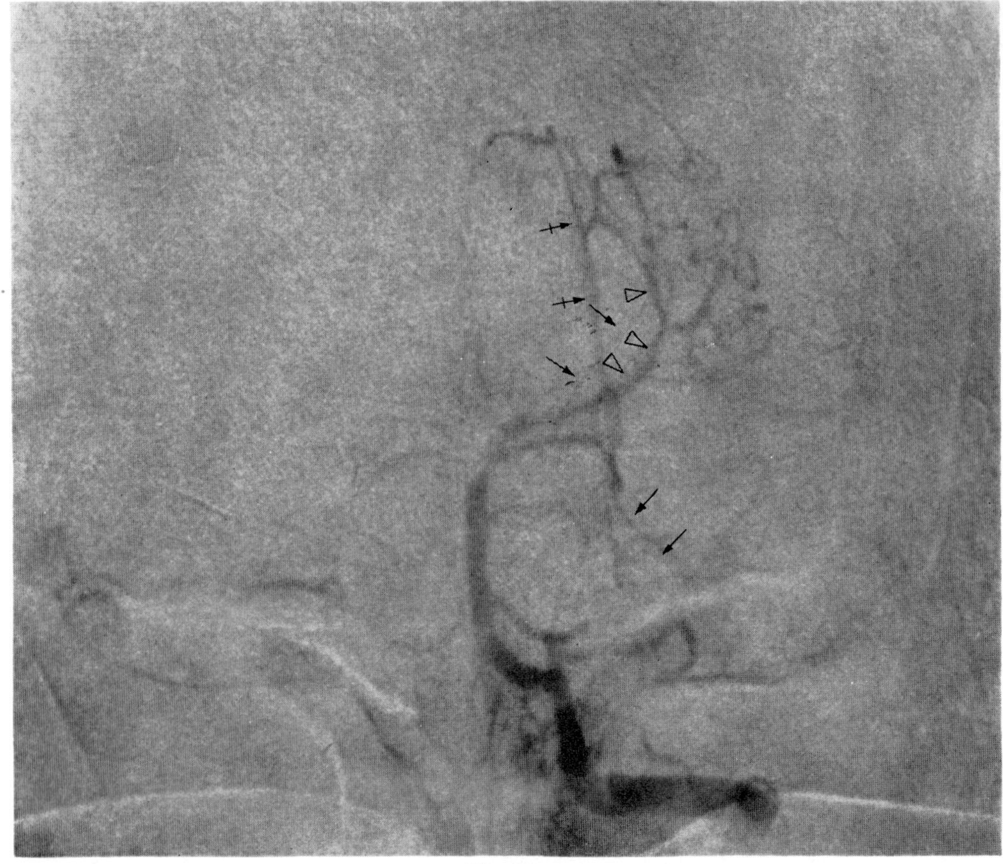

Fig. 90

CEREBELLAR TONSILLAR HERNIATION

Herniations, of the tonsils may be suspected when there is downward displacement of the caudal loop of the posterior inferior cerebellar artery. However, downward displacement of this loop is not a reliable indication of herniated cerebellar tonsils. The loop may course below the foramen magnum in normal cases as well as in cases with a tonsillar herniation or Arnold-Chiari malformation. This loop is located above the foramen magnum in 60%, while the caudal loop is at the line of the foramen magnum in 5% and extends below the foramen magnum in 35% (Margolis and Newton, 1971). It is only when small tonsillar branches arising from the posterior inferior cerebellar artery are seen below the foramen magnum that a diagnosis of a tonsillar herniation can be made in the lateral projection of a vertebral angiogram.

In addition, there may be associated angiographic findings. There are usually arteriographic and venographic findings of increased intracranial pressure. In particular, the inferior vermian vein is diffusedly depressed downward with inferior displacement of the copular point.

Margolis and Newton (1971) emphasized a new finding of the tonsillar herniation observed on the hemispheric branches of the posterior inferior cerebellar artery. They state that the most proximal portion of the hemispheric branches of the posterior inferior cerebellar artery are stretched and pulled downward toward the edge of the foramen magnum by herniated tonsils as seen best on the straight anteroposterior projections.

Tonsillar Herniation in Medulloblastoma

A 9-year-old male: Figs. 91–94

Fig. 91 Arterial phase in the lateral projection. The basilar artery is compressed against the clivus and the thalamoperforate arteries are stretched, indicating increased intracranial pressure in the posterior fossa. The caudal loop of the posterior inferior cerebellar artery is depressed below the foramen magnum bilaterally (2 arrows). The cranial loop and vermian branch of this artery is also displaced inferiorly. The findings suggest bilateral tonsillar herniation.

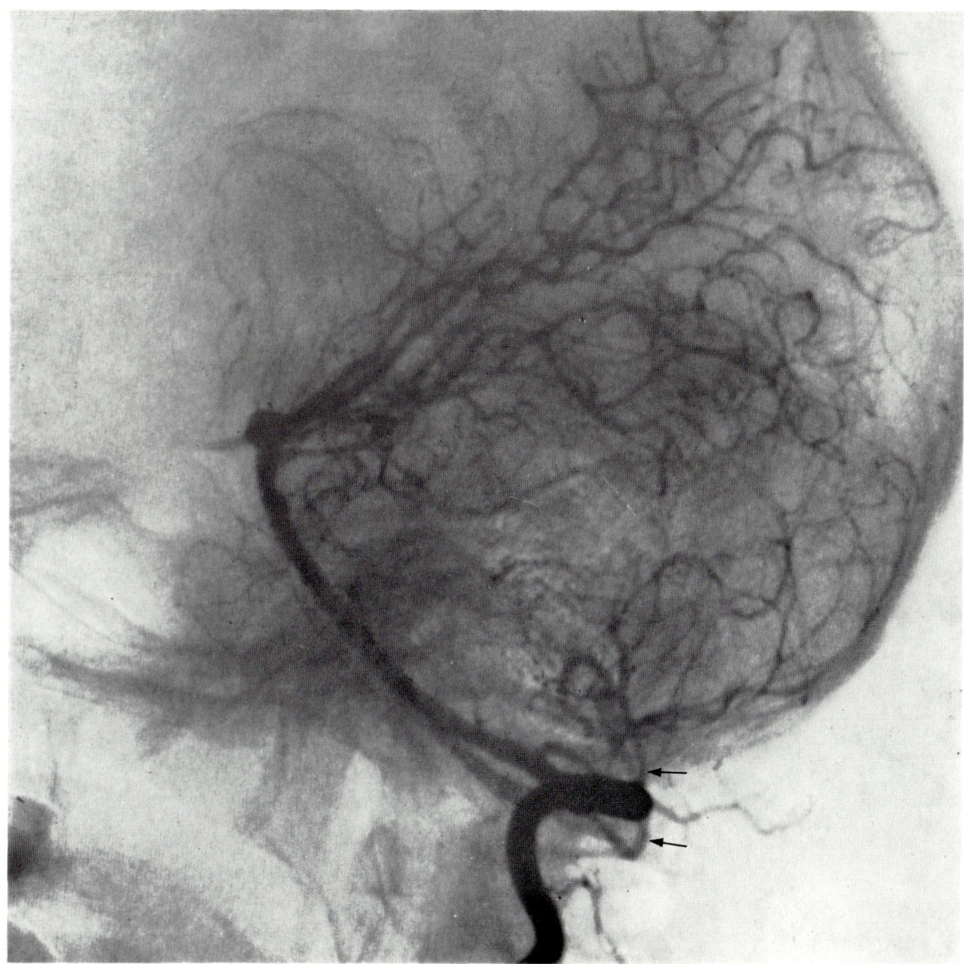

Fig. 91

Fig. 92 Venous phase in the lateral projection. The inferior retrotonsillar tributary of the inferior vermian vein is depressed downwards bilaterally (2 arrows).

Fig. 93 Arterial phase in the Towne projection. Arterial branches in the posterior fossa are very small, probably due to increased intracranial pressure. The vermian branch of the posterior inferior cerebellar artery is slightly stretched and displaced laterally (2 arrows). The caudal loop is displaced inferiorly.

Fig. 94 Venous phase in the Towne projection. The inferior retrotonsillar tributary of the inferior vermian vein is stretched and depressed downwards (2 arrows).

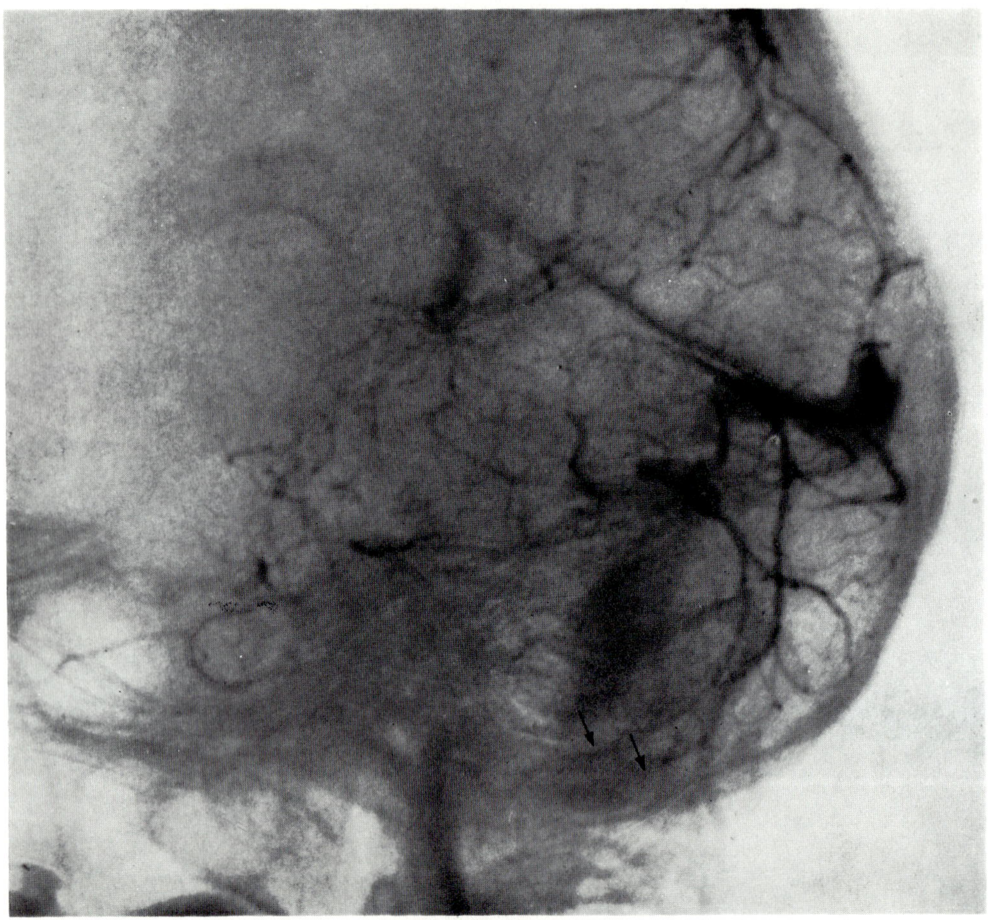

Fig. 92

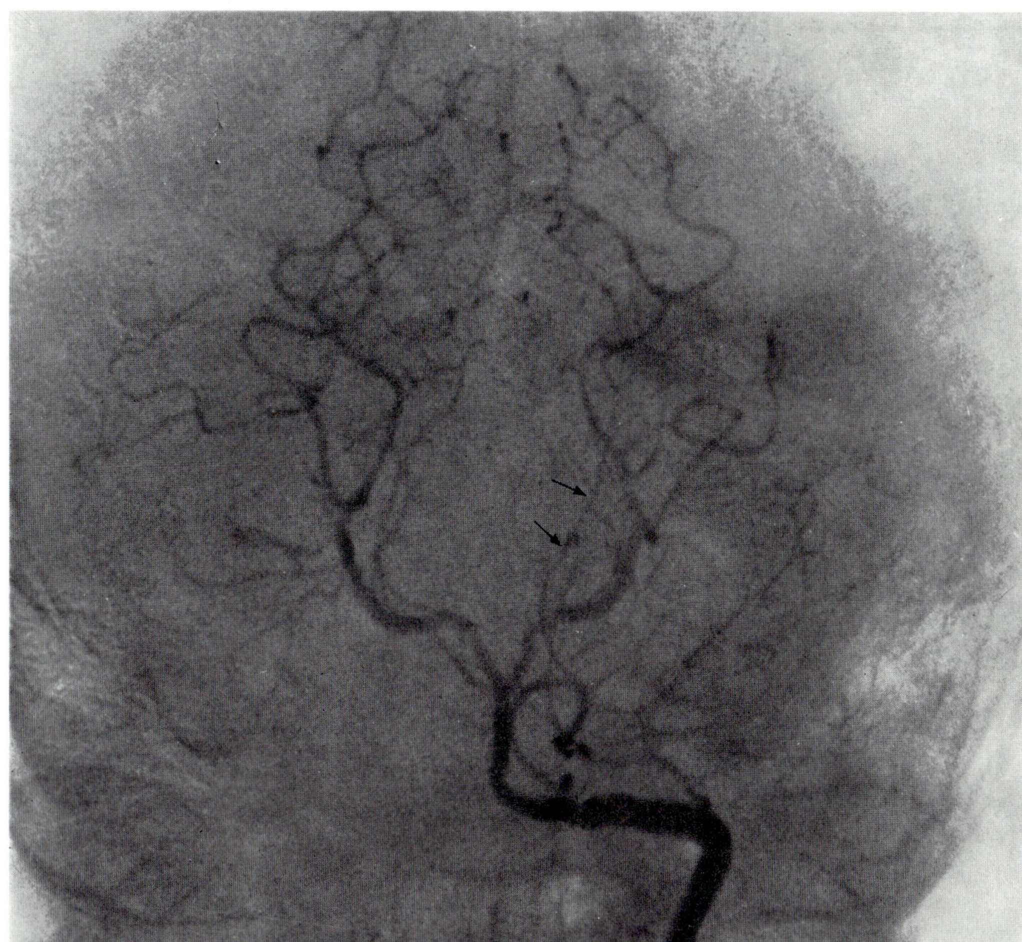

Fig. 93

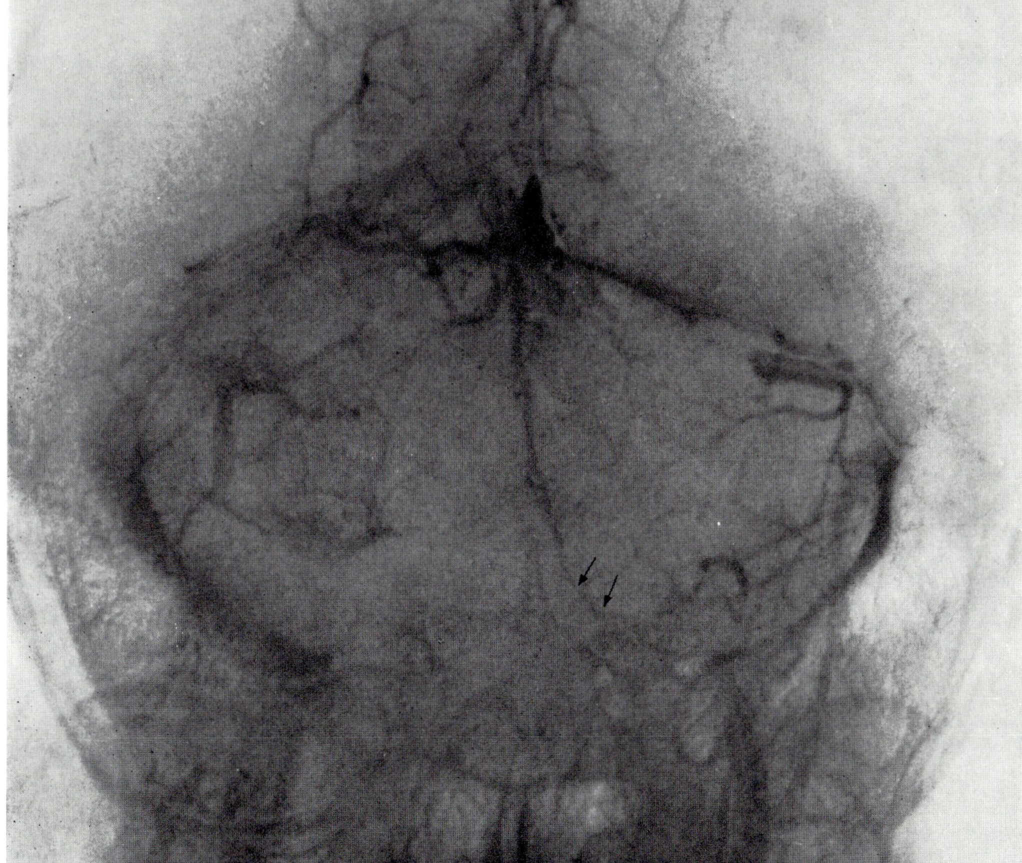

Fig. 94

DILATATION OF THE SUPRATENTORIAL VENTRICLES

Arteriographic features

With enlargement of the posterior portion of the third ventricle, the medial posterior choroidal artery is displaced posteriorly and superiorly, while the lateral posterior choroidal artery is depressed and takes a straight course as the lateral ventricle enlarges. Therefore, there is superimposition or crossing of the medial and posterior choroidal arteries. The posterior pericallosal artery shows stretching and increased curvature due to enlargement of the lateral ventricles.

The thalamoperforate arteries are separated by the enlarged third ventricle in the Towne projection, since these arteries run along the walls of the third ventricle.

Venographic features

When there is visualization of the choroid plexus and the internal cerebral vein, there is reduction of the distance between the choroid plexus and the internal cerebral veins (Takahashi and Okudera, 1972). This is due to the fact that the choroid plexus moves inferiorly with enlargement of the lateral ventricles. The course of the internal cerebral vein is flattened and the basal vein is displaced backwards and downwards.

The subependymal veins such as the direct atrial vein may be stretched and outline the wall of the enlarged lateral ventricles.

Intracerebellar Cyst in the Right Inferior Hemisphere and the Inferior Vermis

A one-year and 10-month-old female: Figs. 95–98

There was no neoplastic mural nodule.

Fig. 95 Arterial phase in the lateral projection. The medial and lateral choroidal arteries are depressed (2 arrows) and the posterior pericallosal artery is displaced posteriorly (2 crossed arrows), producing considerably increased distance between these arteries. There is straightening and depression of the main segments of the posterior cerebral artery, while there is posterior and inferior displacement of the parieto-occipital artery (3 open arrowheads). These findings are indicative of dilatation of the lateral ventricles. The basilar artery is compressed against the clivus. The posterior inferior cerebellar artery is faintly visualized and appears to be depressed downwards bilaterally (closed arrowheads), suggesting a mass lesion in the posterior fossa.

Fig. 96 Arterial phase in the Towne projection. The thalamoperforate arteries are visualized and appear to be separated, probably due to dilatation of the third ventricle (2 arrows). The quadrigeminal and anterior culminate segments of the superior cerebellar arteries are displaced laterally (2 crossed arrows), indicating tendency of upward transtentorial herniation. The enlarged occipital horns displace the parieto-occipital and calcarine arteries medially on both sides (2 arrowheads).

Fig. 97 Venous phase in the lateral projection. There is reduction of distance between the choroid plexus and internal cerebral veins (2 opposing arrows). The basal vein of Rosenthal is straightened and depressed downwards (3 arrows). The interpeduncular segment of the anterior pontomesencephalic vein is depressed inferiorly (a crossed arrow).

Fig. 98 Venous phase in the Towne projection. Venous filling in the right posterior fossa is poor compared with the left, secondary to compression of the veins by the tumor.

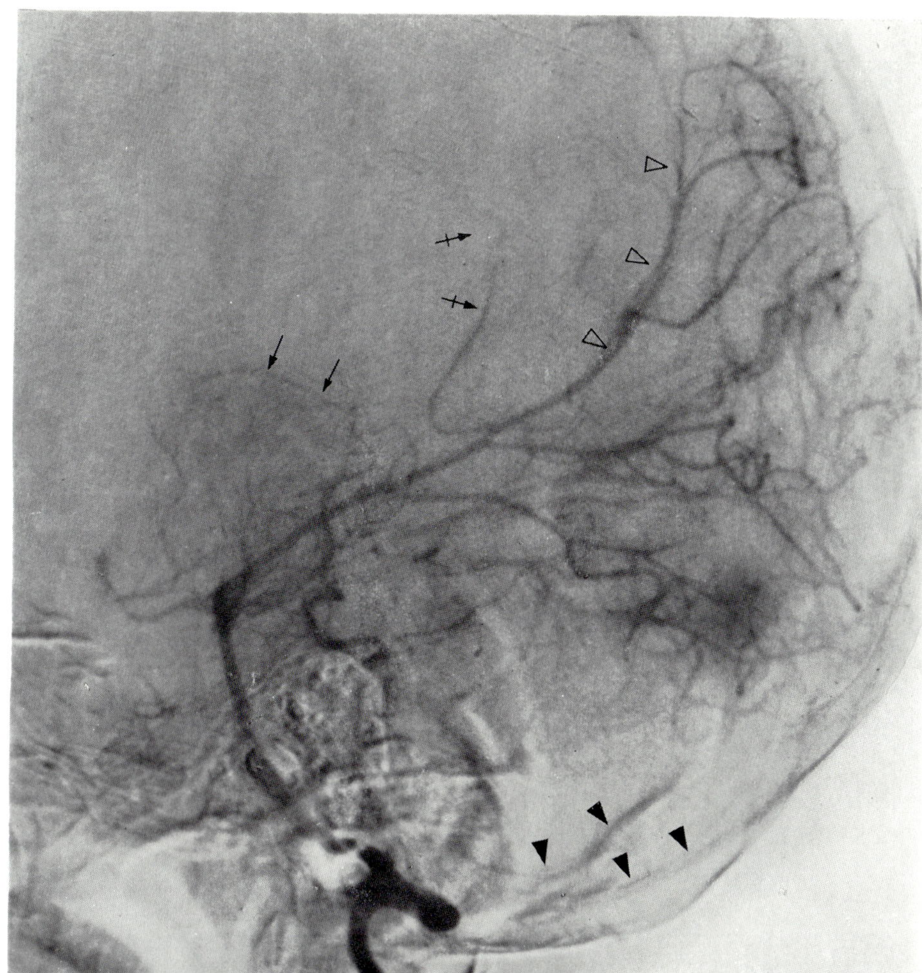

Fig. 95

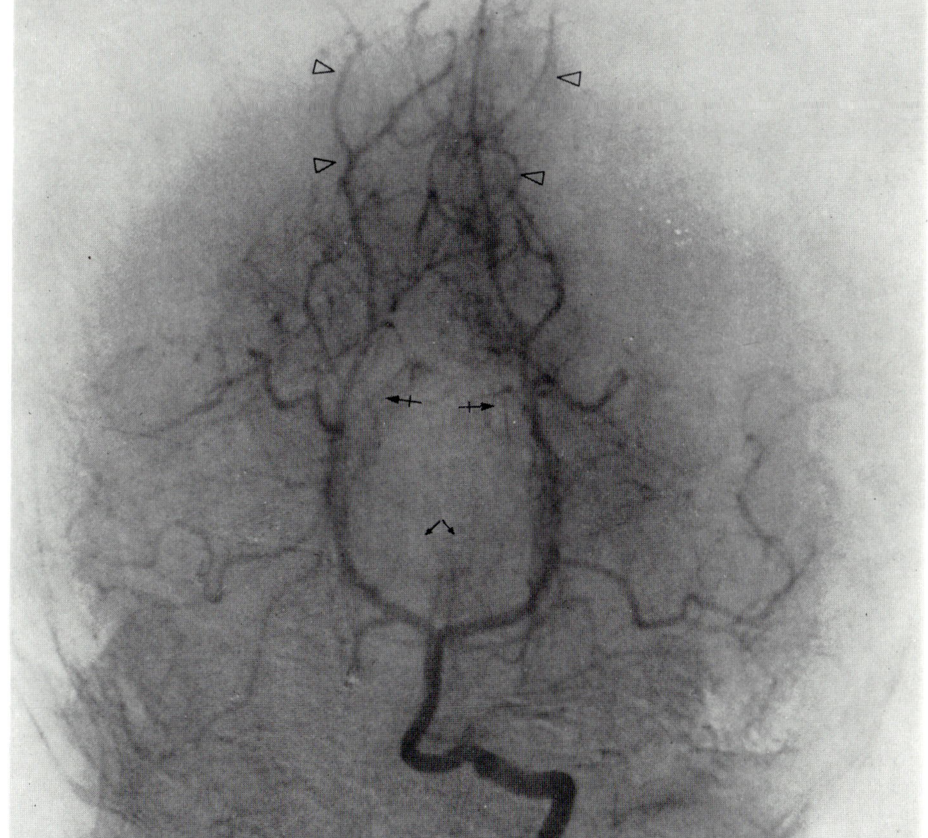

Fig. 96

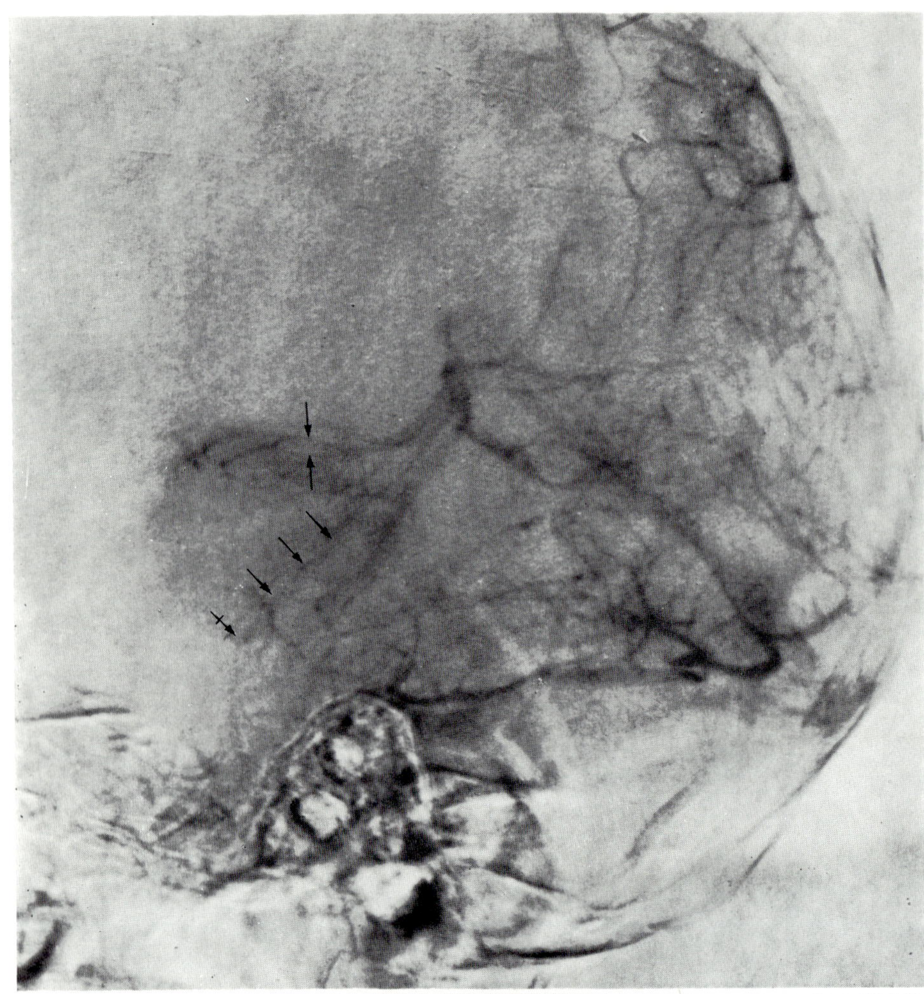

Fig. 97

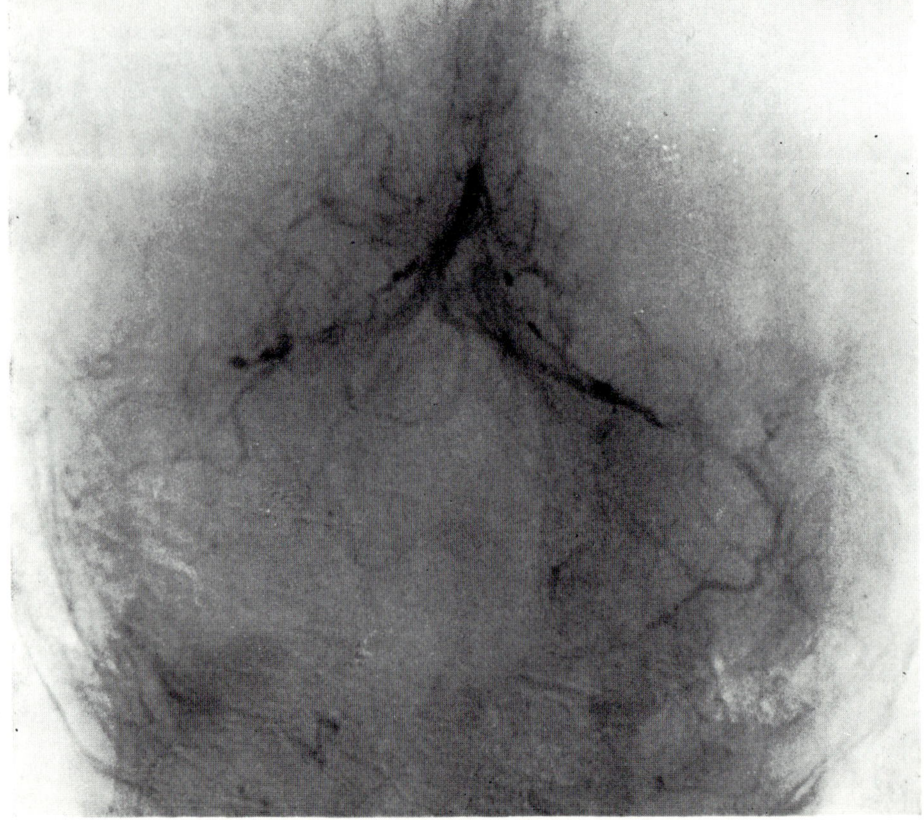

Fig. 98

MIDLINE SHIFT IN THE POSTERIOR FOSSA

Arteriographic features

The vermian branches of both the superior cerebellar and posterior inferior cerebellar arteries run in the paramedian sulcus within the interhemispheric fissure, forming abundant anastomoses between their terminal arterial branches. Angiographically, these vermian branches are localized in the midline as a single vessel or in pairs, providing an important sign of midline shift in the posterior fossa. These vermian branches should be differentiated from other midline arteries such as the posterior pericallosal, medial posterior choroidal, thalamoperforate and posterior meningeal arteries. Differentiation is easily done if lateral views are considered together.

The precentral cerebellar artery may be used to localize the midline, but this artery is infrequently visualized in the anteroposterior or Towne projections.

The thalamoperforate arteries may be shifted to the normal side by a supratentorial expanding lesion.

Venographic features

The precentral cerebellar vein is localized in the midline and is shifted to the opposite side by a posterior fossa tomor. It should be noted that only one of the brachial tributaries of the precentral cerebellar vein is often visualized and may be mistaken for a midline shift.

The inferior vermian veins running in the paramedian sulcus may be displaced to the normal side by an expanding lesion of the posterior fossa.

Metastatic Fibrosarcomas of the Left Occipital Lobe and Left Cerebellar Hemisphere

A 2-year-old female: Figs. 99–102

A fibrosarcoma of the right thigh was removed 2 years previously.

Fig. 99 Arterial phase in the Towne projection. The parieto-occipital (3 arrows) and calcarine (3 crossed arrows) branches of the left posterior cerebral artery are stretched and displaced laterally by the tumor in the left occipital lobe. The posterior inferior cerebellar artery on the left is markedly displaced to the right of the midline (3 open arrowheads). The quadrigeminal segments of the superior cerebellar arteries are also shifted to the right (2 closed arrowheads), indicating a mass in the left cerebellar hemisphere.

Fig. 100 Venous phase in the Towne projection. The left inferior vermian vein is markedly displaced across the midline in an arcuate fashion with stretching of the superior and inferior retrotonsillar tributaries (4 arrows). The right inferior vermian vein is also displaced to the right. The petrosal vein is compressed against the petrous bone (a crossed arrow).

Fig. 101 Arterial phase in the lateral projection. The parieto-occipital branch of the posterior cerebral artery is straightened and displaced superiorly (3 arrows). The proximal segment of the calcarine branch of the same artery is accordioned (2 open arrowheads) and the distal segment is stretched and displaced superiorly (3 crossed arrows). There is arcuate stretching of the anterior culminate and vermian segments of the superior cerebellar artery (2 closed arrowheads), suggesting presence of a tumor in the posterior fossa. The posterior medullary and supratonsillar segments of the posterior inferior cerebellar artery are displaced anteriorly (2 long arrows). The vermian segment (a double-crossed arrow) as well as the tonsillo-hemispheric branch (a triple-crossed arrow) of this artery is stretched.

Fig. 102 Venous phase in the lateral projection. Venous filling of the occipital area is poor due to compression by the tumor. The inferior vermian veins and their copular points are displaced superiorly with elevation of the retrotonsillar tributary (arrows). The distance between the choroid plexus and the internal cerebral vein is reduced by enlagement of the lateral ventricle (2 opposing arrows).

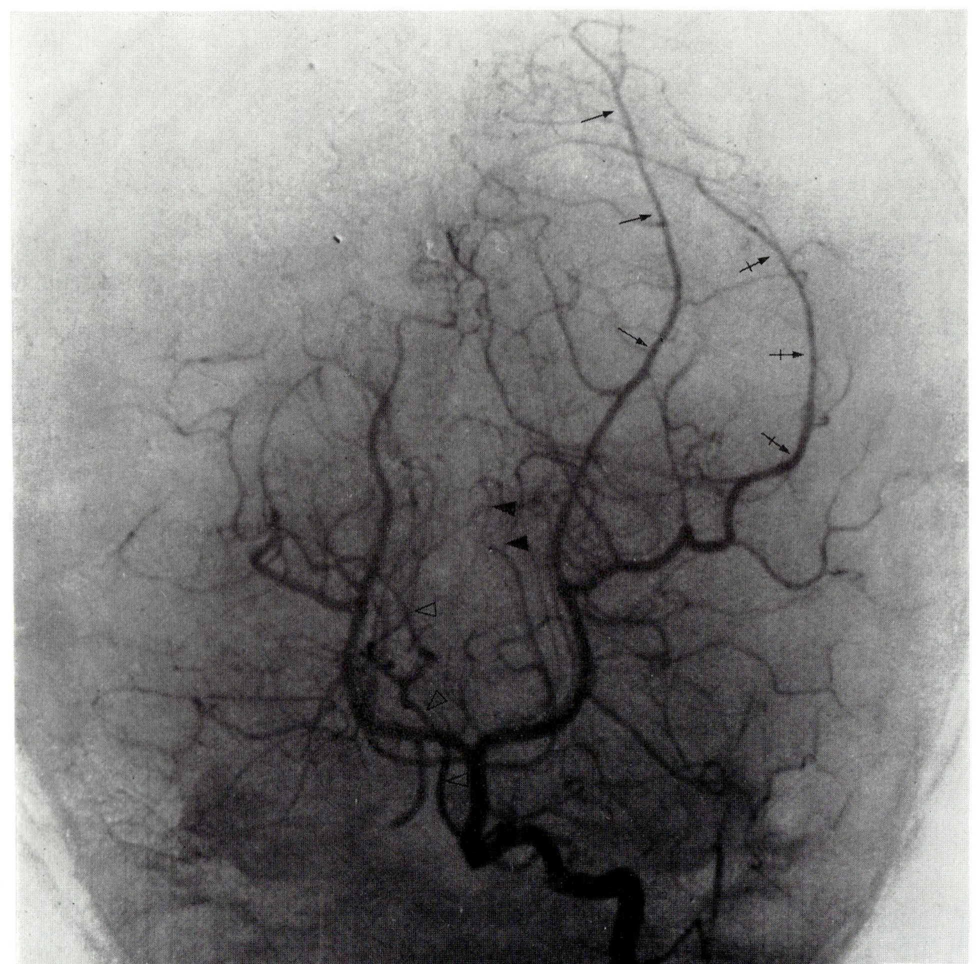

Fig. 99

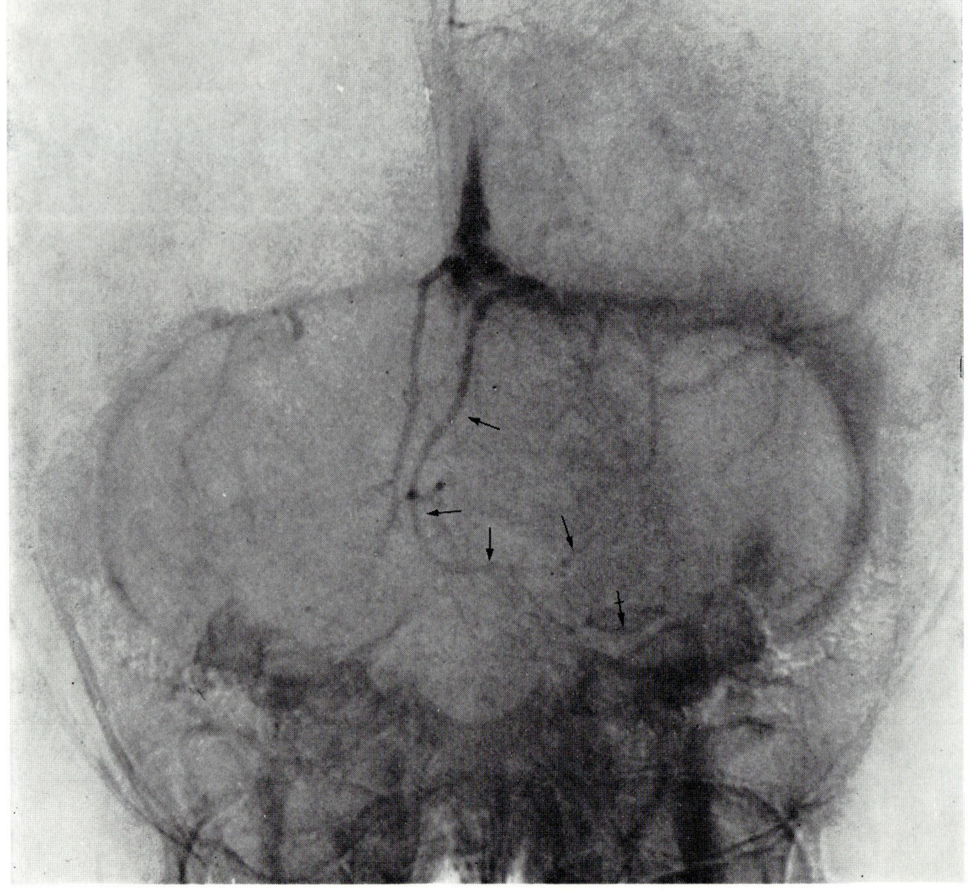

Fig. 100

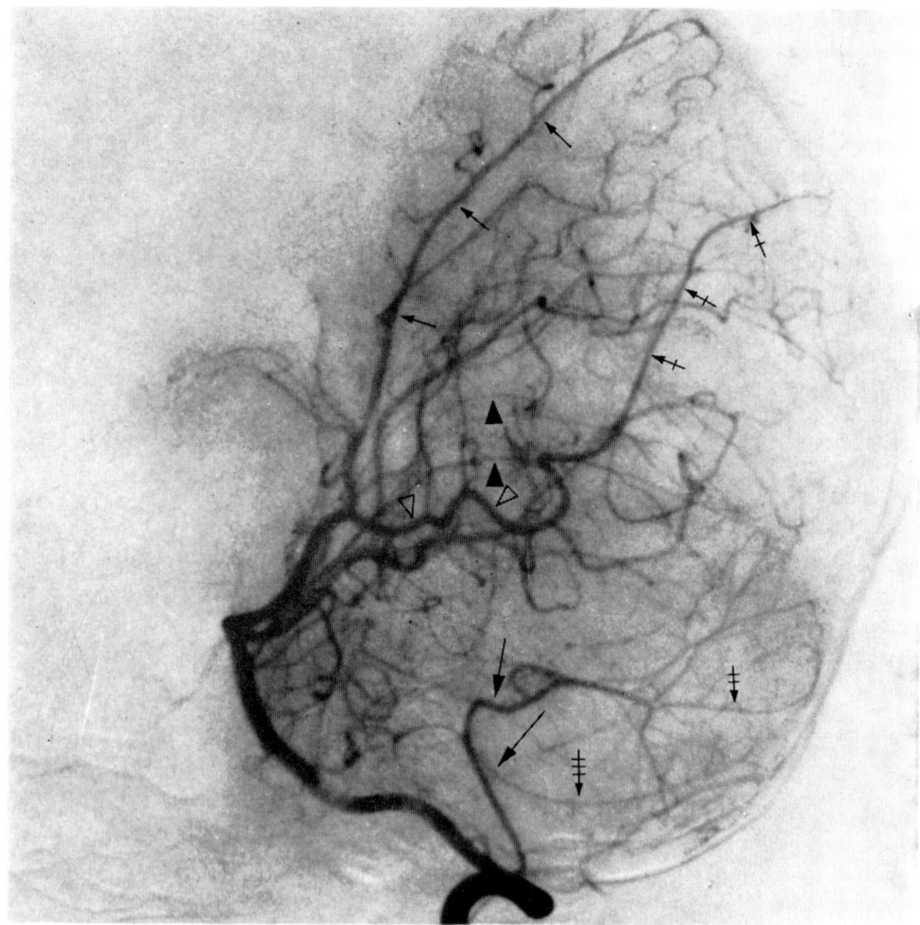

Fig. 101

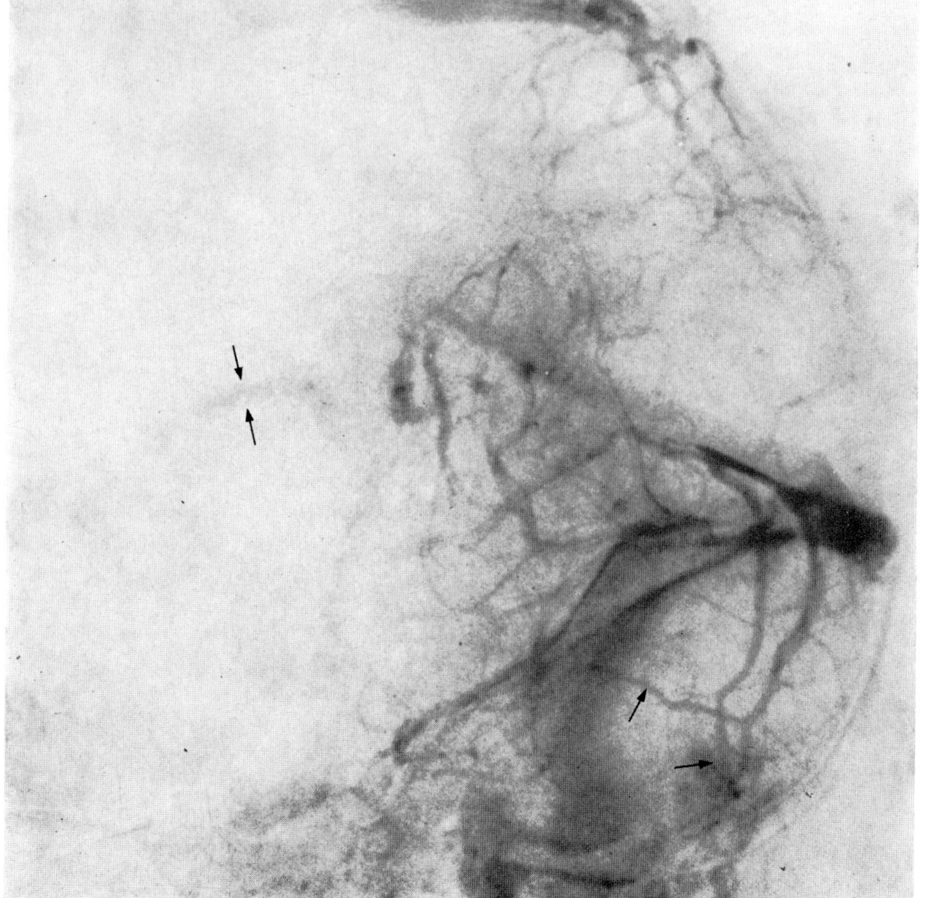

Fig. 102

Left Acoustic Neurinoma

A 20-year-old female: Figs. 103–105

Fig. 103 Arterial phase in the Towne projection. There are two superior cerebellar arteries on the left. The lower artery is displaced medially in an arcuate fashion, suggesting a mass lesion in the cerebellopontine angle (2 arrowheads). The posterior medullary and supratonsillar segments of the posterior inferior cerebellar artery is displaced across the midline, as are the vermian segments (3 arrows).

Fig. 104 Venous phase in the Towne projection. The inferior vermian vein on the left is slightly displaced to the right across the midline (2 arrows). The petrosal vein is displaced laterally (a crossed arrow) and an abnormal vein is displaced superiorly in an arched fashion (3 arrowheads).

Fig. 105 Arterial phase in the lateral projection. The basilar artery is compressed against the clivus. The posterior medullary segment of the posterior inferior cerebellar artery is displaced backwards (2 arrows).

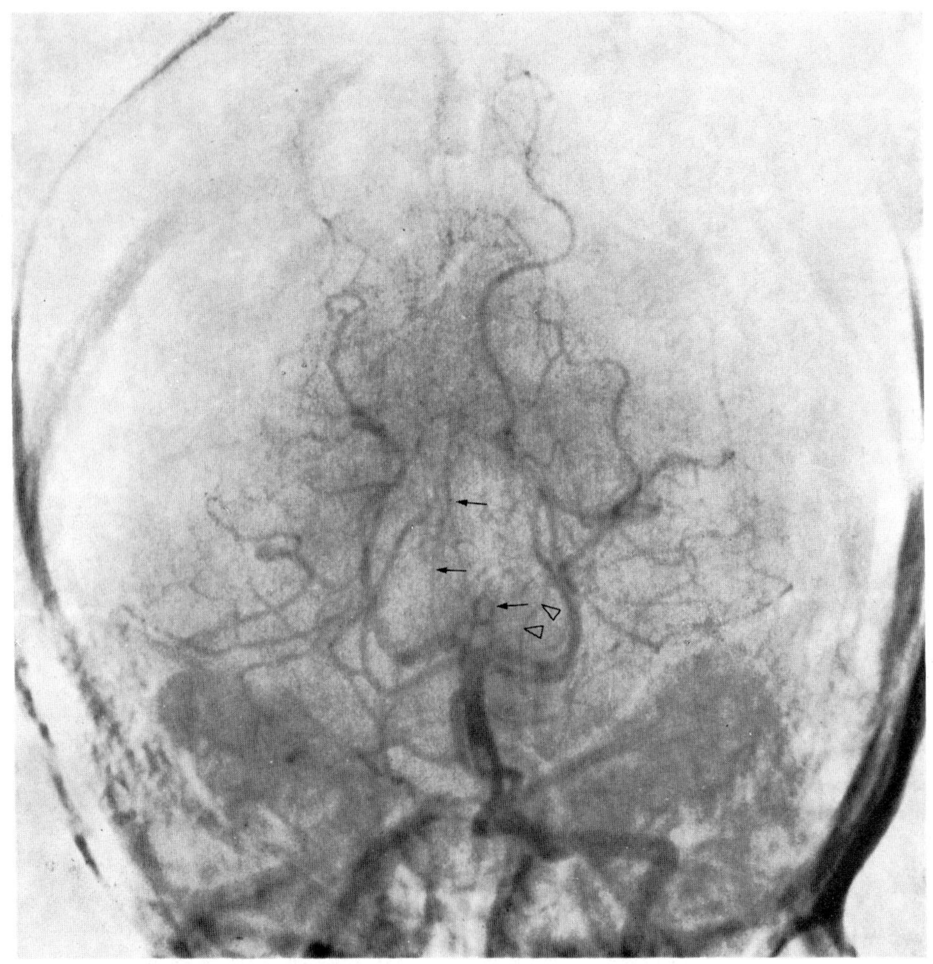

Fig. 103

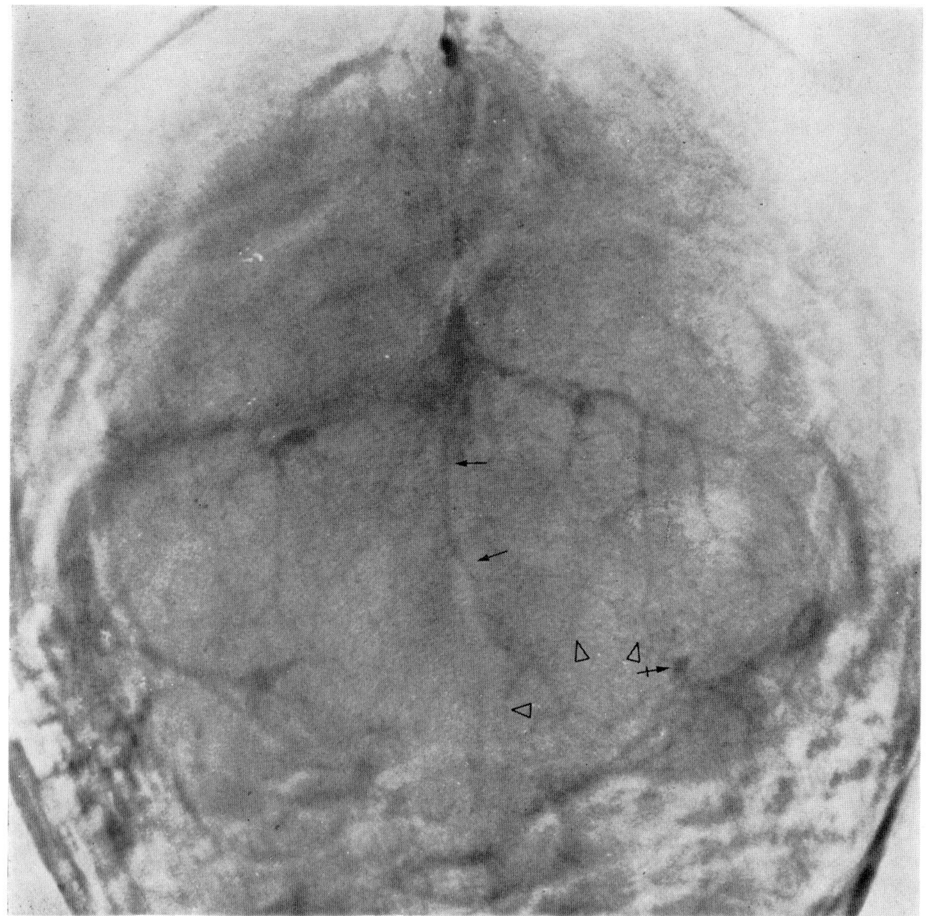
Fig. 104

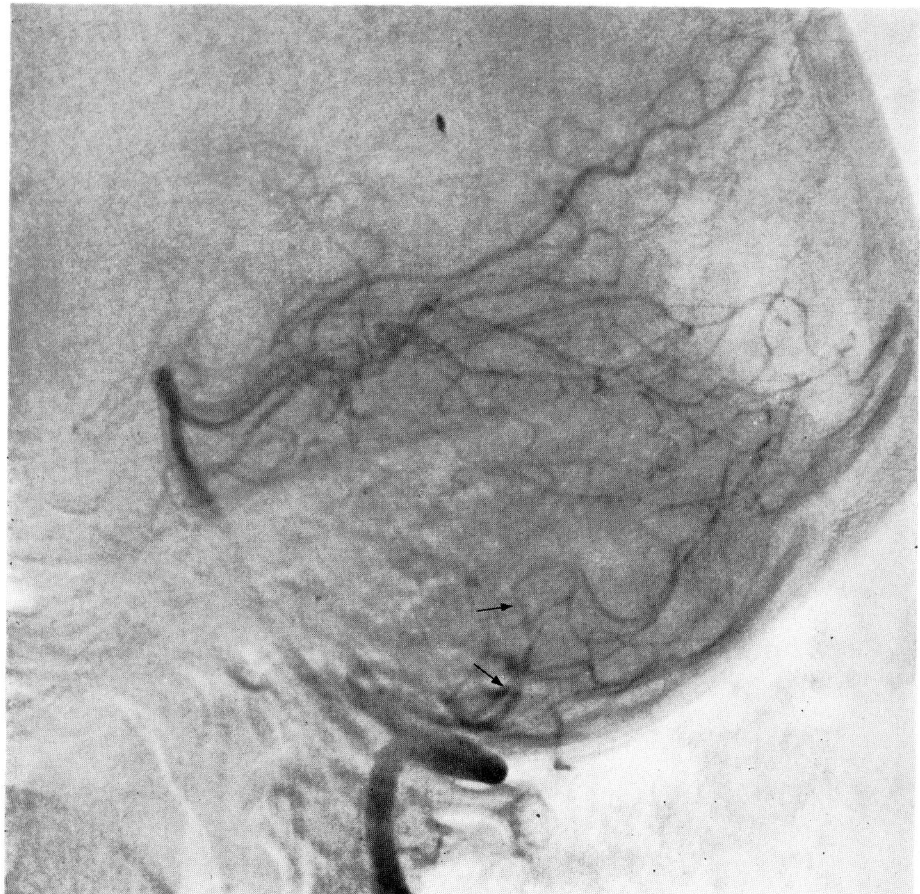
Fig. 105

Recurrent Neurinoma of the Left Accessory Nerve

A 60-year-old female: Figs. 106–109

A neurionoma of the left accessory nerve was removed 3 years previously.

Fig. 106 Arterial phase in the Towne projection. The vermian branch of the left posterior inferior cerebellar artery is markedly displaced to the right (3 arrows) together with the same branch on the right (3 crossed arrows). Because of the absence of displacements of the superior cerebellar artery a mass is localized in the inferior portion of the posterior fossa.

Fig. 107 Venous phase in the Towne projection. There is poor visualization of the left petrosal vein (an arrow) compared with the right (a crossed arrow).

Fig. 108 Arterial phase in the lateral projection. The anterior, lateral and posterior medullary segments of the posterior inferior cerebellar artery are crowded and anteriorly displaced (an arrow). The vermian branch and the supratonsillar segments are displaced superiorly (3 arrowheads). The hemispheric branch is displaced downward (2 crossed arrows).

Fig. 109 Venous phase in the lateral projection. The inferior vermian vein is posteriorly displaced (2 arrows) and the pontine segment of the anterior pontomesencephalic vein is compressed against the clivus (2 crossed arrows). There is reduced distance between the choroid plexus and the internal cerebral vein (2 opposing arrows).

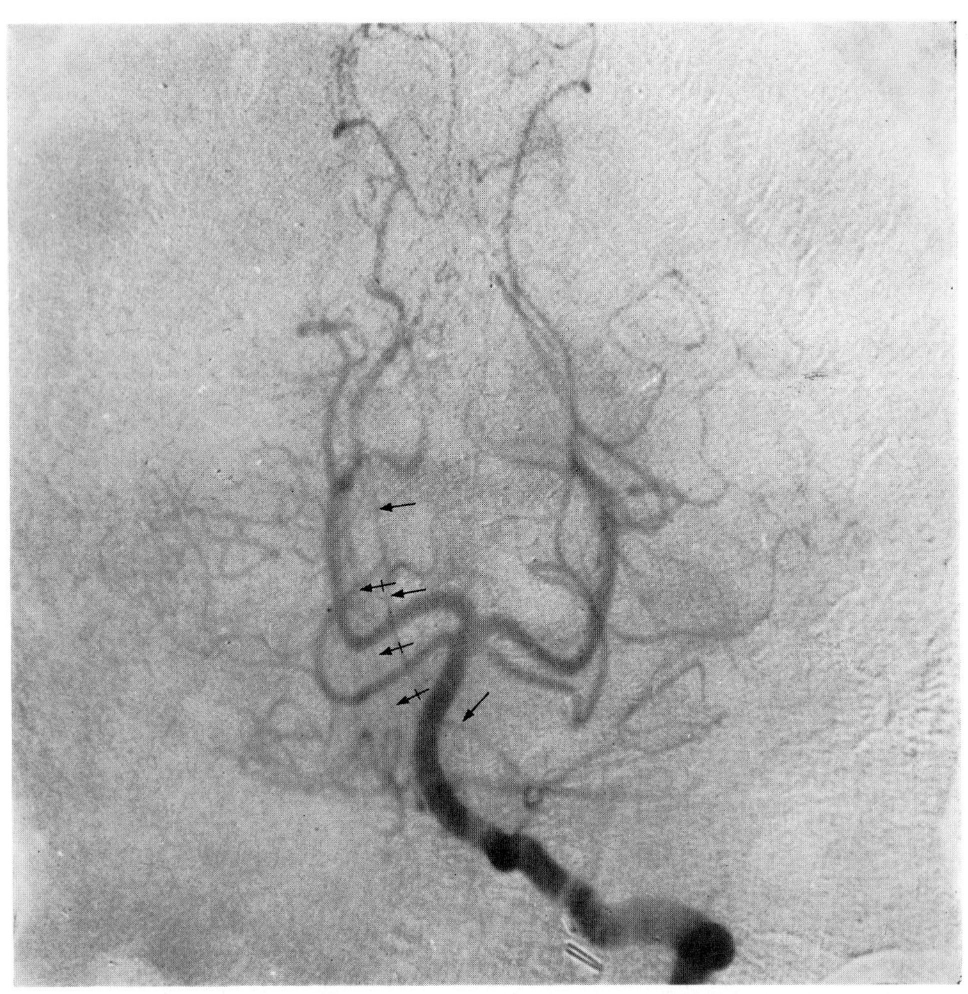

Fig. 106

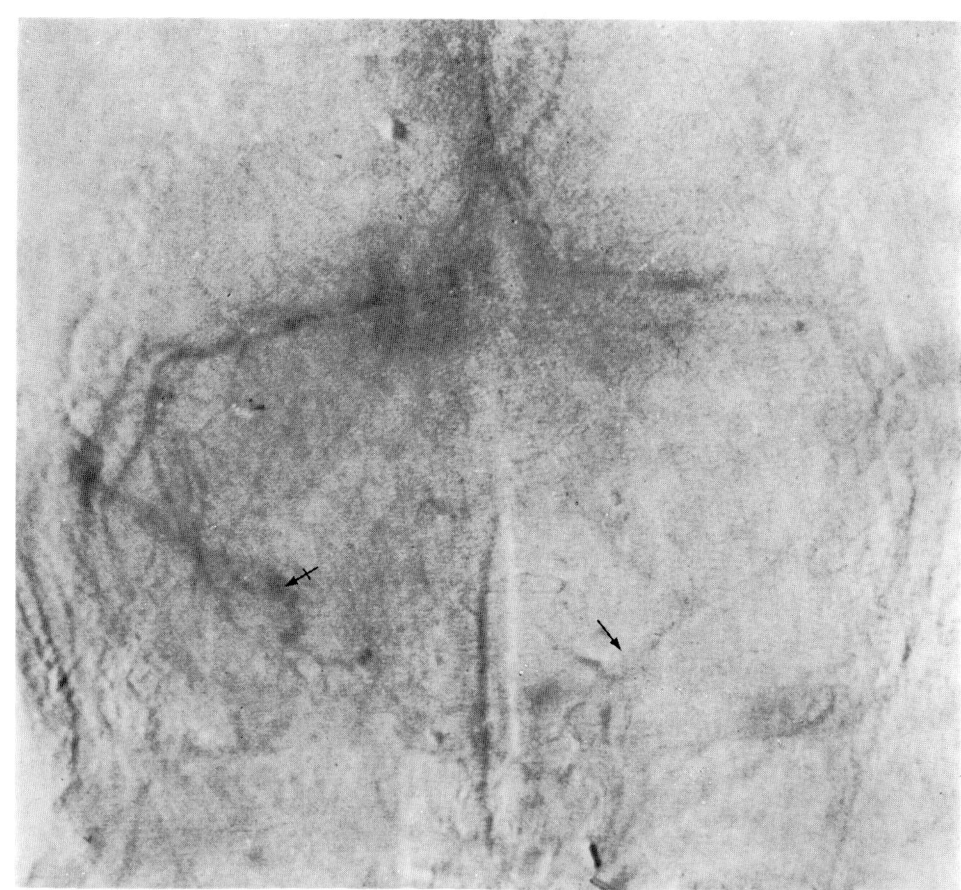

Fig. 107

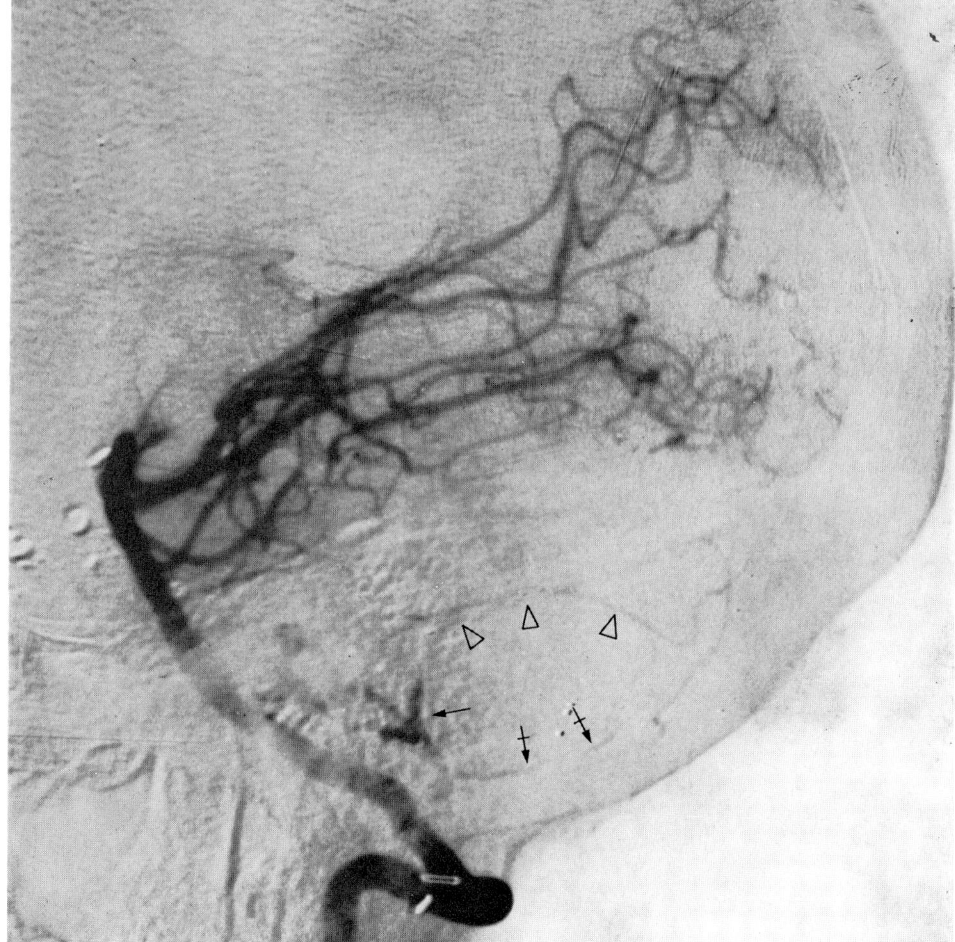

Fig. 108

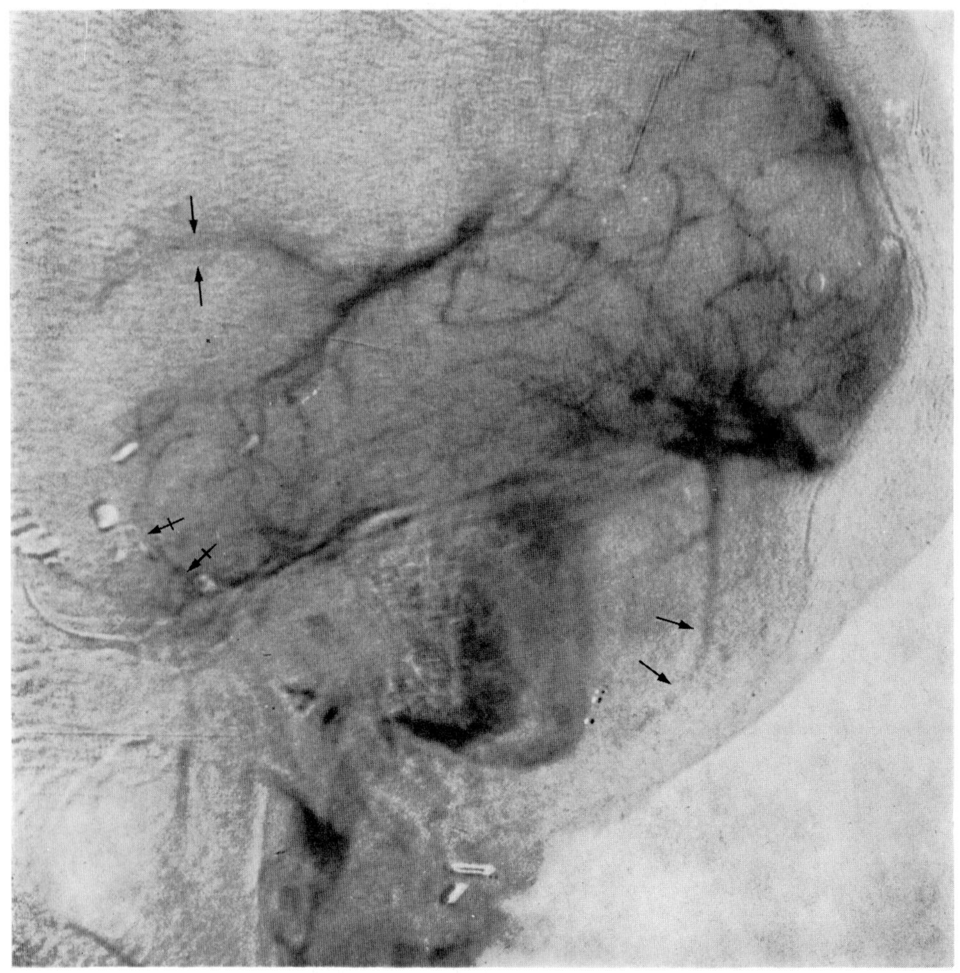

Fig. 109

6

Posterior Fossa Tumors

CEREBELLAR HEMISPHERIC TUMORS

Arteriographic features

The posterior inferior cerebellar artery

One of the most important findings in the diagnosis of cerebellar hemispheric tumors is displacement of the midline vermian branches of the posterior inferior cerebellar artery towards the normal side. This finding indicates lateralization of the tumor. The hemispheric branches may be stretched taut over the surface of the tumor. The retrotonsillar segment may be displaced anteriorly with shortening of the supratonsillar segment. The posterior medullary segment may be displaced anteriorly. These arteriographic features are more marked in the presence of inferior hemispheric tumors than with superior hemispheric masses.

The superior cerebellar artery

The hemispheric branches of the superior cerebellar artery are stretched taut over the surface of the tumors. The marginal artery may be markedly stretched anteriorly and superiorly. The anterior culminate and quadrigeminal segments may be displaced to the opposite side. More prominent findings are observed in this artery in the presence of superior hemispheric masses.

The basilar artery

The basilar artery normally bows away from the side of the dominant vertebral artery. Lateral displacement of this artery by a hemispheric mass should be evaluated in the light of such course of the artery. This finding is not reliable unless displacement is marked. Anterior displacement of the basilar artery is a non-specific sign of an expanding lesion in the posterior fossa.

The anterior inferior cerebellar artery

This artery is straightened and compressed against the petrous bone, but no specific changes useful for localization of these tumors are present.

Venographic features

The posterior group

The inferior vermian vein may be displaced to the opposite side. This vein is also displaced posteriorly with posterior and inferior displacement of the copular point. The copular angle may be widened. The hemispheric cerebellar veins, which drain into the lateral sinus or sinus confluence, are frequently stretched and arched by a hemispheric mass. Venous filling on the side of the mass is usually poor due to compression of the veins by the tumors. This finding is valuable in lateralization of a mass. However, this should be evaluated in the light of good filling of both posterior inferior cerebellar arteries, since these arteries vascularize most of the area drained by the petrosal veins, inferior vermian veins and hemispheric veins.

The anterior group

The petrosal vein and its tributaries are compressed against the petrous bone. The distance between the transverse pontine vein and the petrous bone is markedly reduced. The superior and inferior hemispheric veins and the vein of the great horizontal fissure may be stretched by the tumor. Poor filling of the petrosal vein and its tributaries is also demonstrated on the side of the tumor and this should also be evaluated in the light of the degree of filling of both posterior inferior cerebellar arteries.

The superior group

The precentral cerebellar vein is usually displaced anteriorly and to the opposite side. There is an increased colliculocentral angle with anterior displacement of the colliculocentral point. The superior vermian vein is also displaced to the opposite direction with occasional foreshortening. The supraculminate vein may be compressed against the straight sinus.

Cystic Astrocytoma with a Mural Nodule

A 3-year-old male: Figs. 110–112

A 3×3 cm tumor was arising from the superior vermis and extending into the left cerebellar hemisphere. There was bilateral tonsillar herniation

Fig. 110 Arterial phase in the Towne projection. The ambient and quadrigeminal segments of both superior cerebellar arteries are slightly displaced to the right (3 arrows). Separation of the quadrigeminal segments is noted, indicating upward transtentorial herniation. There is a displaced arterial branch from the ambient segment of the left superior cerebellar artery (3 crossed arrows), probably running over the surface of the tumor. Vermian and hemispheric segments of the left posterior inferior cerebellar artery are stretched (3 arrow heads). The most proximal portion of this artery is displaced across the midline (a double-crossed arrow). The anterior inferior cerebellar artery on the right is stretched (2 arrows). The findings suggest a large tumor in the left superior cerebellar hemisphere.

Fig. 111 Venous phase in the Towne projection. The inferior vermian vein on the left is stretched and slightly shifted towards the midline (3 arrows). The petrosal vein is compressed against the petrous apex on both sides (a crossed arrow).

Fig. 112 Arterial phase in the lateral projection. The basilar artery is compressed against the clivus. The quadrigeminal, anterior culminate and vermian segments of the superior cerebellar artery are displaced upward in an arcuate fashion (3 arrows; 4 arrows). These vessels are projected above the posterior cerebral arteries. The posterior inferior cerebellar artery is depressed downwards: its tonsillohemispheric branch is located below the foramen magnum (2 crossed arrows), suggesting a tonsillar herniation. The vermian branch of this artery is also stretched and depressed downward (3 arrowheads).

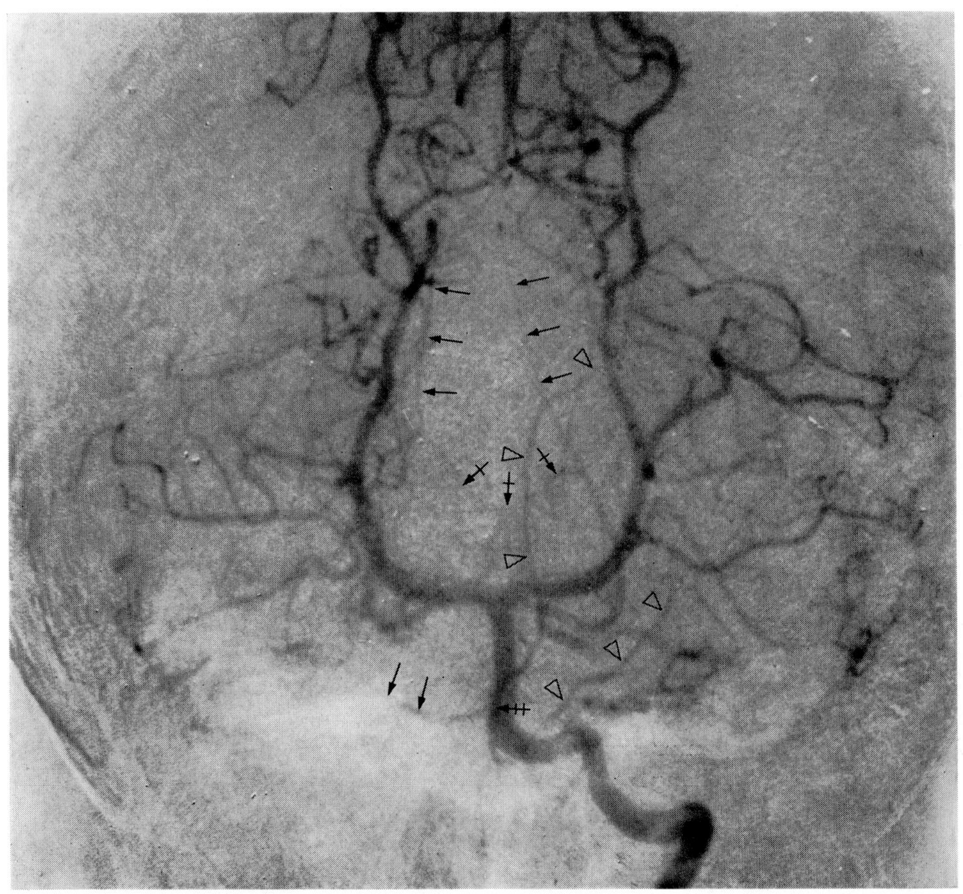

Fig. 110

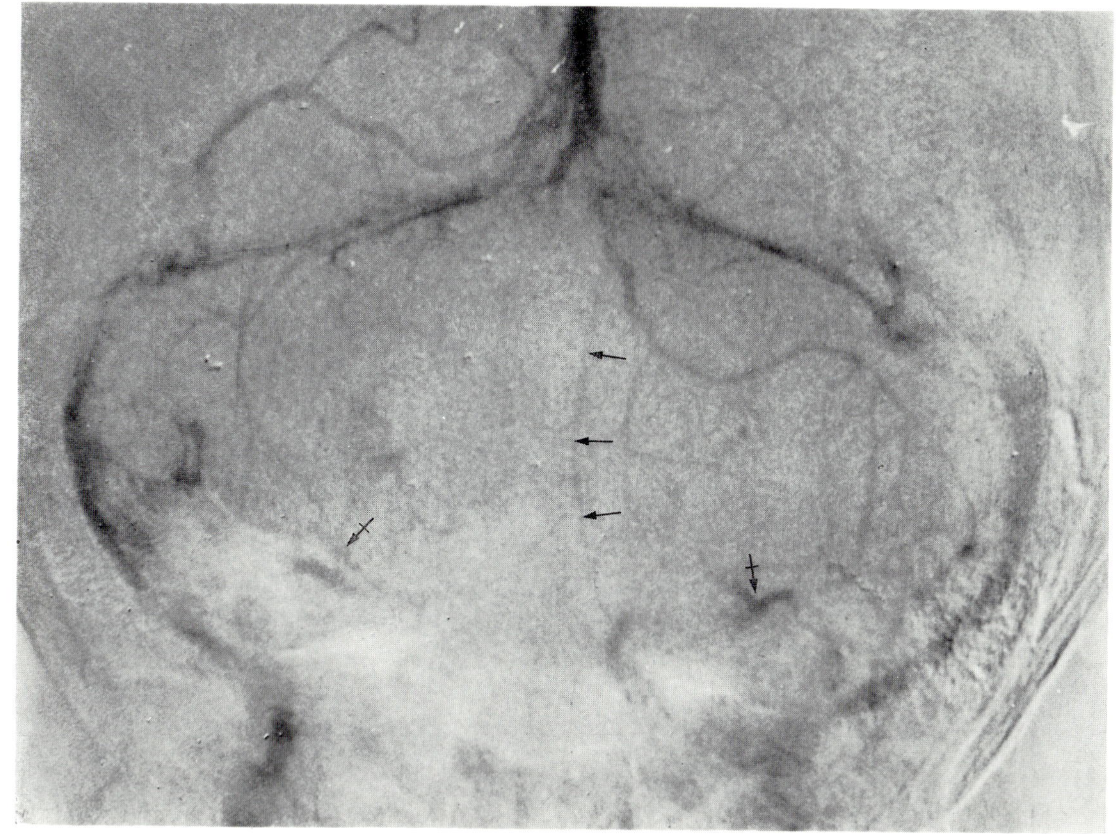

Fig. 111

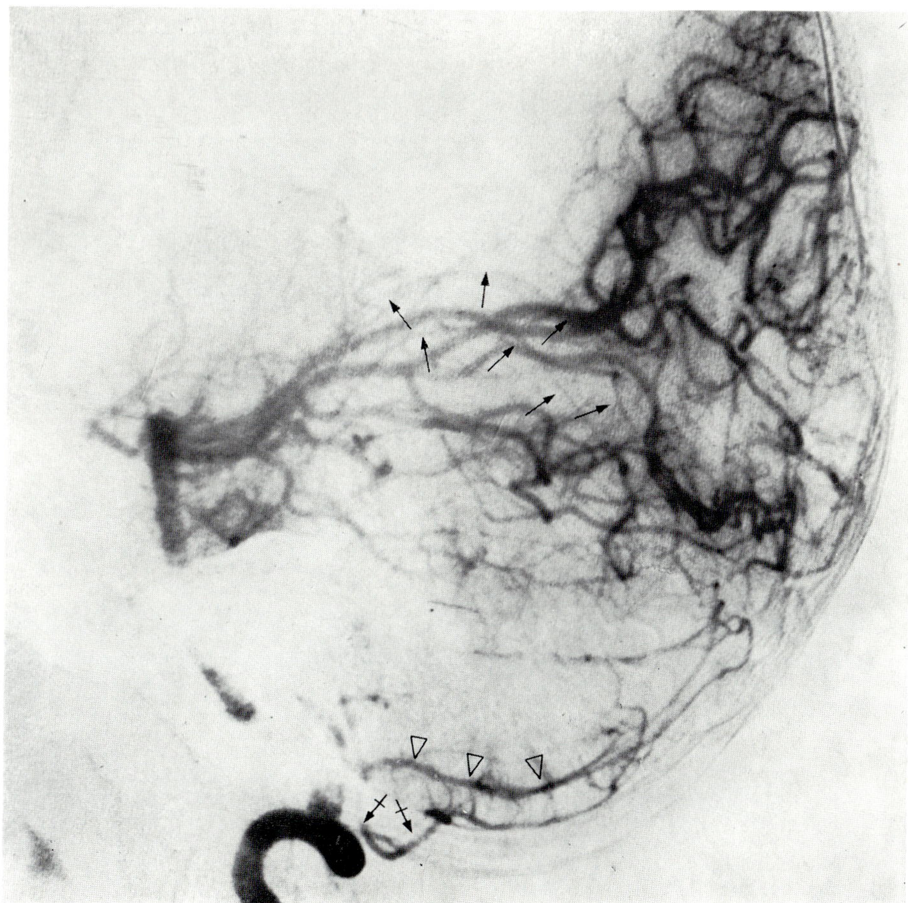

Fig. 112

Astrocytoma of the Right Inferior Cerebellar Hemisphere

A 2-year-old male: Figs. 113–115

Fig. 113 Arterial phase in the Towne projection. A branch of the posterior inferior cerebellar artery is markedly displaced medially in an arcuate fashion (3 arrows). A hemispheric branch of this artery is displaced laterally (3 open arrowheads). The superior cerebellar artery on the left is displaced laterally (3 crossed arrows). The quadrigeminal segments of both the superior cerebellar arteries are separated (2 closed arrowheads), indicating upward transtentorial herniation. The ambient segments of the posterior cerebral arteries are also separated. The findings indicate a large mass in the right inferior cerebellar hemisphere.

Fig. 114 Arterial phase in the lateral projection. There are changes due to increased intracranial pressure: anterior displacement of the basilar artery, straightening of the thalamoperforate arteries, and depression of the posterior choroidal arteries. Both the hemispheric (3 arrows) and vermian (3 crossed arrows) branches of the left posterior inferior cerebellar arteries are stretched and the undivided portion is anteriorly displaced (an arrowhead). In particular, the vermian branch is compressed against the occipital bone.

Fig. 115 Venous phase in the lateral projection. The anterior pontomesencephalic vein is displaced anteriorly. Its interpeduncular segment is depressed (an arrow). The distance between the internal cerebral vein and the choroid plexus is reduced due to dilatation of the lateral ventricles (2 opposing arrows). The precentral cerebellar and inferior vermian veins are not visualized.

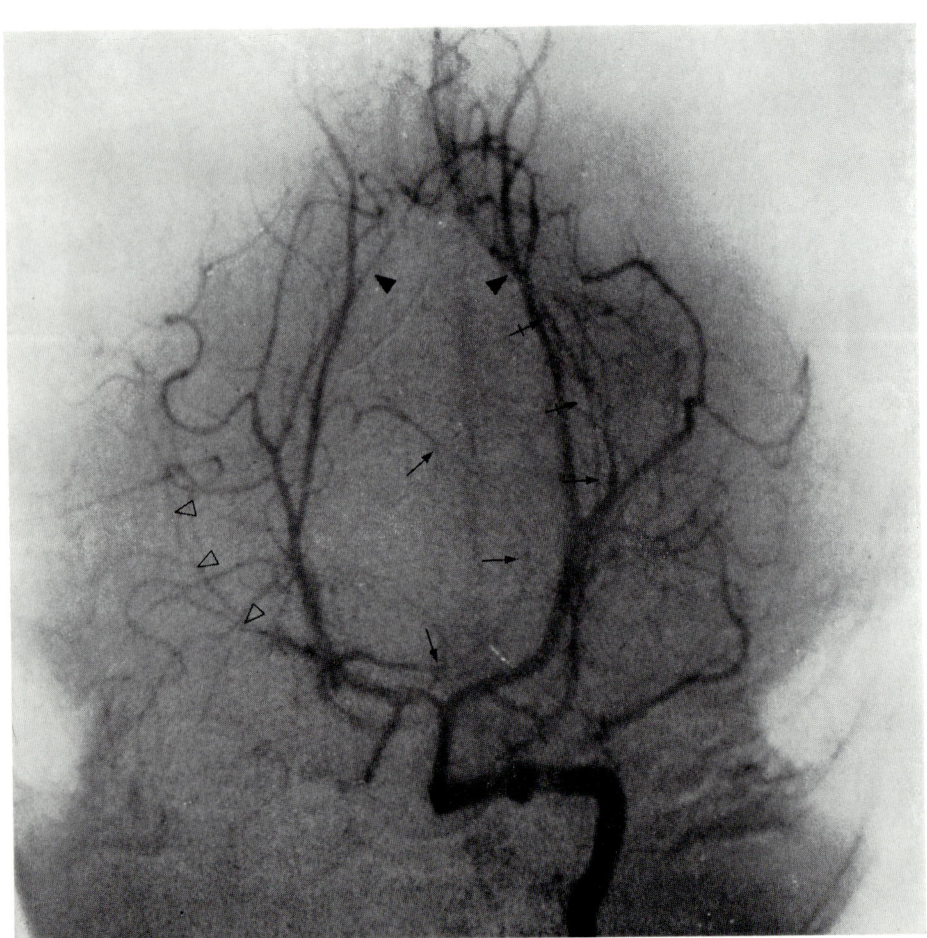

Fig. 113

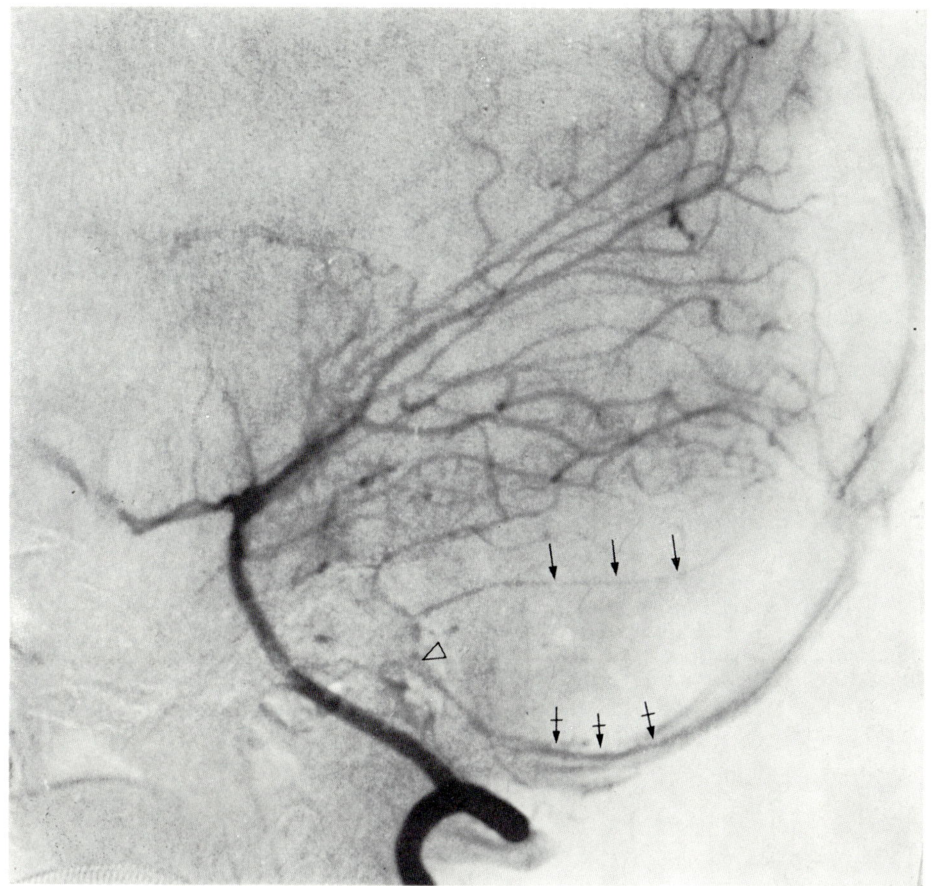

Fig. 114

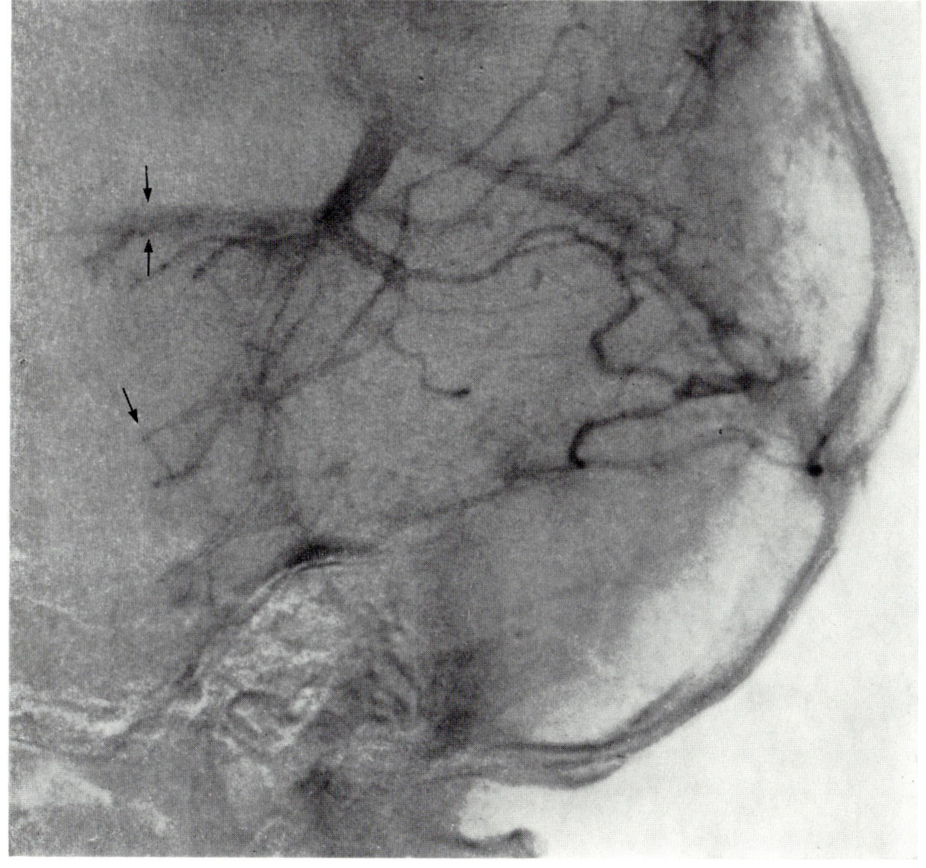

Fig. 115

Hemangioblastoma of the Right Inferior Cerebellar Hemisphere

A 19-year-old female: Figs. 116–121

Fig. 116 Arterial phase in the Towne projection. There is an extensively vascular lesion in the inferior portion of the right posterior fossa. Three arterial branches from the distal portion of the right vertebral artery are considerably enlarged and participate in the blood supply of the tumor. Distal two branches are probably the posterior and anterior inferior cerebellar arteries (an arrow; a crossed arrow). The proximal branch is probably the posterior meningeal artery (2 arrows). The superior cerebellar artery on the right is enlarged and supplies the tumor. There is displacement of the right superior cerebellar artery towards the left (3 arrows), while vermian segments are moderately separated (2 closed arrowheads), suggesting upward transtentorial herniation. The proximal portion of the left posterior inferior cerebellar artery is displaced to the left (3 open arrowheads).

Fig. 117 Capillary phase in the Towne projection. There is a 4.5 cm cystic tumor with multiple nodular staining. The stains are homogeneous and their contour is smooth. These findings are characteristic of a hemangioblastoma. Drainage is to the lateral sinus near the sinus confluence (an arrow). Tumor vessels noted on the arterial phase are not visualized any more.

Fig. 118 Venous phase in the Towne projection. Veins in the right posterior fossa are displaced in an arcuate fashion by the tumor (3 arrows). Veins surrounding the tumor are noted (3 crossed arrows). The petrosal vein is poorly visualized on the right. Mural nodules and abnormal veins visualized on capillary phase are not seen.

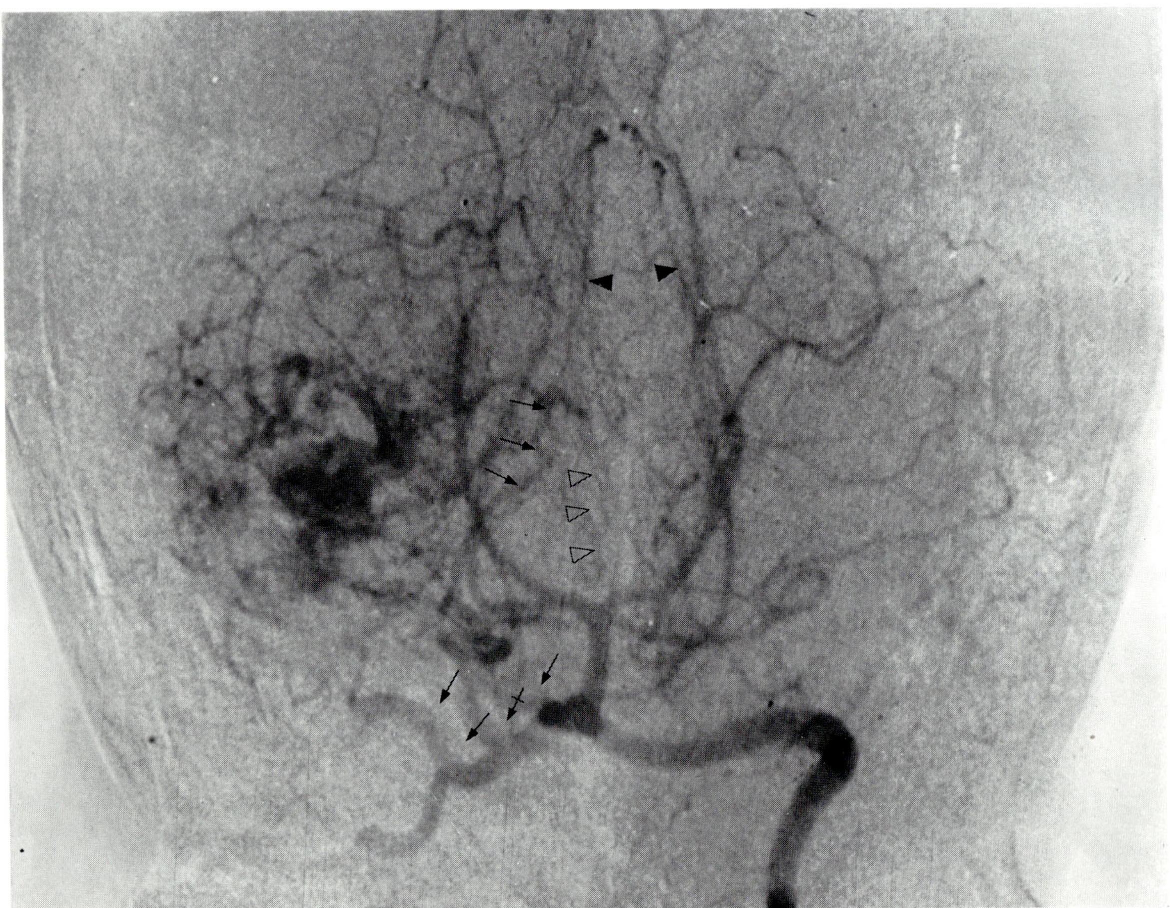

Fig. 116

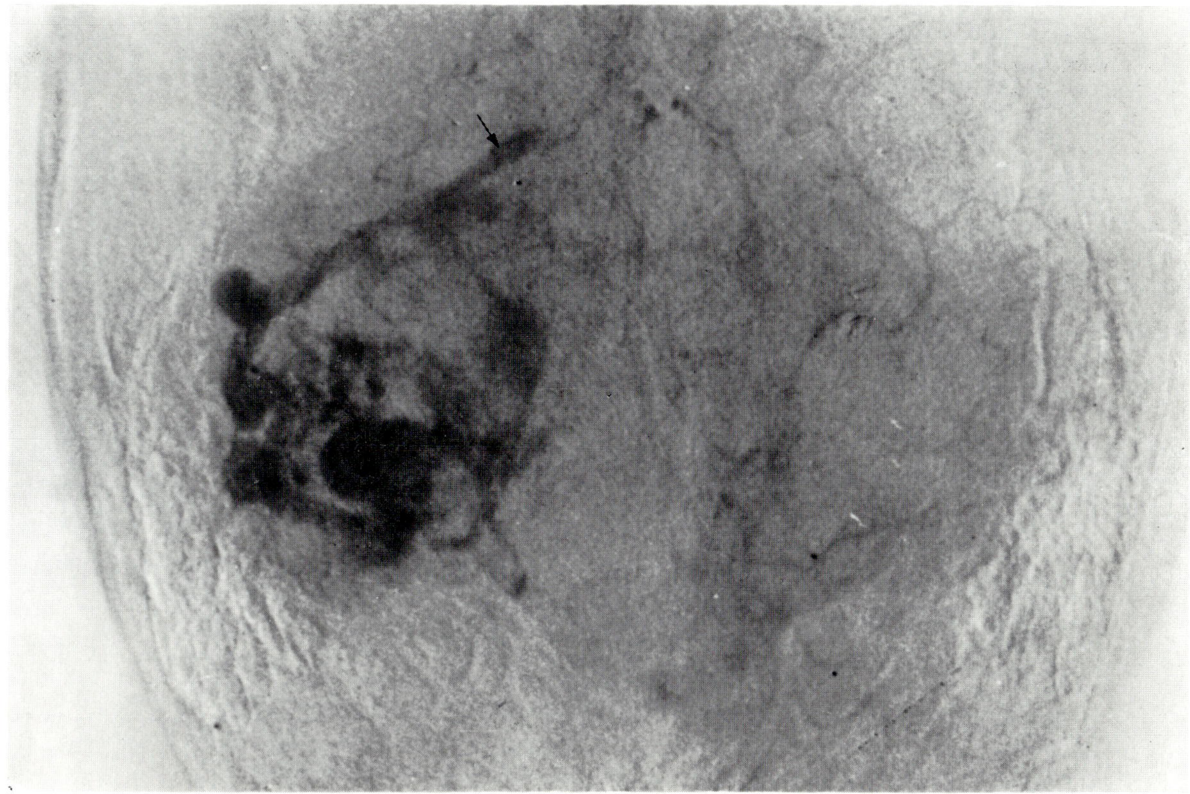

Fig. 117

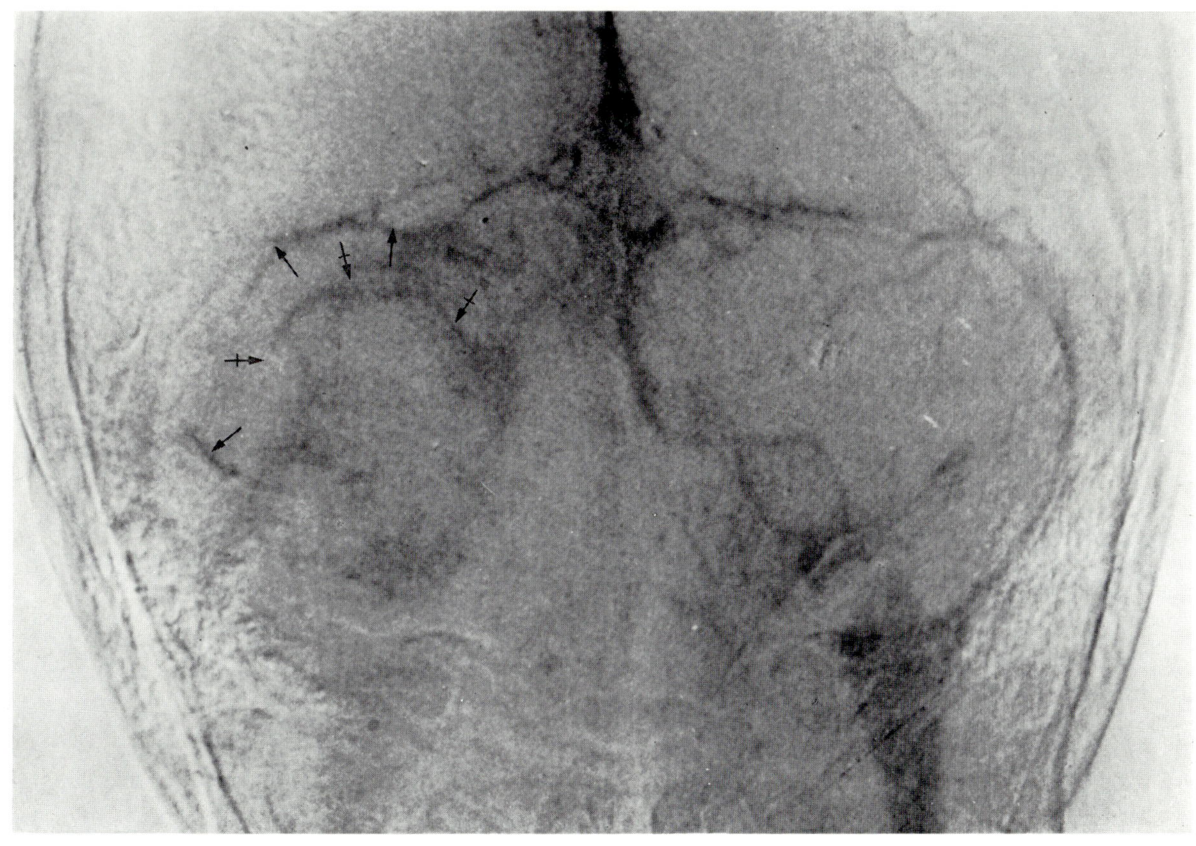

Fig. 118

Fig. 119 Arterial phase in the lateral projection. The extensively vascular lesion is again noted with blood supply from the right vertebral artery (5 open arrowheads). Individual feeding arteries are not well shown. The basilar artery is compressed against the clivus and the anterior culminate and vermian segments of the superior cerebellar arteries are stretched (4 arrows). Dilatation of the lateral ventricle is shown by straightening of the thalamoperforate arteries (2 crossed arrows), flattening of the posterior choroidal arteries (2 closed arrowheads) and unrolling of the anterior cerebral arteries (2 double crossed arrows).

Fig. 120 Capillary phase in the lateral projection. The mural nodules are well shown with homogeneous stains and smooth contour. An abnormal vein drains into the lateral sinus (an arrow).

Fig. 121 Venous phase in the lateral projection. The precentral cerebellar vein is displaced anteriorly (an arrow) and the superior vermian vein is compressed against the straight sinus, indicating superior tumor extension (3 crossed arrows). The inferior vermian vein is depressed downward (3 arrows). The interpeduncular segment of the anterior pontomesencephalic vein is depressed (a crossed arrow) and the distance between the superior choroid vein and the internal cerebral vein is reduced (2 opposing arrows), indicating the presence of hydrocephalus.

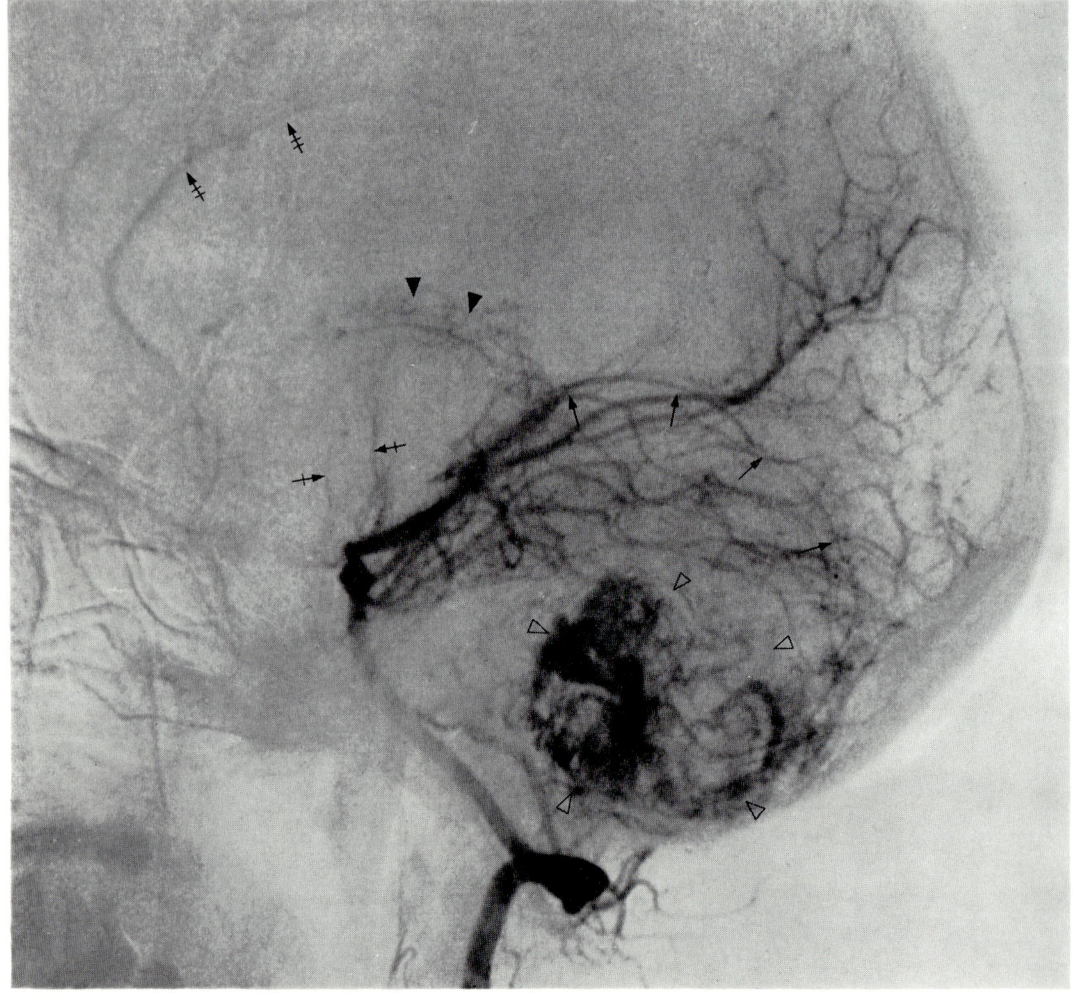

Fig. 119

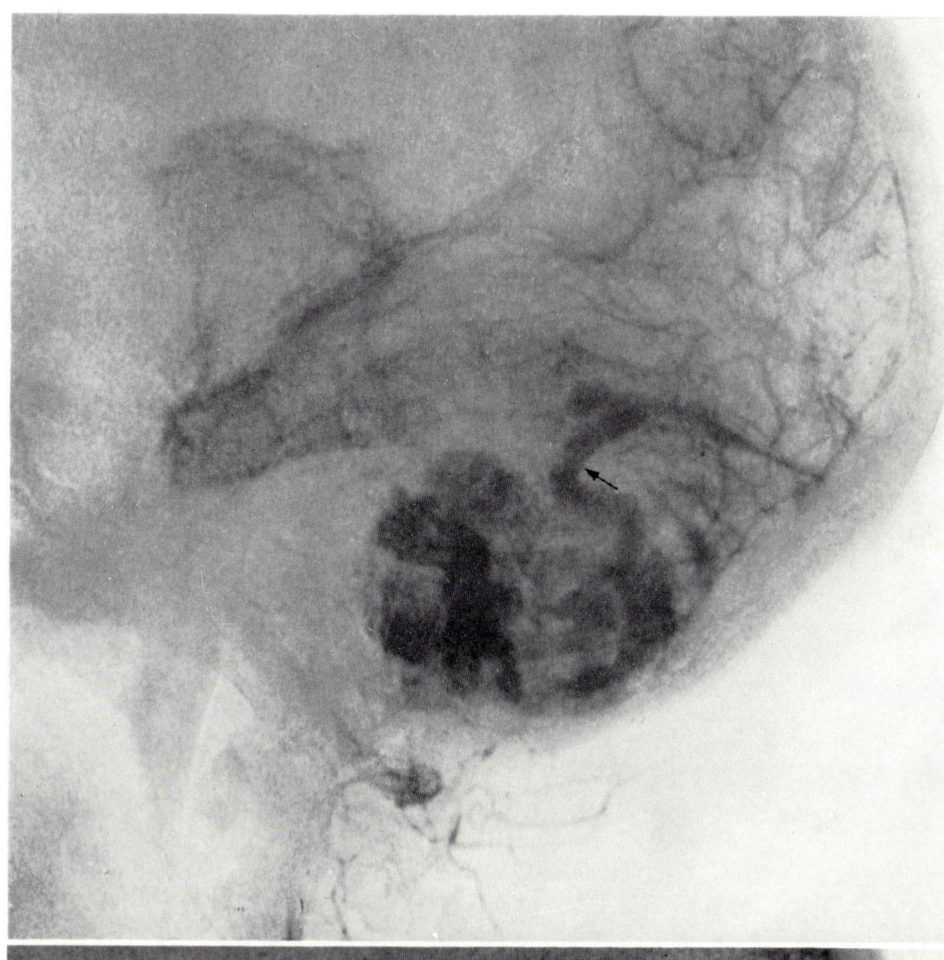
Fig. 120

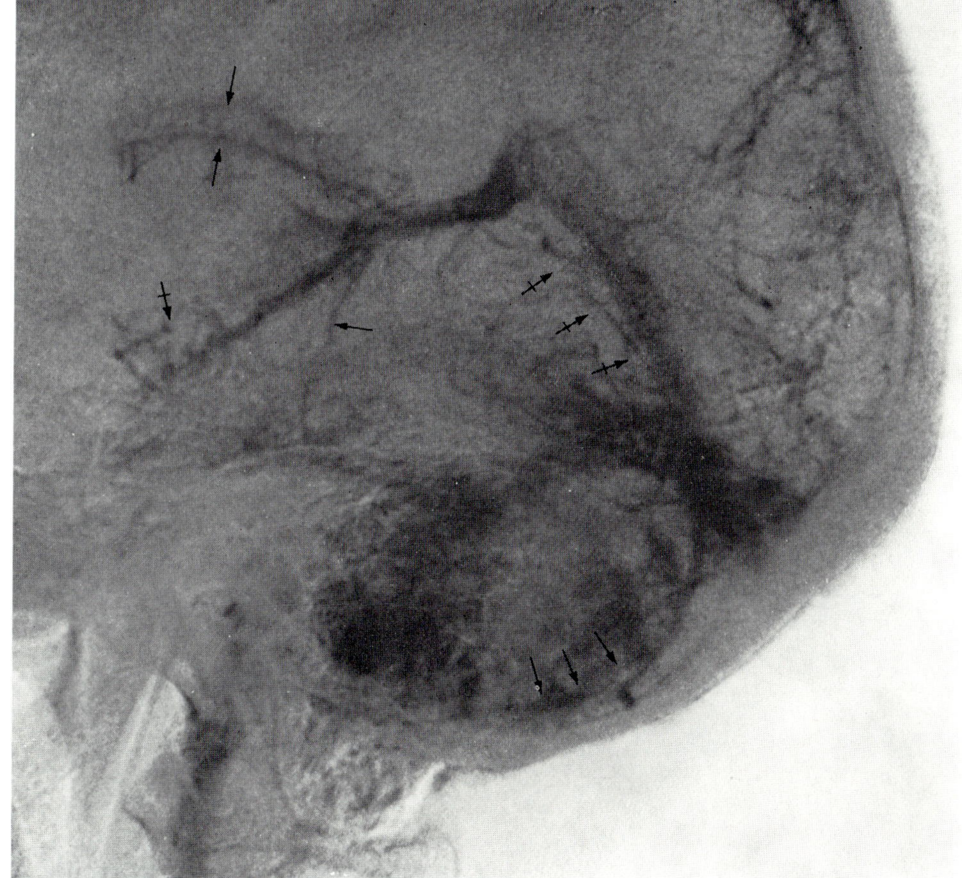
Fig. 121

Hemangioblastoma of the Left Inferior Cerebellar Hemisphere

A 36-year-old female: Figs. 122–126

The tumor was a 3×4 cm cyst with a small mural nodule.

Fig. 122 Arterial phase in the Towne projection. There is a 1.0×1.0 cm tumor stain on the left with little vascular displacement (2 arrowheads). The quadrigeminal segments of the superior cerebellar arteries are slightly separated and displaced to the right (2 arrows). The hemispheric and vermian segments of the posterior inferior cerebellar arteries are not displaced.

Fig. 123 Capillary phase in the Towne projection. The tumor stain is now well demonstrated (2 arrowheads). There is a feeding artery arising from the posterior inferior cerebellar artery (3 arrows).

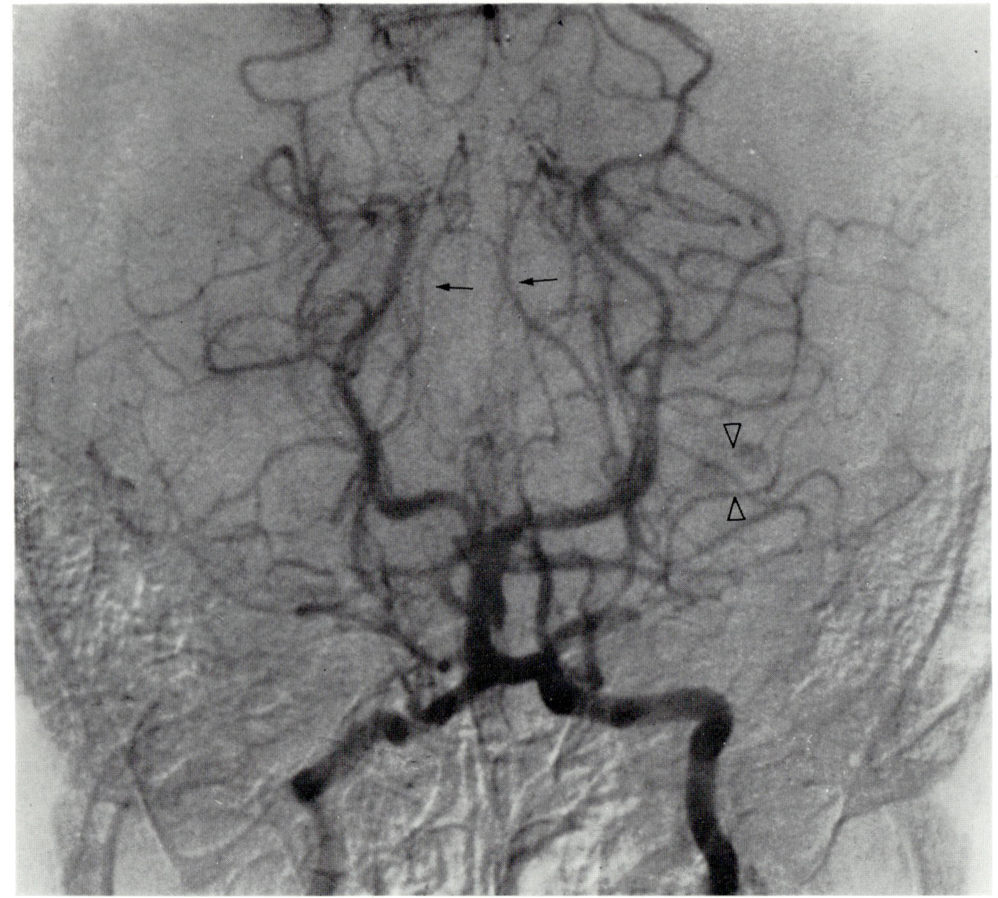

Fig. 122

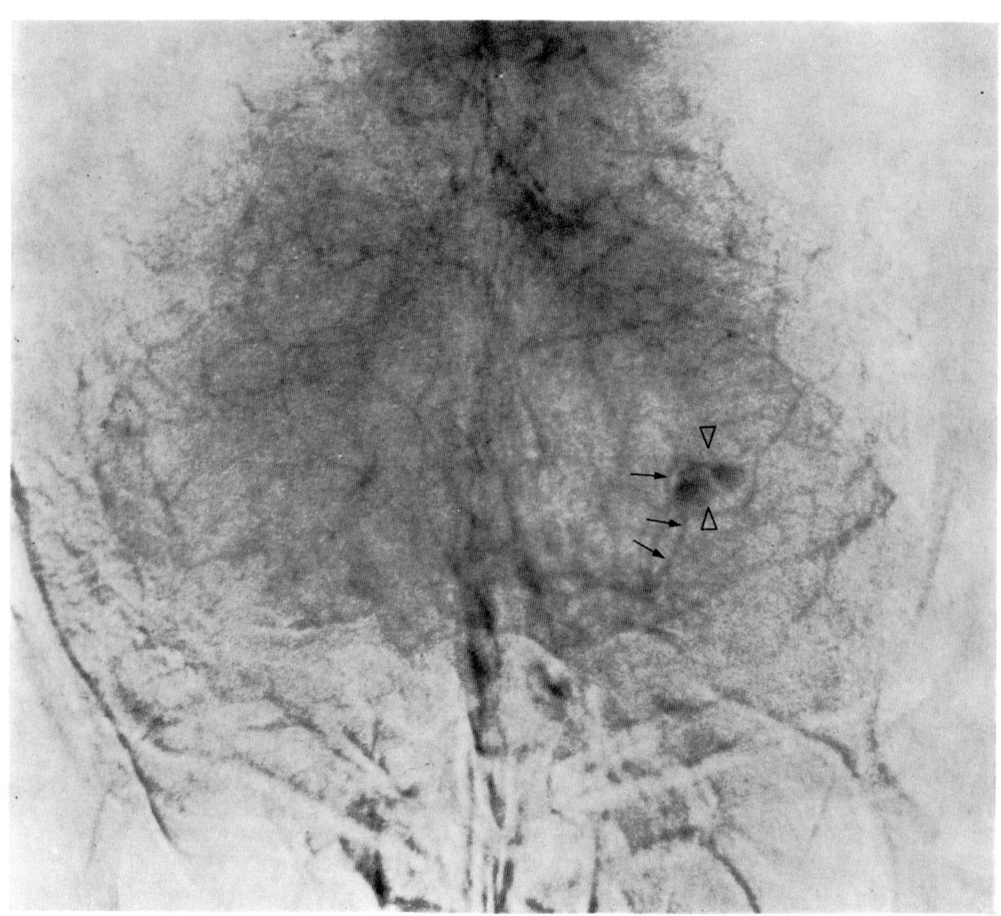

Fig. 123

Fig. 124 Venous phase in the Towne projection. The tumor stain is now faintly seen (2 arrowheads). The inferior vermian vein is displaced across the midline (4 arrows). The anterior pontomesencephalic vein is superimposed over this vein. There is compression of the petrosal vein against the petrous bone (a crossed arrow). Venous displacements indicate a large cystic component to the tumor.

Fig. 125 Arterial phase in the lateral projection. There are arterial changes due to increased intracranial pressure in the posterior fossa. Anterior displacement of the basilar artery, arcuate superior displacement of the anterior culminate segment of the superior cerebellar artery (4 arrows), and stretching of the thalamoperforate arteries. In addition, the supratonsillar segment of the posterior inferior cerebellar artery is angulated and anteriorly displaced (a crossed arrow). The superior retrotonsillar segment is markedly displaced anteriorly (2 open arrowheads). The hemispheric and vermian segments are considerably depressed (3 arrows) with visualization of faint tumor stains (2 double-crossed arrows). The findings are those of a large avascular tumor with a mural nodule in the inferior cerebellar hemisphere. The hemispheric branch on the left is depressed below the foramen magnum (a closed arrowhead).

Fig. 126 Early venous phase in the lateral projection. The tumor stain is well shown (2 arrowheads) with a draining vein towards the lateral sinus (2 arrows). The precentral cerebellar vein is anteriorly displaced (an arrow). The anterior pontomesencephalic vein is compressed against the clivus (2 crossed arrows). There is decreased distance between the superior choroid vein and the internal cerebral vein (2 opposing arrows).

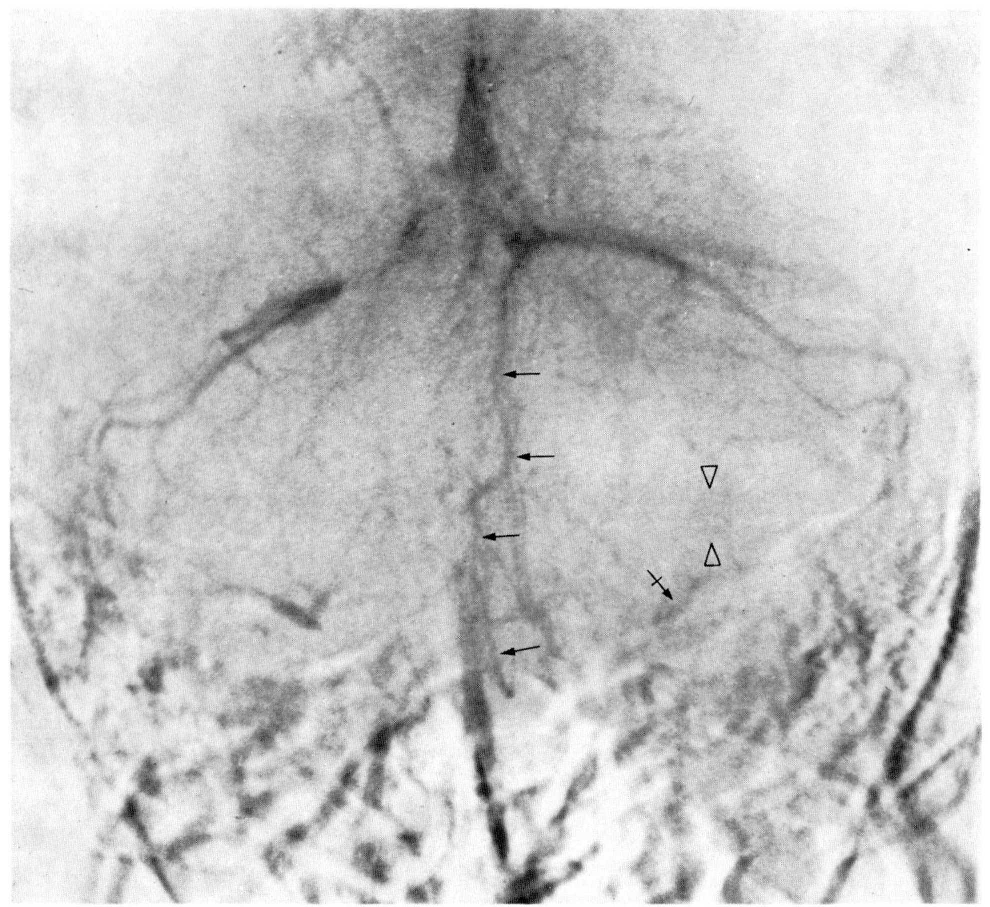

Fig. 124

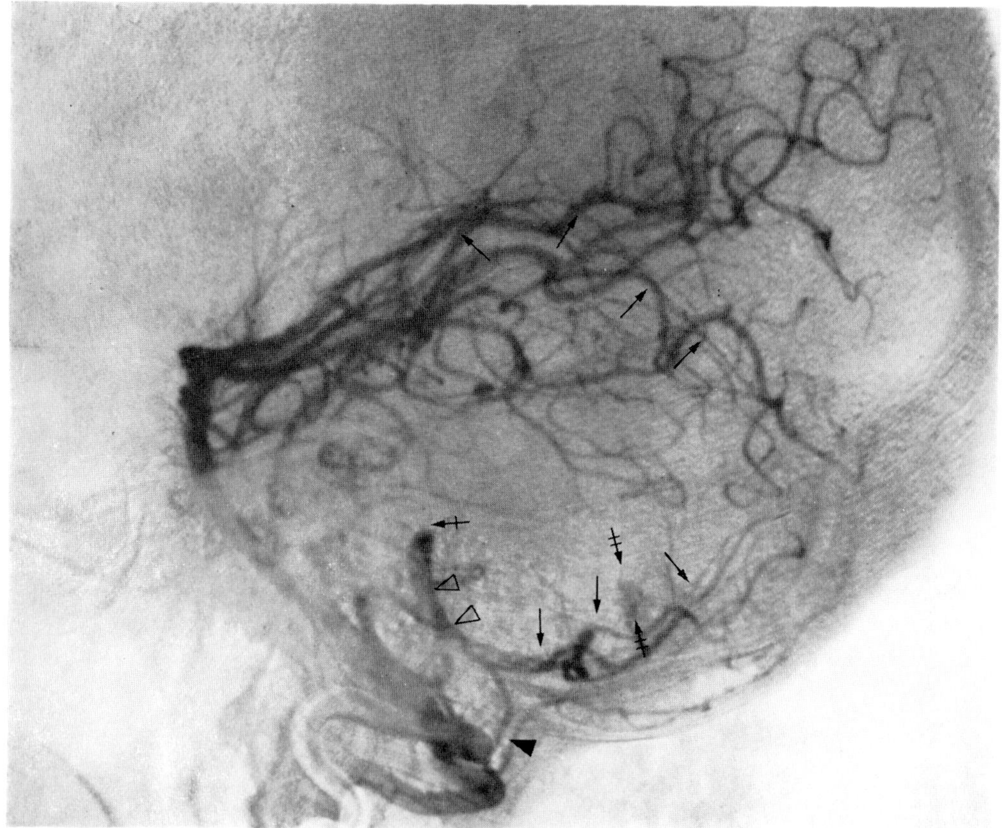

Fig. 125

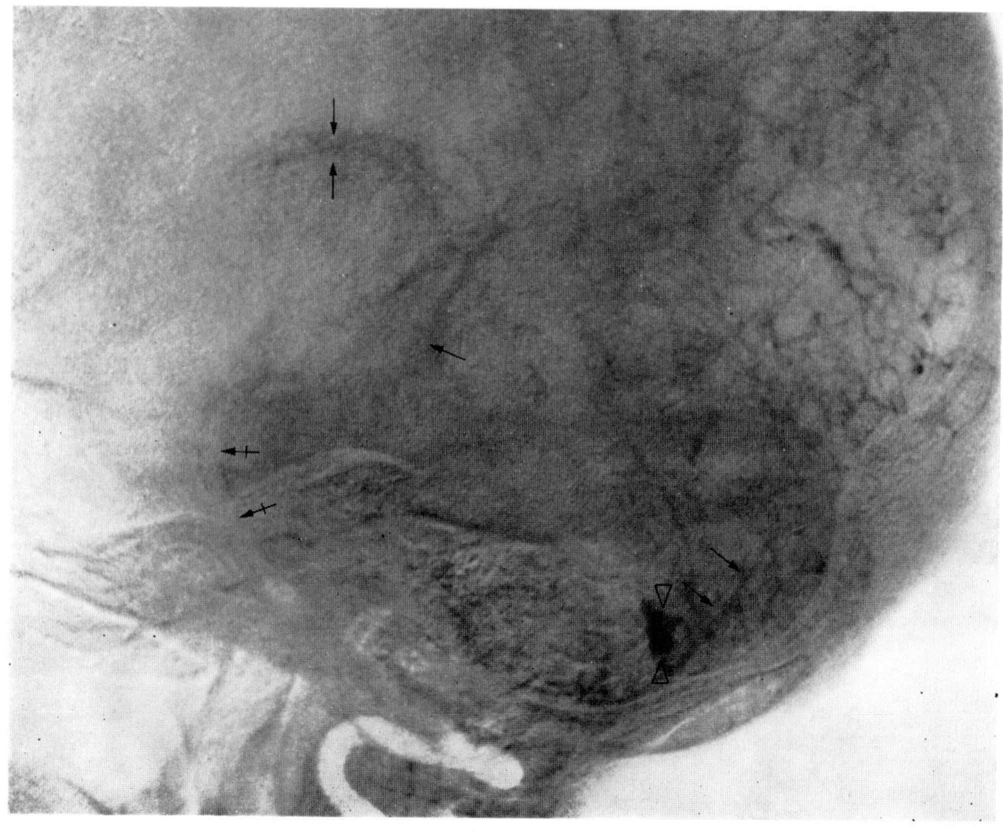

Fig. 126

Left Inferior Cerebellar Astrocytoma

A 7-year-old male: Figs. 127–129

A 3 cm solid astrocytoma was found in the left inferior cerebellar hemisphere, extending into the cerebellar nuclei. There was tonsillar herniation on the left.

Fig. 127 Arterial phase in the Towne projection. The lateral and posterior medullary segments of the left posterior inferior cerebellar artery are markedly displaced to the right of the midline (3 arrows). The vermian segment of this artery returns towards the midline (2 crossed arrows). The superior cerebellar arteries on both sides are slightly shifted to the right with distortion of their branches (2 arrowheads). These findings strongly suggest a mass lesion in the left cerebellar hemisphere near the undivided portion of the posterior inferior cerebellar artery. The course of the posterior cerebral arteries are anomalous with marked separation.

Fig. 128 Venous phase in the Towne projection. The left inferior vermian vein is displaced to the normal side (3 arrows), while the hemispheric tributaries of the inferior vermian vein (an arrowhead and a crossed arrow), are stretched. The petrosal vein is not well visualized on the left, probably due to compression of this vein. The right petrosal vein is not filled since the right posterior inferior cerebellar artery is not opacified.

Fig. 129 Arterial phase in the lateral projection. The basilar artery is compressed against the clivus. There is minimal distortion in the course of posterior medullary and supratonsillar segments of the left posterior inferior cerebellar artery. The hemisphere branches appear to be stretched (arrows) and the tonsillar branch is depressed downward (a crossed arrow).

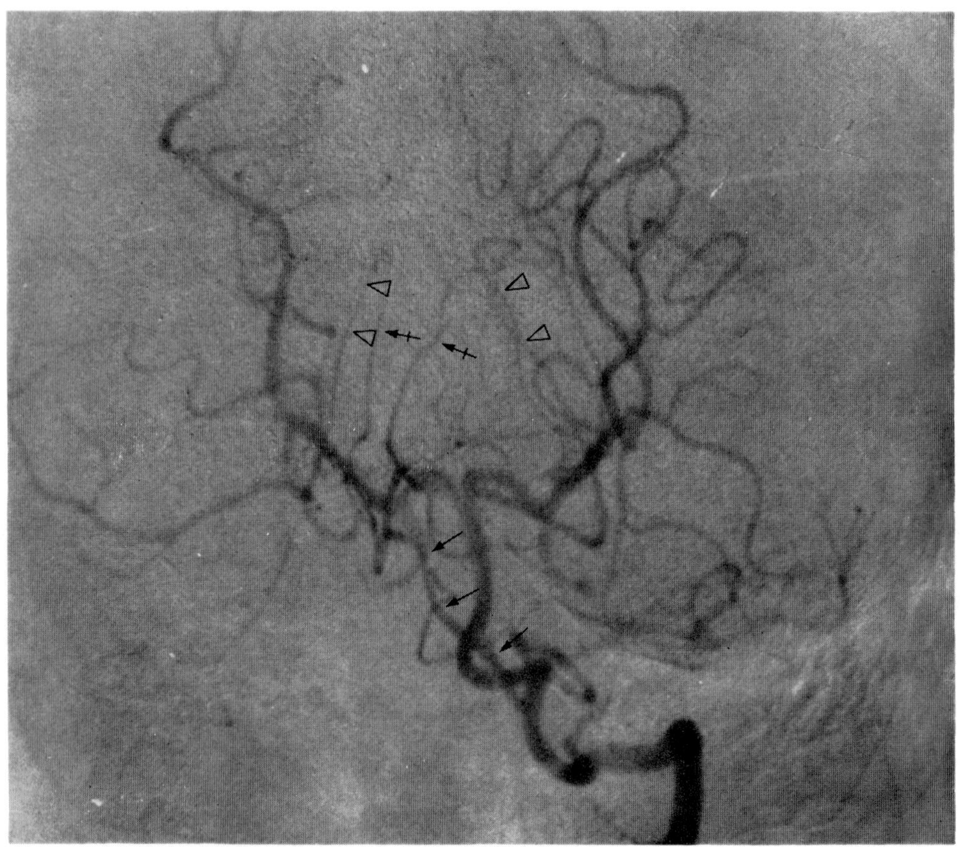

Fig. 127

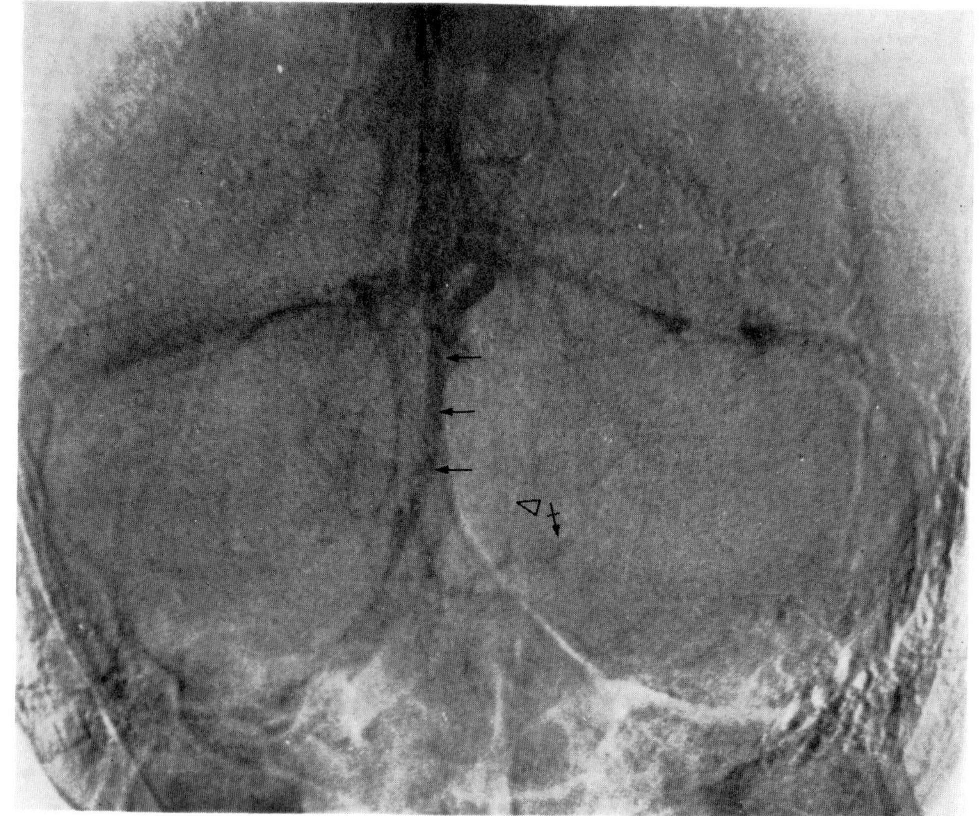

Fig. 128

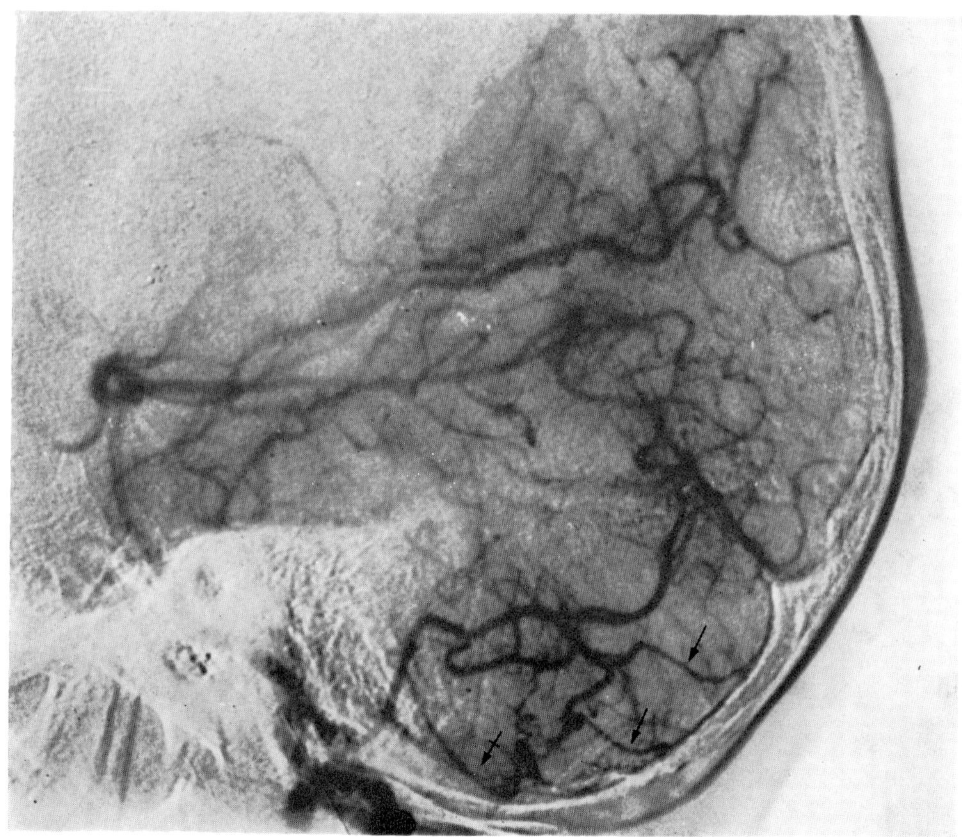

Fig. 129

Cystic Hemangioblastoma with a Mural Nodule

A 13-year-old male: Figs. 130–132

Fig. 130 Arterial phase in the Towne projection. There is a 1.5×1.0 cm homogeneous tumor stain superimposed over the right petrous apex (3 arrowheads). Blood supply appears to come from the right anterior inferior cerebellar artery (3 arrows). In add tion, the vermian segment of the posterior inferior cerebellar artery on the left is displaced to the left (3 crossed arrows). There is marked separation on the quadrigeminal segments of the superior cerebellar arteries (2 arrows), strongly suggesting that the tumor is very large. Therefore, a cystic hemangioblastoma with a mural nodule arising from the left inferior cerebellar hemisphere is strongly considered.

Fig. 131 Venous phase in the Towne projection. A midline vein, probably the inferior vermian vein on the left, is displaced across the midline (3 arrows). An abnormal vein is faintly visualized (2 crossed arrows), probably indicating draining vein into the sinus confluence. The veins in the right posterior fossa are poorly visualized partly due to compression by tumor and partly due to poor reflux of contrast media into the right vertebral artery. The tumor stain is not demonstrated.

Fig. 132 Arterial phase in the lateral projection. The basilar and intracranial vertebral arteries are markedly compressed against the clivus. The posterior medullary segment of the posterior inferior cerebellar artery is displaced anteriorly (2 arrows). The supratonsillar segment is elongated and displaced superiorly (3 crossed arrows). There is a 1.0×1.0 cm tumor stain superimposed over the hemispheric branch of the posterior inferior cerebellar artery (2 arrowheads).

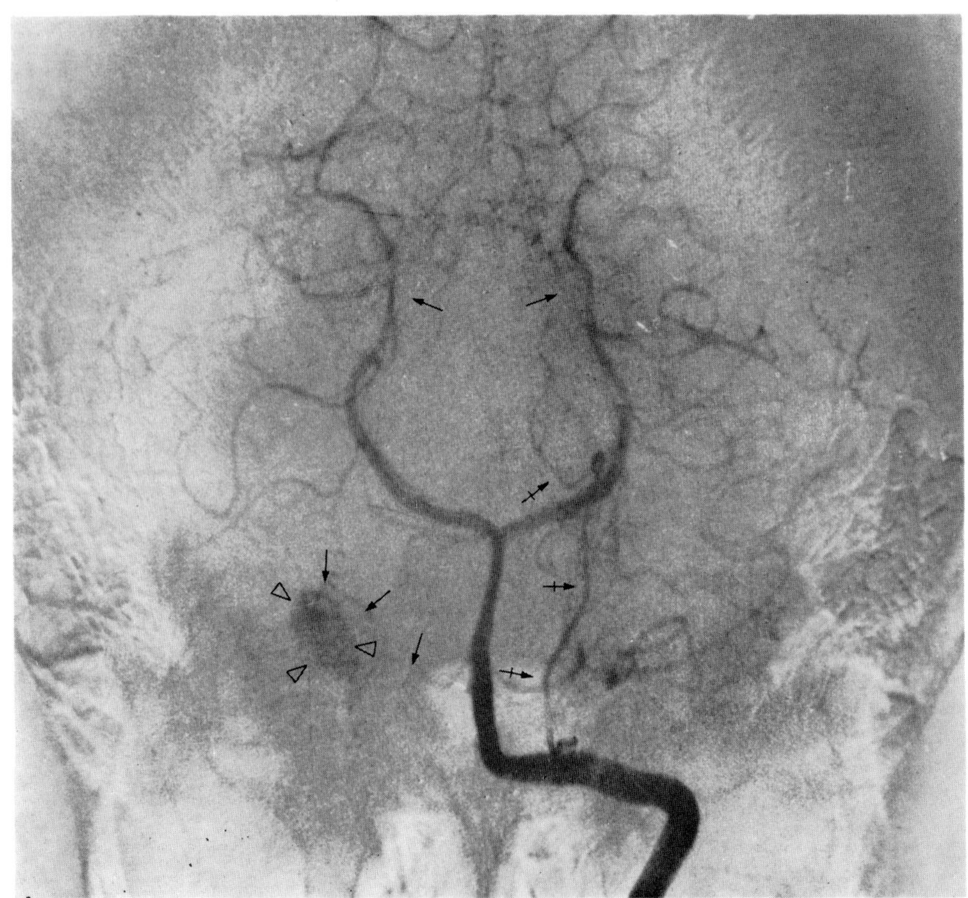

Fig. 130

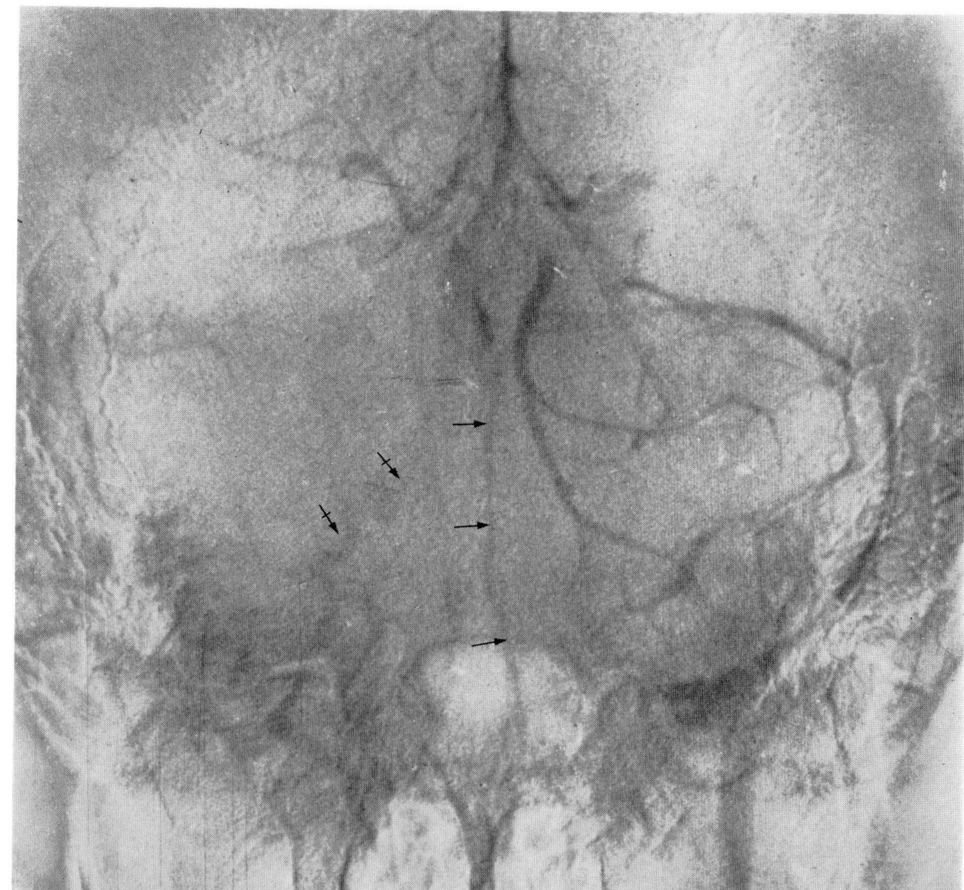

Fig. 131

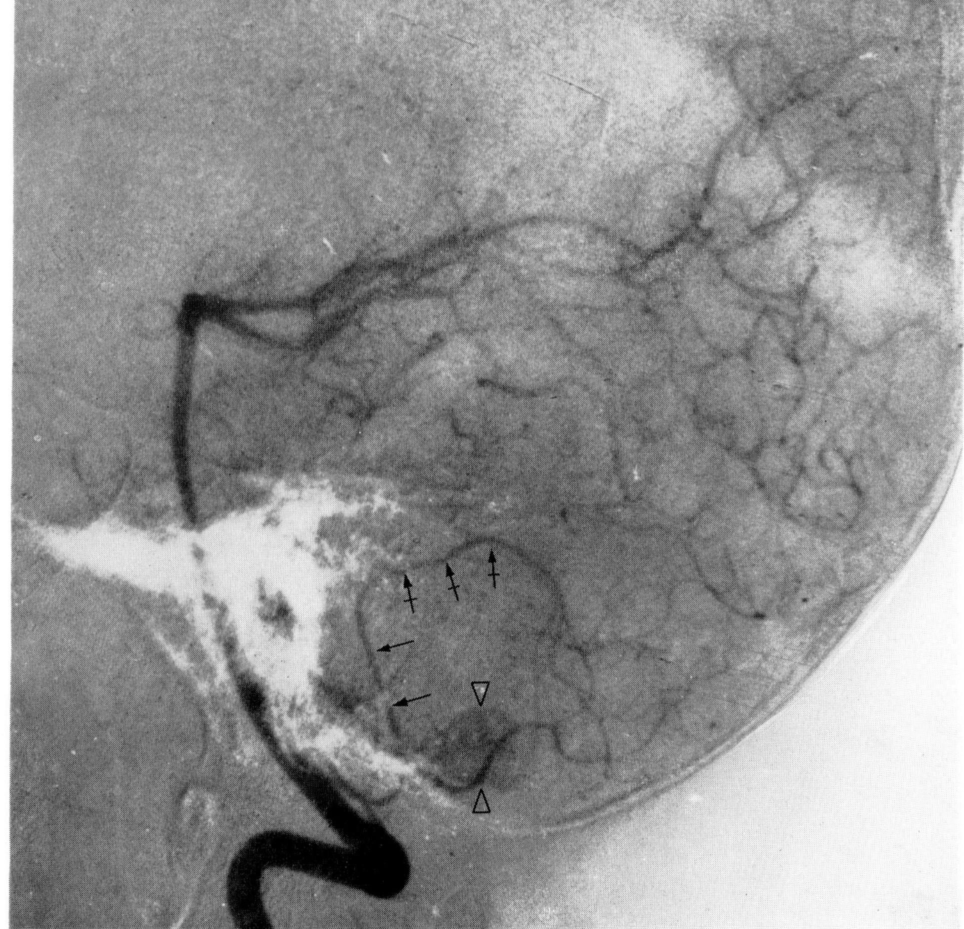

Fig. 132

TUMORS OF THE VERMIS WITH EMPHASIS ON MEDULLOBLASTOMA

Tumors of the vermis extend into the cerebellar heimsphere and the fourth ventricle at the early stage. Therefore, characteristic angiographic features are not present. Astrocytomas and hemangioblastomas in the vermis frequently involve the cerebellar hemisphere, while medulloblastomas extend into the fourth ventricle with obstruction of the cerebrospinal fluid pathways. In this chapter angiographic findings of medulloblastomas will be discussed in detail and tumors with hemispheric extension will be considered in the chapter of cerebellar hemispheric tumors.

Arteriographic features

The posterior inferior cerebellar artery

Medulloblastomas have tendency to balloon the fourth ventricle with the major bulk of tumor remaining within the fourth ventricle. Tumors do not usually form a large mass in the vallecula. Therefore, the supratonsillar segment is usually markedly displaced downward against the occipital bone, while the posterior medullary segment is displaced anteriorly. The copular point and pyramidal branches are displaced downward and backward. In contradistinction to fourth ventricle tumors, the supratonsillar and posterior medullary segments are not dislocated laterally, indicating minimal or no tumor extension into the vallecula. There is usually no midline shift of the vermian branches.

The superior cerebellar artery

Compression or invasion of the superior vermis is indicated by arcuate stretching of the anterior culminate and vermian segments of the superior cerebellar artery. The distal portion of the precentral cerebellar artery is displaced posteriorly and superiorly when the fourth ventricle is enlarged with elevation of the roof of the fourth ventricle. This artery may be displaced anteriorly when a tumor originates in the superior vermis. The quadrigeminal segments of these arteries are frequently laterally displaced indicating upward transtentorial herniation of the superior vermis.

The anterior inferior cerebellar artery

Straightening and compression against the petrous bone are frequently noted due to increased intracranial pressure, but localizing signs are not obtained from this artery.

The choroidal and nodular branches of the posterior inferior cerebellar artery

These arterial branches originate from the supratonsillar segments of the posterior inferior cerebellar artery, supplying the choroid plexus of the fourth ventricle and the nodule of the inferior vermis. In the presence of intraventricular extension the choroidal branches are enlarged and visualized on angiograms. The nodular branches are enlarged and displaced posteriorly in the presence of tumors in the inferior vermis. These arterial branches are not usually visualized unless they are enlarged in the presence of tumors (Takahashi et al., 1972).

Venographic features

The posterior group

The inferior vermian vein is compressed against the occipital bone. The copular angle is reduced and the copular point is displaced inferiorly or posteriorly. These changes are quite prominent in contradistinction to fourth ventricle tumors with vallecular extension, in which superior displacement of the copular point is more frequently observed.

The anterior group

The petrosal vein and its tributaries are frequently stretched and compressed against the petrous bone. These findings are observed in the course of the transverse pontine vein and the main trunk of the petrosal vein. The vein of the lateral recess of the fourth ventricle is poorly visualized. When this vein is visualized in the Towne projection, there is lateral displacement, being projected lateral to the brachial tributary of the petrosal vein. In the lateral projection, the vein of the lateral recess may be straightened.

The superior group

The fissural portion of the precentral cerebellar vein is poorly visualized due to compression or invasion of the superior vermis. When this segment is visualized, there is usually posterior displacement with decreased colliculocentral angle and elevation of the colliculocentral point. This vein may be anteriorly displaced in the presence of early invasion of the anterior medullary velum and the superior vermis. There is usually no midline shift of this vein, but the brachial tributaries may be separated. The superior vermian vein is frequently foreshortened and the supraculminate vein running over the superior vermis is stretched and compressed against the straight sinus. The posterior mesencephalic and lateral anastomotic mesencephalic veins are displaced laterally in the majority of medulloblastomas.

Large Medulloblastoma Filling and Ballooning the Fourth Ventricle

A 6-year-old male: Figs. 133–136

A small tumor was extending into the vallecula. There was infiltration of right lateral recess of the fourth ventricle and the inferior vermis. Two metastatic nodules were noted over the right cerebeller hemisphere.

Fig. 133 Arterial phase in the Towne projection. The arterial branches are all slightly diminished in caliber. The vermian segment of the posterior inferior cerebellar artery is straightened, but localized in the midline (3 crossed arrows). The quadrigeminal segments of the superior cerebellar arteries are separated (2 arrows), suggesting upward transtentorial herniation.

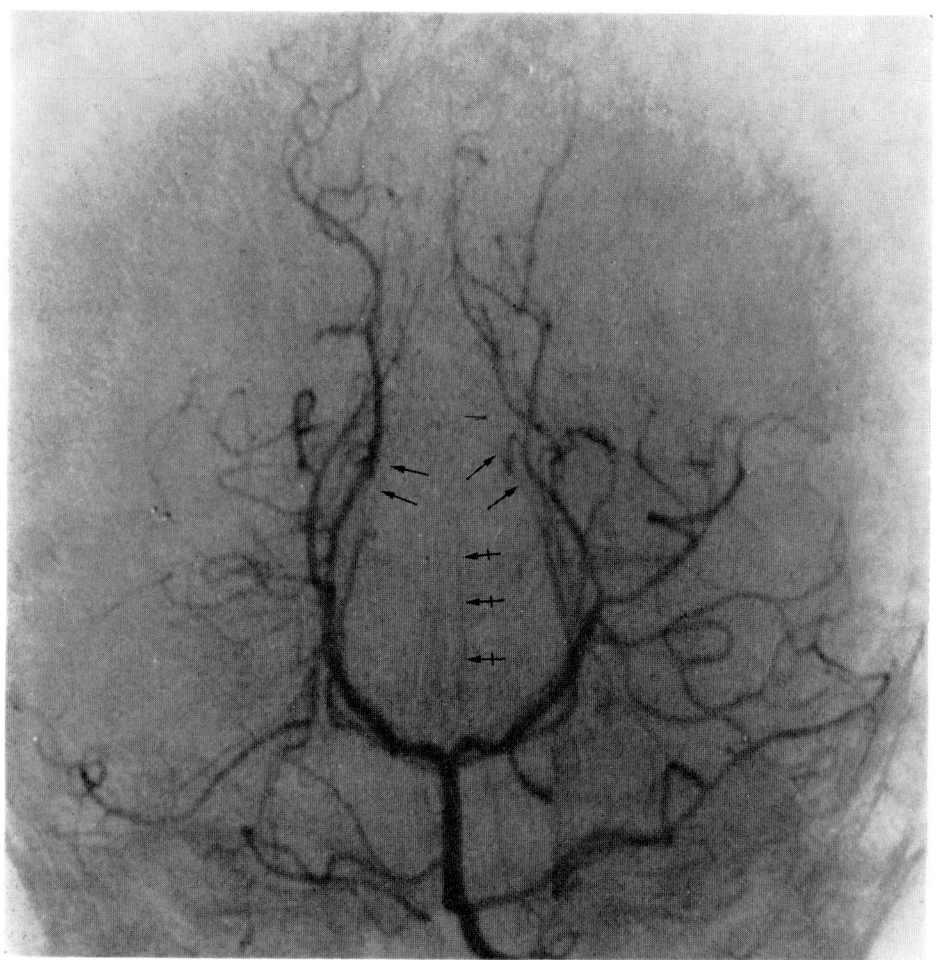

Fig. 133

Fig. 134 Venous phase in the Towne projection. The veins in the posterior fossa are small and appear to be stretched. The copular angle is widened bilaterally (an arrow on each side) and the vein of the lateral recess of the fourth ventricle shows arcuate course (2 arrowheads). There is medial displacement of both inferior vermian veins (2 opposing arrows).

Fig. 135 Arterial phase in the lateral projection. The basilar artery is compressed against the clivus and the thalamoperforate arteries are stretched, indicating increased intracranial pressure in the posterior fossa. There is arcuate displacement of the anterior culminate and vermian segments of the superior cerebellar artery (3 arrows). The posterior inferior cerebellar arteries are depressed bilaterally (crossed arrows). The anterior and inferior cerebellar arteries have a common origin on the left (2 arrowheads).

Fig. 136 Venous phase in the lateral projection. Distance between the internal cerebral vein and the choroid plexus is reduced, indicating ventricular dilatation (2 opposing arrows). The precentral cerebellar vein is superiorly displaced (an arrow). The inferior vermian vein is compressed against the occipital bone (3 arrows).

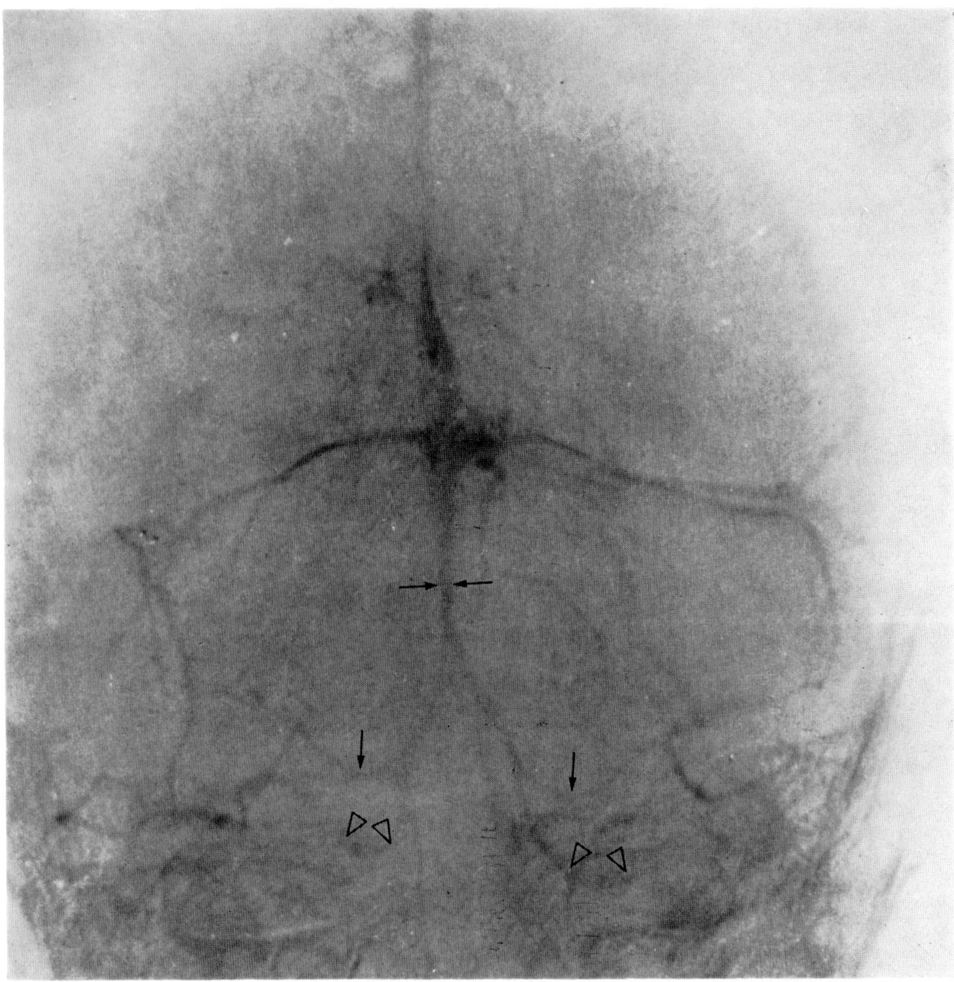

Fig. 134

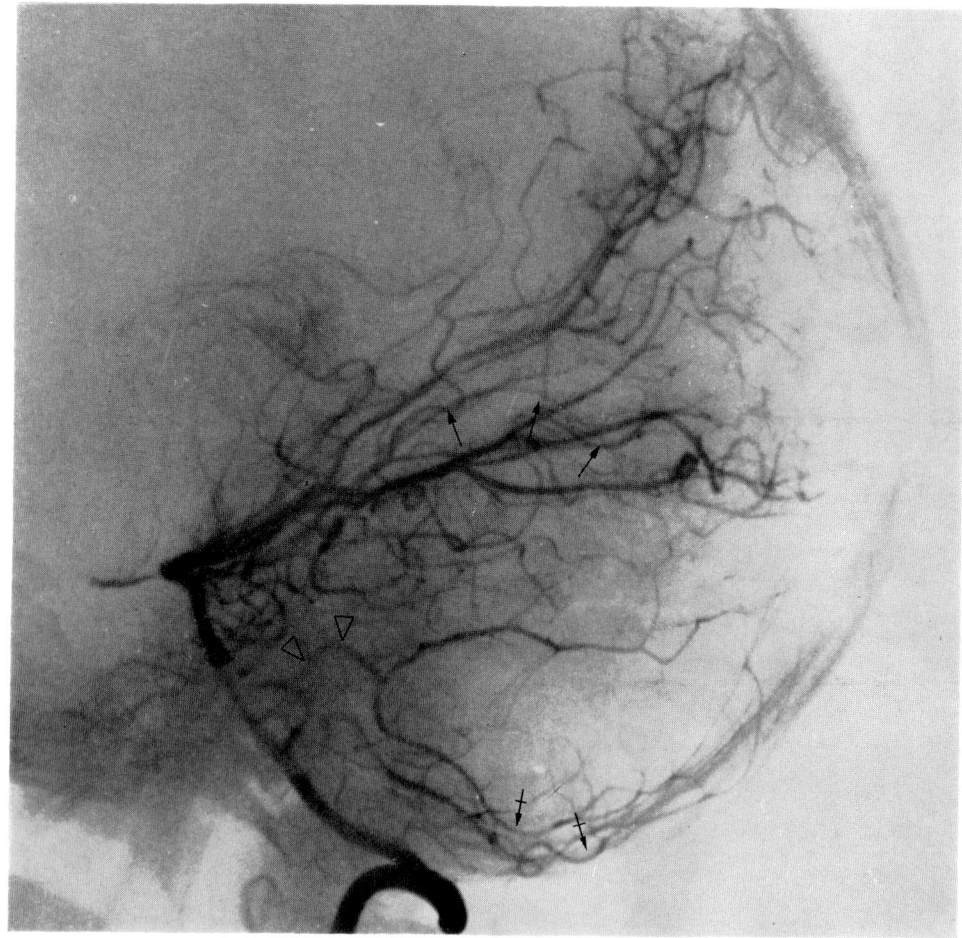

Fig. 135

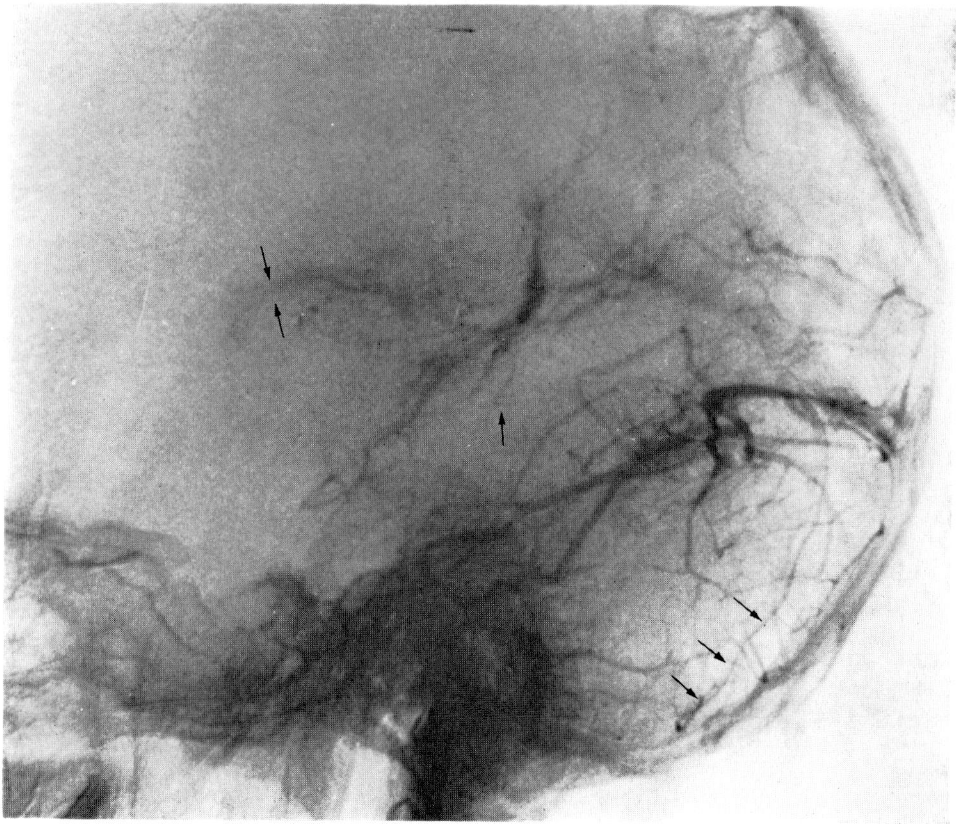

Fig. 136

Medulloblastoma Filling an Enlarged Fourth Ventricle with Infiltration of the Inferior Vermis

A 10-year-old male: Figs. 137–140

Fig. 137 Arterial phase in the lateral projection. There are arteriographic findings of increased intracranial pressure. The basilar artery is compressed against the clivus and the thalamoperforate arteries are straightened. The anterior culminate and vermian segments of the superior cerebellar arteries are displaced in an arcuate fashion simulating a stepladder (arrows). The posterior inferior cerebellar artery is faintly visualized and appears to be depressed downward (3 crossed arrows). The findings are consistent with a large midline tumor, but not diagnostic.

Fig. 138 Venous phase in the lateral projection. The interpeduncular segment of the anterior pontomesencephalic vein is depressed (an arrow). The distance between the superior choroid vein and the internal cerebral vein is reduced secondary to enlarged lateral ventricles (2 opposing arrows). There is posterior displacement of the fissural portion of the precentral cerebellar vein (an arrowhead). The inferior vermian veins are compressed against the occipital bone (crossed arrows).

Fig. 139 Arterial phase in the Towne projection. The vermian segment of the posterior inferior cerebellar artery is minimally displaced to the right (2 arrows), but the proximal main portion is in the midline. This finding on the vermian segment strongly suggests a midline mass lesion with more involvement of the left hemisphere. There is separation of the quadrigeminal segments of the superior cerebellar arteries (2 crossed arrows).

Fig. 140 Venous phase in the Towne projection. The left petrosal vein is compressed against the clivus (crossed arrows), probably indicating extension of the tumor into the left cerebellar hemisphere. The posterior mensencephalic veins are not stretched or displaced (arrows).

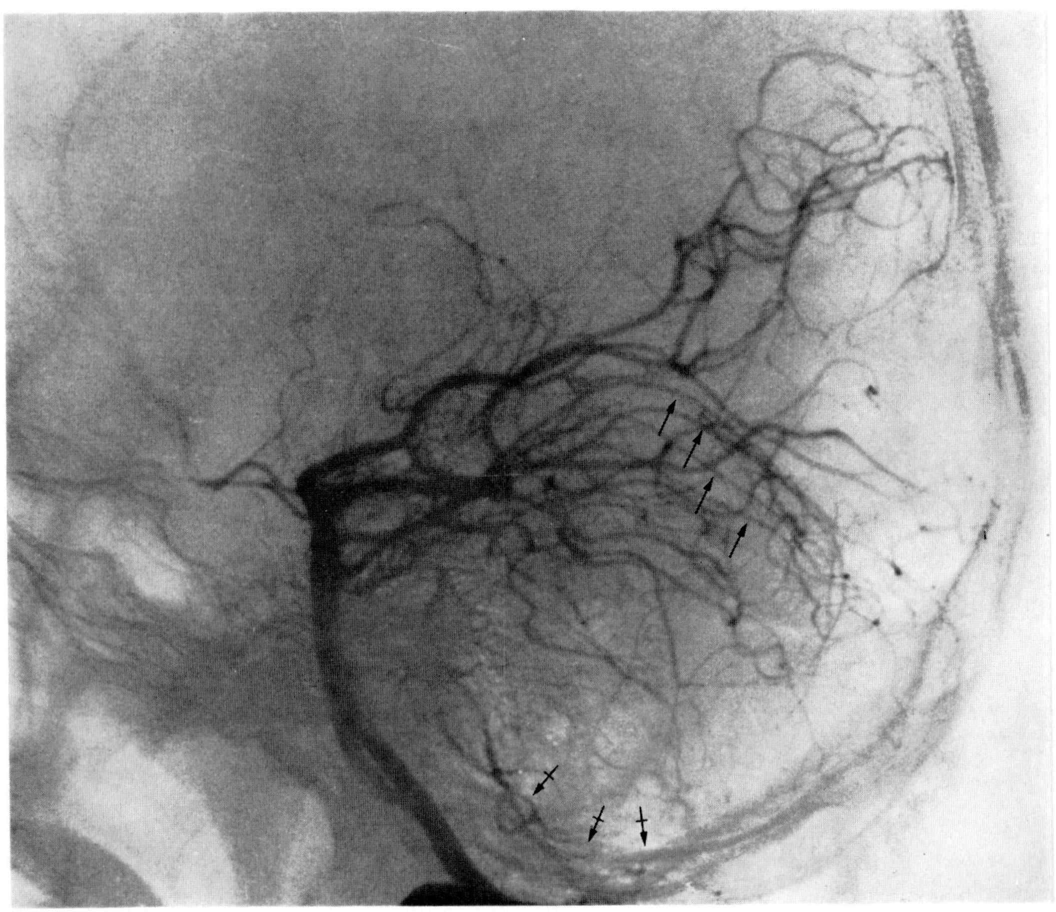

Fig. 137

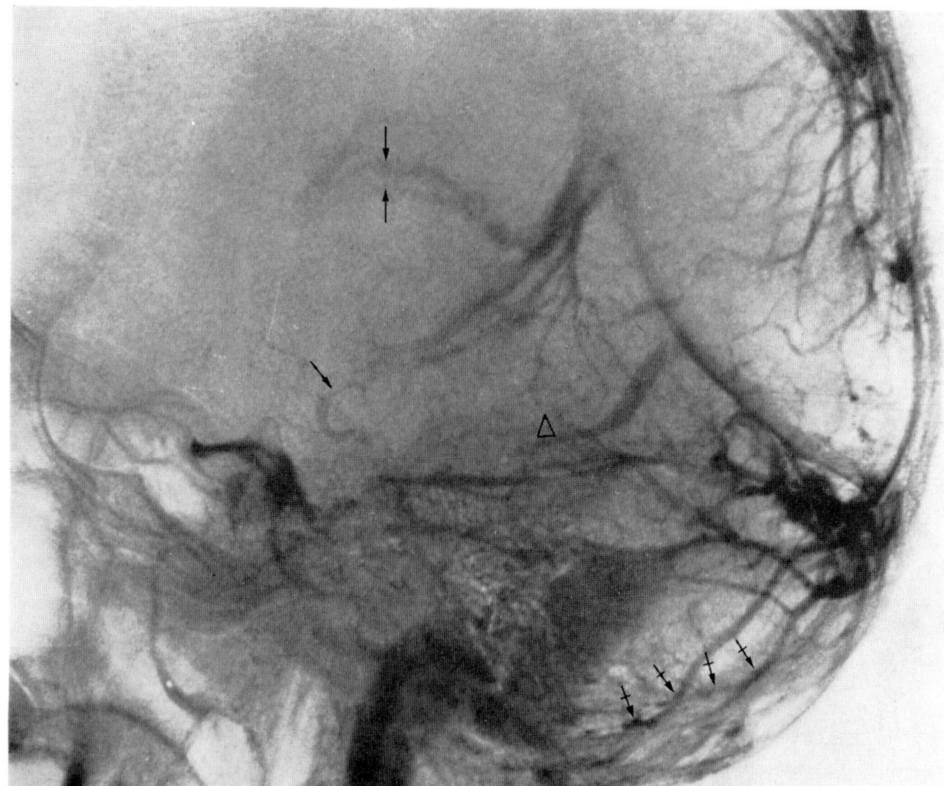

Fig. 138

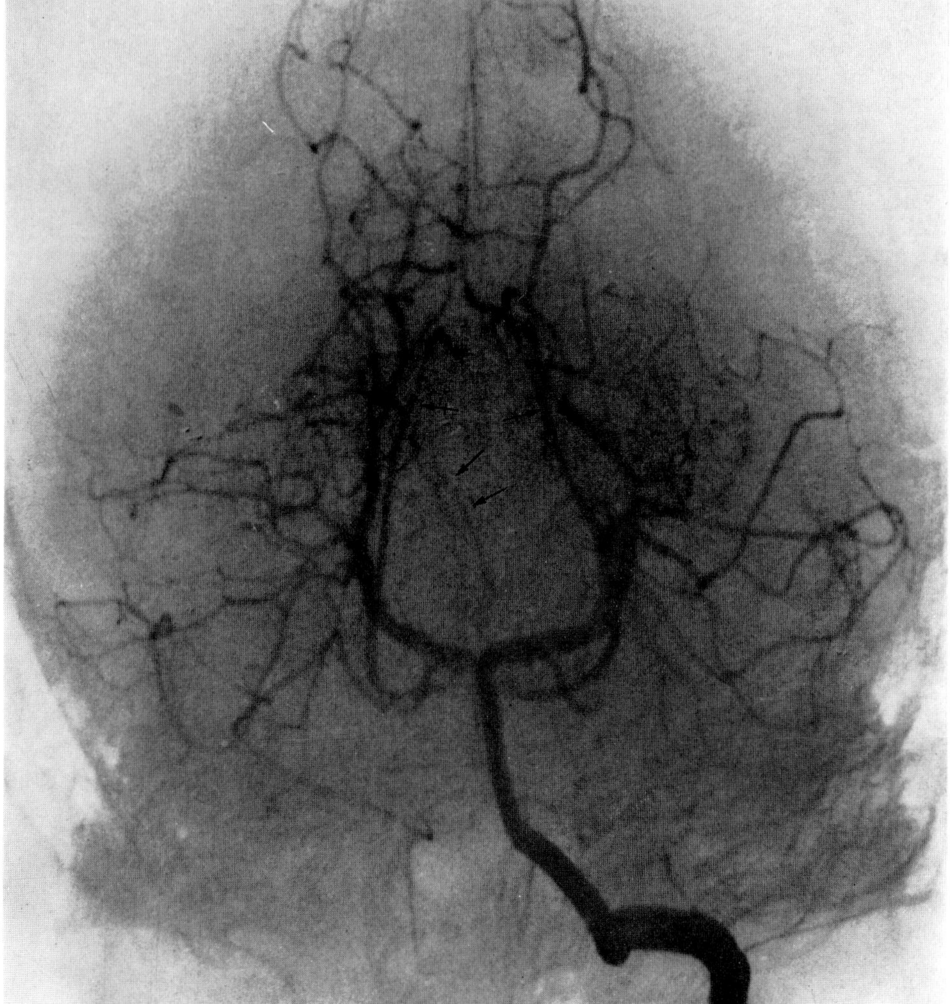

Fig. 139

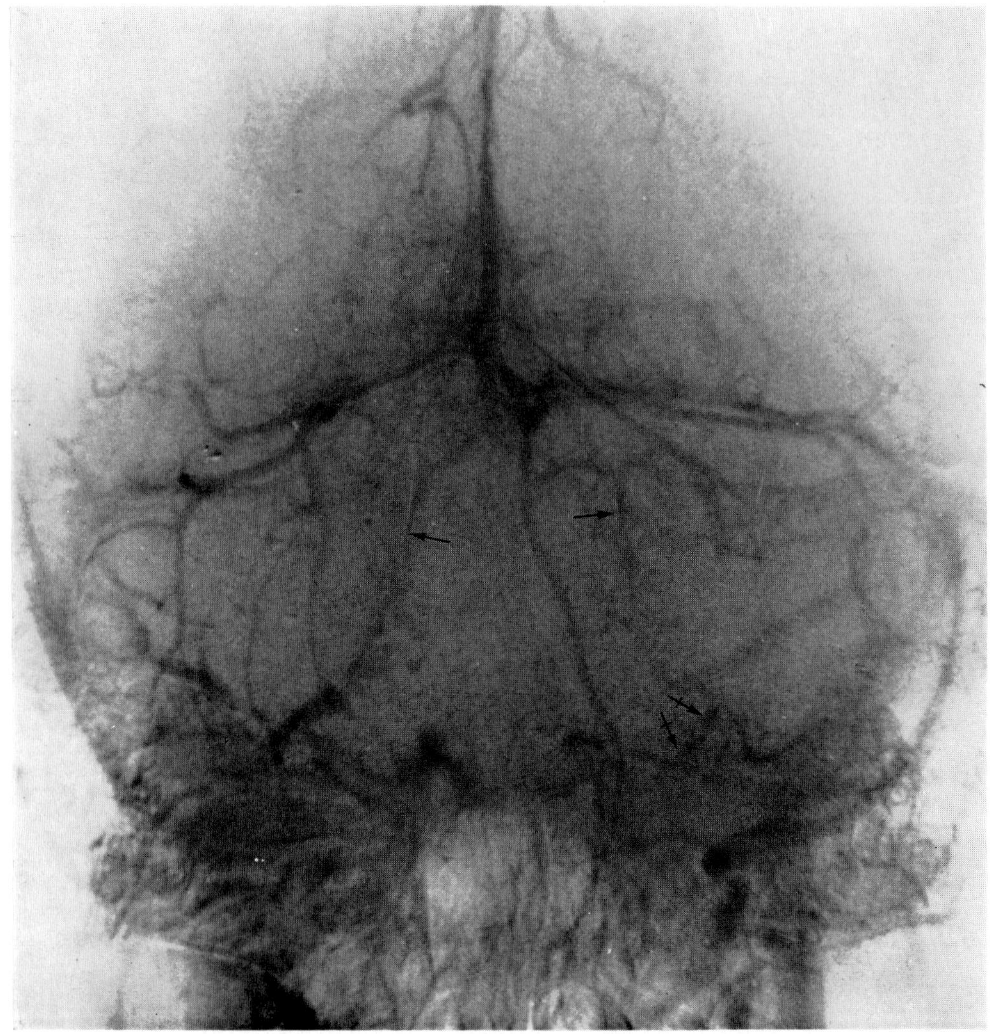

Fig. 140

Medulloblastoma Filling the Entire Fourth Ventricle

A 14-year-old female: Figs. 141–143

There was involvement of the inferior vermis with slight extension into the vallecula. The left tonsil was herniated.

Fig. 141 Arterial phase in the Towne projection. The lateral and posterior medullary segments of the posterior inferior cerebellar artery are slightly displaced laterally together with separation of the supratonsillar and vermian segments, indicating tumor extension into the vallecula (arrows). The quadrigeminal segments of the superior cerebellar arteries are separated, probably due to upward transtentorial herniation (2 crossed arrows).

Fig. 142 Venous phase in the Towne projection. The veins in the posterior fossa are all diminished in caliber due to increased intracranial pressure. The petrosal veins and their tributaries are compressed against the clivus (arrows).

Fig. 143 Arterial phase in the lateral projection. There are changes due to increased intracranial pressure: anterior displacement of the basilar artery and straightening of the thalamoperforate arteries (3 closed arrowheads). The arterior culminate and vermian segments of the superior cerebellar arteries are displaced in an arcuate fashion (3 arrows). The supratonsillar and superior retrotonsillar segments of the posterior inferior cerebellar arteries are displaced inferiorly on both sides (2 open arrowheads), while there is anterior displacement of the lateral and posterior medullary segments (crossed arrows).

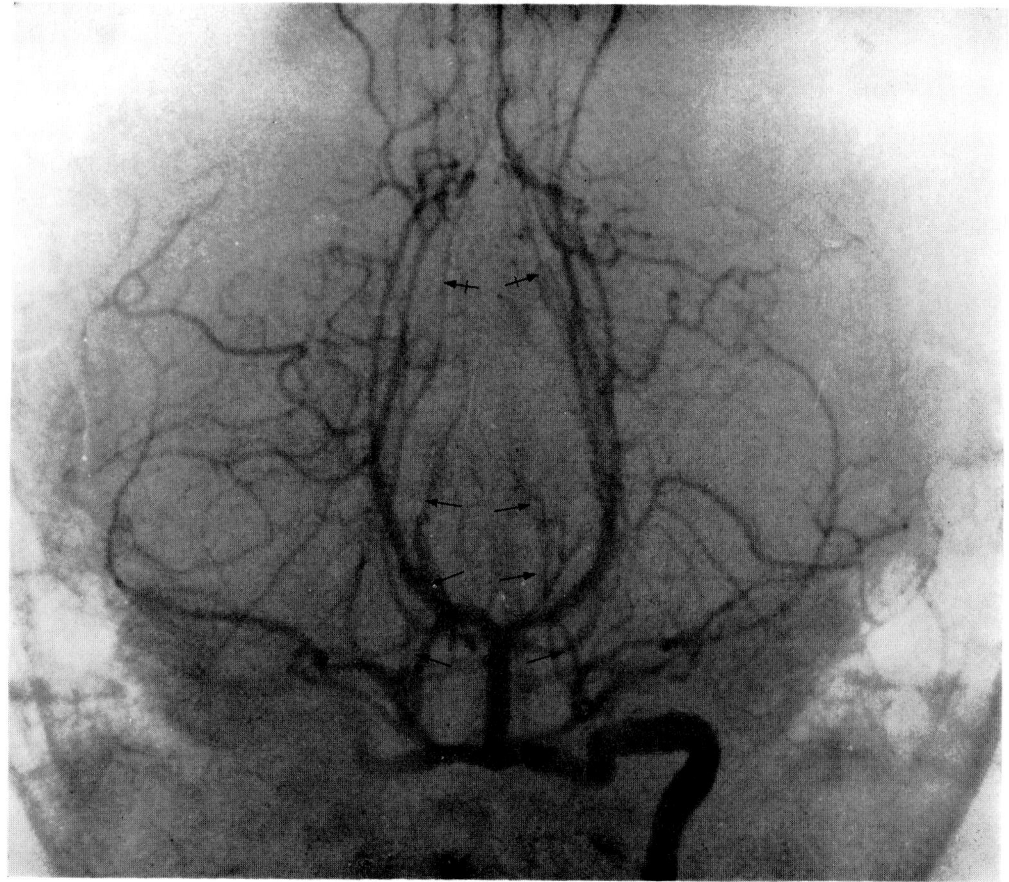

Fig. 141

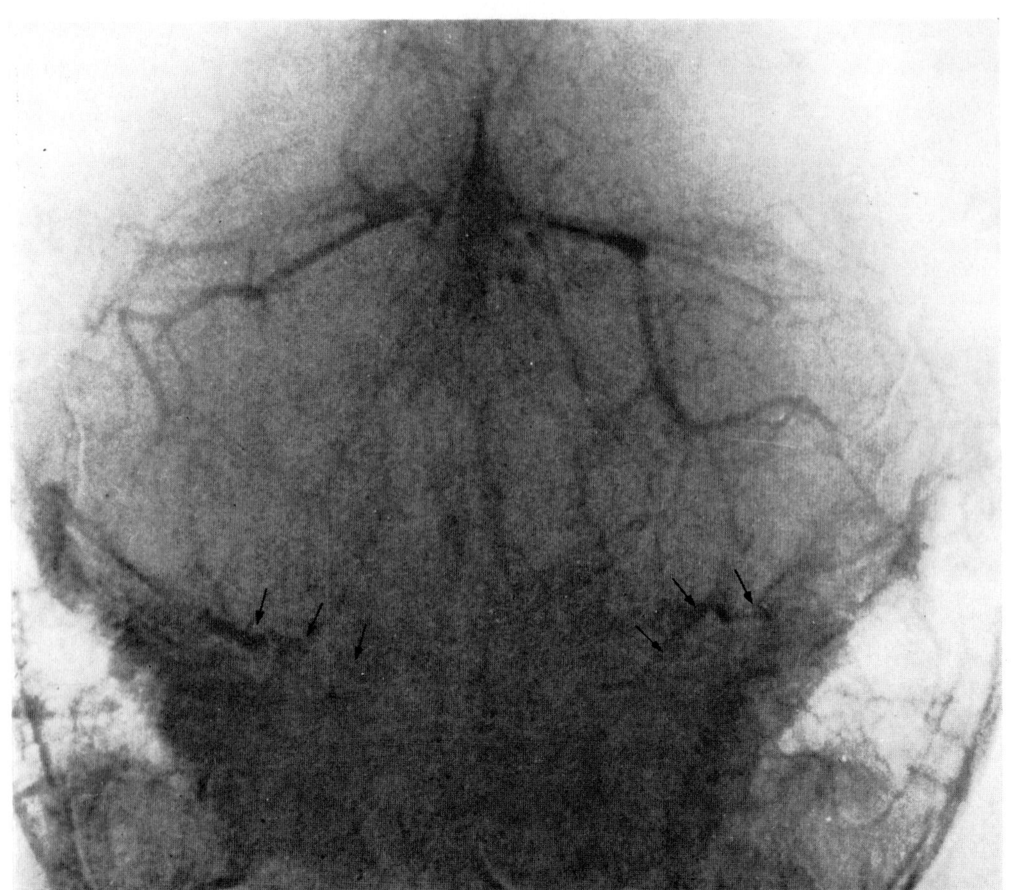

Fig. 142

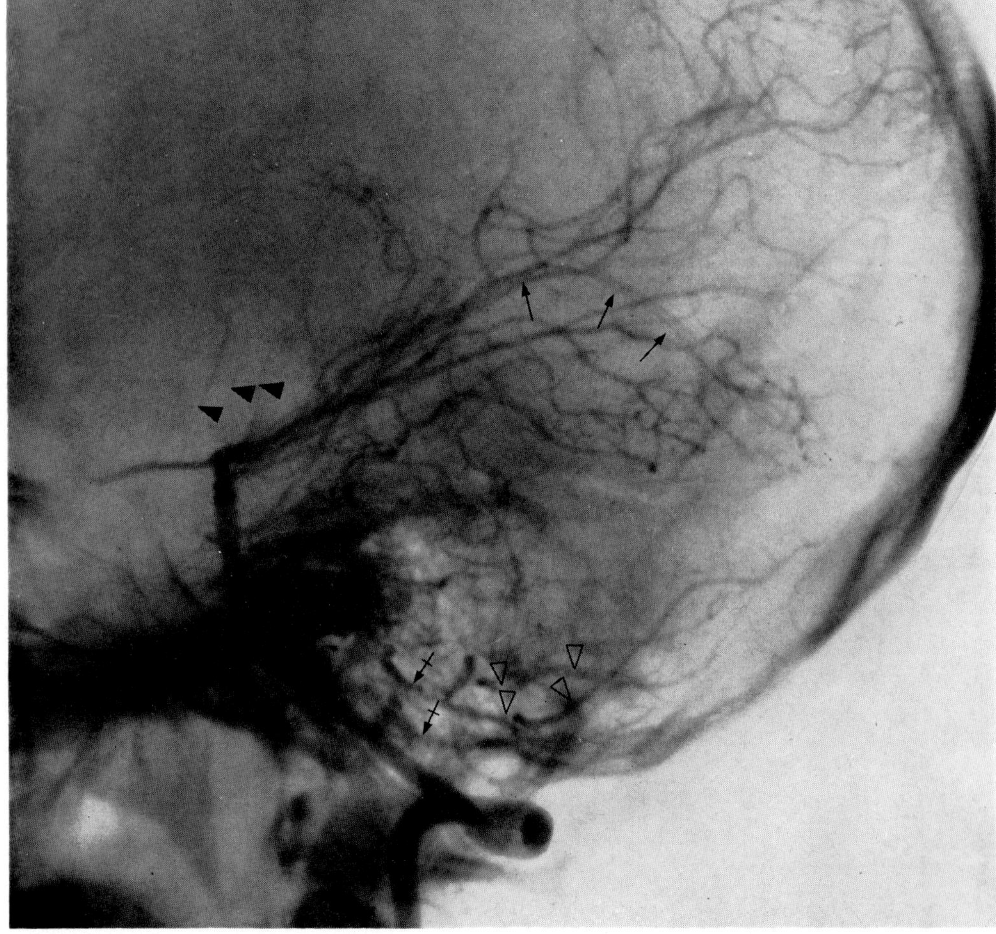

Fig. 143

Medulloblastoma of the Inferior Vermis with Involvement of the Entire Fourth Ventricle

A 3-year-old male: Figs. 144 and 145

Fig. 144 Arterial phase in the lateral projection. The nodular branches, originating from the supratonsillar segment of the posterior inferior cerebellar artery, are displaced posteriorly and superiorly in an arcuate fashion (3 arrows). There is also a tortuous choroidal branch (2 open arrowheads). These arterial branches are rarely seen on vertebral angiogram unless there is a tumor in the fourth ventricle and the inferior vermis. The supratonsillar segment is elongated and displaced inferiorly (3 crossed arrows). The vermian segment and the copular point (2 closed arrowheads) are displaced posteriorly. The tonsillohemispheric branches on both sides are elongated and displaced inferiorly (2 double-crossed arrows). The basilar artery is compressed against the clivus, while there is stretching of the anterior culminate segment of the superior cerebellar artery and the thalamoperforate arteries.

Fig. 145 Arterial phase in the Towne projection. The supratonsillar segment of the posterior inferior cerebellar artery is superimposed on the small arterial branches, probably the choroidal and nodular branches (2 opposing arrows). The superior cerebellar arteries are separated at the tentorial incisura (2 crossed arrows) and the tonsillohemispheric branches of the posterior inferior cerebellar artery are elongated and stretched on the left side (arrowheads).

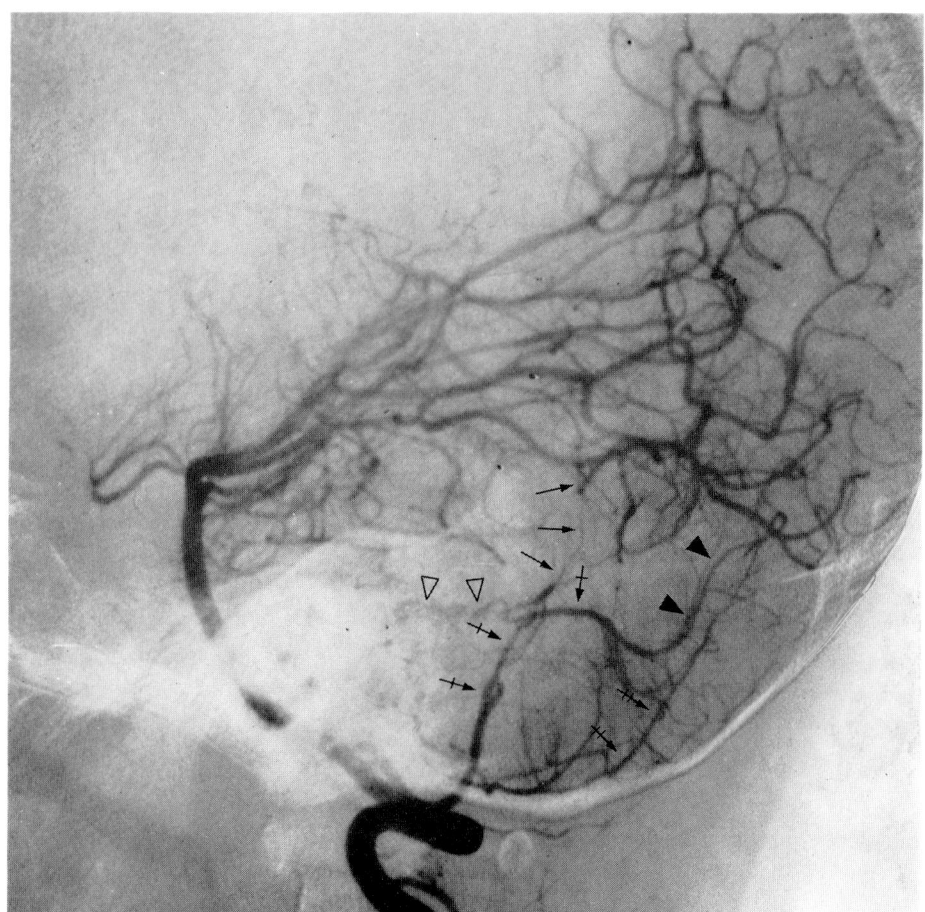

Fig. 144

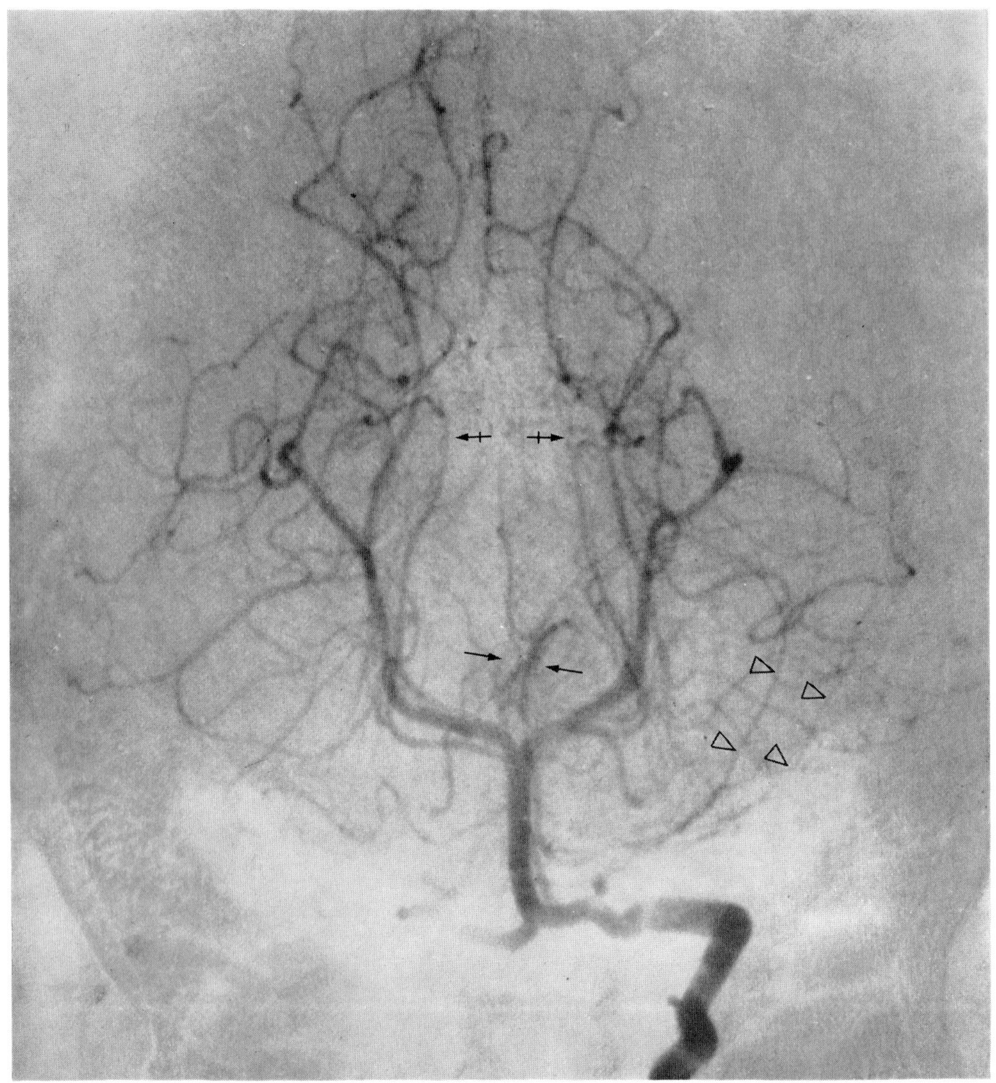

Fig. 145

Medulloblastoma with Involvement of the Fourth Ventricle

A 5-year-old female: Figs. 146–148

At surgery, the fourth ventricle was ballooned and occupied by a large tumor. There was bilateral tonsillar herniation, but no extension of tumor into the vallecula.

Fig. 146 Arterial phase in the lateral projection. The supratonsillar segment of the posterior inferior cerebellar artery is diffusely displaced inferiorly (3 arrows) with posterior displacement of the copular point (a double-crossed arrow). The nodular branch is enlarged and displaced posteriorly (3 crossed arrows). The choroidal branch is enlarged and tortuous (3 closed arrowheads). Anterior displacement of the basilar artery and arcuate stretching of the vermian segments are demonstrated (open arrowheads). The thalamoperforate arteries are straightened (2 opposing arrows).

Fig. 147 Capillary phase in the lateral projection. There is early opacification of the vein of the lateral recess of the fourth ventricle (3 arrows) and the inferior vermian vein (2 arrowheads). The copular point is displaced posteriorly (crossed arrow). The anterior pontomesencephalic vein is compressed against the clivus.

Fig. 148 Arterial phase in the Towne projection. The vermian segments of the left posterior inferior cerebellar artery appear to be in the midline. There is minimal separation of the quadrigeminal segments of the superior cerebellar arteries (2 arrows).

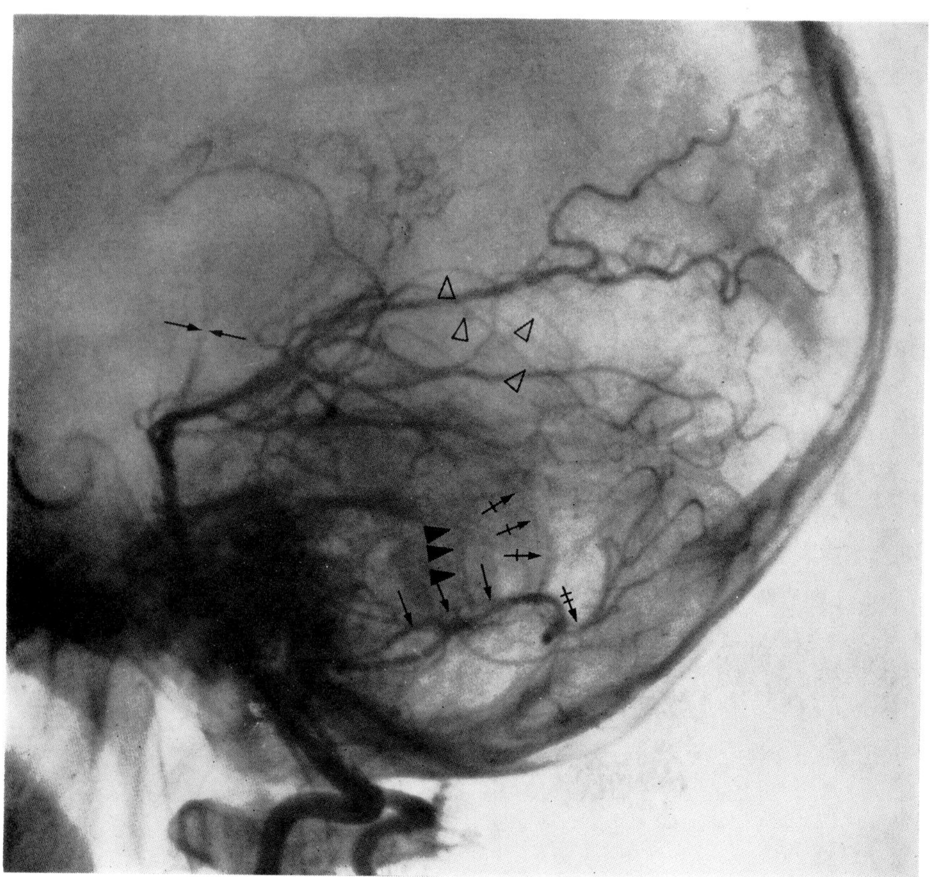

Fig. 146

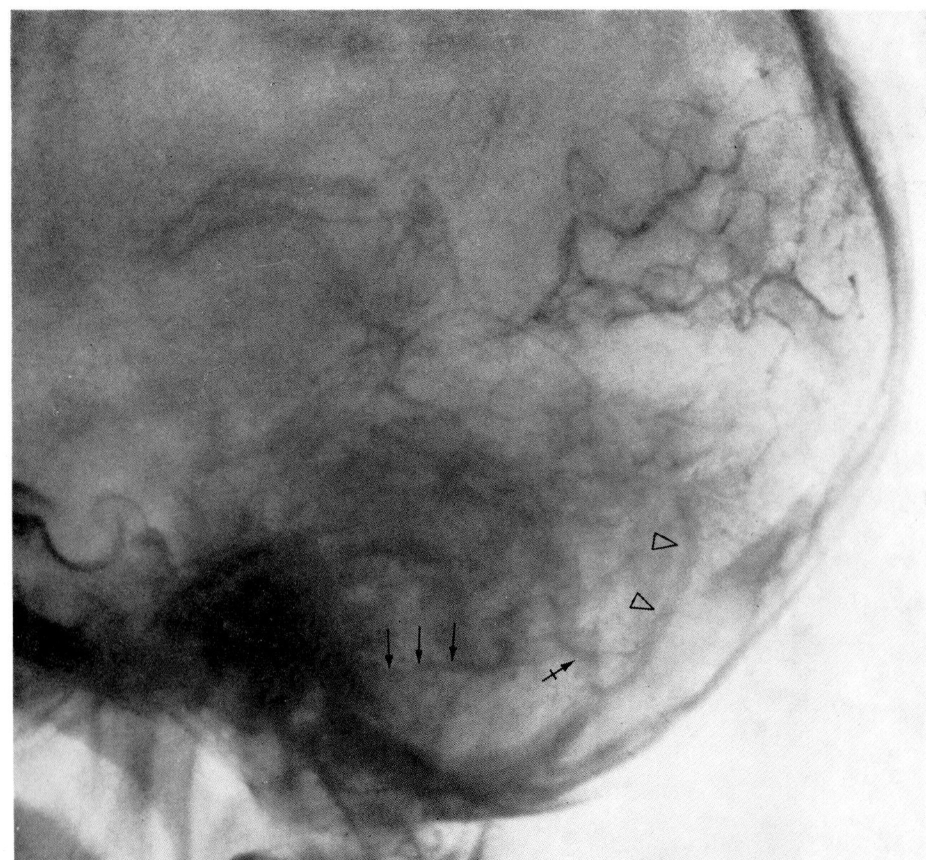

Fig. 147

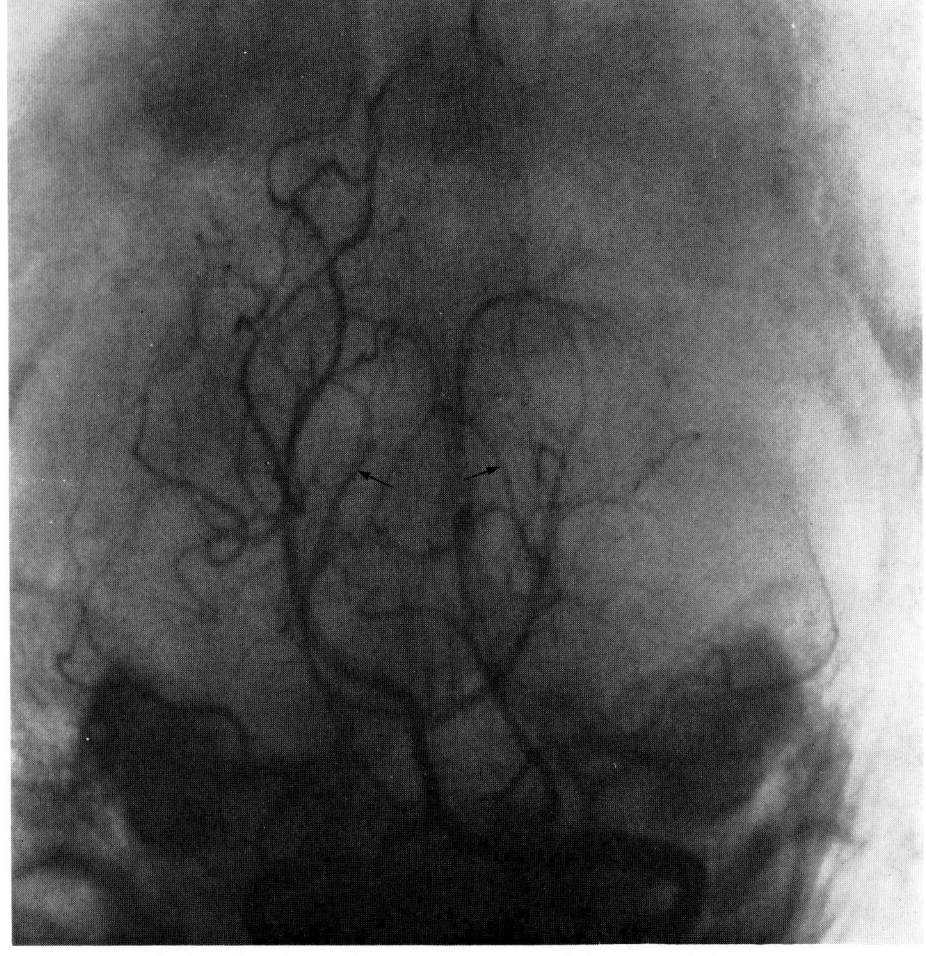

Fig. 148

Medulloblastoma of the Left Inferior Vermis Filling the Enlarged Fourth Ventricle

A 4-year-old male: Figs. 149 and 150

There was infiltration of both tonsils. No mass was formed in the vallecula.

Fig. 149 Arterial phase in the lateral projection. The basilar artery is compressed against the clivus. The thalamoperforate arteries are stretched. The posterior inferior cerebellar artery is displaced in the inferior direction bilaterally (2 arrows). There are small nodular branches arising from the supratonsillar segments. Most of these arterial branches are displaced posteriorly (3 crossed arrows). There is also an enlarged branch coursing anteriorly (2 arrowheads). The latter indicates a choroidal branch.

Fig. 150. Arterial phase in the Towne projection. There are small arterial branches superimposed over the supratonsillar segment of the posterior inferior cerebellar artery, probably representing nodular and choroidal branches of the supratonsillar segment (2 opposing arrows). The quadrigeminal segment of the superior cerebellar artery is laterally displaced on both sides (2 crossed arrows).

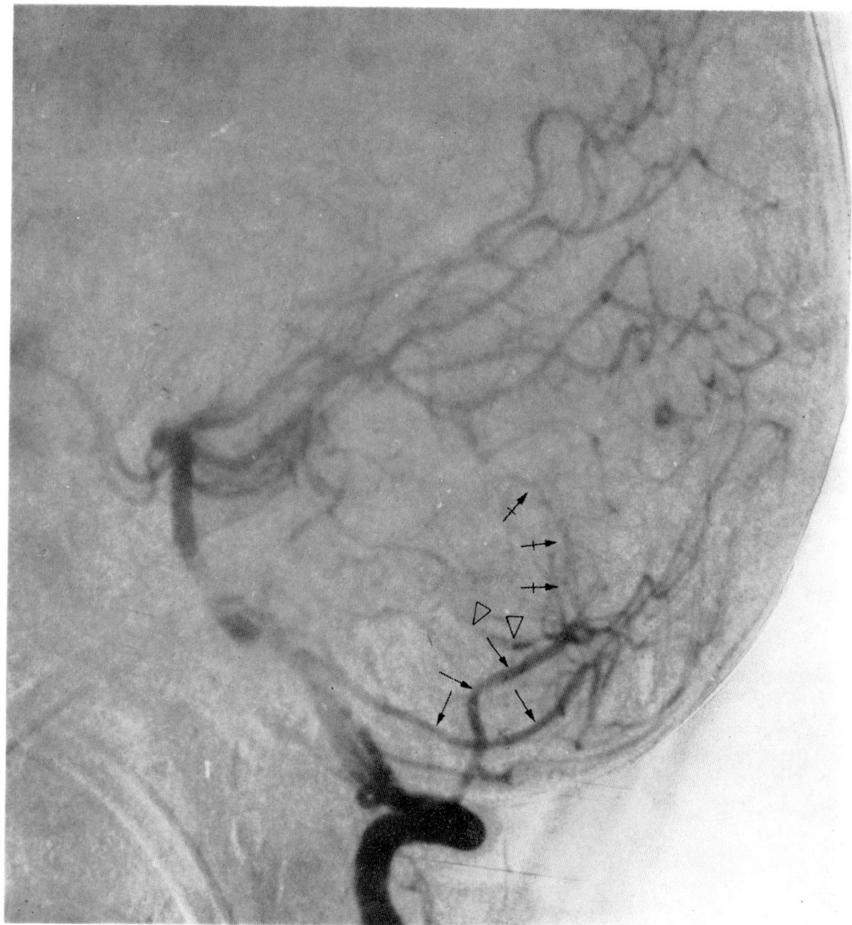

Fig. 149

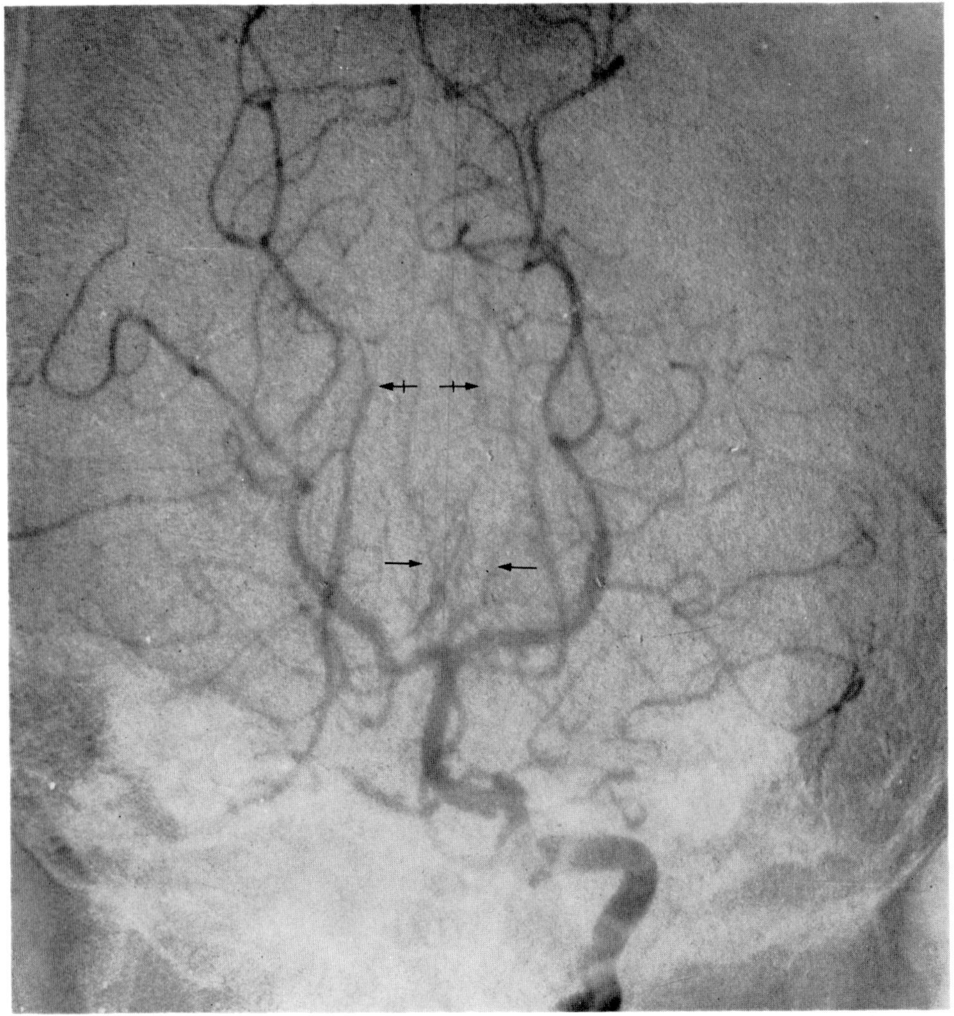

Fig. 150

Hemangioblastoma Arising from the Left Inferior Vermis and Extending into the Vallecula

A 35-year-old male: Figs. 151–153

Fig. 151 Arterial phase in the lateral projection. There is a 3.0 cm homogeneous density with smooth margins in the area of the vallecula. The posterior inferior cerebellar artery is slightly enlarged and participates in the blood supply (5 arrows). The supratonsillar segment is displaced superiorly (a crossed arrow). The draining vein, probably the inferior vermian vein, arises from the superior and posterior aspect of the tumor and drains into the sinus confluence (2 arrowheads). There are no other arterial changes except for anterior displacement of the basilar artery and stretching of the superior cerebellar arteries.

Fig. 152 Arterial phase in the Towne projection. The homogeneous density is noted in the midline (5 arrowheads). The supratonsillar segments of the left posterior inferior cerebellar artery are enlarged and displaced to the right (4 arrows), suggesting origin of the tumor on the left.

Fig. 153 Capillary phase in the Towne projection. The homogeneous tumor stain is well shown with drainage to the sinus confluence via the inferior vermian vein.

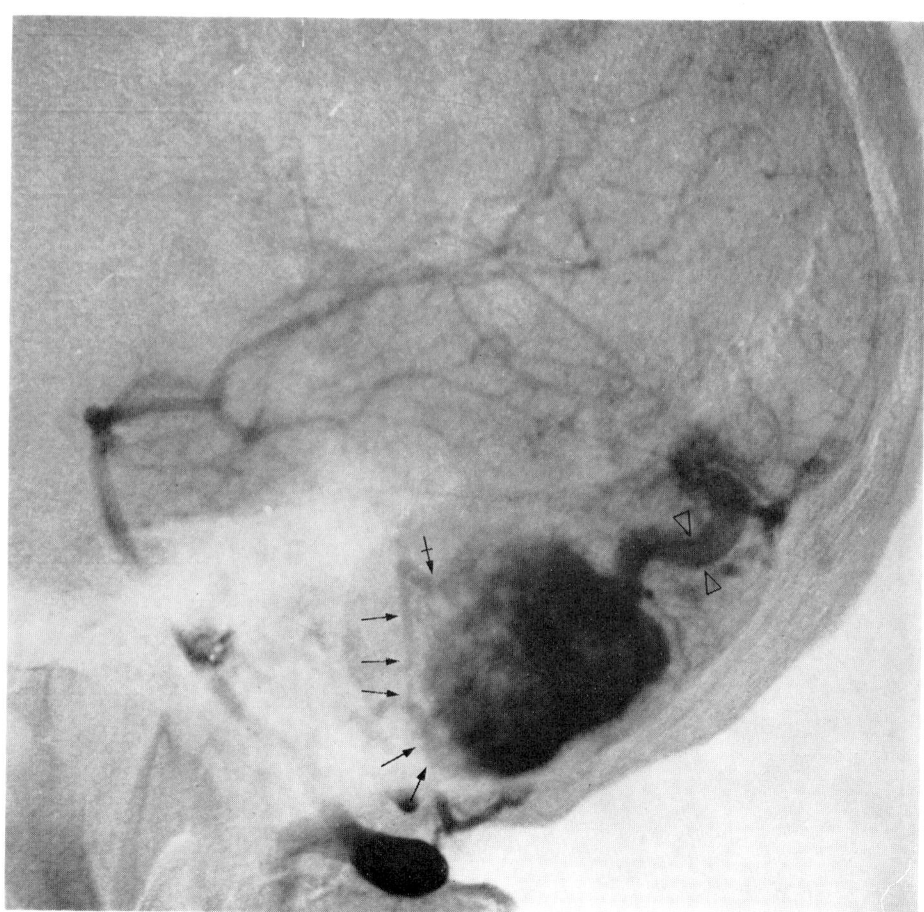

Fig. 151

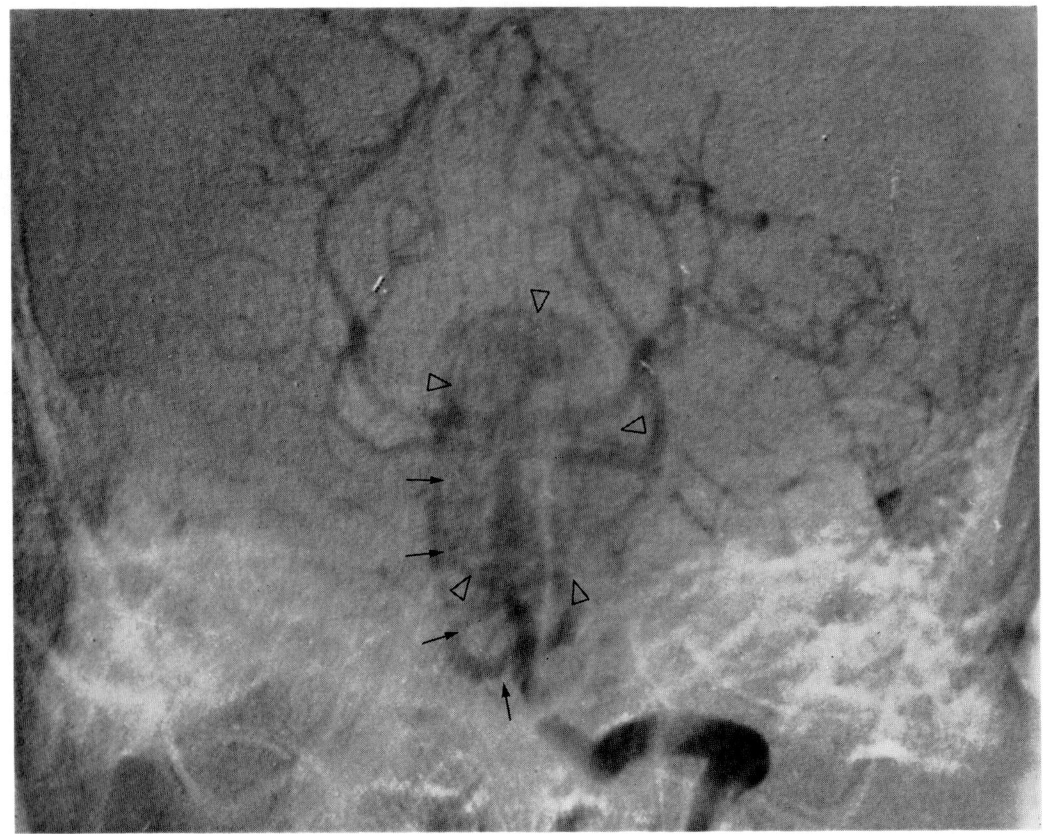

Fig. 152

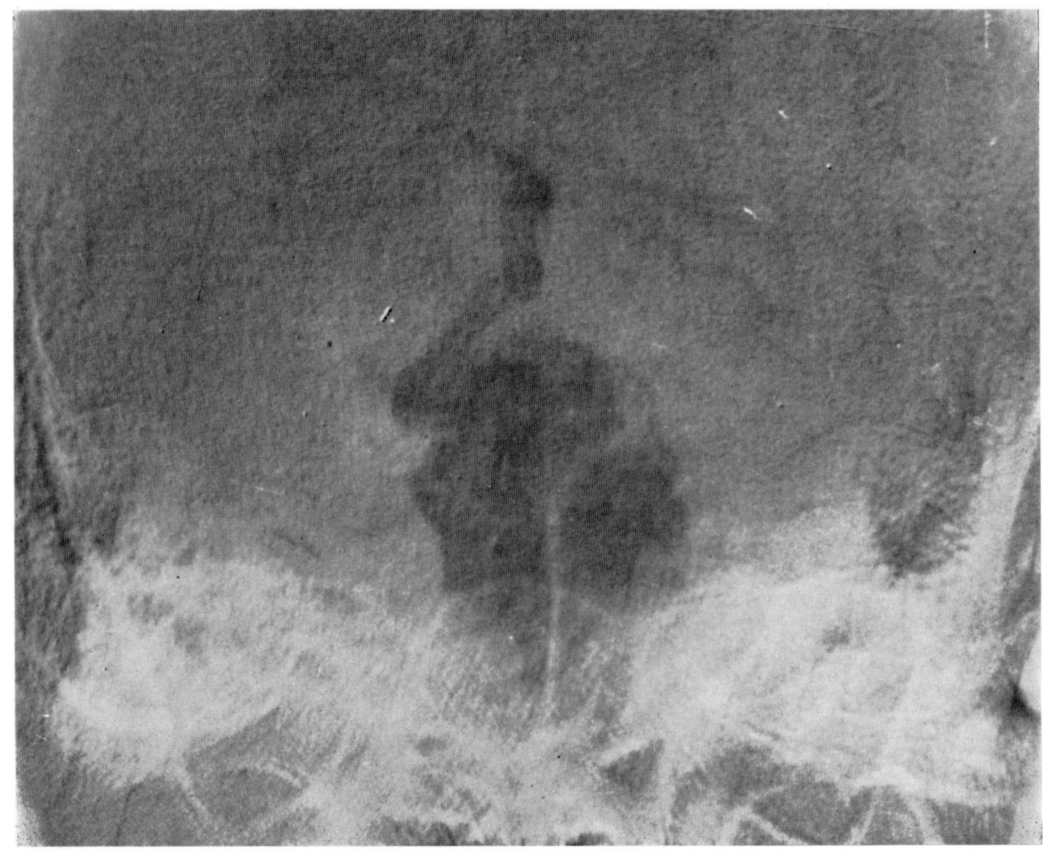

Fig. 153

BRAIN STEM TUMORS

Arteriographic features

Posterior inferior cerebellar artery

Brain stem tumors displace the fourth ventricle backward with decreased anteroposterior diameter of the tonsils. In the lateral projection there is marked posterior displacement of the posterior medullary segment as well as minimal to moderate posterior dislocation of the supratonsillar, superior retrotonsillar and vermian segments. The anterior and lateral medullary segments appear to be stretched and elongated. In the Towne projection, the posterior medullary and supratonsillar segments usually take normal courses in brain stem tumors, but there may be arcuate lateral displacement of the lateral medullary segment in the presence of medullary extension.

Superior cerebellar artery

The aqueduct and the floor of the fourth ventricle are posteriorly displaced, forming a continuous arch. The quadrigeminal plate and the upper part of the cerebellum are displaced backward.

Therefore, the precentral cerebellar artery is displaced backward with straightening. The colliculocentral point is displaced posteriorly and the colliculocentral angle is markedly increased. The vermian segments of the superior cerebellar artery may be compressed against the straight sinus. In the Towne projection, the ambient segments may be laterally displaced by the tumor extending into the midbrain.

Basilar artery

The basilar artery is displaced anteriorly and compressed against the clivus. The distance between the clivus and the basilar artery is more or less reduced. Transverse pontine arteries, minute arterial branches of the basilar artery, may be bowed anteriorly in the lateral projection. When these transverse pontine branches run over an anteriorly lobulated mass, there is arcuate stretching of these branches, frequently projected anterior to the basilar artery. In the Towne or straight anteroposterior projections, the basilar artery may lose the undulated course secondary to elongation.

In rare instances, lobulated tumor nodules are formed from the enlarged pons and displace the pons in the posterior direction upon reaching the clivus. The basilar artery and often the anterior pontomesencephalic vein are encased in the lobulated tumor nodules and become displaced posteriorly. Therefore, there is increased distance between the clivus and the basilar artery. The transverse pontine branches are usually displaced anteriorly if visualized. This finding has been called a paradoxical phenomenon and reported only in the presence of brain stem tumors.

Thalamoperforate arteries

Usually upward displacement of the upper brain stem is present in brain stem tumors with resultant stretching and straightening of the thalamoperforate arteries. The thalamoperforate arteries are more or less bowed anteriorly in contrast to straightening without bowing in the presence of hydrocephalus.

Posterior cerebral arteries

The ambient segment may be laterally displaced or lose its undulating course in the Towne projection. In the lateral projection there are usually no significant changes, but the ambient segment may be superiorly displaced.

Anterior inferior cerebellar artery

The anterior inferior cerebellar artery is frequently displaced downward in an arcuate fashion, but this finding is non-specific for brain stem tumors.

Venographic features

Anterior group

There is a marked posterior dislocation of the junction of the supratonsillar and medial tonsillar tributaries of the vein of the lateral recess of the fourth ventricle. The peduncular segment of this vein may be elongated and displaced downward in arcuate fashion. The junction of the first and second segments of this vein is frequently widened. The medial posterior spinal vein and the vein of the restiform body are displaced posteriorly. The petrosal vein and the transverse pontine veins are compressed against the petrous apex. The brachial vein may be displaced laterally in an arcuate fashion.

Superior group

The pontine segment of the anterior pontomesencephalic vein is anteriorly displaced with marked stretching. Not infrequently, these veins may be encased by lobulated pontine tumor and displaced posteriorly, while laterally located pontine veins such as the transverse pontine vein may be displaced anteriorly. These findings may be called the "paradoxical phenomenon" of the veins. There may also be a discrepancy in the location of the anterior aspect of the brain stem outlined by the veins and arteries.

The precentral cerebellar vein is displaced backward and runs parallel to the clivus. The colliculocentral point is displaced backward and its angle is decreased. The supraculminate vein may be compressed against the straight sinus.

The interpeduncular segment of the anterior pontomesencephalic vein, outlining the interpeduncular fossa, is displaced superiorly since there is upward displacement of the upper brain stem.

Posterior group

The angle formed by the superior retrotonsillar tributary and the inferior retrotonsillar tributary is widened with backward displacement of the junction. The copular point is displaced posteriorly and the copular angle is narrowed. In the Towne projection there is no lateral displacement of the inferior vermian vein and its tributaries.

Large Pontine Tumor Extending into the Medulla and the Midbrain

A 7-year-old female: Figs. 154–157

Fig. 154 Arterial phase in the lateral projection. The posterior medullary segment of the posterior inferior cerebellar artery is markedly displaced posteriorly (2 arrows) with angulation of the supratonsillar segment (a crossed arrow). The lateral medullary segment is stretched and the copular point is dislocated backward (an open arrowhead). The basilar artery is straightened and displaced backward, while pontine branches of this artery are projected anteriorly (2 closed arrowheads). This finding of the basilar artery may be called the "paradoxical phenomenon". The thalamoperforate arteries are stretched (2 double-crossed arrows). The posterior choroidal arteries, especially one of the lateral branches, are displaced superiorly in an arcuate fashion (4 arrows).

Fig. 155 Venous phase in the lateral projection. The precentral cerebellar vein is markedly displaced posteriorly (3 arrows) and the anastomotic lateral mesencephalic vein is bowed backward, probably due to a lobulated tumor in this area (3 crossed arrows). The interpeduncular segment of the anterior pontomesencephalic vein is elevated (2 open arrowheads). There is posterior displacement of the inferior vermian vein (3 closed arrowheads).

Fig. 156 Arterial phase in the Towne projection. The mesencephalic segments of the superior cerebellar artery and the posterior cerebral arteries are displaced laterally in an arcuate fashion on both sides (2 arrows). The lateral medullary and supratonsillar segments of the right posterior inferior cerebellar artery are displaced to the right (3 crossed arrows). The vermian segments of the posterior inferior cerebellar artery are straightened and localized in the midline (2 arrowheads).

Fig. 157 Venous phase in the Towne projection. The petrosal vein and the transverse pontine vein are compressed against the petrous bone (2 arrows). The copular angle of the inferior vermian vein is slightly widened (crossed arrows).

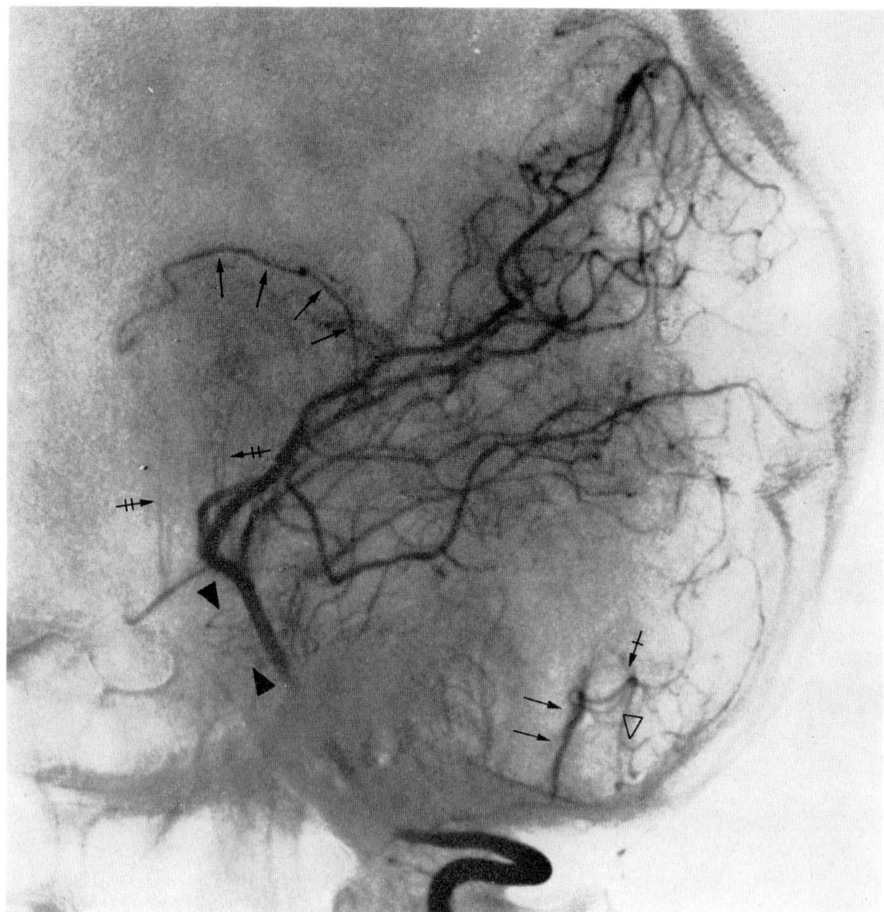

Fig. 154

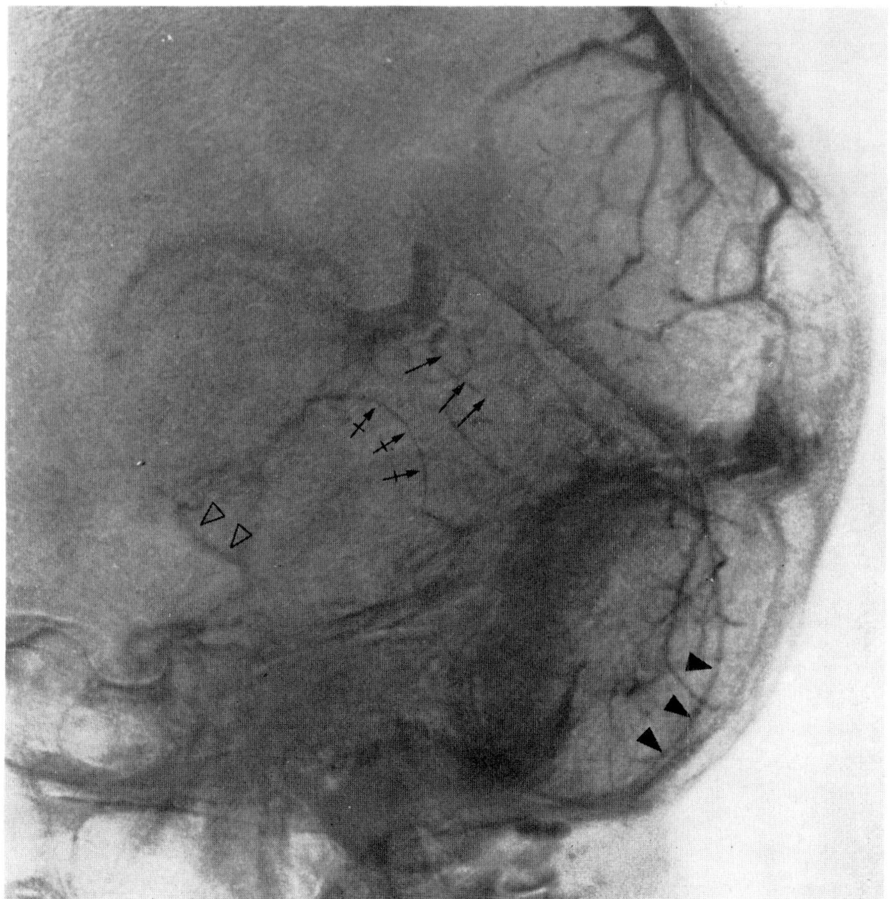

Fig. 155

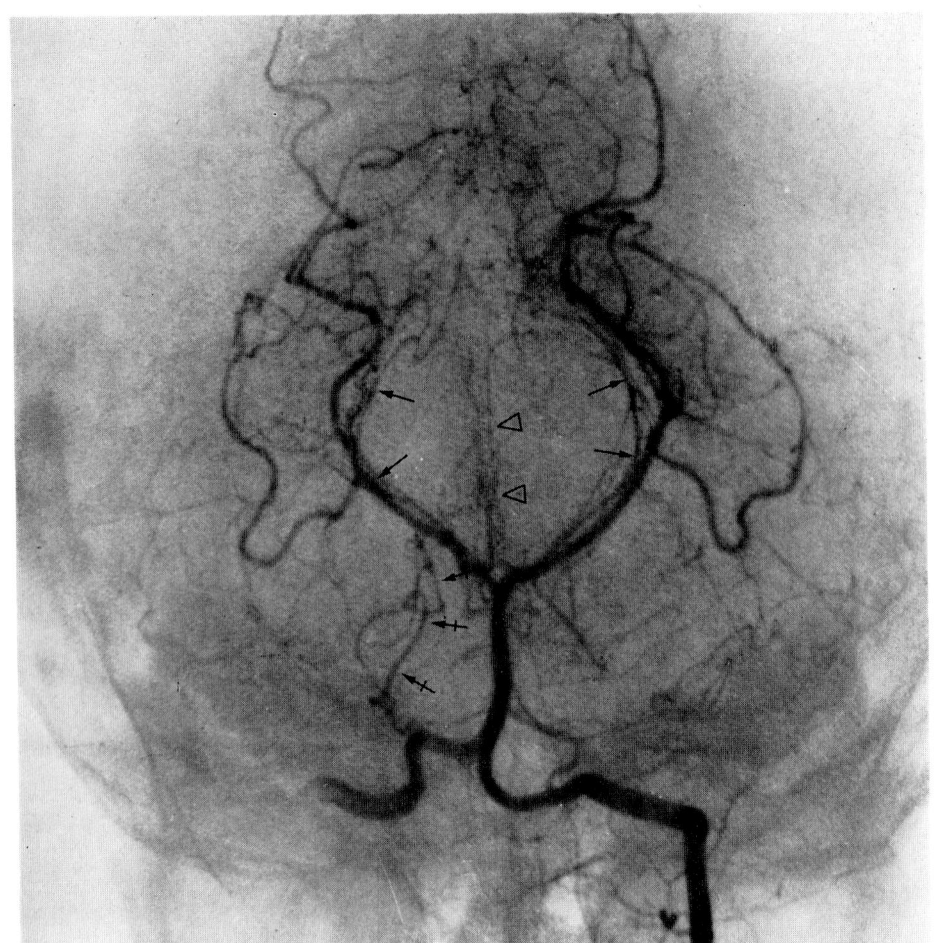

Fig. 156

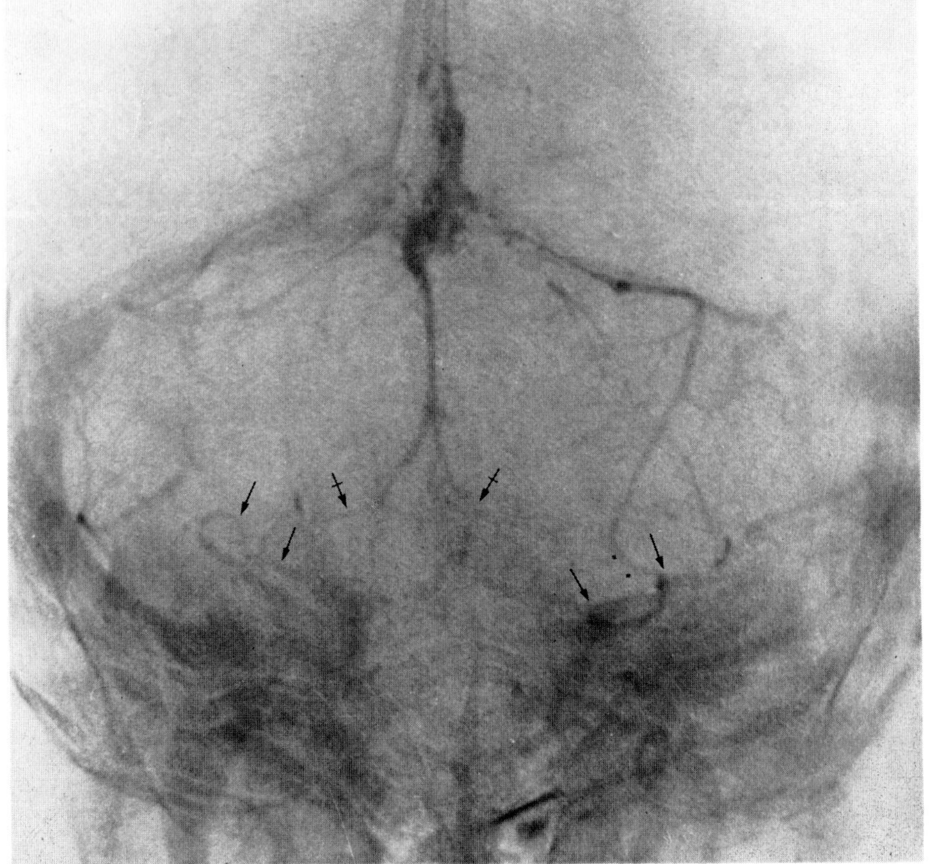

Fig. 157

Pontine Tumor

A 32-year-old male: Figs. 158–161

There was tumor extension into the medulla, cervical spinal cord and the midbrain.

Fig. 158 Arterial phase in the lateral projection. The basilar artery is compressed against the clivus (2 arrows). The supratonsillar segment (a crossed arrow) and posterior medullary segment (3 arrowheads) of the posterior inferior cerebellar artery are slightly displaced posteriorly. The caudal loop is below the foramen magnum, but this is probably not a significant finding.

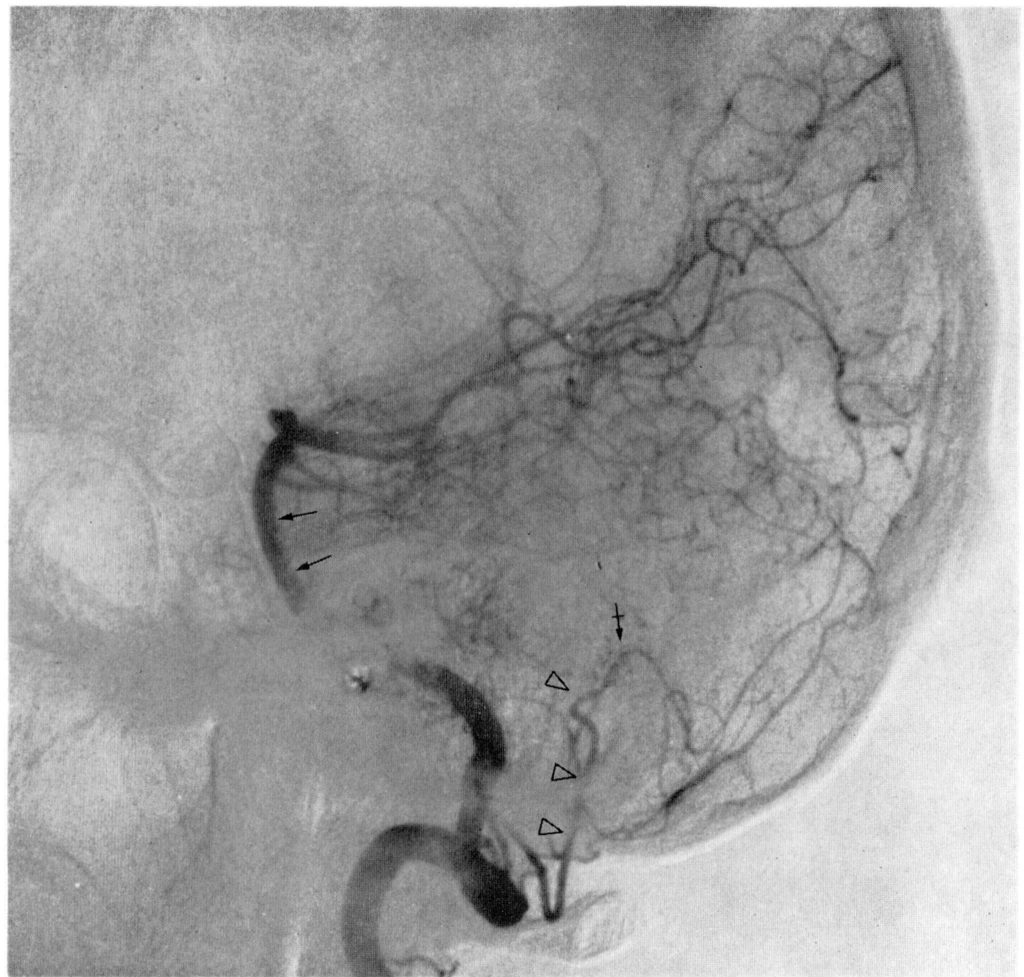

Fig. 158

Fig. 159 Venous phase in the lateral projection. The anterior pontomesencephalic vein is compressed against the clivus (3 arrows) and the precentral cerebellar vein is displaced posteriorly (3 crossed arrows).

Fig. 160 Arterial phase in the Towne projection. The anterior inferior cerebellar artery is displaced downwards in an arcuate fashion on the right (3 arrows). The superior cerebellar artery shows around, wide sweep, bilaterally. The interpeduncular-crural segment of this artery is slightly elevated on the right (2 crossed arrows).

Fig. 161 Venous phase in the Towne projection. The petrosal vein is displaced laterally with compression of the transverse pontine vein on the right (2 crossed arrows). The brachial vein is displaced laterally in an arcuate fashion on both sides (3 arrows).

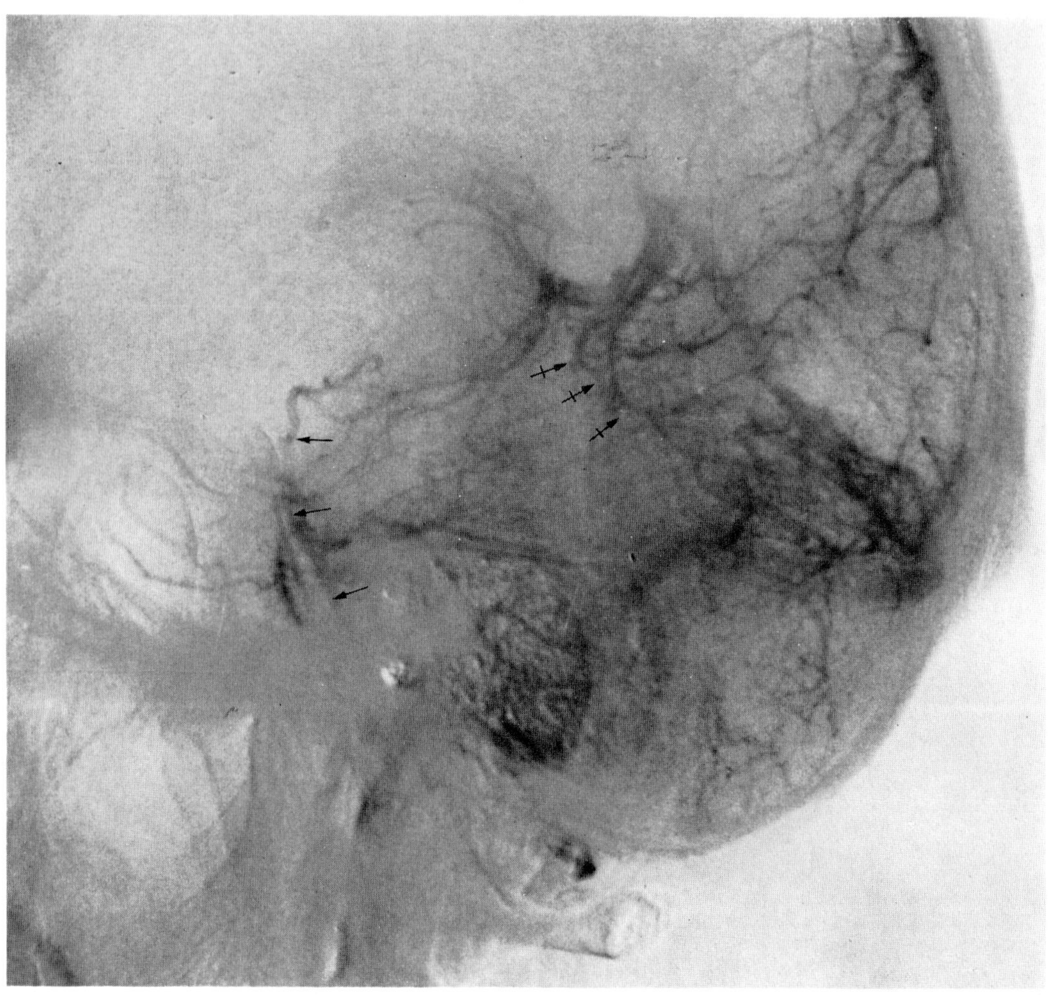

Fig. 159

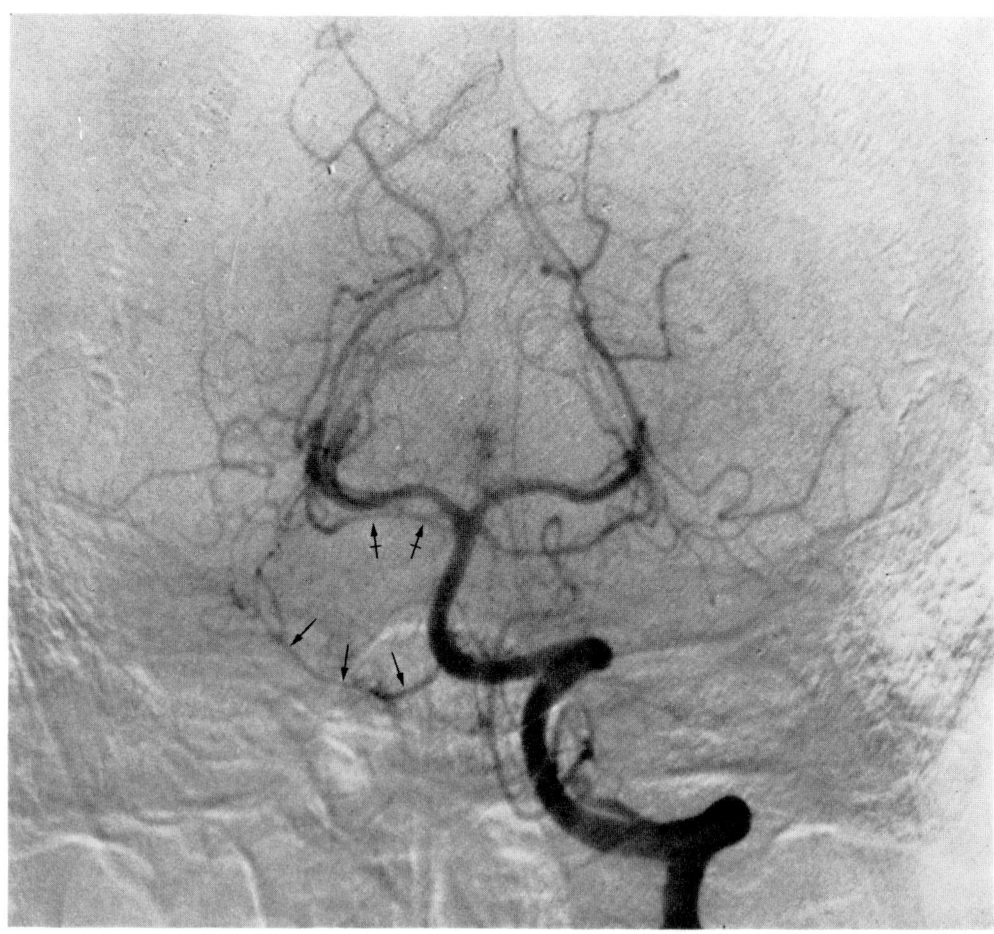

Fig. 160

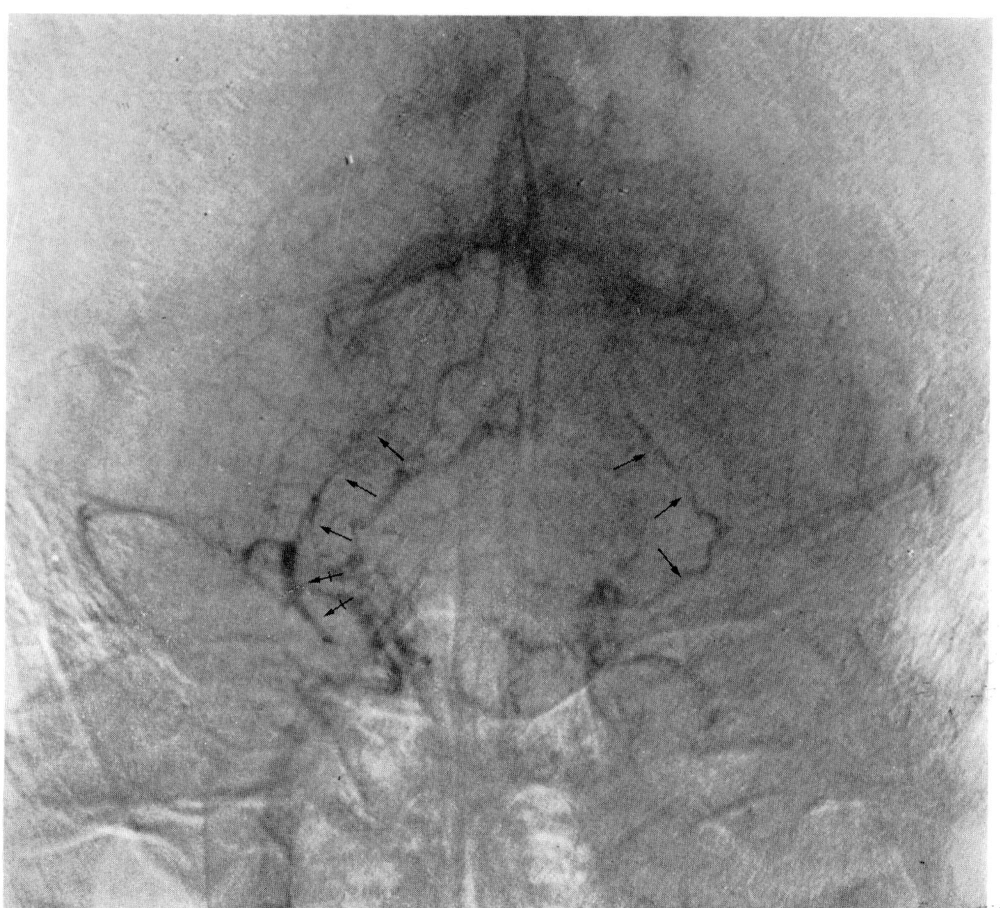

Fig. 161

Pontine Tumor

A 7-year-old male: Figs. 162–164 (with the courtesy of Dr. Greitz, Karolinska Institute, Stockholm)

There was fungating tumor of the pons. The tumor was encasing the basilar artery with posterior displacement.

Fig. 162 Arterial phase in the lateral projection. The basilar artery is displaced posteriorly with increased distance between the clivus and the basilar artery. However, the pontine branches of this artery are projected anteriorly (3 arrows), indicating paradoxical phenomenon. The terminal segment of the basilar artery is elongated superiorly and the posterior communicating arteries are considerably stretched (2 closed arrowheads). The posterior medullary segment of the posterior inferior cerebellar artery is displaced posteriorly together with supratonsillar segment (3 crossed arrows). The distal segments of the superior cerebellar artery are displaced posteriorly (3 open arrowheads).

Fig. 163 Arterial phase in the Towne projection. The basilar artery is straightened and elongated secondary to encasement by the tumor. There is lateral displacement of the superior cerebellar artery and the posterior cerebral artery (3 arrows).

Fig. 164 Venous phase in the Towne projection. The petrosal vein and the transverse pontine vein are compressed against the petrous apex bilaterally (2 arrows). There is arcuate lateral displacement of the posterior mesencephalic vein bilaterally (2 crossed arrows).

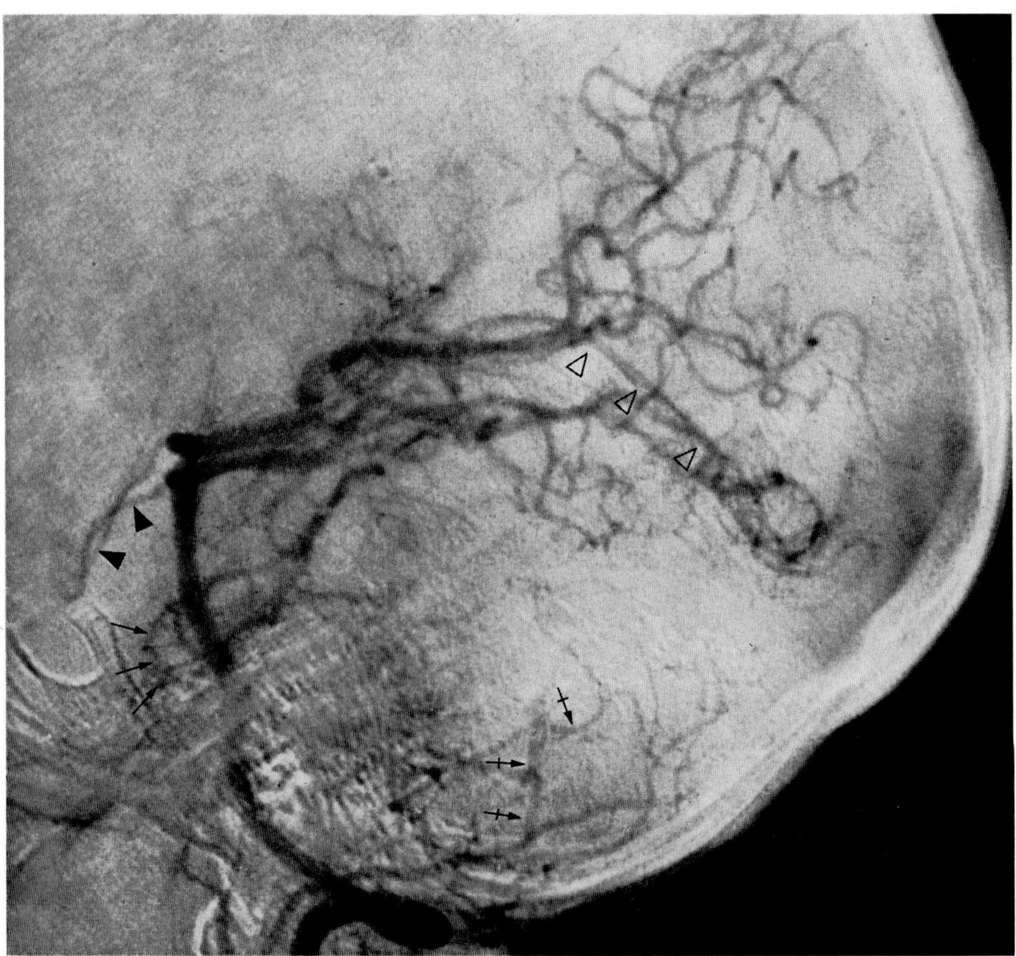

Fig. 162

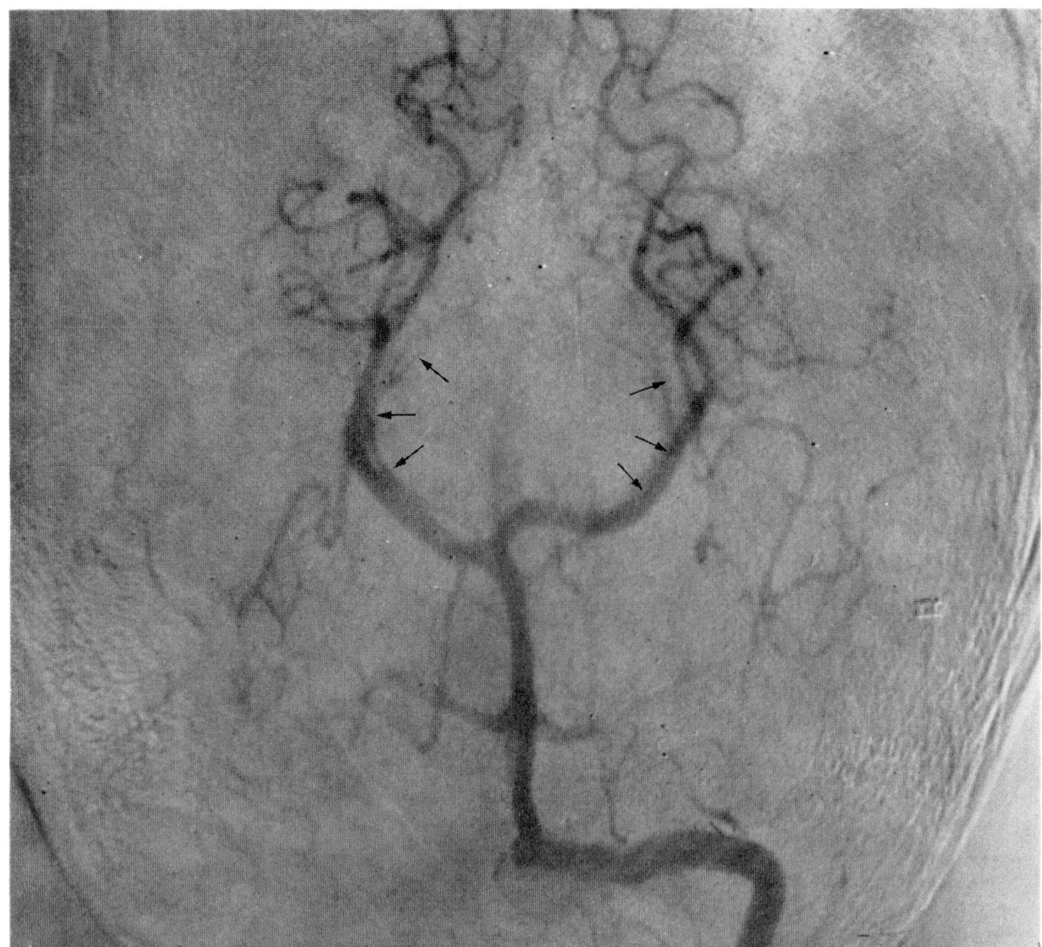

Fig. 163

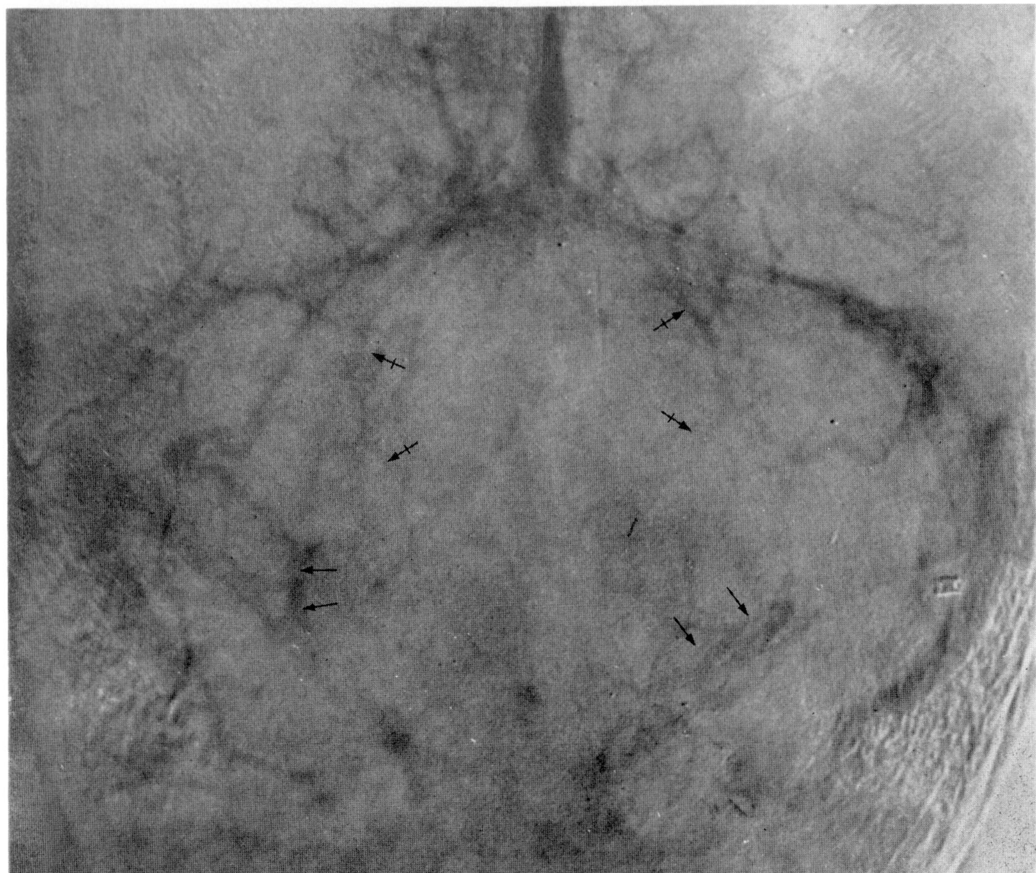

Fig. 164

FOURTH VENTRICLE TUMORS

Arteriographic features

The posterior inferior cerebellar artery

Fourth ventricle tumors usually extend into the vallecula. The brain stem is flattened anteriorly, while the tonsils are elongated in the anteroposterior direction and displaced markedly laterally. In the lateral projection, the posterior medullary segment is displaced forward and the supratonsillar segment is elongated with minimal downward displacement. The retrotonsillar segment is displaced backward. In the Towne projection the posterior medullary, supratonsillar and the retrotonsillar segments are displaced laterally in an arcuate fashion. The copular point is frequently displaced backward and superiorly in the lateral projection, while the copular point is displaced laterally in the Towne projection. The vermian segments of this artery may be stretched and appear to be compressed against the occipital bone.

In fourth ventricle tumors, the choroidal branches arising from the supratonsillar segment may be enlarged and stretched so as to be demonstrated angiographically. Normally, the choroidal branches are fine, tortuous vessels which are not usually seen on vertebral angiograms. If the tumor involves the nodule of the inferior vermis, there may be enlargement of the nodular branches arising from the supratonsillar segment.

The superior cerebellar artery

Fourth ventricle tumors produce extensive enlargement of the fourth ventricle and dilatation of the aqueduct. The roof of the fourth ventricle is considerably elevated. The superior vermis is squeezed and compressed against the straight sinus and tentorium.

Therefore, the superior culminate and vermian segments of the superior cerebellar artery are displaced superiorly and posteriorly in an arcuate fashion. The fissural portion of the precentral cerebellar artery, if optimally visualized, is elevated and runs horizontally. The colliculocentral point is displaced upward with decreased colliculocentral angle. The quadrigeminal segments of the superior cerebellar arteries are frequently separated in the Towne projection, indicating tendency of upward transtentorial herniation of the superior vermis.

The anterior inferior cerebellar artery

This artery is frequently straightened and compressed against the clivus, but no significant localizing signs can be attached to this artery.

The basilar artery

This artery is compressed against the clivus with decreased distance between this artery and the clivus.

Venographic features

Posterior group

A large extension of fourth ventricle tumors into the vallecula produces significant changes on the inferior vermian vein and its tributaries. In the lateral projection, the superior retrotonsillar tributary is displaced posteriorly with separation of superior and inferior retrotonsillar tributaries. The copular point is displaced in the posterior and superior direction and the copular angle is reduced. The main trunk of the inferior vermian vein is compressed against the occipital bone. In the Towne projection, there may be lateral displacements of the superior retrotonsillar tributary.

Anterior group

The supratonsillar and medial tonsillar tributaries of the vein of the lateral recess of the fourth ventricle are stretched and their junction is displaced anteriorly and laterally to a considerable degree.

The peduncular segment of the vein of the lateral recess of the fourth ventricle is displaced anteriorly in the lateral projection, while there is a lateral displacement of this vein in the Towne projection. The median spinal vein and the vein of the restiform body are usually displaced forward. The petrosal veins are frequently stretched and compressed against the clivus. The transverse pontine vein is compressed against the clivus and the anastomotic lateral mesencephalic vein is frequently displaced laterally.

Superior group

The superior vermian vein is foreshortened and the supraculminate vein over the superior vermis is compressed against the straight sinus secondary to compression of the superior vermis. The fissural portion of the precentral cerebellar vein is displaced posteriorly and superiorly with elevation of the colliculocentral point. The colliculocentral angle is reduced considerably. These changes on the precentral cerebellar vein are produced by elevation of the roof of the fourth ventricle or a direct displacement by a tumor.

In the Towne projection, the precentral cerebellar vein is localized in the midline, but the brachial tributaries may be separated by the enlarged fourth ventricle.

Large Ependymoma in the Fourth Ventricle

A 24-year-old male: Figs. 165–168

The tumor extended into the vallecula with formation of a large mass. The medulla was surrounded by the tumor.

Fig. 165 Arterial phase in the lateral projection. The basilar artery is compressed against the clivus and the thalamoperforate arteries are straightened. The anterior culminate segment of the superior cerebellar artery is stretched in an arcuate fashion. These findings are those of increased intracranial pressure in the posterior fossa. The lateral and posterior medullary segments of the posterior inferior cerebellar artery are displaced anteriorly (long arrows) with elongated supratonsillar segment (3 arrows). The superior retrotonsillar segment is displaced posteriorly with backward displacement of the copular point (a crossed arrow). The choroidal and nodular branches are not observed.

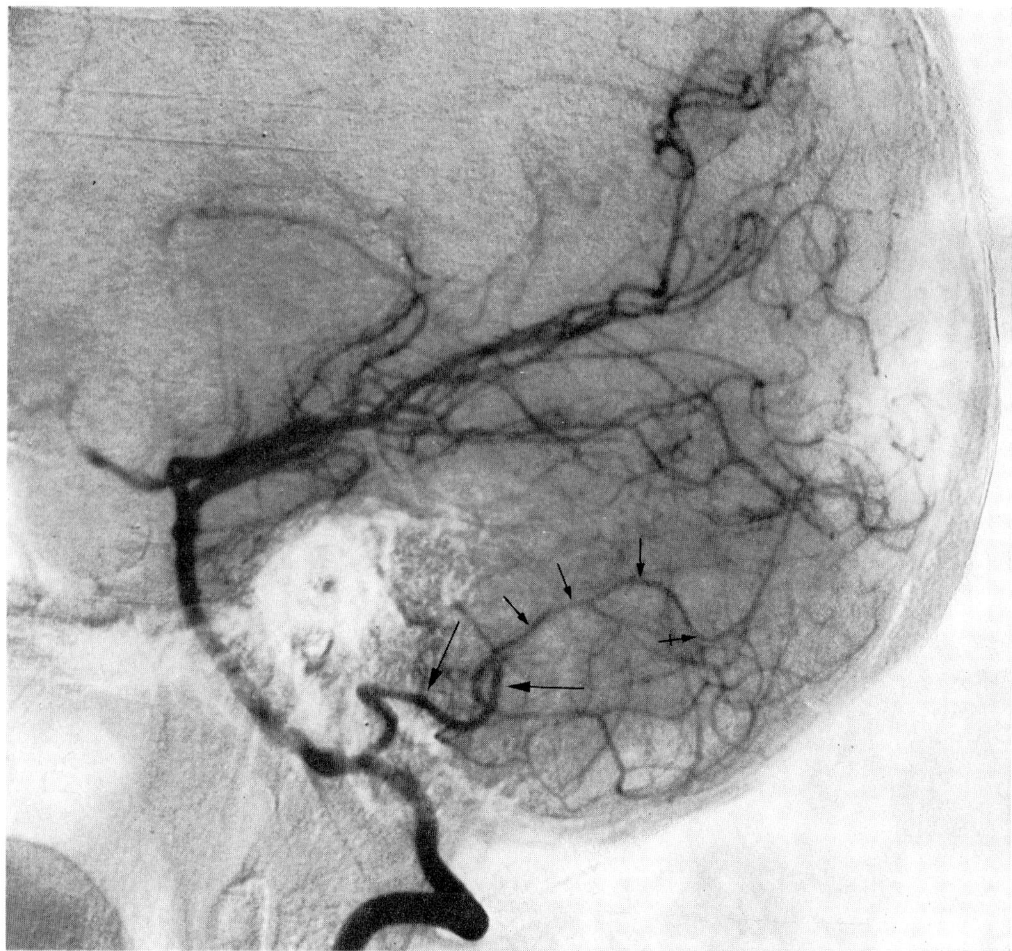

Fig. 165

Fig. 166 Arterial phase in the Towne projection. The lateral medullary, posterior medullary, and supratonsillar segments are all displaced laterally (3 arrows), indicating tumor extension into the vallecula. The quadrigeminal segments are separated due to upward transtentorial herniation of the superior vermis (2 crossed arrows).

Fig. 167 Venous phase in the lateral projection. There are venographic changes of increased intracranial pressure in the posterior fossa. The superior vermian and anterior pontomesencephalic veins are compressed against the straight sinus and the clivus, respectively. The interpeduncular segment of the anterior pontomesencephalic vein is depressed (an arrow), while there is decreased distance between the superior choroid vein and the internal cerebral vein (2 opposing crossed arrows). Only the main portion of the precentral cerebellar vein is visualized due to compression of the fissural portion (2 arrowheads). There is elevation of the copular point (2 arrows) with the redundant inferior vermian vein.

Fig. 168 Venous phase in the Towne projection. The left inferior vermian vein is superiorly displaced by a large tumor in the vallecula (an arrow). The transverse pontine vein is compressed against the clivus (2 crossed arrows).

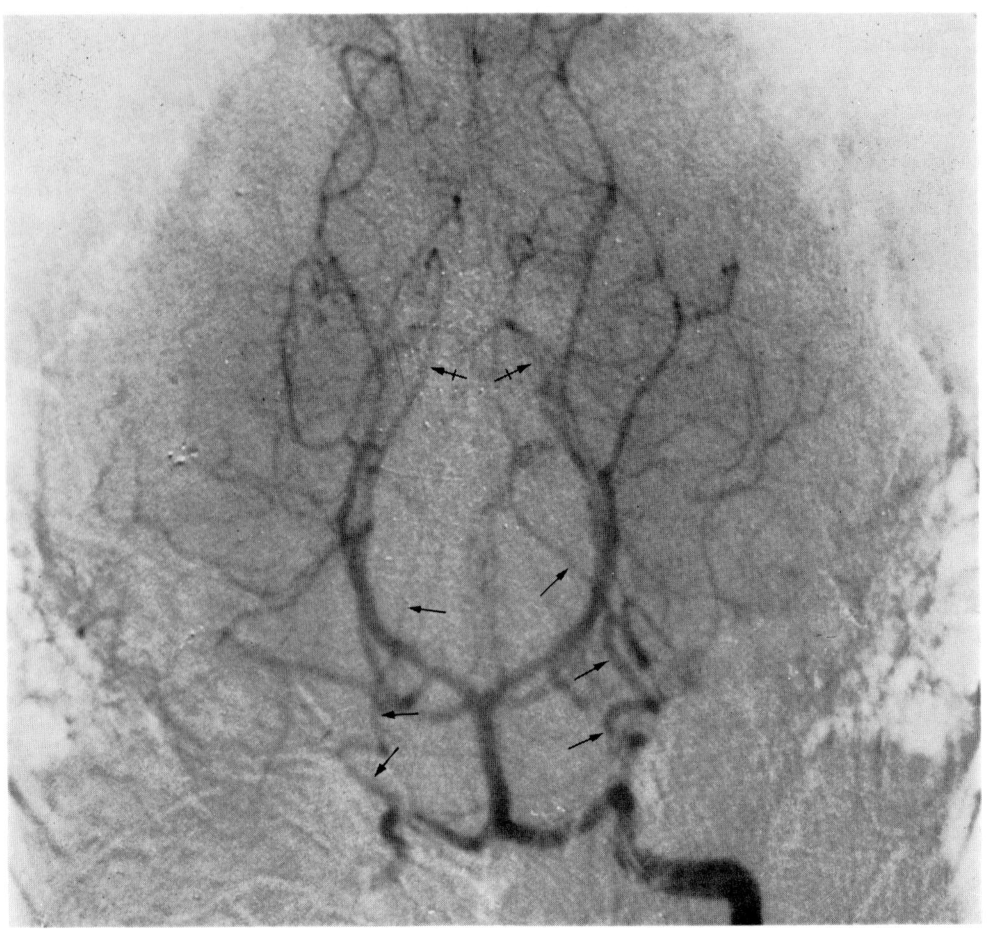

Fig. 166

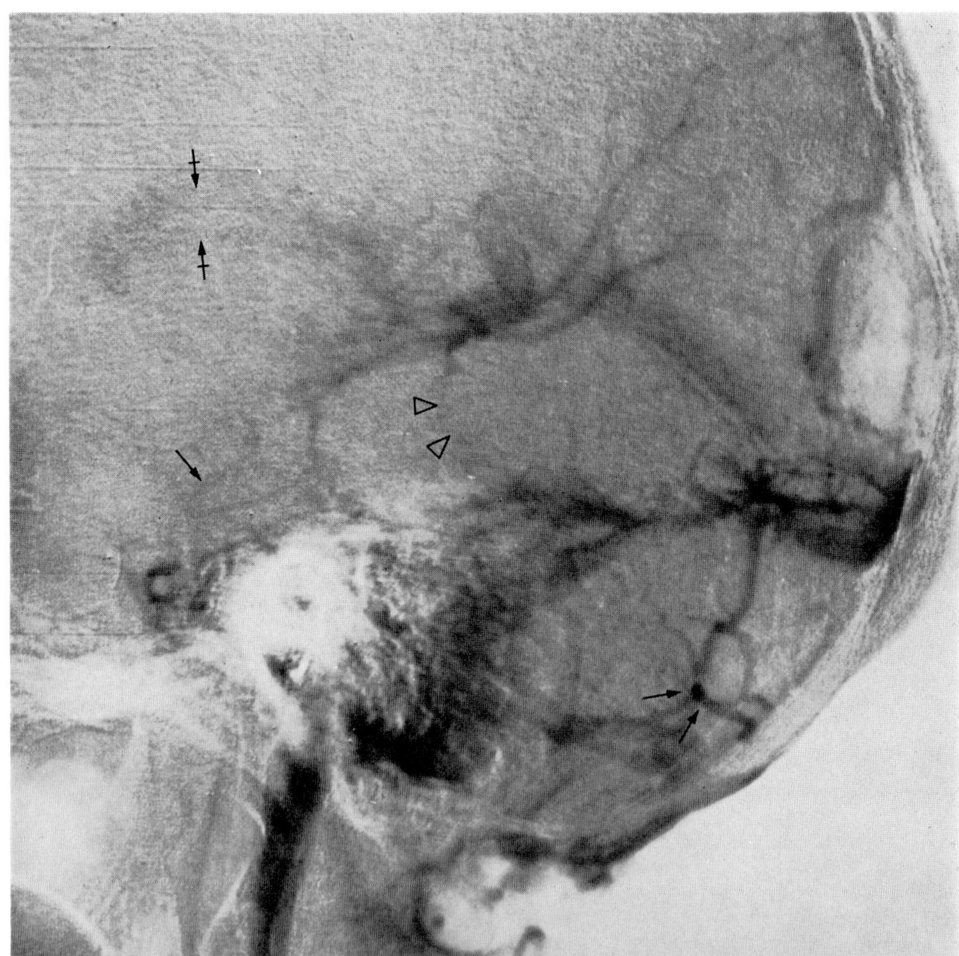

Fig. 167

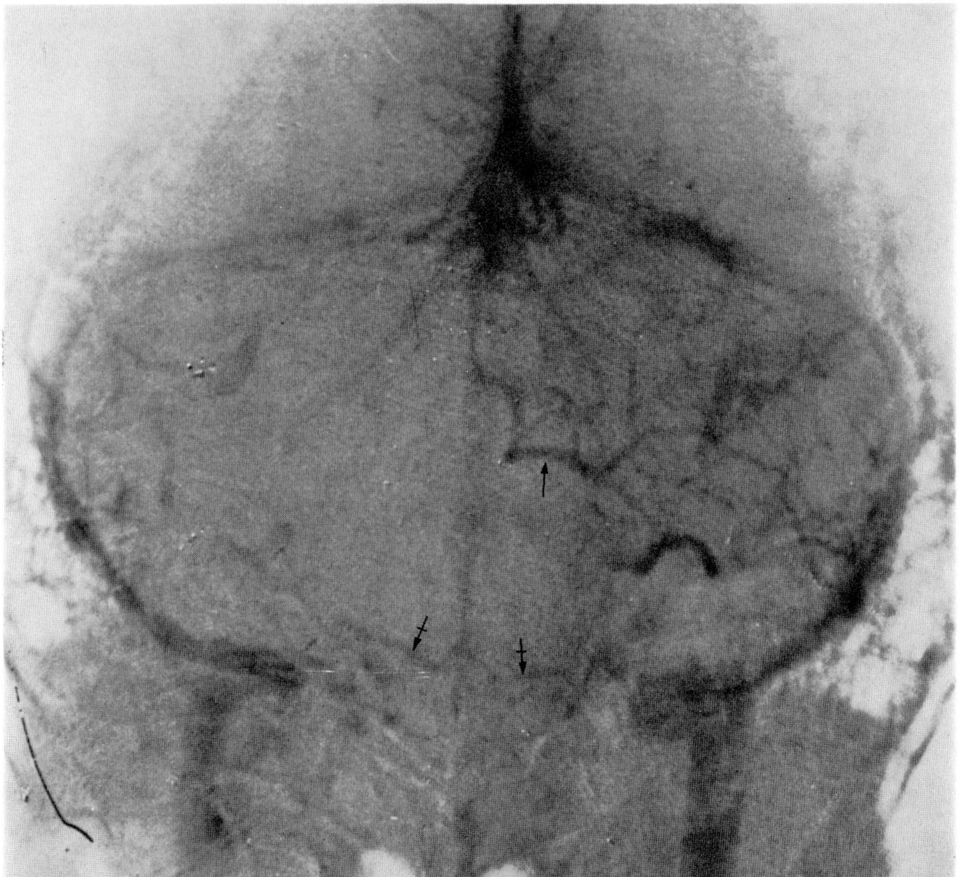

Fig. 168

Large Papilloma of the Fourth Ventricle with Extension into the Vallecula

A 2-year-old female: Figs. 169–172

Fig. 169 Arterial phase in the lateral projection. There are no arteriographic features of increased intracranial pressure in the posterior fossa except for the slightly stretched anterior culminate segment of the superior cerebellar artery (3 closed arrowheads) and anteriorly displaced basilar artery. The supratonsillar segment of the posterior inferior cerebellar artery is elongated in the anteroposterior direction (3 arrows). The nodular branch is stretched posteriorly (3 open arrowheads). The copular point is markedly displaced posteriorly (a crossed arrow), suggesting tumor extension into the vallecula.

Fig. 170 Venous phase in the lateral projection. The distance of the internal cerebral vein and the superior choroid vein is reduced (2 opposing arrows), and the anterior pontomesencephalic vein is displaced anteriorly (2 crossed arrows), suggesting slightly increased intracranial pressure. Other posterior fossa veins are not visualized to good advantage.

Fig. 171 Arterial phase in the Towne projection. The lateral medullary, posterior medullary and the supratonsillar segments of the left posterior inferior cerebellar artery are markedly displaced laterally in an arcuate fashion (4 arrows), secondary to a large tumor extension into the vallecula. The same segments of the right posterior inferior cerebellar artery are visualized faintly and displaced to the right (3 arrowheads). There is no separation of the quadrigeminal segments of the superior cerebellar artery (2 crossed arrows).

Fig. 172 Venous phase in the Towne projection. The anastomotic lateral mesencephalic and brachial veins (2 arrows) are laterally displaced on both sides, probably due to tumor extension into the aqueduct. The petrosal vein is compressed against the clivus bilaterally (crossed arrows).

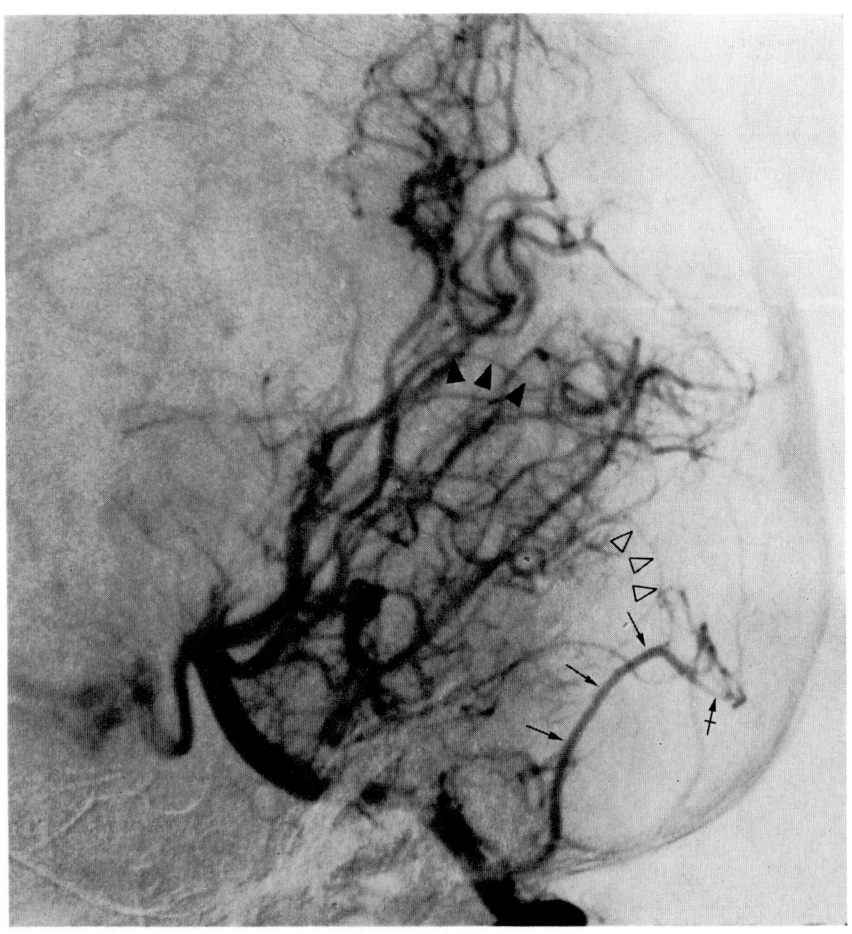

Fig. 169

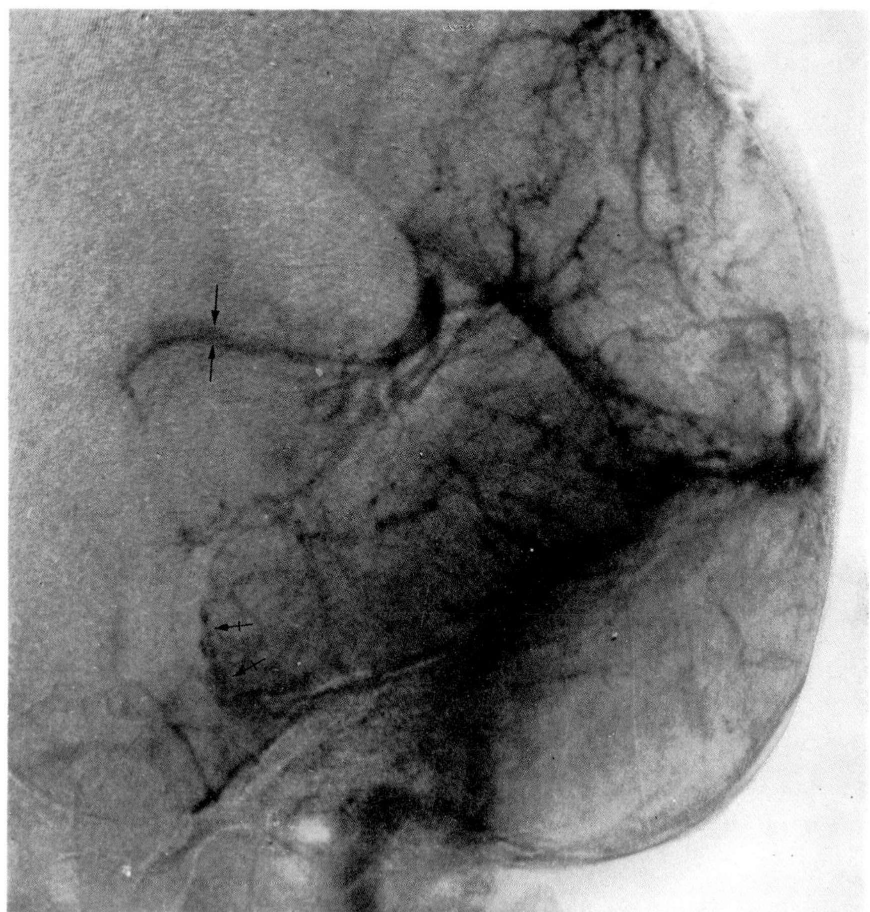

Fig. 170

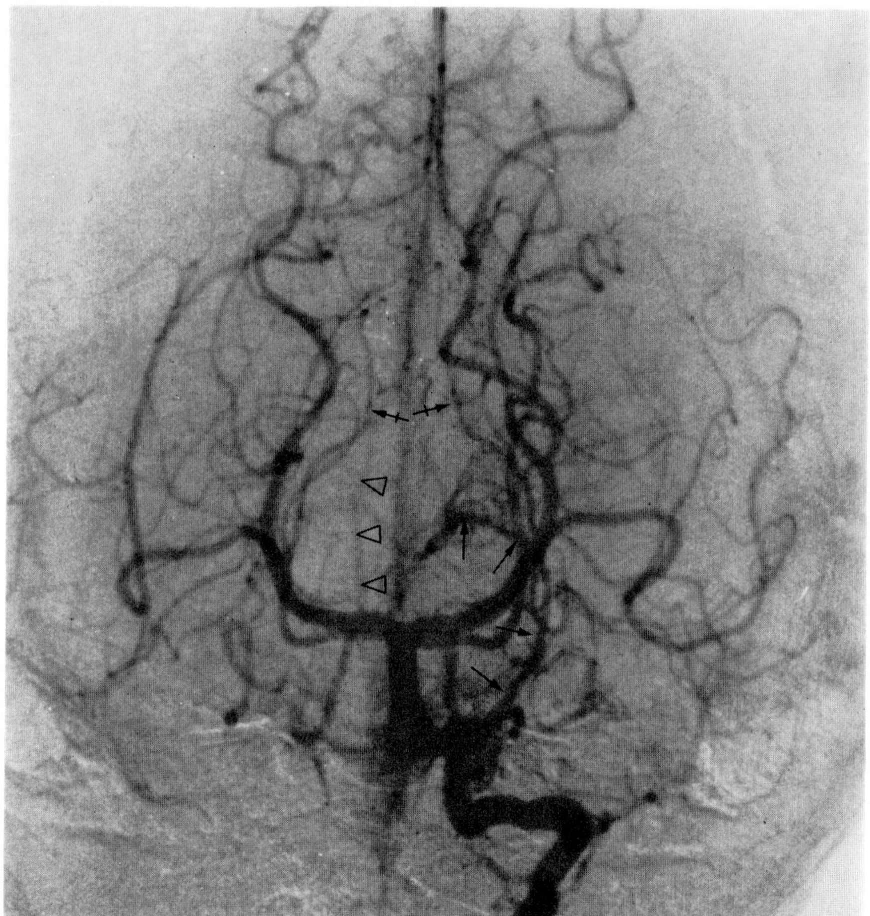

Fig. 171

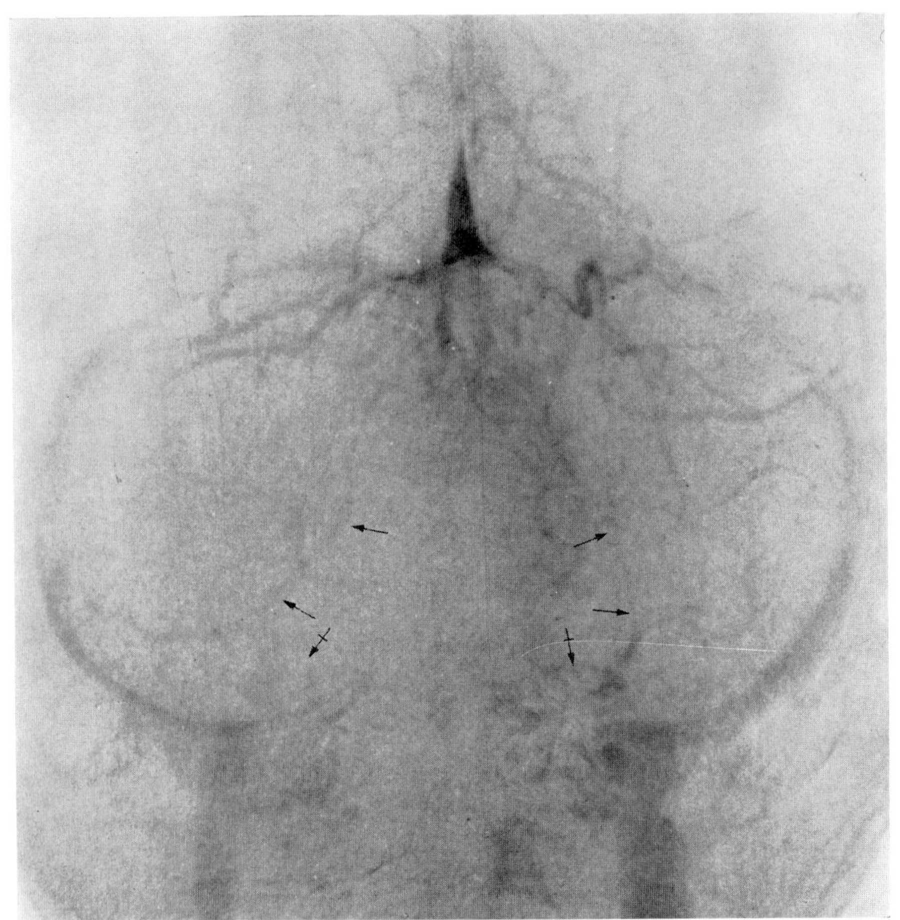

Fig. 172

TUMORS OF THE CEREBELLOPONTINE ANGLE

Arteriographic features

The superior cerebellar artery

The lateral portion of the interpeduncular-crural and the ambient segment is diffusely elevated with blunting of the angle formed by these two segments usually secondary to rotation or contralateral displacement of the brain stem. Large cerebellopontine angle tumors may encroach upon the anterior portion of the ambient segment and produce arched arterial displacements. The marginal artery, arising from the anterior portion of the ambient segment, may be displaced superiorly and laterally by larger cerebellopontine angle tumors. The precentral cerebellar artery may be displaced backward with posterior dislocation of the brain stem.

The anterior inferior cerebellar artery

Cerebellopontine angle tumors displace this artery in either the superior, posterior, or inferior direction depending upon the origin of the lesions and the course of the artery. Superior displacement of this artery can easily be appreciated in the anteroposterior projection, while inferior displacement is somewhat difficult to appreciate since this artery normally takes a downward course. Straightening of this artery in the anteroposterior projection is frequently associated with posterior displacement.

The posterior inferior cerebellar artery

Large tumors in the cerebellopontine angle rotate the medulla oblongata posteriorly and to the opposite side. Therefore, the caudal loop may be displaced backward and downward with frequent angulation. The supratonsillar segment is displaced posteriorly and foreshortened, forming a smaller circle over the superior portion of the tonsils. The vermian branch of the posterior inferior cerebellar artery may be displaced to the contralateral side, while tonsillohemispheric branches of the involved side may be stretched.

The basilar artery

Because of wide variations in the course of the basilar artery, it is quite difficult to appreciate dislocations of this artery. Nevertheless, large cerebellopontine angle tumors displace the basilar artery to the opposite side. Posterior displacement may be seen by rotation of the brain stem or extension of tumors into the prepontine cistern.

The posterior cerebral artery

The ambient segment of the posterior cerebral artery is occasionally elevated in the presence of large cerebellopontine angle tumors. Since the artery is supratentorial, the elevation is usually secondary to rotation of the brain stem. With this arterial change there are usually associated arterial displacements of the superior cerebellar, the basilar and the anterior inferior cerebellar arteries.

Venographic features

The anterior group

The petrosal vein receives blood from many tributaries in the cerebellopontine angle and drains into the superior petrosal sinus above the internal auditory meatus.

The petrosal vein and its tributaries are frequently displaced by the cerebellopontine angle tumors. The main trunk of the petrosal vein is usually displaced laterally and superiorly. The transverse pontine vein may be elevated by medial extension of the tumor. The brachial tributary may be displaced laterally. The vein of the lateral recess of the fourth ventricle is usually displaced medially and posteriorly. Other tributaries of the petrosal vein are frequently displaced.

There is frequently development of an abnormal vein in acoustic neurinomas. This vein is enlarged to a diameter of 2 to 3 mm. It usually originates from the posterior, inferior and medial aspect of the tumor, and circumvents the mass from above with drainage into the petrosal vein. This vein is arched with superior convexity on both lateral and anteroposterior projections. This finding is not usually observed in other cerebellopontine angle tumors beside acoustic neurinomas.

Non-visualization or poor visualization of the petrosal vein occurs when the cerebellopontine angle tumors compress the petrosal veins. Since this vein primarily drains the cerebellum which receives blood supply from the posterior inferior cerebellar artery, this finding is significant only when the posterior inferior cerebellar artery is well opacified on the side of the tumors.

The superior group

The precentral cerebellar vein is displaced backward with increased colliculocentral angle. The anterior pontomesencephalic vein may be displaced posteriorly and the posterior mesencephalic vein is occasionally elevated. These findings are observed when the tumors rotate the brain stem or extend into the prepontine cistern.

The posterior group

The inferior vermian vein may be displaced posteriorly and to the normal side in the presence of large cerebellopontine angle tumors.

Other venographic findings

Circulation time is delayed and visualization of the posterior fossa veins is poor on the side of the tumors.

Left Acoustic Neurinoma

A 43-year-old female: Figs. 173–178.

Fig. 173 Arterial phase in the Towne projection. The left anterior inferior cerebellar artery is displaced superiorly in an arcuate fashion (3 arrows). There may be minimal tumor vessels in the course of this artery. The left superior cerebellar artery is also slightly elevated (2 crossed arrows) with faintly visualized left posterior cerebral artery. There is minimal midline shift of supratonsillar segment of the posterior inferior cerebellar artery (a double-crossed arrow). The marginal artery (2 closed arrowheads) and hemispheric branches of the posterior inferior cerebellar artery are slightly stretched (2 open arrowheads). There is common origin of the anterior and posterior inferior cerebellar arteries on both sides. Differentiation of the anterior inferior cerebellar artery and the marginal artery was difficult with this projection.

Fig. 174 Early venous phase in the Towne projection. There are tumor stains within the medial aspect of the tumor (5 arrows). Visualization of the veins in the left posterior fossa is poor, while there is good visualization of the inferior vermian and petrosal veins on the right. Circulation time is delayed on the left. The left inferior vermian vein is not demonstrated. The left petrosal vein is not well seen.

Fig. 175 Venous phase in the Towne projection. There is now visualization of the left inferior vermian vein 2 seconds later than Fig. 174 with medial displacement (3 arrows). An abnormal vein is present with posterior and lateral displacement (2 arrowheads). The petrosal vein is poorly visualized due to compression by the tumor (a crossed arrow).

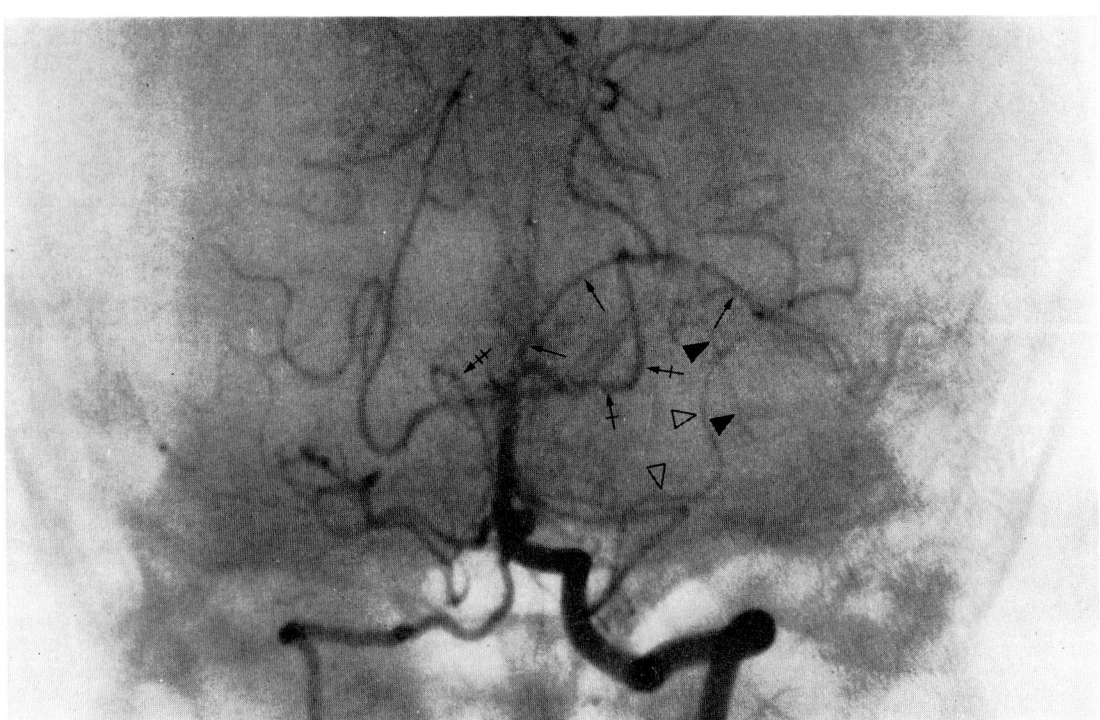

Fig. 173

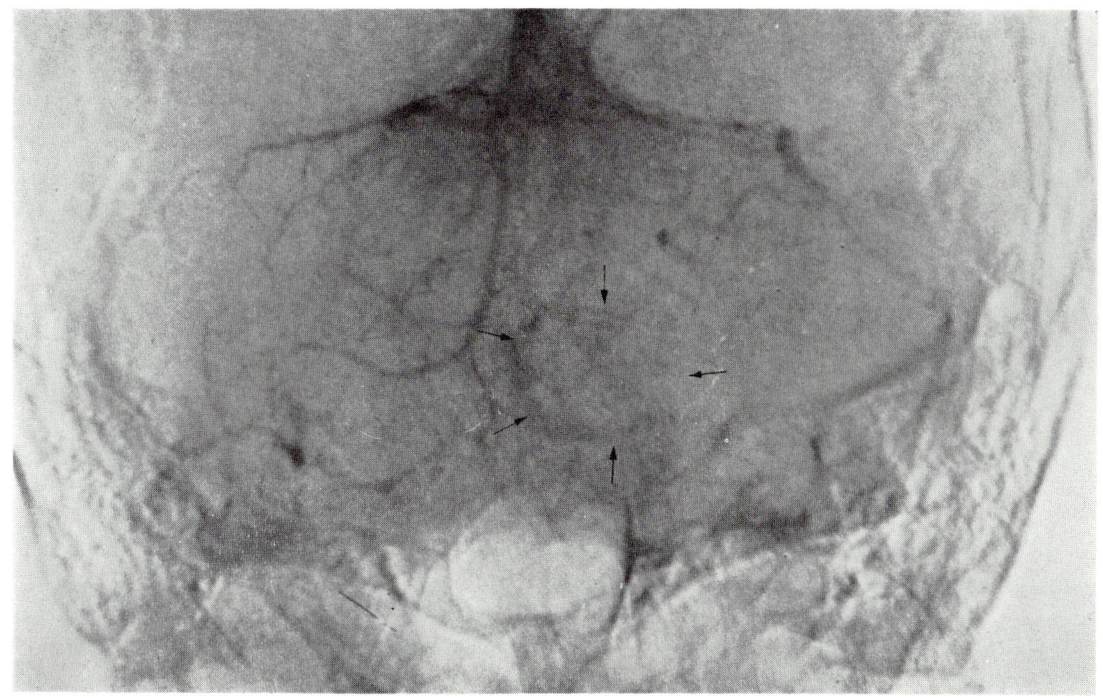

Fig. 174

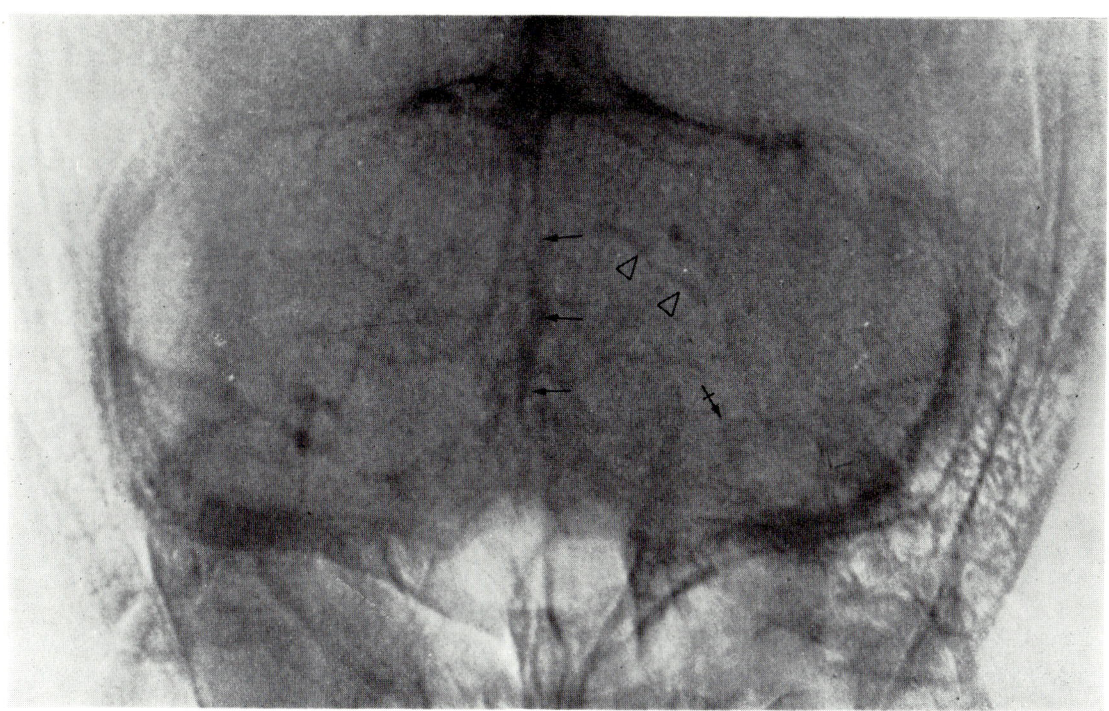

Fig. 175

Fig. 176 Arterial phase in the anteroposterior projection. There is an arcuate, superior displacement of the left anterior inferior cerebellar artery (3 arrows) with diffuse elevation of the superior cerebellar and posterior cerebral arteries (2 arrowheads). The hemispheric branch of the left posterior inferior cerebellar artery is stretched (2 crossed arrows). Note the posterior inferior cerebellar artery arising from the anterior inferior cerebellar arteries bilaterally.

Fig. 177 Arterial phase in the lateral projection. The left anterior inferior cerebellar artery is displaced superiorly and posteriorly (4 arrows), supplying irregular tumor vessels. There is diffuse inferior displacement of the posterior inferior cerebellar artery on the left, which has common origin with the displaced anterior inferior cerebellar artery (3 crossed arrows). The posterior medullary and supratonsillar segments on the right are displaced posteriorly (3 arrowheads). The tonsillar branches on both sides are also displaced below the foramen magnum, suggesting a tonsillar herniation (2 arrowheads). There are angiographic changes of increased intracranial pressure: anterior displacement of the basilar artery and straightening of the thalamoperforate arteries.

Fig. 178 Venous phase in the lateral projection. There is an abnormal vein displaced superiorly and posteriorly in an arcuate fashion (4 arrows). The vein appears to have communication with the inferior vermian vein and drains into the petrosal vein. The copular point is displaced posteriorly (a crossed arrow).

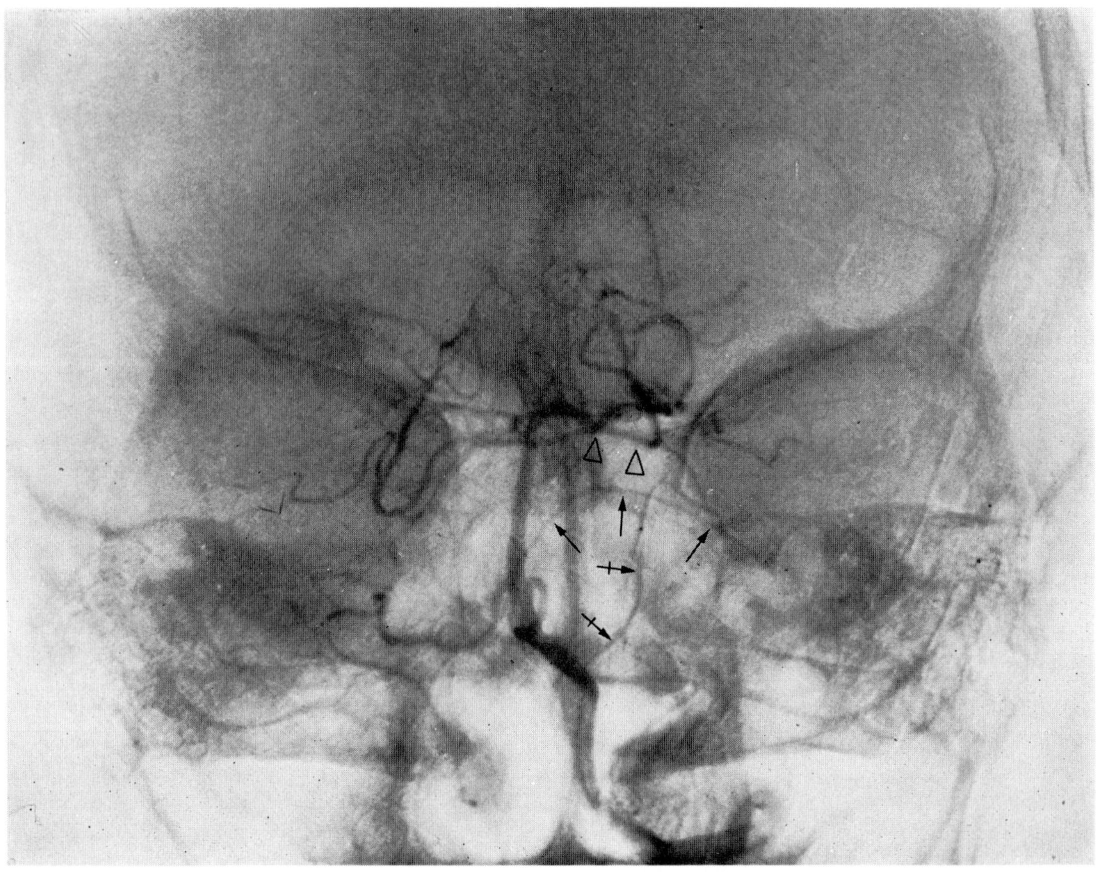

Fig. 176

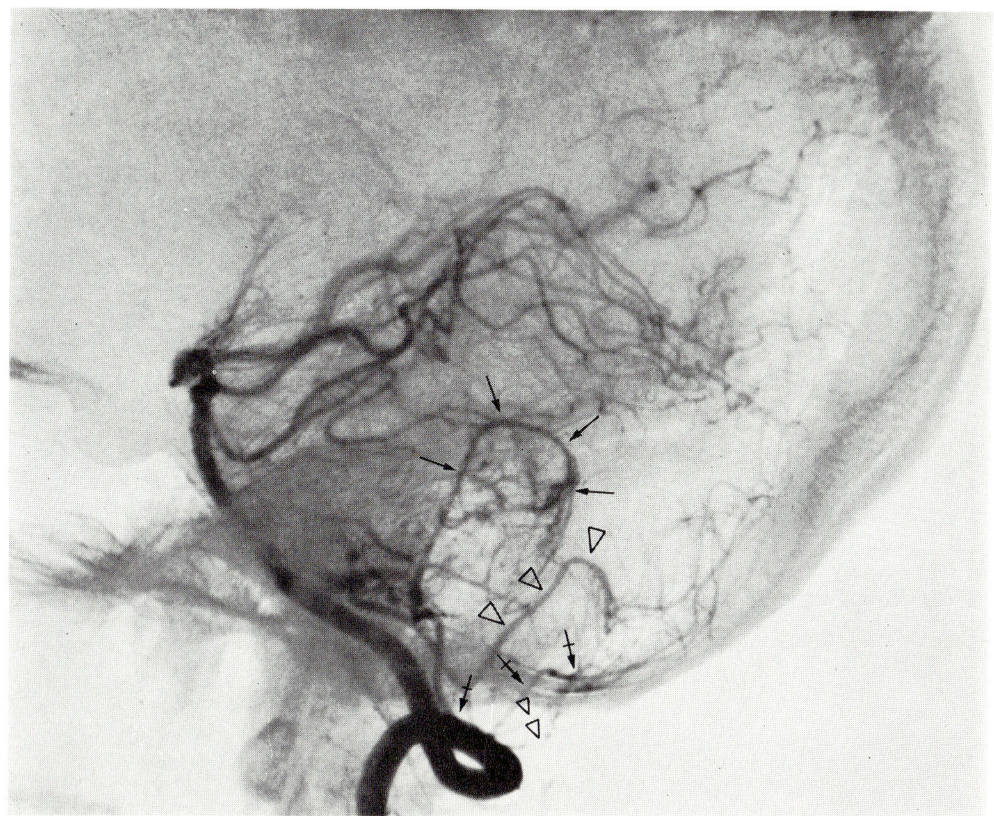

Fig. 177

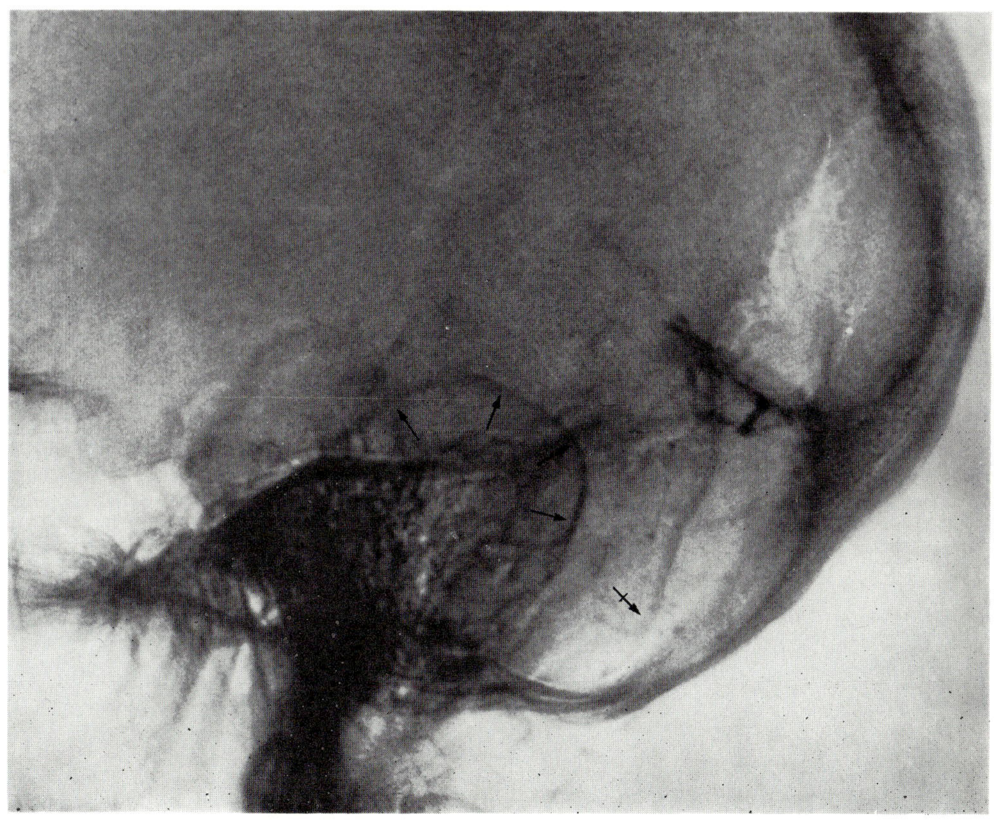

Fig. 178

Right Acoustic Neurinoma with Extension into the Prepontine Cistern and Rotation of the Brain Stem

A 42-year-old male: Figs. 179–183

Fig. 179 Arterial phase in the lateral projection. The basilar artery is displaced posteriorly with 2 cm distance between the clivus (2 long arrows) and the artery. The cranial and caudal loops (short arrows) of the posterior inferior cerebellar artery are angulated with minimal posterior displacement. The precentral cerebellar artery is displaced posteriorly (an arrow).

Fig. 180 Venous phase in the lateral projection. The transverse pontine vein is displaced superiorly and posteriorly (a long arrow). There is also posterior dislocation of the precentral cerebellar vein (an arrow).

Fig. 181 Arterial phase in the Towne projection. The basilar artery is displaced to the normal side. The superior cerebellar artery is generally elevated (2 short arrows). There is straightening of the anterior inferior cerebellar artery (3 long arrows), suggesting a displacement in the posterior direction. The marginal artery is questionably displaced laterally (an arrow).

Fig. 182 Early venous phase in the Towne projection. There is an avascular lesion in the cerebellopontine angle with arched displacement of the superficial veins (3 arrows). The cerebellum and the brain stem are diffusely stained in contrast to the avascular tumor. The tumor extends across the midline. The petrosal vein is laterally displaced (an arrowhead) and a small vein, probably an inferior hemispheric vein, is stretched (2 crossed arrows).

Fig. 183 Venous phase in the Towne projection. The transverse pontine vein is displaced posteriorly and laterally and drains into the medial portion of the superior petrosal sinus (3 long arrows). The petrosal vein and its tributary are also displaced laterally (an arrow). Visualization of the posterior fossa veins on the right is less marked probably secondary to compression by the large tumor.

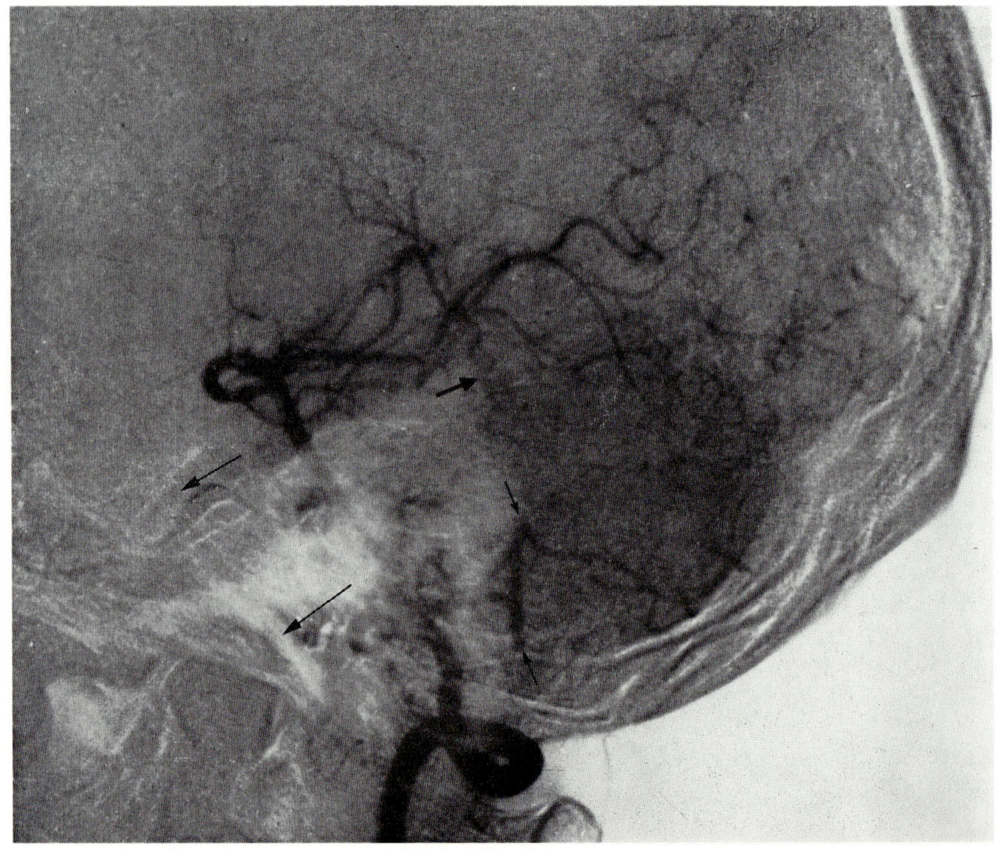

Fig. 179

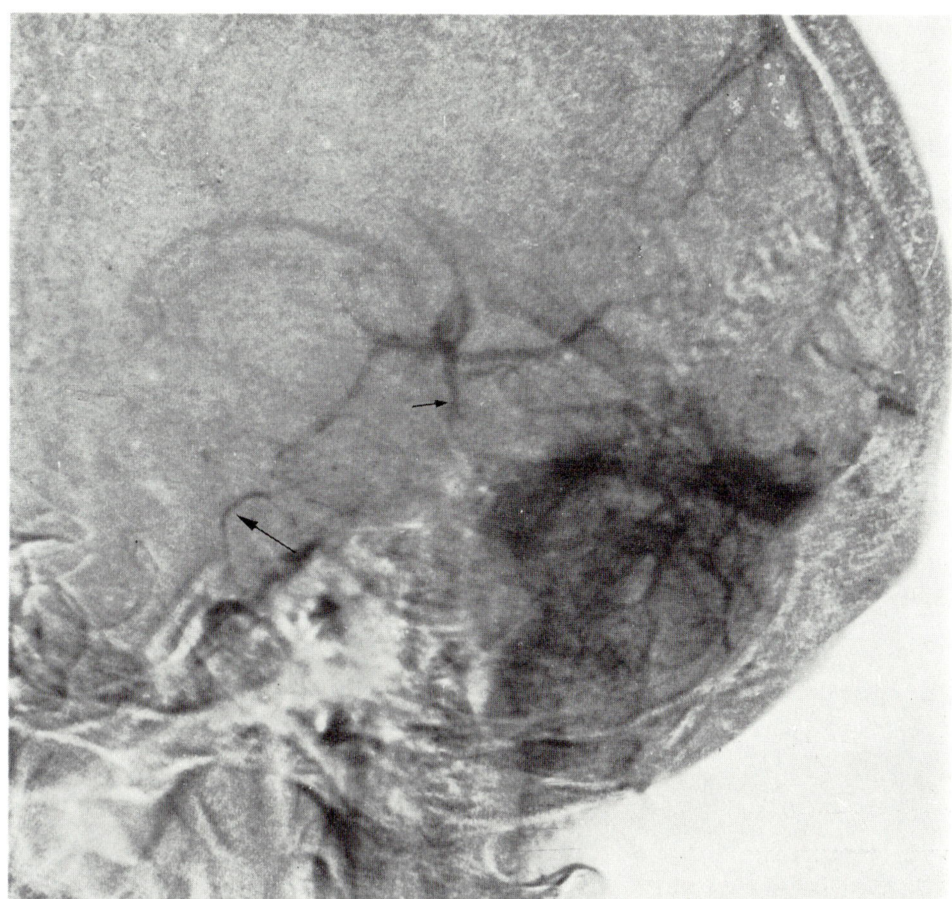

Fig. 180

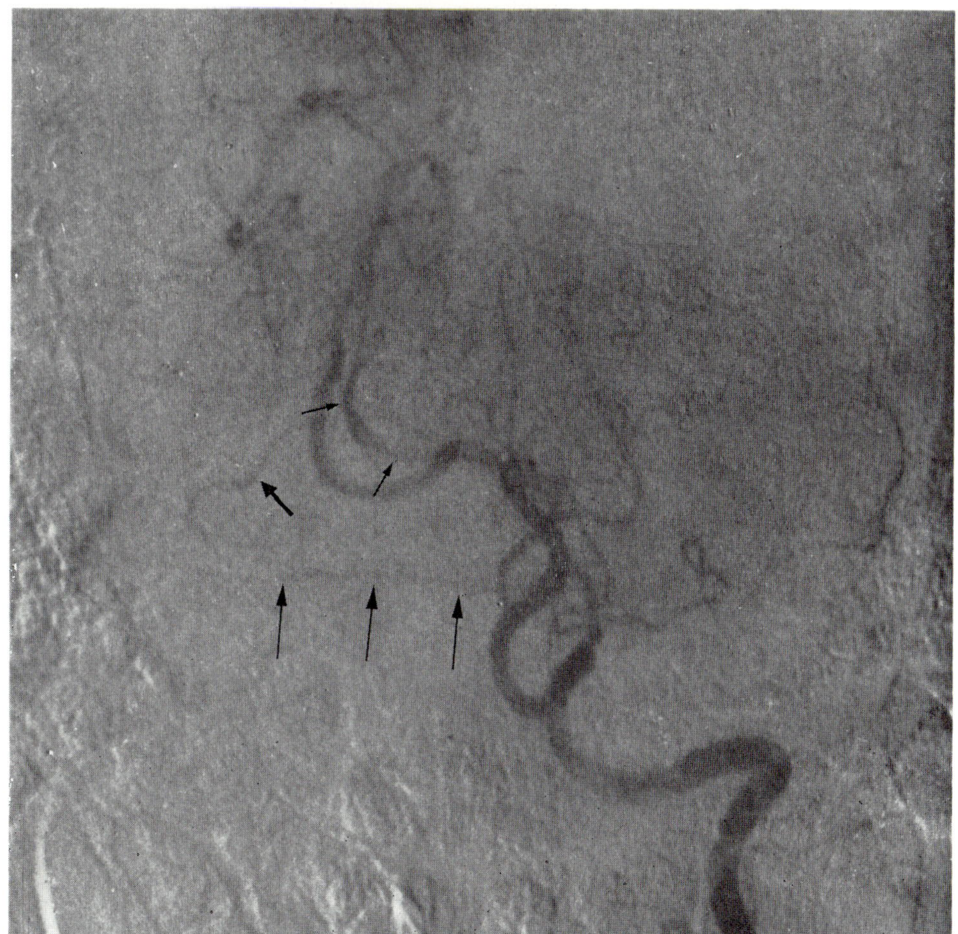

Fig. 181

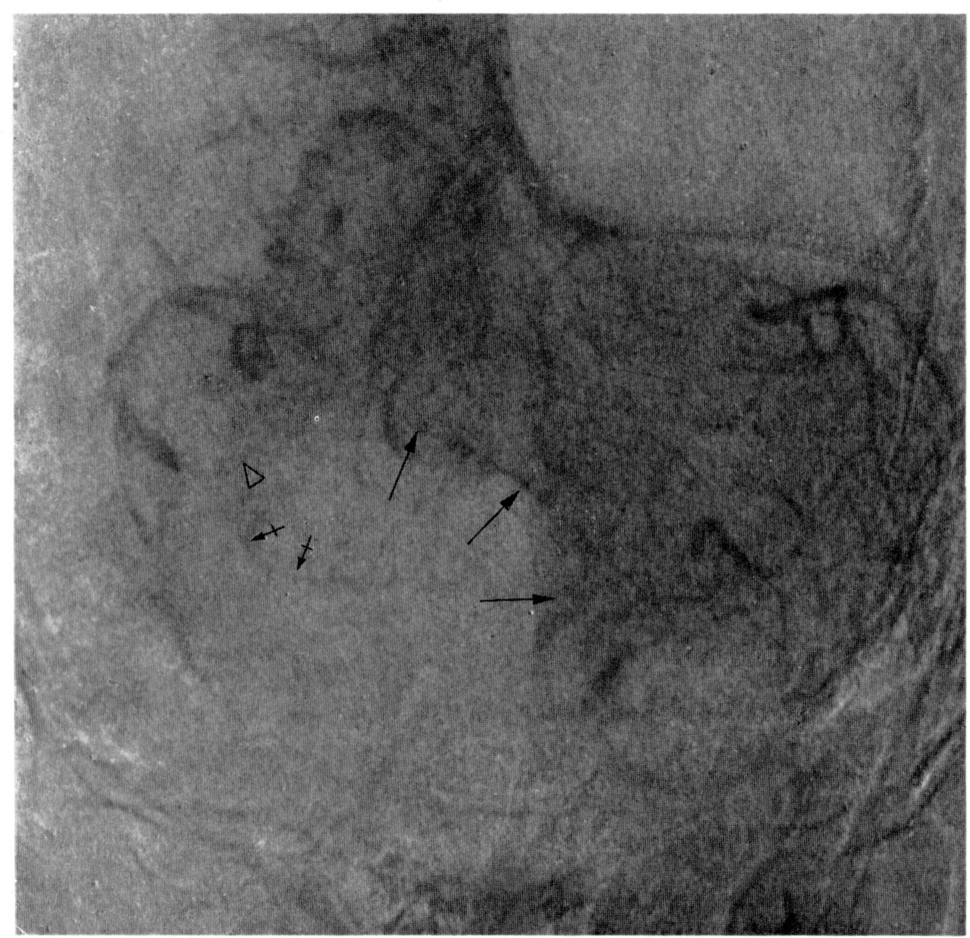

Fig. 182

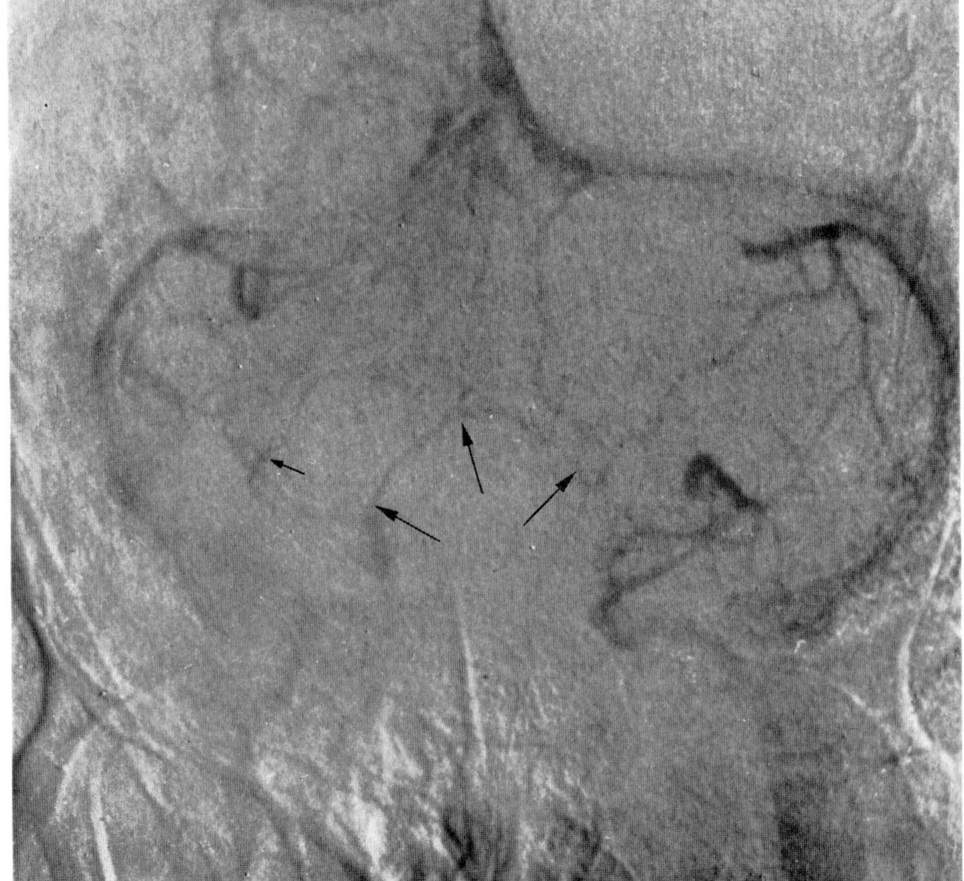

Fig. 183

Left Acoustic Neurinoma

A 49-year-old female: Figs. 184–187

Fig. 184 Arterial phase in the Towne projection. There is arched displacement of the ambient segment of the superior cerebellar artery (a large arrow). Distal portion of this artery is duplicated. The marginal artery is displaced superiorly and laterally in an arcuate fashion (3 long arrows). There is displacement of vermian branch of the posterior inferior cerebellar artery across the midline (2 short arrows). The basilar artery is displaced to the right. There is not a good visualization of the anterior inferior cerebellar artery.

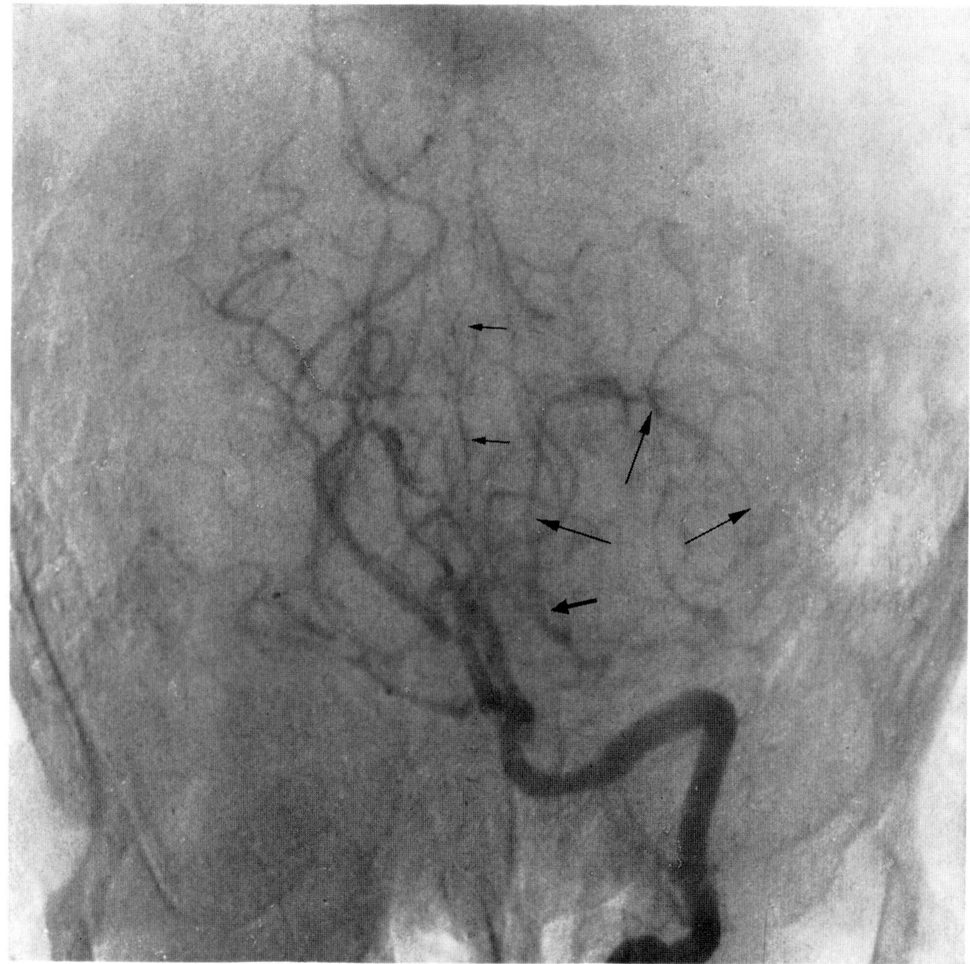

Fig. 184

Fig. 185 Venous phase in the Towne projection. The petrosal vein on the left is poorly visualized, but there is faint visualization of an abnormal vein which is displaced superiorly (a large arrow). The left inferior vermian vein is slightly shifted to the right (2 short arrows).

Fig. 186 Arterial phase in the lateral projection. The basilar artery is compressed against the clivus and the caudal loop of the posterior inferior cerebellar artery is displaced below the foramen magnum (a large arrow). There is increased distance between the posterior pericallosal and posterior choroidal arteries (2 arrows), suggesting moderate hydrocephalus.

Fig. 187 Venous phase in the lateral projection. There is anterior displacement of the anterior pontomesencephalic vein (2 arrows). The inferior vermian vein is displaced posteriorly (2 crossed arrows). All of these venous findings are suggestive of a space-taking lesion in the posterior fossa. There is reduction of the distance between the superior choroid vein and internal cerebral vein (2 opposing arrows).

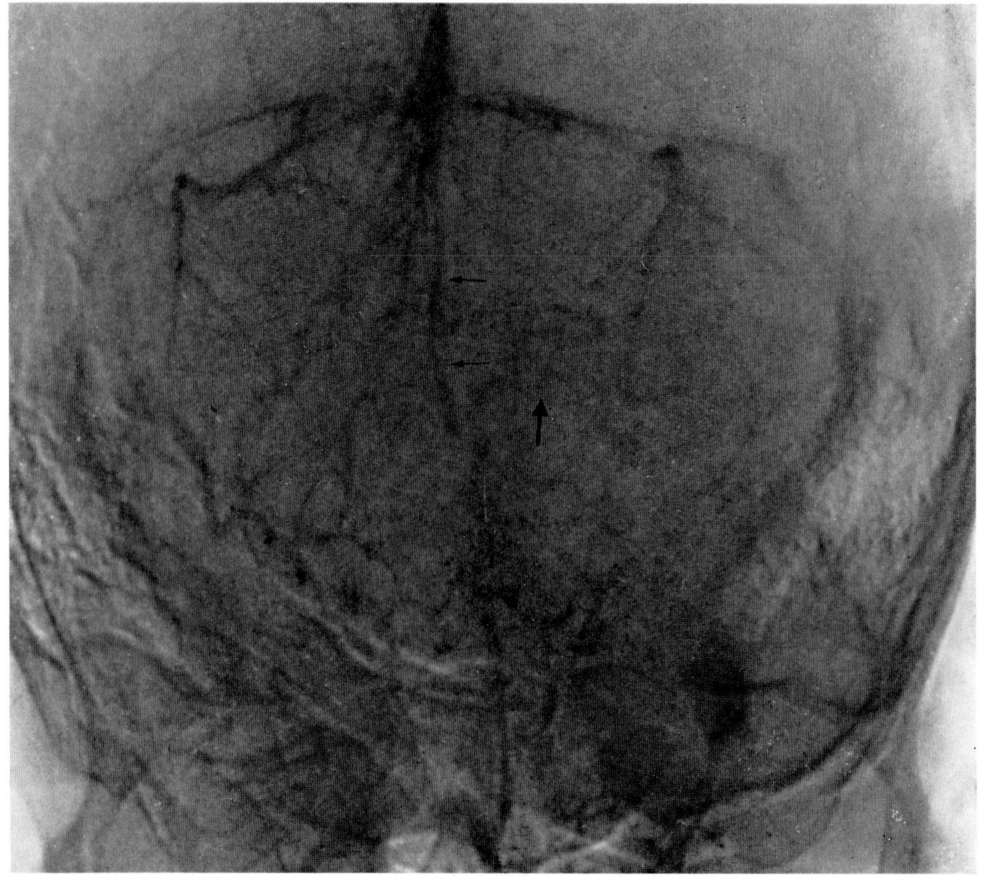

Fig. 185

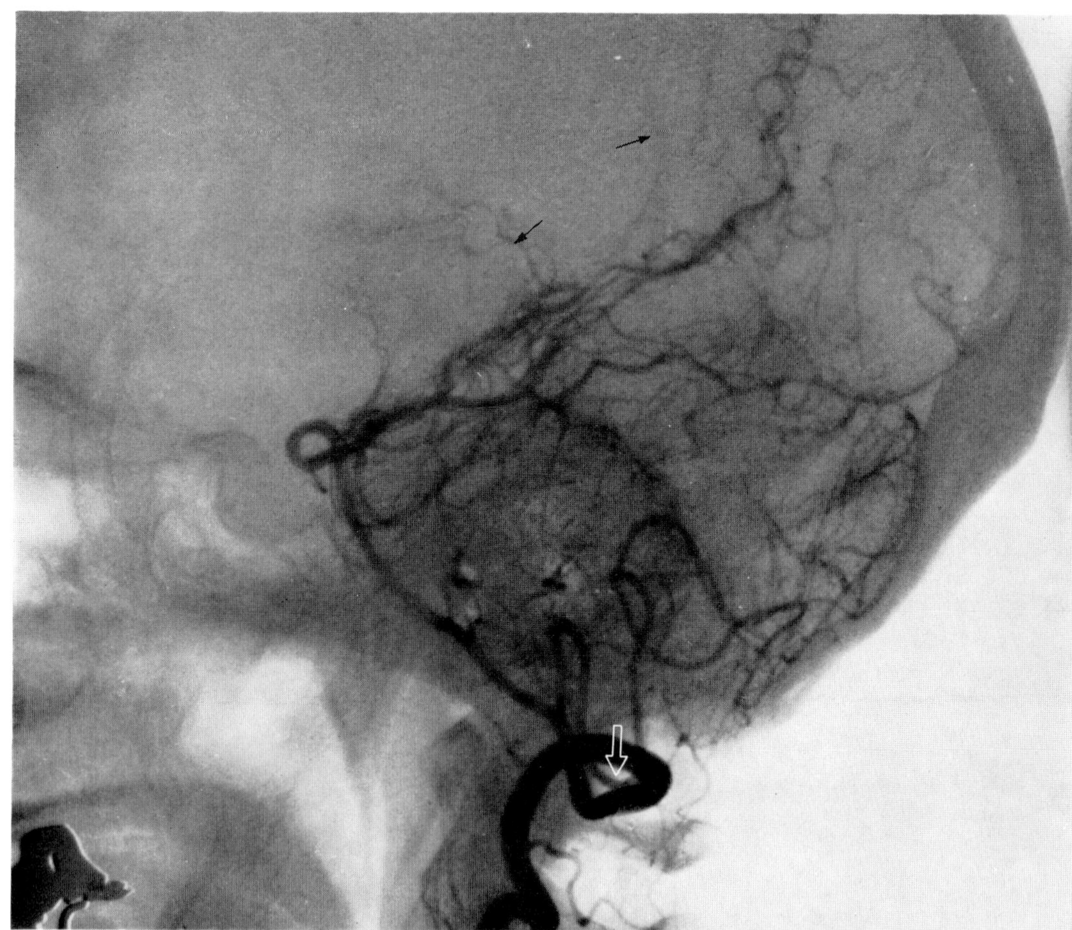

Fig. 186

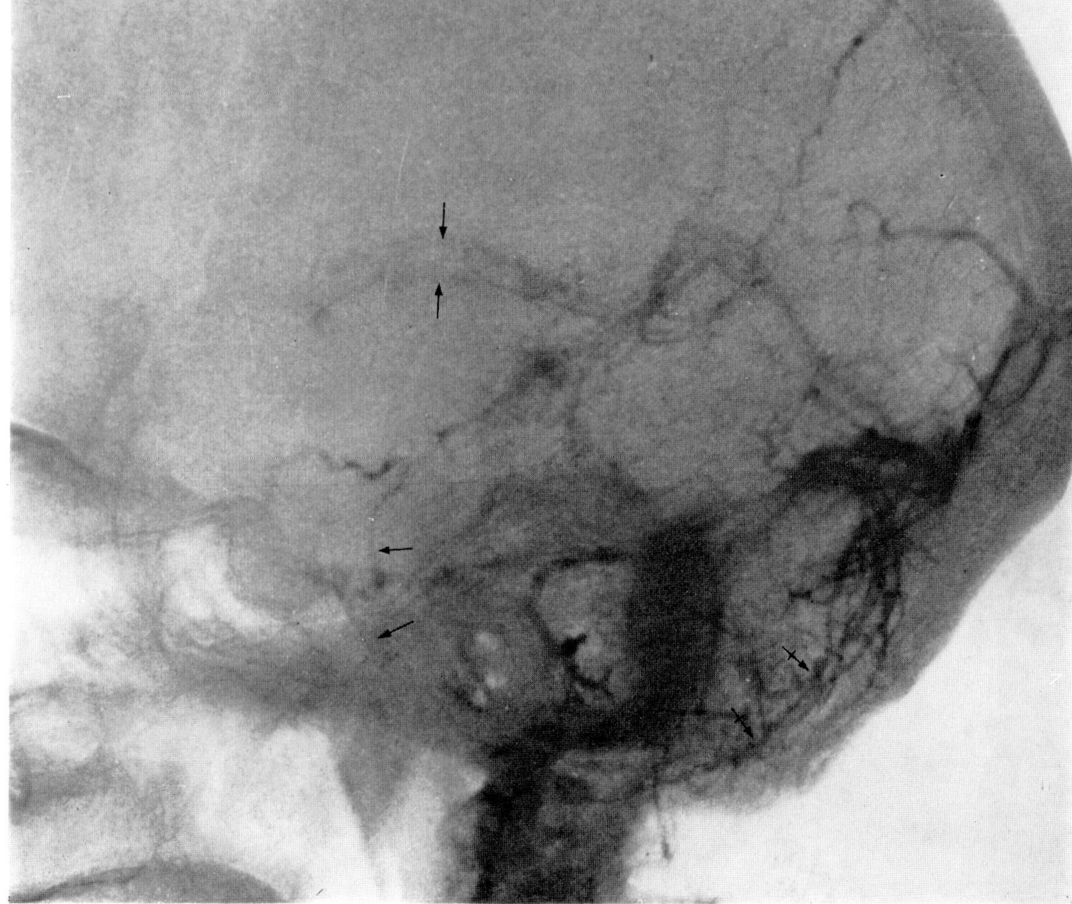

Fig. 187

Right Acoustic Neurinoma

A 38-year-old female: Figs. 188 and 189

Fig. 188 Arterial phase in the Towne projection. The ambient segment of the superior cerebellar artery is diffusely elevated (2 short arrows). The marginal artery is displaced superiorly and laterally in an arcuate fashion (3 long arrows). The vermian segment of the posterior inferior cerebellar artery is slightly shifted across the midline (3 crossed arrows).

Fig. 189 Venous phase in the Towne projection. There is lateral displacement of the petrosal vein (a short arrow). A tributary of the petrosal vein is displaced in the lateral direction (2 long arrows). Visualization of the veins on the right is poor compared with the left.

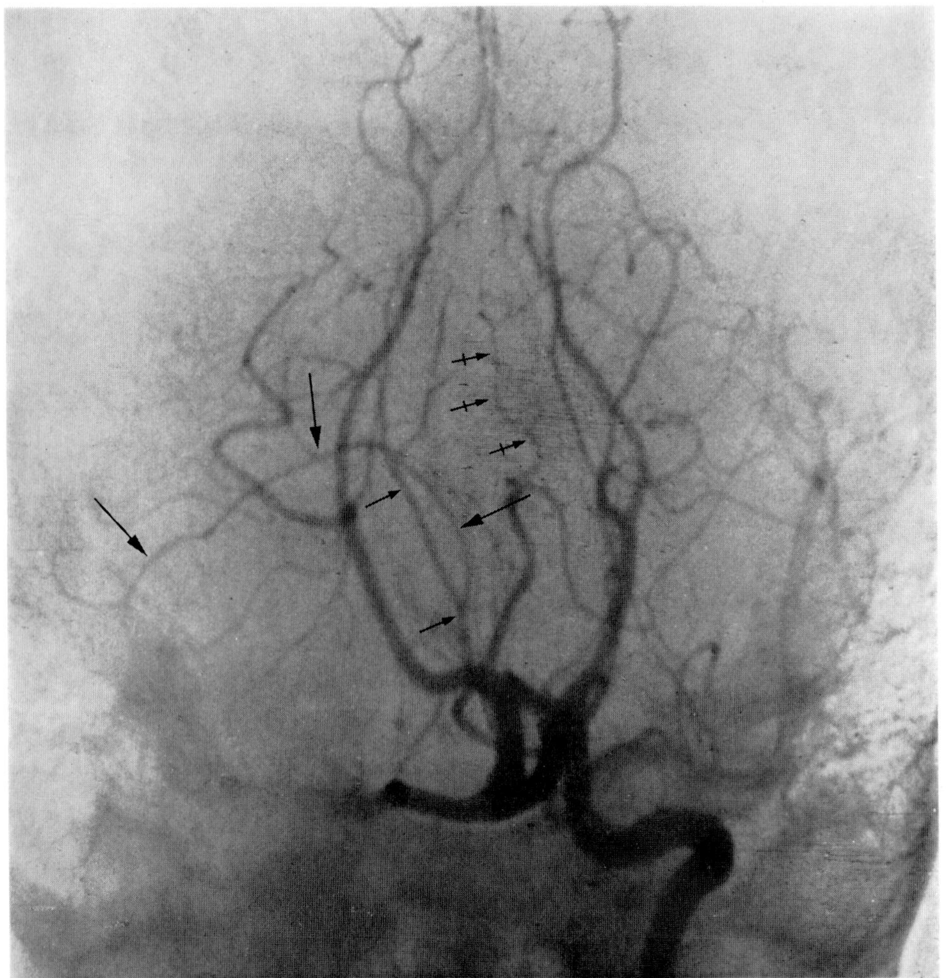

Fig. 188

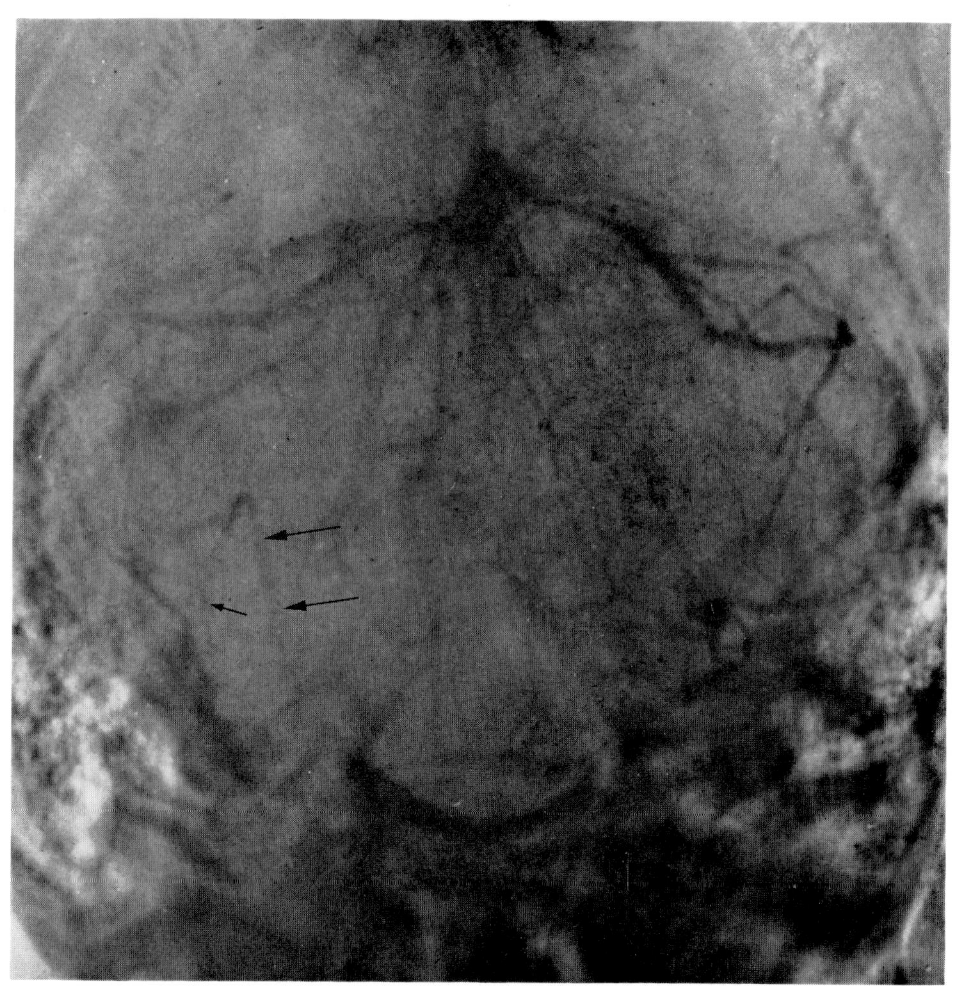

Fig. 189

Left Acoustic Neurinoma

A 41-year-old female: Figs. 190 and 191

Fig. 190 Arterial phase in the Towne projection. There is an arched displacement of the superior cerebellar artery (2 short arrows). The marginal artery is displaced in an arcuate fashion (3 long arrows). The anterior inferior cerebellar artery originates from the posterior inferior cerebellar artery and is displaced downward (2 large arrows). The vermian branch of the right posterior inferior cerebellar artery is displaced across the midline (a large arrow).

Fig. 191 Venous phase in the Towne projection. The tributaries of the petrosal vein are poorly visualized on the left. The petrosal vein is displaced laterally (a large arrow). There is flattening of the anterolateral aspect of the posterior mesencephalic vein (2 arrows).

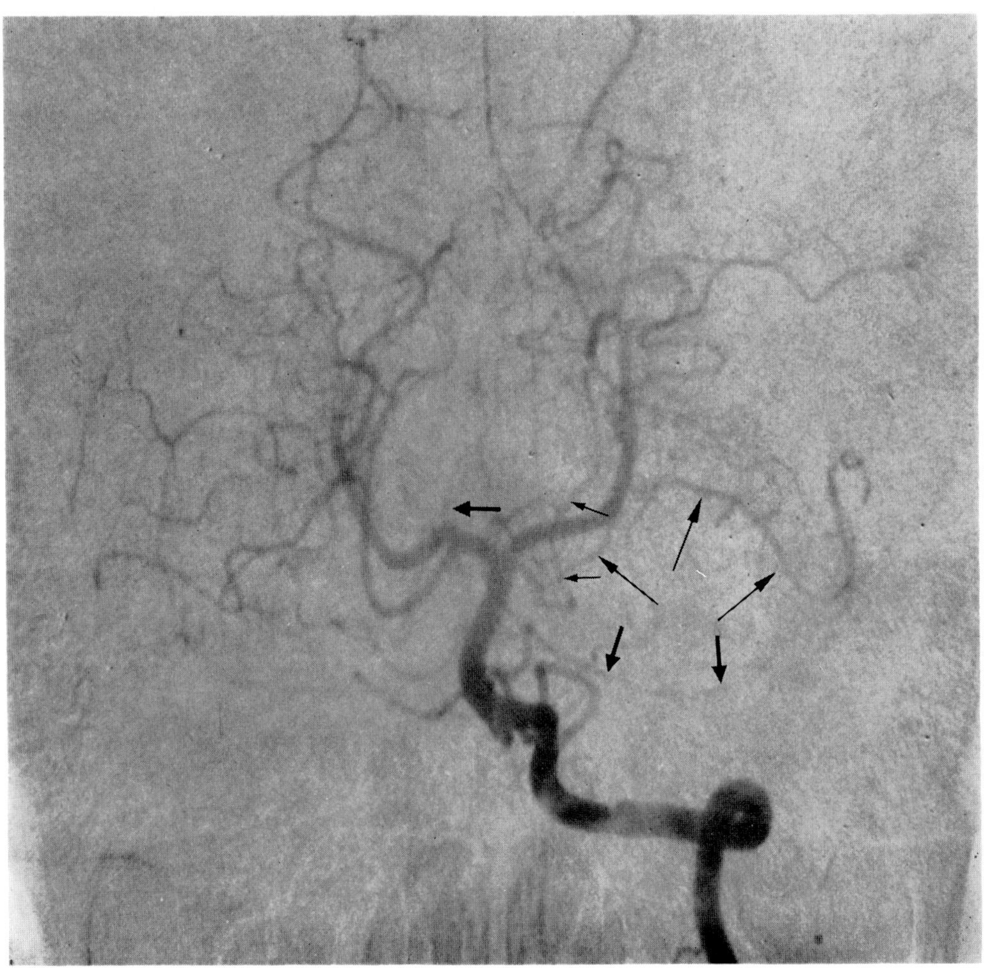

Fig. 190

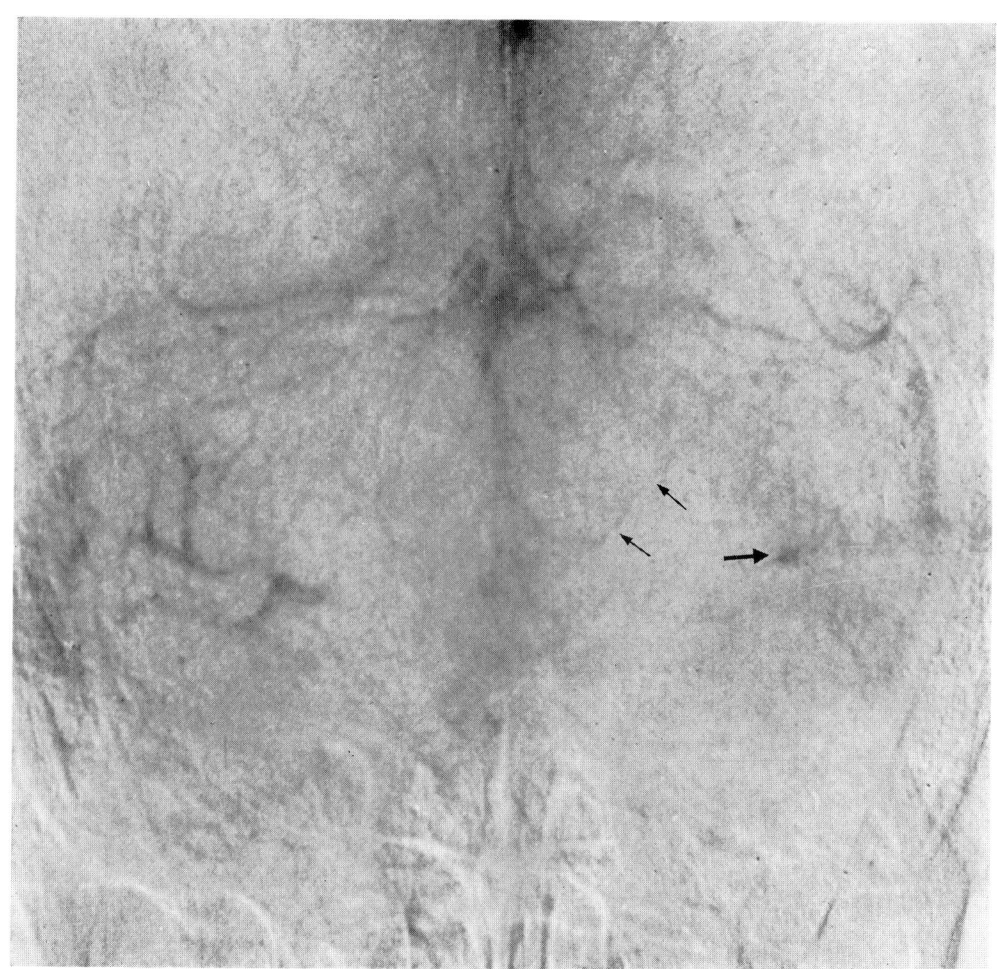

Fig. 191

Left Acoustic Neurinoma

A 25-year-old female: Figs. 192–195

Fig. 192 Arterial phase in the lateral projection. There are angiographic changes due to increased intracranial pressure. The basilar artery is compressed against the clivus and the vermian and anterior culminate segments of the superior cerebellar arteries are elevated in an arcuate fashion (3 arrows). The thalamoperforate arteries are stretched (2 arrowheads). The posterior inferior and anterior inferior cerebellar arteries arising from the common trunk are displaced inferiorly and posteriorly. The posterior medullary segment is displaced backwards (2 crossed arrows). The supratonsillar segment is angulated and dislocated posteriorly (a long arrow).

Fig. 193 Venous phase in the lateral projection. An abnormal vein originates in the area of the tonsil and courses over the tumor with drainage into the superior petrosal sinus (4 arrows).

Fig. 194 Arterial phase in the Towne projection. The left superior cerebellar arteries are medially displaced (2 arrows) together with medial displacement of the posterior cerebral artery (2 crossed arrows).

Fig. 195 Venous phase in the Towne projection. The abnormal vein (3 short arrows) is superimposed over the stretched petrosal vein (3 long arrows). The course of the abnormal vein simulates that of the vein of the lateral recess of the fourth ventricle.

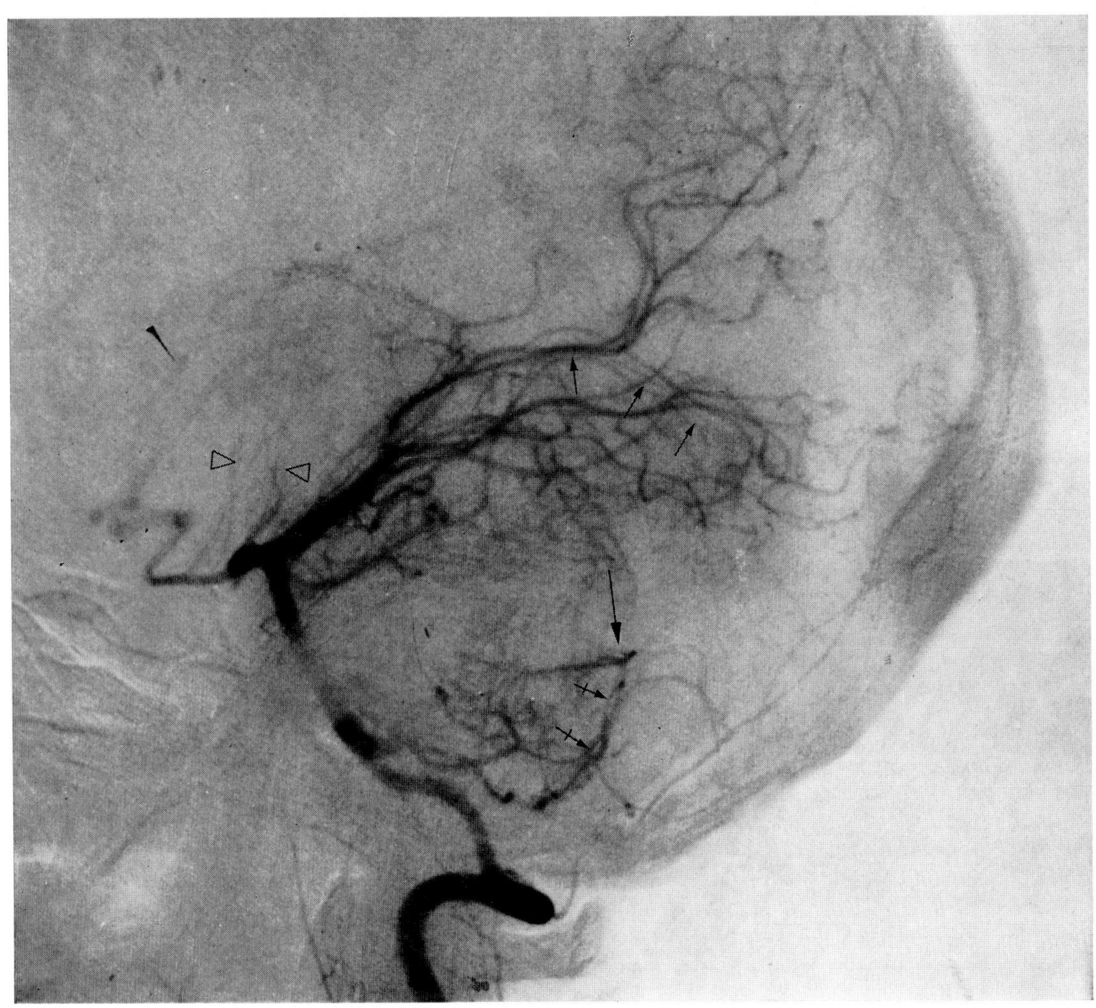

Fig. 192

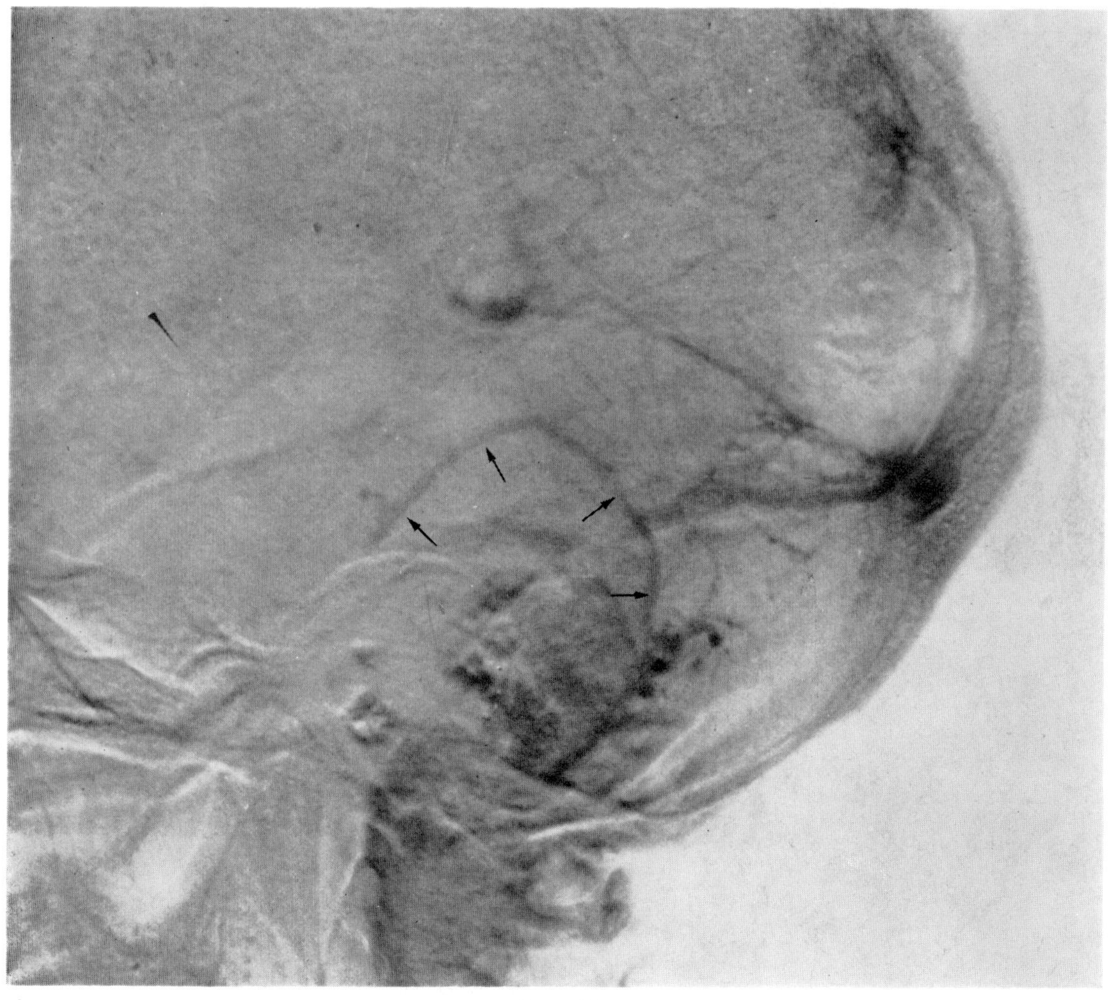

Fig. 193

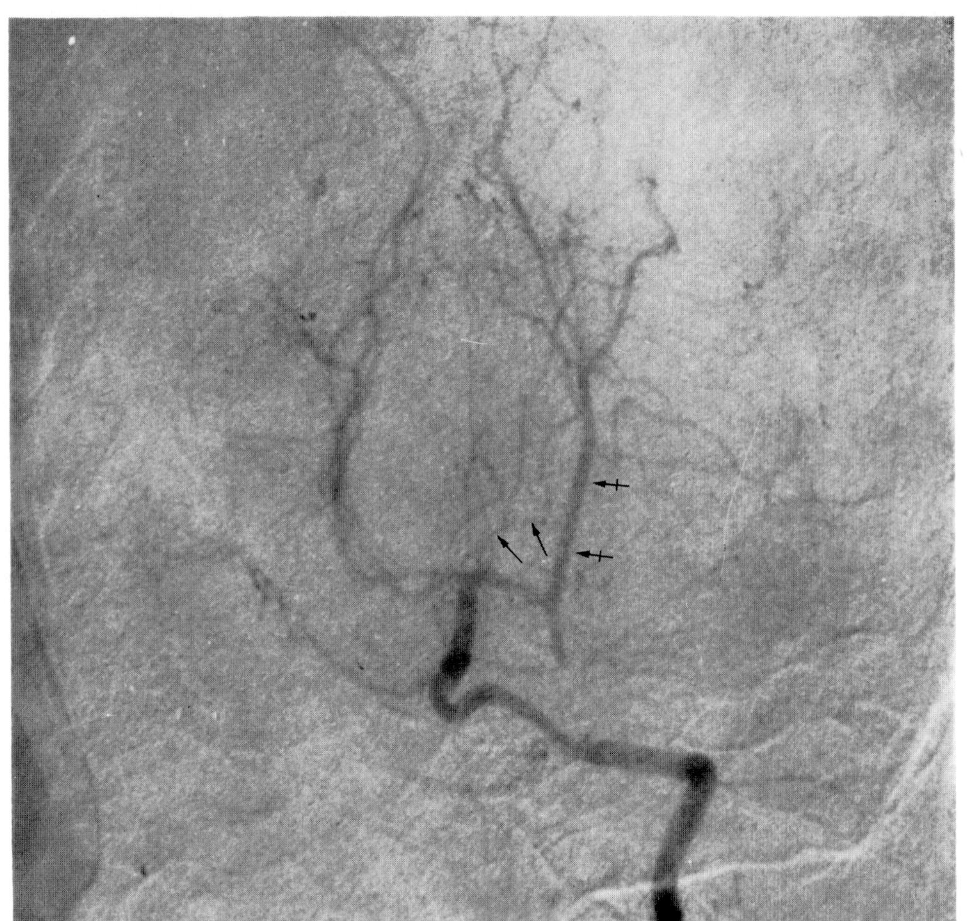

Fig. 194

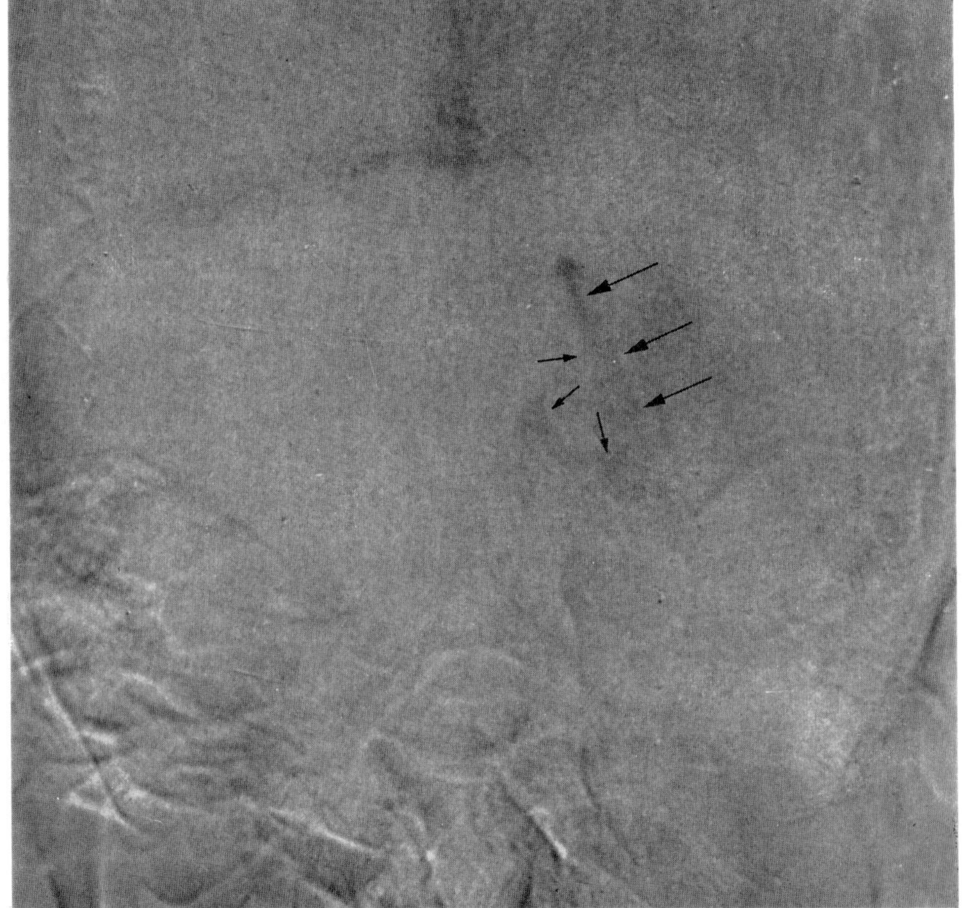

Fig. 195

Right Acoustic Neurinoma

A 44-year-old female: Figs. 196 and 197

Fig. 196 Arterial phase in the Towne projection. The superior cerebellar artery is displaced medially (a large arrow) and the anterior inferior cerebellar artery is elevated in an arcuate fashion (3 short arrows). Arched displacement of an unnamed artery is noted (4 long arrows). These were presumed to be networks of minute arterial branches on the tumor surface at surgery. The posterior cerebral artery is not visualized on the right.

Fig. 197 Venous phase in the Towne projection. An abnormal vein is visualized. The vein originates from the medial, inferior portion of the posterior fossa and courses over the tumor, eventually draining into the petrosal vein (3 short arrows). The right inferior vermian vein is displaced to the left (2 large arrows).

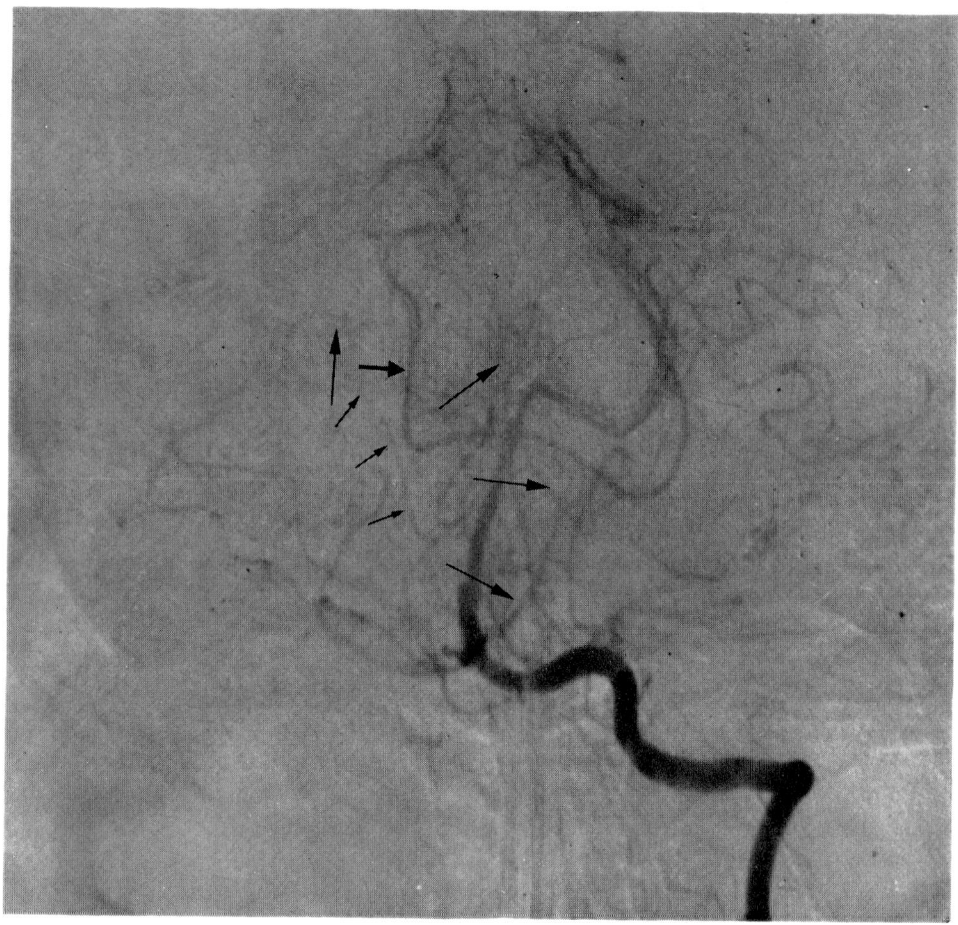

Fig. 196

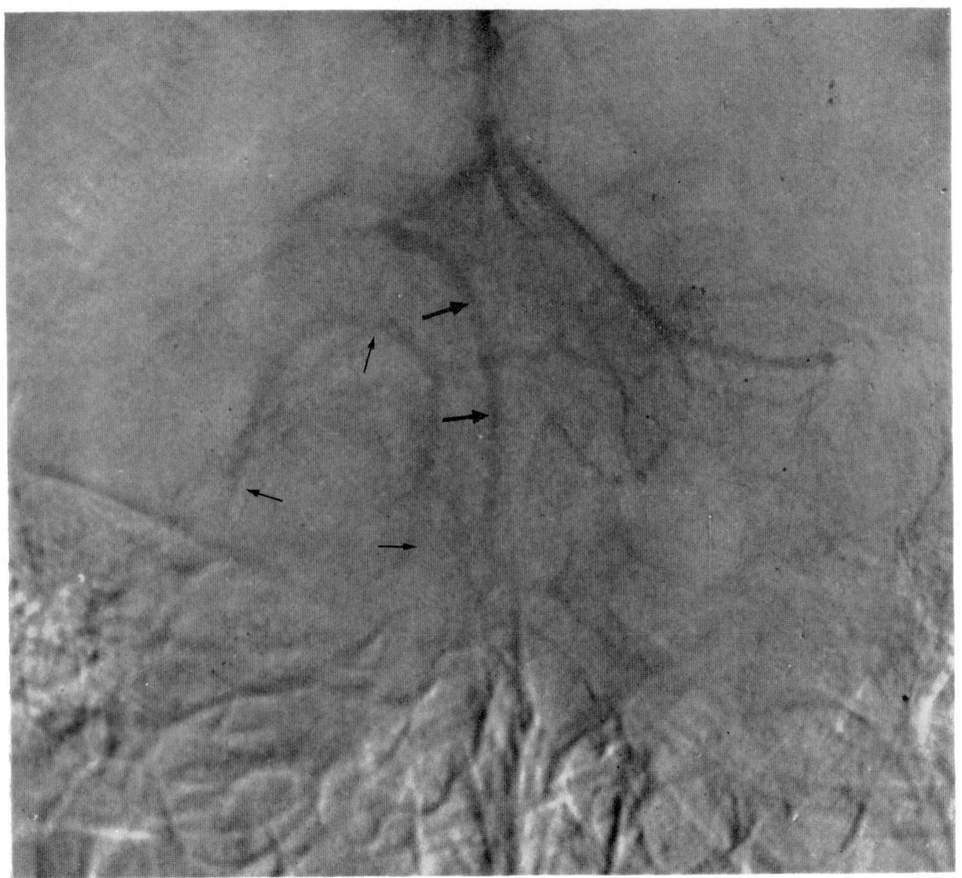

Fig. 197

Meningioma in the Right Cerebellopontine Angle

A 50-year-old female: Figs. 198–200

Fig. 198 Arterial phase in the anteroposterior projection. There is displacement of the basilar artery to the left. The superior cerebellar and posterior cerebral arteries are diffusely elevated on the right (2 arrows). The right anterior inferior cerebellar artery is depressed (2 crossed arrows). All of these findings point to a space-taking lesion in the right cerebellopontine angle. The occipital artery of the right external carotid artery is visualized via the communication with the vertebral artery (3 arrowheads).

Fig. 199 Arterial phase in the lateral projection. The basilar artery is displaced anteriorly. Both the superior cerebellar and the posterior cerebral arteries are elevated on the right (2 crossed arrows). The anterior culminate and the vermian segments of the superior cerebellar artery are compressed against the straight sinus (3 arrows). The anterior inferior cerebellar and anterior meningeal arteries are not identified to good advantage due to superimposition of the arteries. The occipital artery (3 closed arrowheads) and the posterior meningeal artery (4 open arrowheads) are visualized.

Fig. 200 Venous phase in the lateral projection. The interpeduncular segment of the anterior pontomesencephalic vein is superiorly displaced (2 arrows), so is the posterior mesencephalic vein on the right (2 crossed arrows). The left posterior mesencephalic vein is normal (2 closed arrowheads). The precentral cerebellar vein is dislocated posteriorly (a crossed arrow). The copular point and the inferior vermian vein (3 open arrowheads) are displaced in the posterior and superior direction.

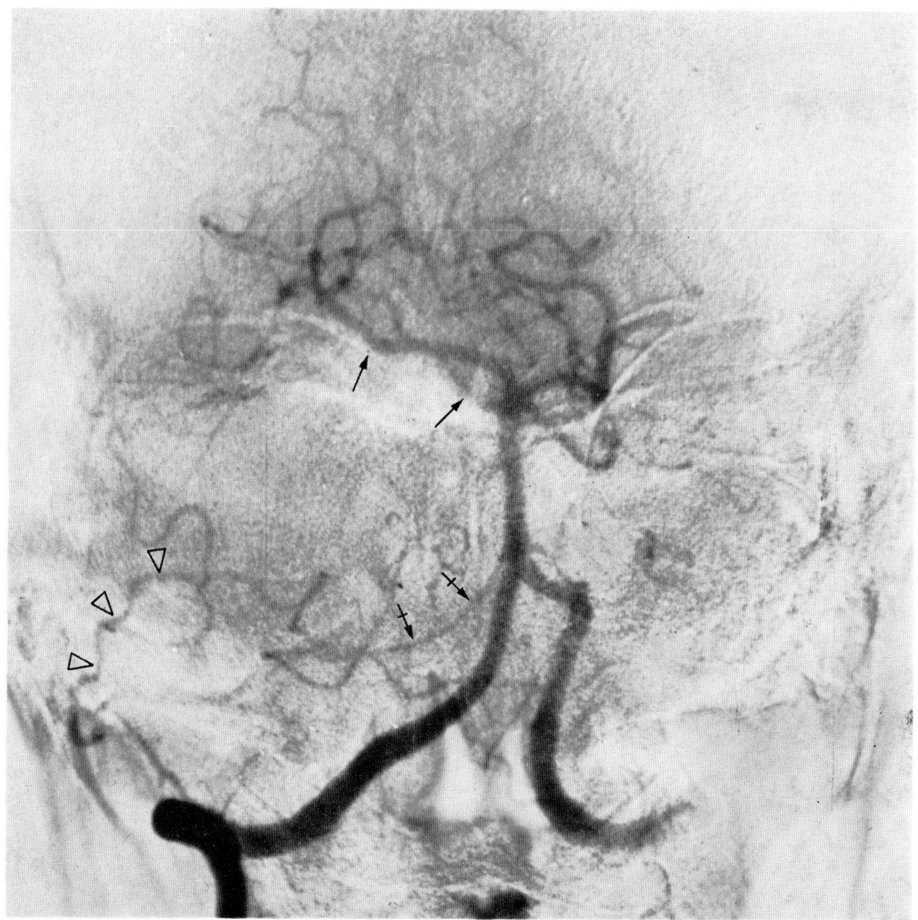

Fig. 198

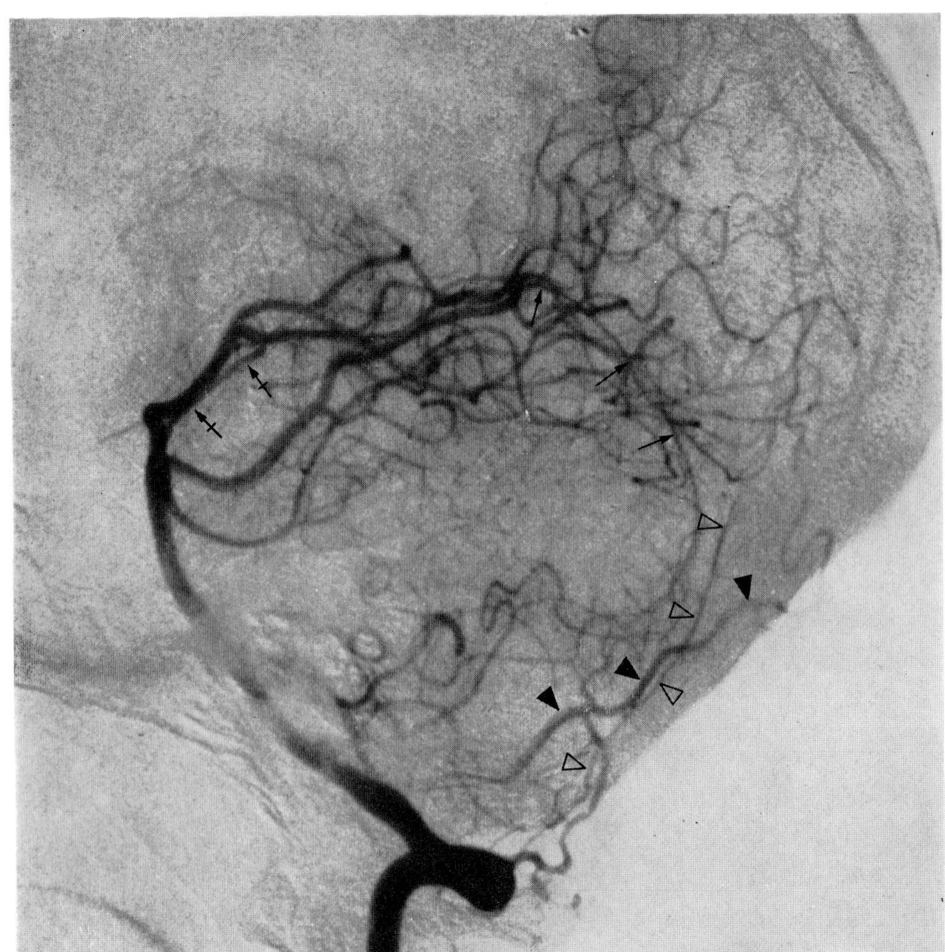

Fig. 199

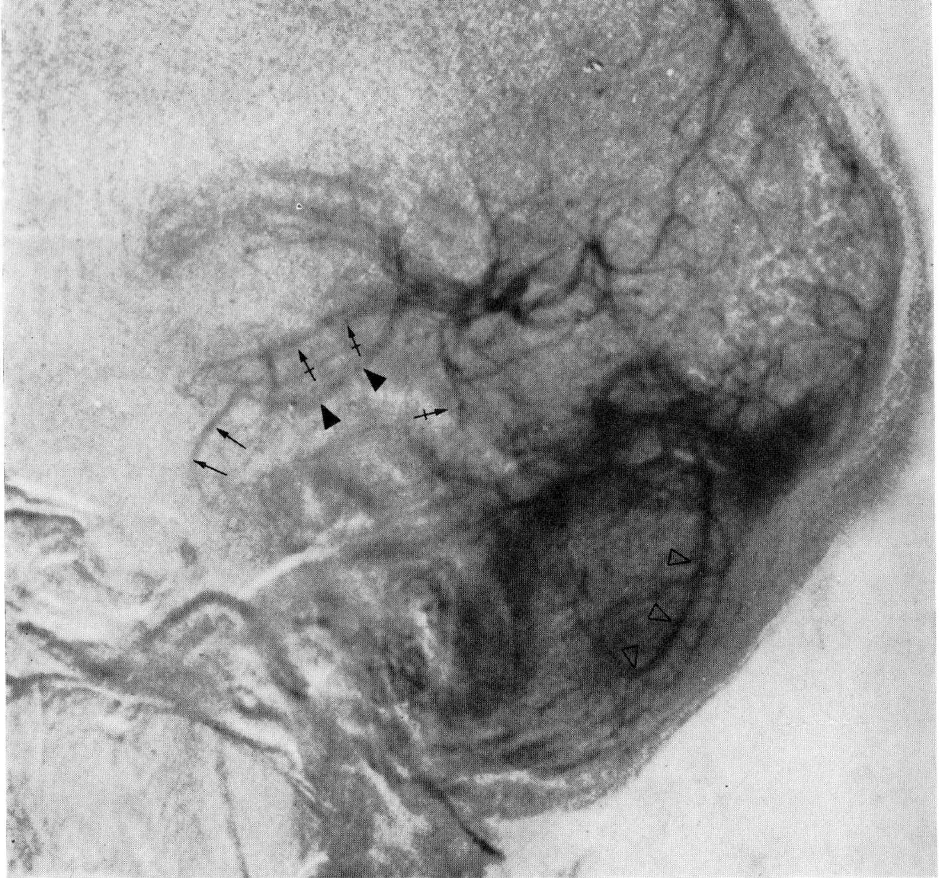

Fig. 200

Neurinoma of the Infratentorial Portion of the Fifth Nerve

A 44-year-old male: Figs. 201–205

The tumor extended towards the cerebellopontine angle.

Fig. 201 Arterial phase in the Towne projection following injection into the left vertebral artery. There is spasm of the distal portion of the left vertebral artery with good filling of the left posterior inferior cerebellar artery (a crossed arrow). The vermian segment is shifted across midline (3 arrows), indicating a mass lesion in the left posterior fossa.

Fig. 202 Right vertebral angiogram in the lateral projection. The tip of the catheter was placed in the right vertebral artery and a successful angiogram was obtained. Arterial phase shows the basilar artery to be displaced posteriorly with increased distance between the dorsum sellae (an arrowhead) and the artery. The marginal artery is displaced superiorly (3 arrows), while the anterior inferior cerebellar artery is depressed in an arcuate fashion (3 crossed arrows).

Fig. 203 Venous phase in the lateral projection. There is posterior displacement of the precentral cerebellar vein (2 arrows). The circumpeduncular segment of the posterior mesencephalic vein is displaced superiorly and posteriorly (2 crossed arrows).

Fig. 204 Arterial phase in the Towne projection. There is displacement of the basilar artery to the right. Superior, arcuate displacement is seen of the proximal superior cerebellar (2 arrows) and marginal arteries (4 crossed arrows). The hemispheric branch of the posterior inferior cerebellar artery is stretched and minimally displaced downwards (3 arrowheads). Arterial displacements suggest a tumor in more anterior, superior and medial location than one would expect in the presence of an acoustic neurinoma.

Fig. 205 Venous phase in the Towne projection. The left petrosal vein is displaced laterally (an arrow).

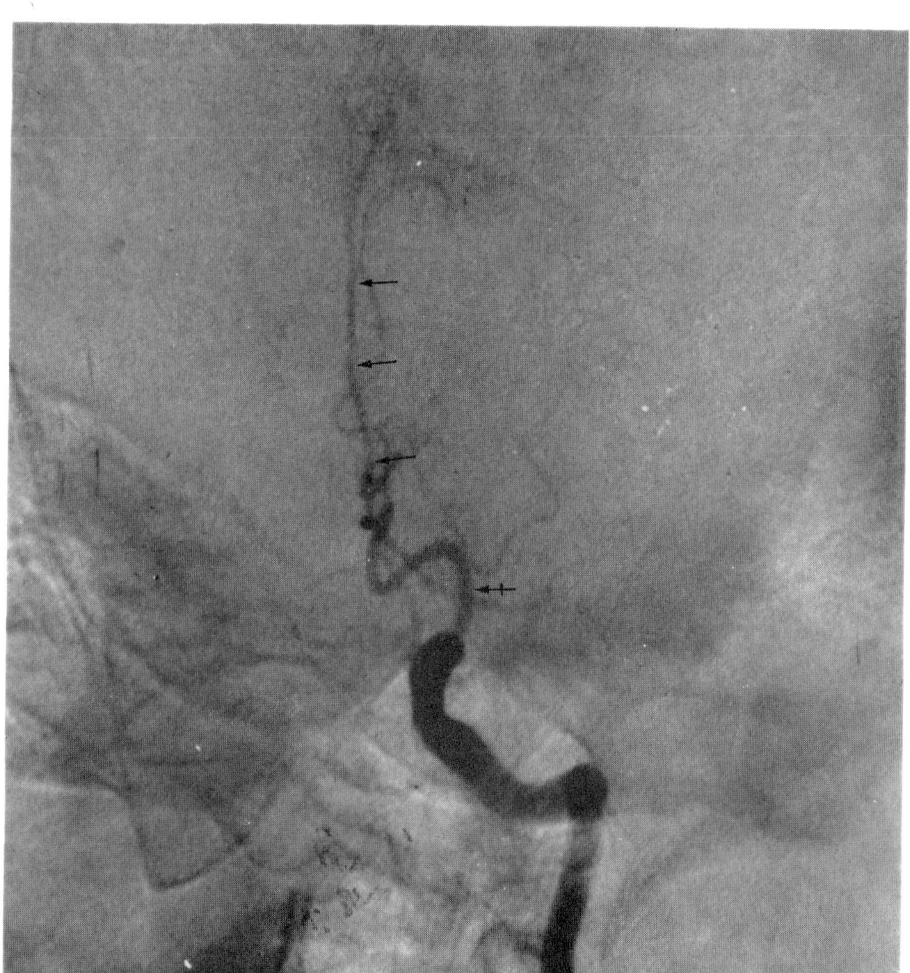

Fig. 201

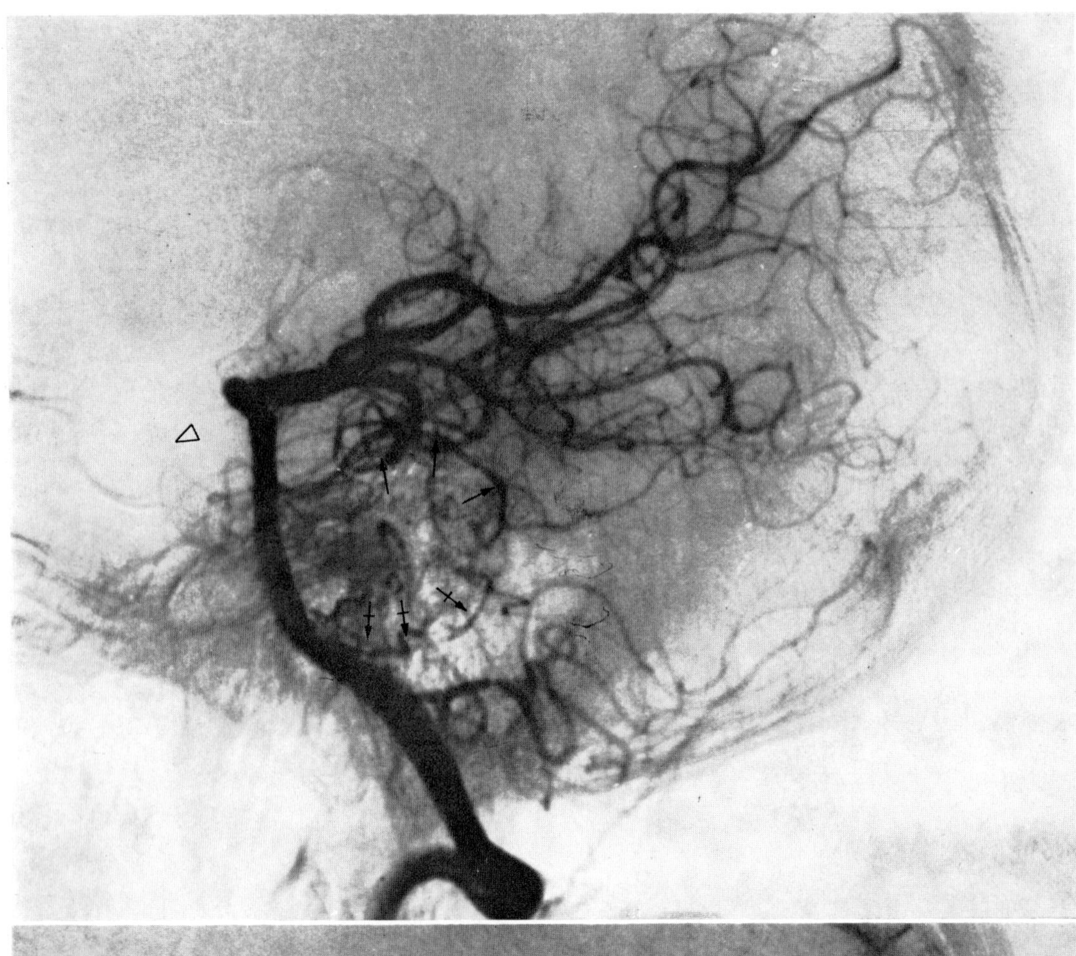

Fig. 202

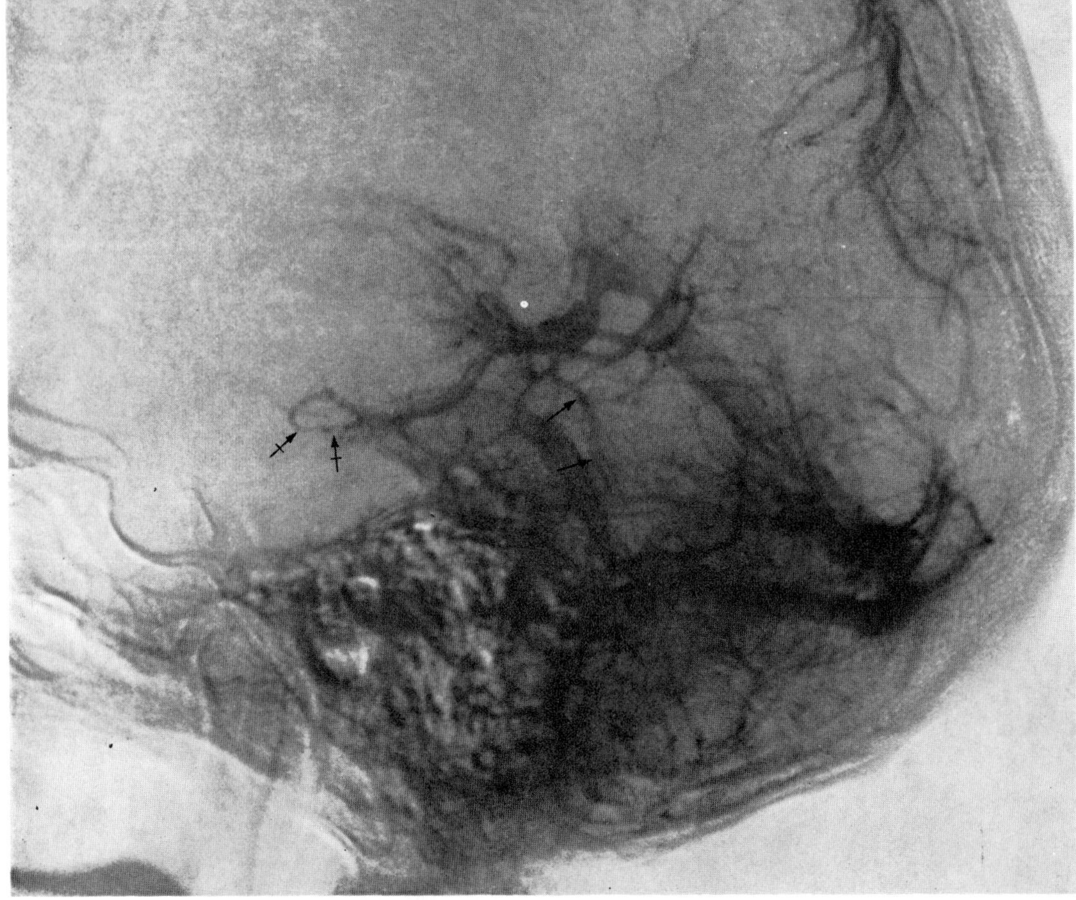

Fig. 203

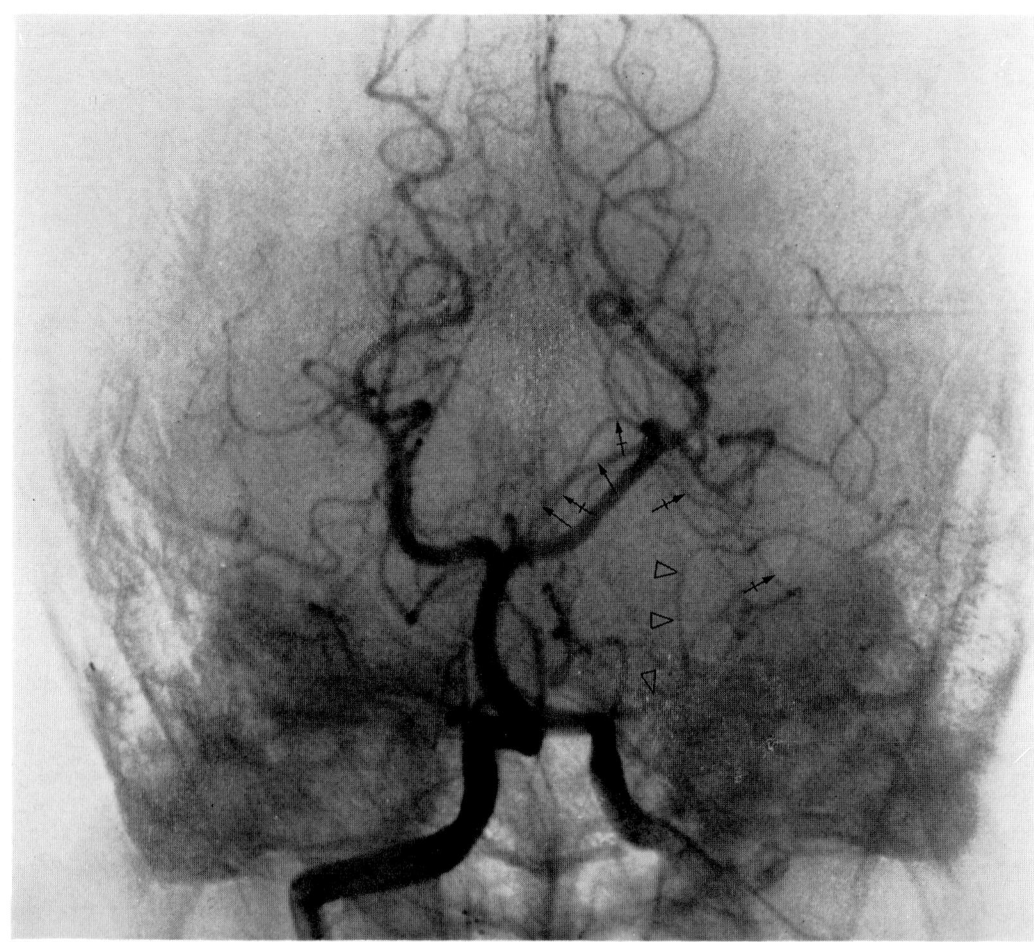

Fig. 204

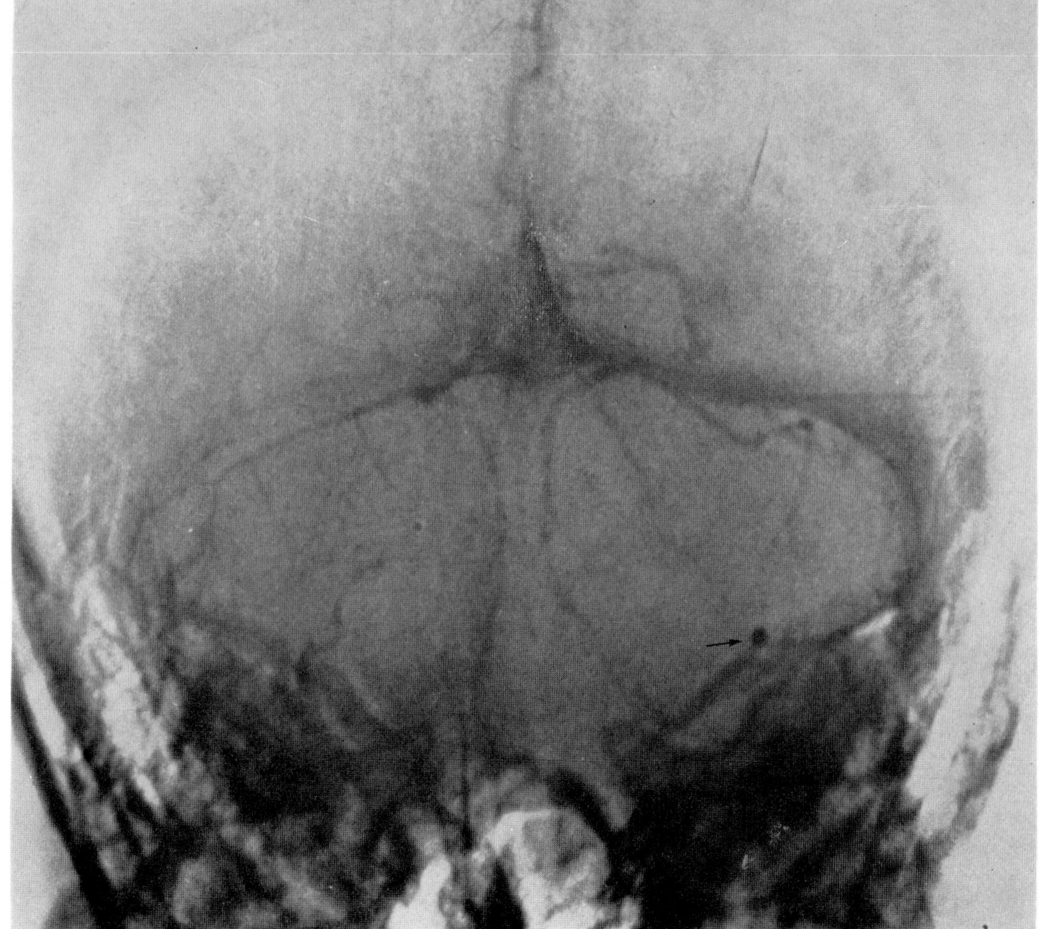

Fig. 205

Direct Extension of Pinealoma into the Left Cerebellopontine Angle

A 21-year-old male: Figs. 206–210

Fig. 206 Arterial phase in the Towne projection. The superior cerebellar and posterior cerebral arteries are diffusely elevated (3 arrows). There is minimal displacement of the distal basilar artery to the right.

Fig. 207 Venous phase in the Towne projection. The petrosal vein is elevated and laterally displaced (2 arrows). These arterial and venous findings suggest presence of a mass lesion in the left cerebellopontine angle.

Fig. 208 Arterial phase in the anteroposterior projection. The common trunk of the anterior inferior and posterior inferior cerebellar arteries is depressed in an arcuate fashion (3 arrows). The superior cerebellar and posterior cerebral arteries are elevated on the left (3 crossed arrows). The distal segment of the basilar artery is displaced across the midline.

Fig. 209 Arterial phase in the lateral projection. The basilar artery is displaced posteriorly, its distal portion being most markedly displaced (3 arrows). The superior cerebellar and posterior cerebral arteries are elevated on the left (open arrowheads). The common trunk of the posterior and anterior inferior cerebellar arteries is seen on each side (a crossed arrow). One of the posterior choroidal arteries appears to be displaced backwards (3 closed arrowheads), secondary to a mass in the pineal region.

Fig. 210 Venous phase in the lateral projection. The anterior pontomesencephalic vein is displaced posteriorly (2 arrows). There is elevation of the petrosal vein (2 crossed arrows). All the angiographic findings are those of a mass in the left cerebellopontine angle, but marked displacement of the upper pons indicates a supratentorial mass extending into the cerebellopontine angle.

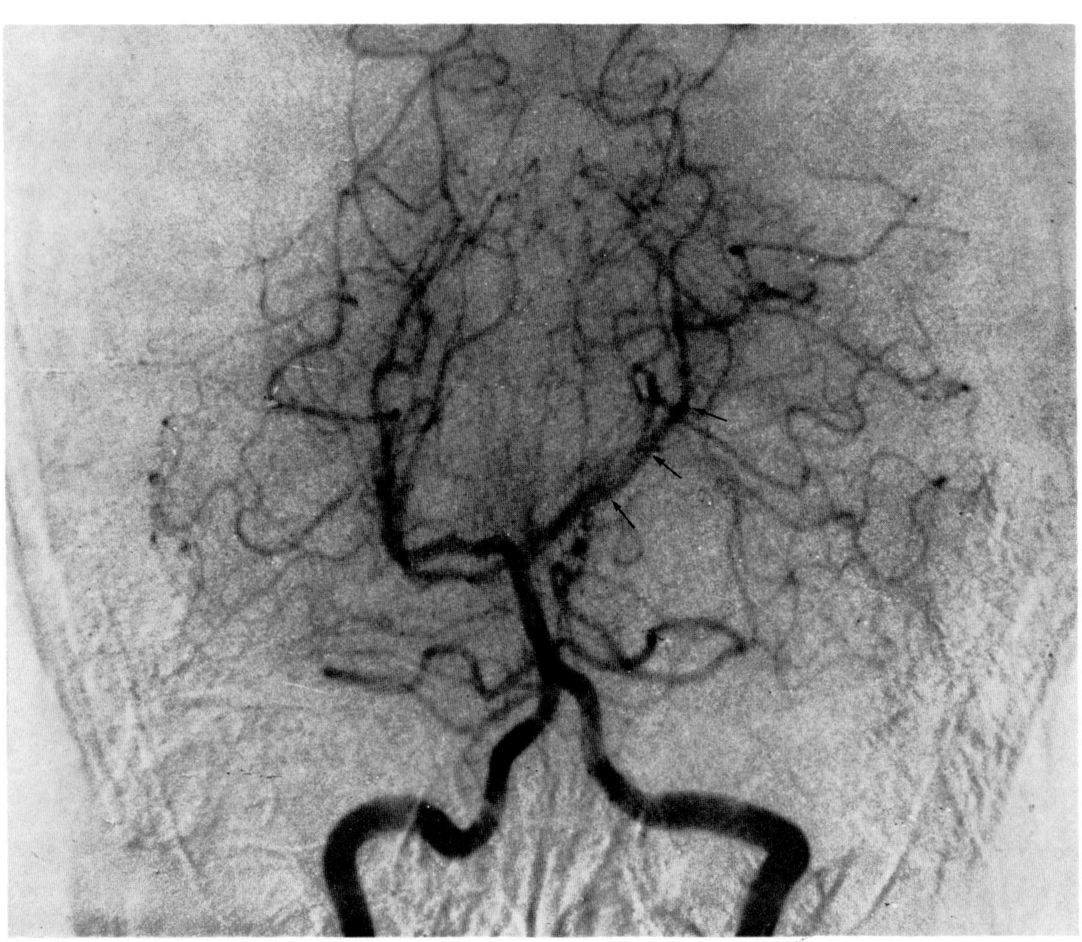

Fig. 206

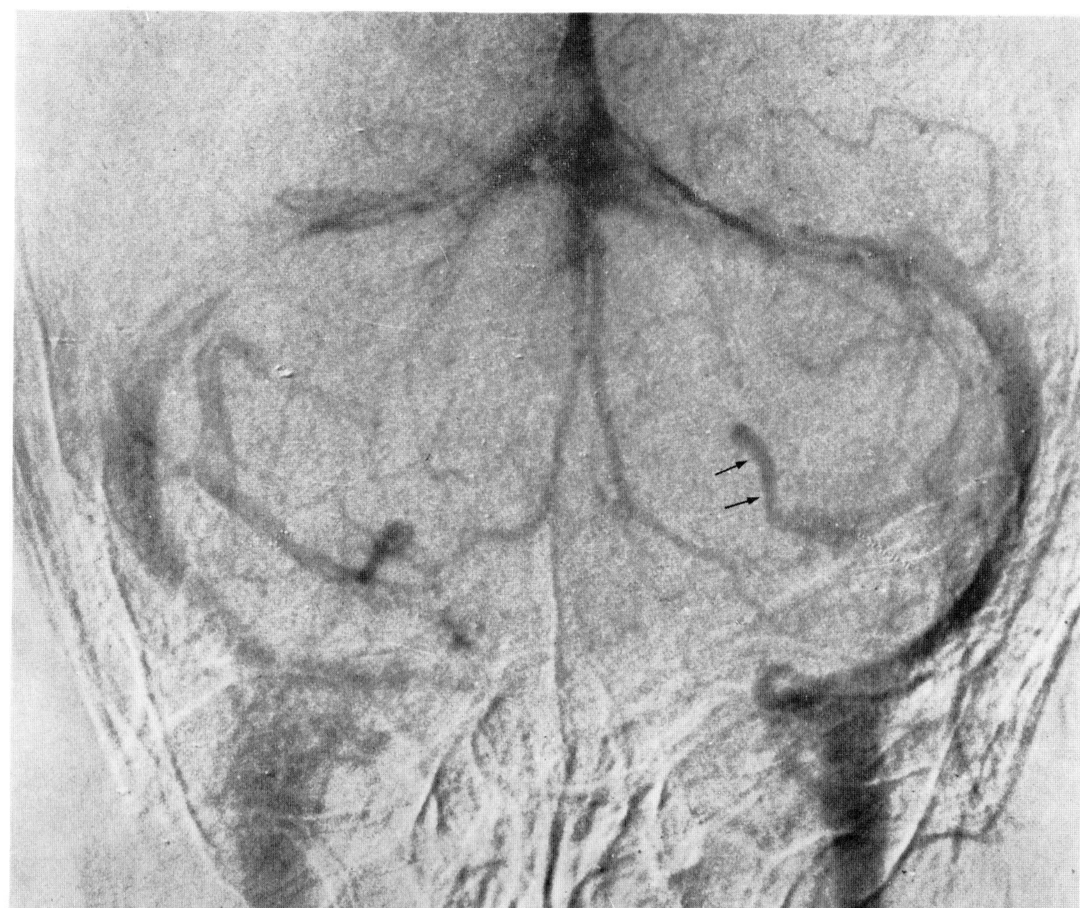

Fig. 207

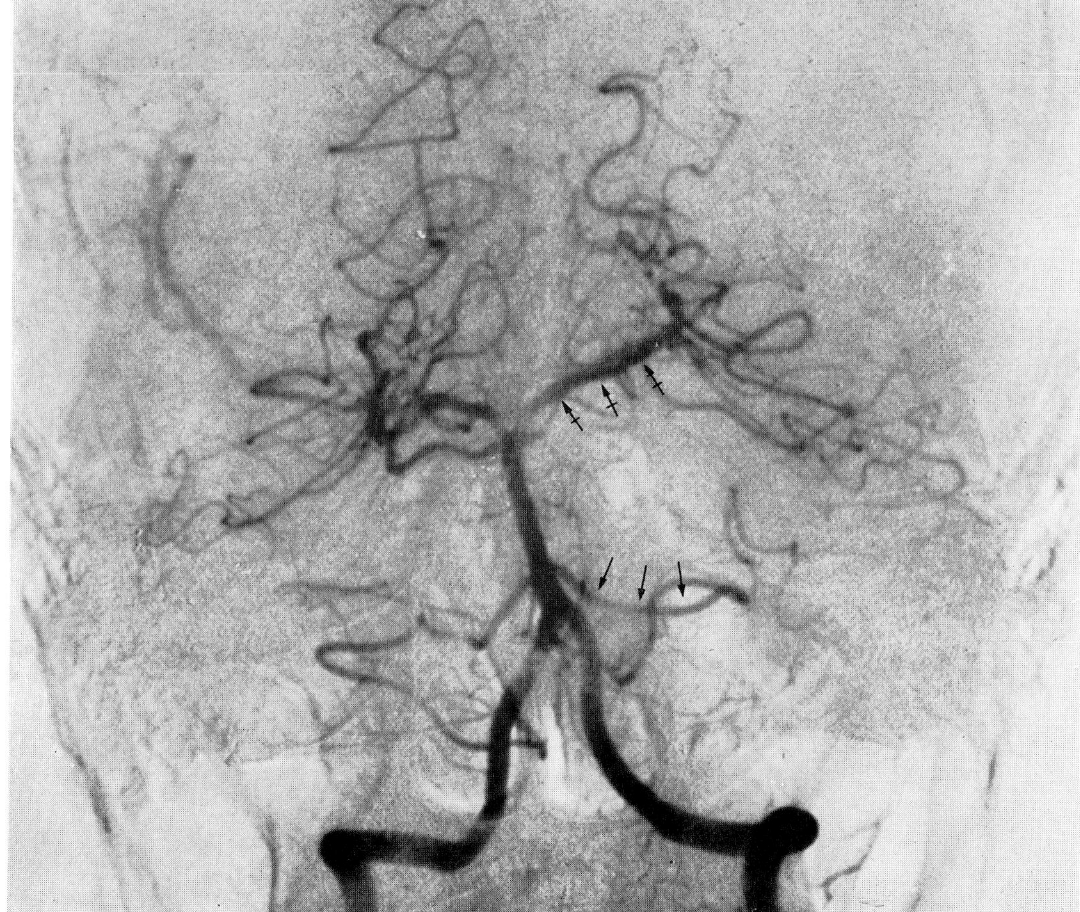

Fig. 208

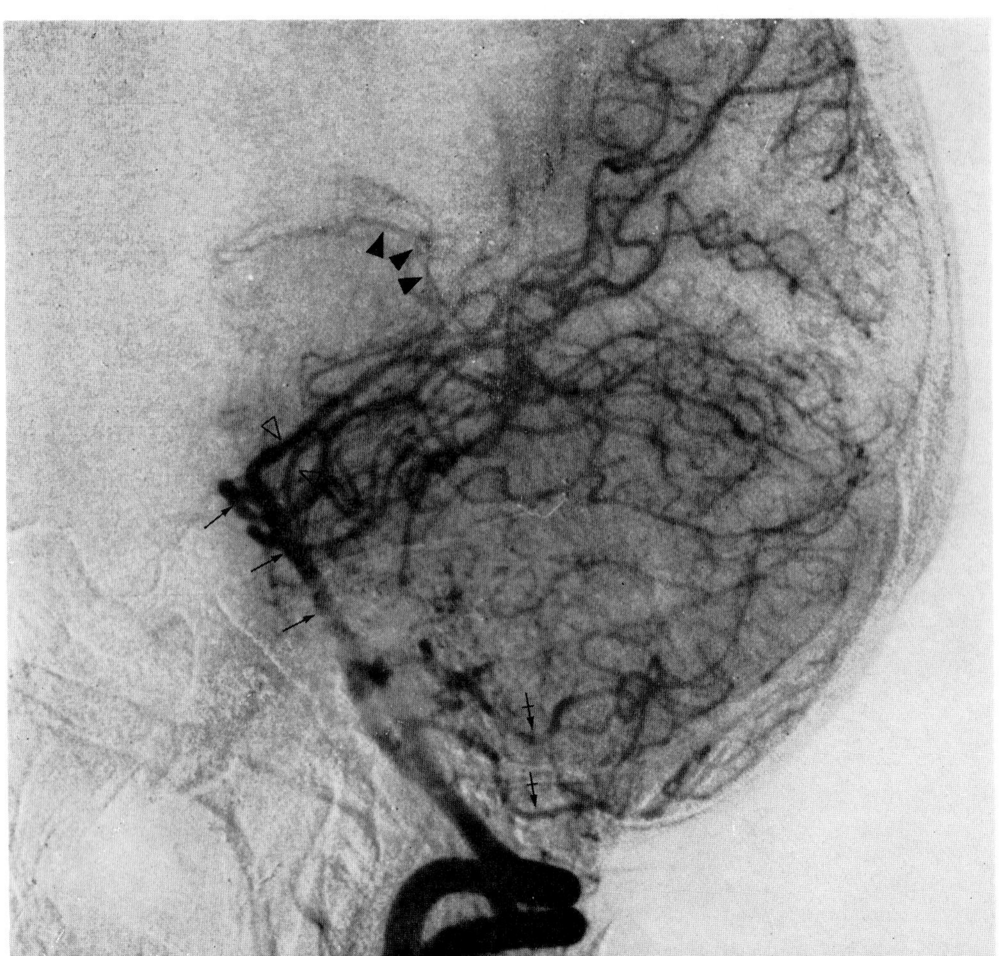

Fig. 209

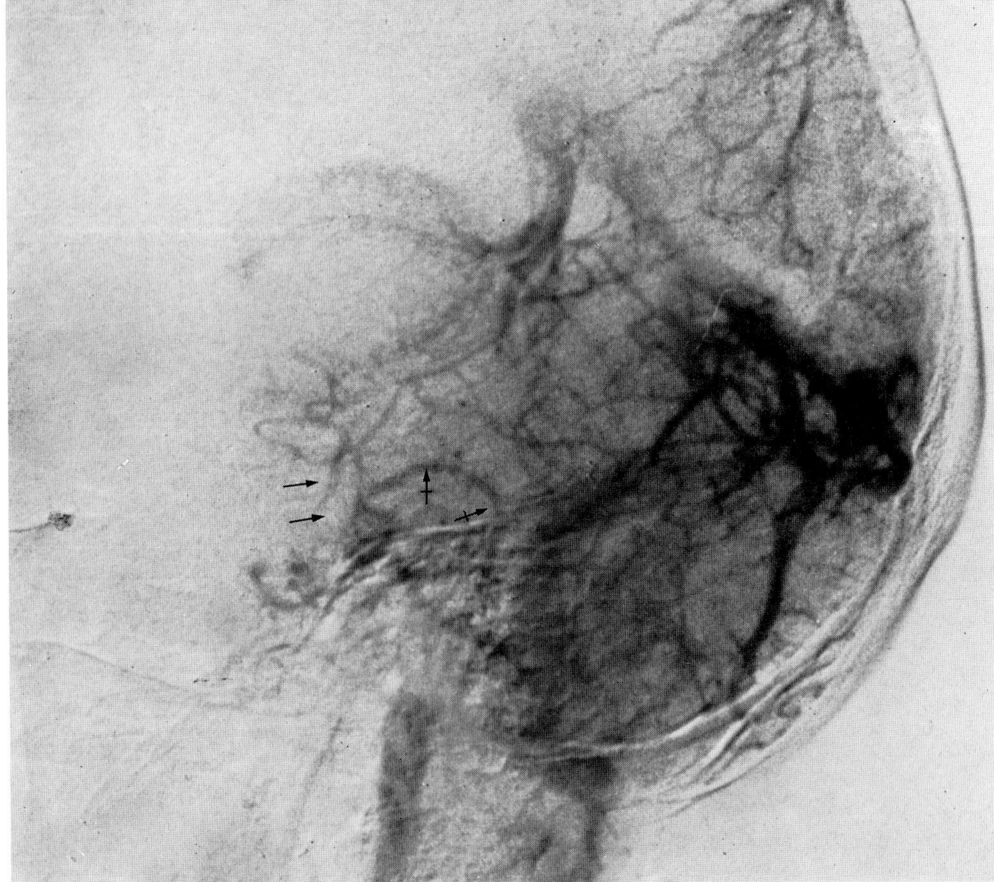

Fig. 210

TUMORS OVER THE CLIVUS

Arteriographic features

Basilar artery

The basilar artery is usually displaced posteriorly and laterally depending upon the origin of the lesion. When posterior displacement of this artery is present, the "paradoxical phenomenon" in the presence of pontine tumors should be differentiated. The pontine branches of the basilar artery are also displaced posteriorly in the presence of clivus tumors.

Anterior inferior cerebellar artery

This artery is usually elevated as seen on the straight anteroposterior projection when the tumor is large or extends into the cerebellopontine angle.

Posterior inferior cerebellar artery

The artery is generally displaced posteriorly due to posterior displacement of the brain stem. The caudal and cranial loops may be displaced posteriorly and are narrowed. The vermian segment may be displaced laterally if the tumor extends primarily to one side.

Superior cerebellar artery

The lateral portion of the interpeduncular-crural segment and the anterior portion of the ambient segment may be diffusely elevated. The angle formed by these two segments is frequently blunted in the Towne projection. When the tumor extends into the cerebellopontine angle, differentiation from cerebellopontine angle tumors is quite difficult.

Venographic features

Anterior group

The main trunk of the petrosal vein is laterally displaced and the transverse pontine veins are lifted away from the clivus in the Towne projection. The lateral projection usually shows posterior displacement of the anterior pontomesencephalic vein.

Superior group

The precentral cerebellar vein is always displaced posteriorly with somewhat decreased colliculocentral angle. The superior vermian vein and the lateral anastomotic mesencephalic vein may be displaced posteriorly.

Posterior group

The superior retrotonsillar and inferior retrotonsillar tributaries may be displaced posteriorly. The copular angle is narrowed and the copular point is displaced posteriorly in the presence of a large clivus tumor.

Nasopharyngeal Carcinoma Extending into the Posterior Fossa

A 55-year-old male: Figs. 211–214

Fig. 211 Arterial phase in the lateral projection. The basilar artery is straightened and displaced posteriorly (3 arrows). The posterior medullary and supratonsillar segments of the posterior inferior cerebellar artery are slightly displaced backwards (3 crossed arrows).

Fig. 212 Venous phase in the lateral projection. The pontine segment of the anterior pontomesencephalic vein is posteriorly dislocated (2 arrows). The inferior vermian veins are also displaced backwards (2 crossed arrows). The precentral cerebellar vein is also displaced backwards (an arrowhead).

Fig. 213 Arterial phase in the Towne projection. The right anterior inferior cerebellar artery is elevated (3 arrows) and the crural and ambient segments of the superior cerebellar artery are displaced upwards (2 crossed arrows), indicating tumor extension into the right cerebellopontine angle. The vermian segment of the right posterior inferior cerebellar artery is displaced across the midline (3 arrowheads).

Fig. 214 Venous phase in the Towne projection. The transverse pontine veins are elevated, outlining the extent of the tumor (2 lateral arrows). The right petrosal vein is dislocated laterally (a crossed arrow). The inferior vermian veins are displaced superiorly and separated (4 arrowheads). The veins over the pons are displaced posteriorly and to the left (2 medial arrows).

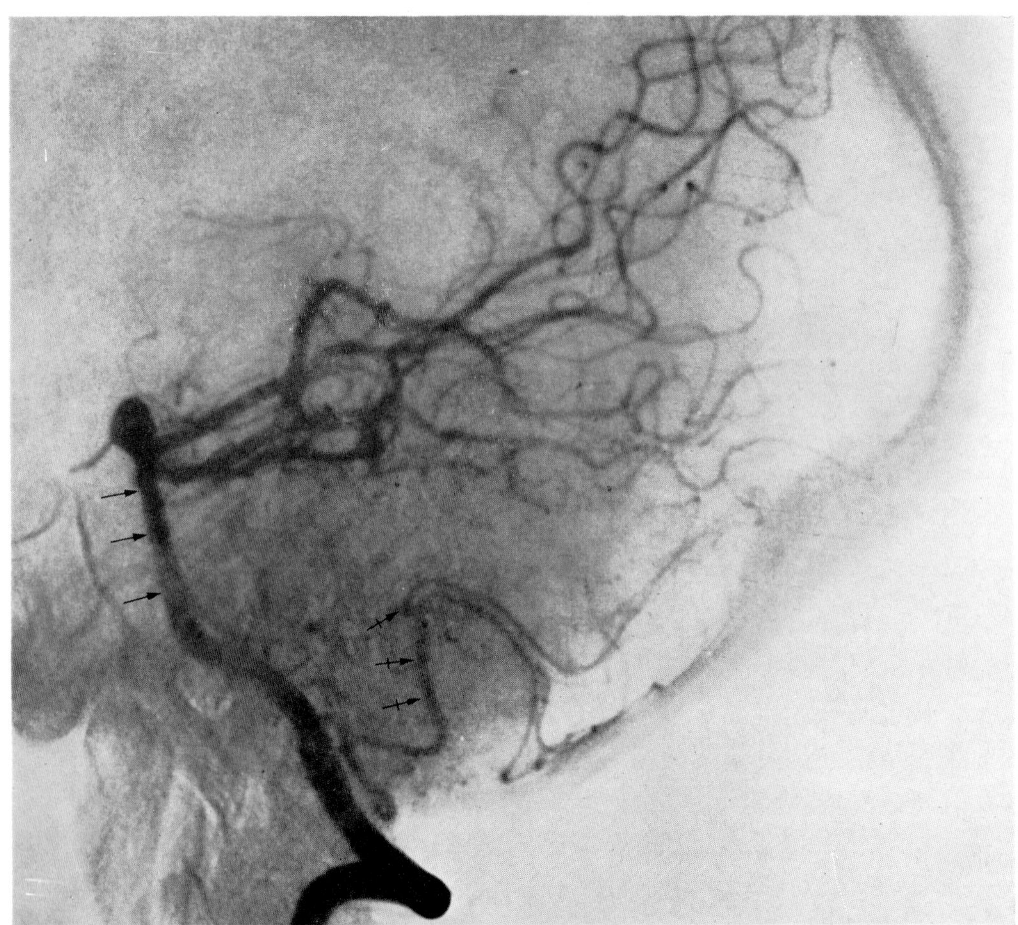

Fig. 211

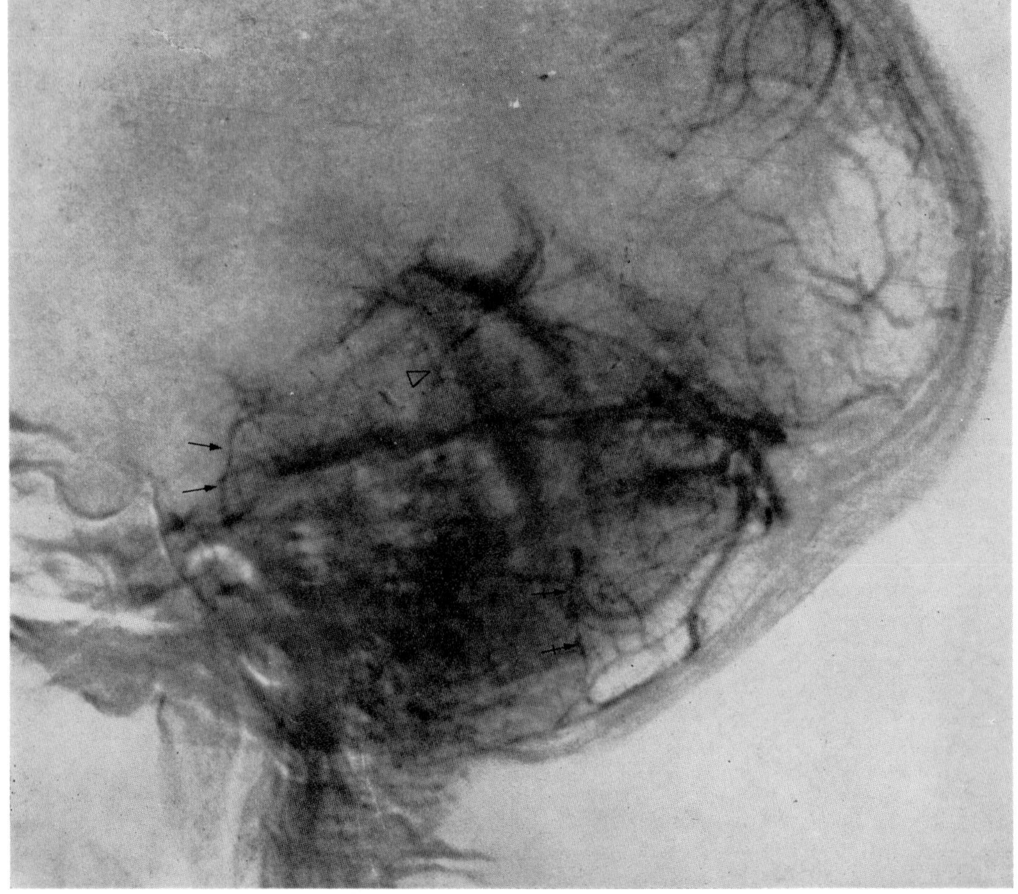

Fig. 212

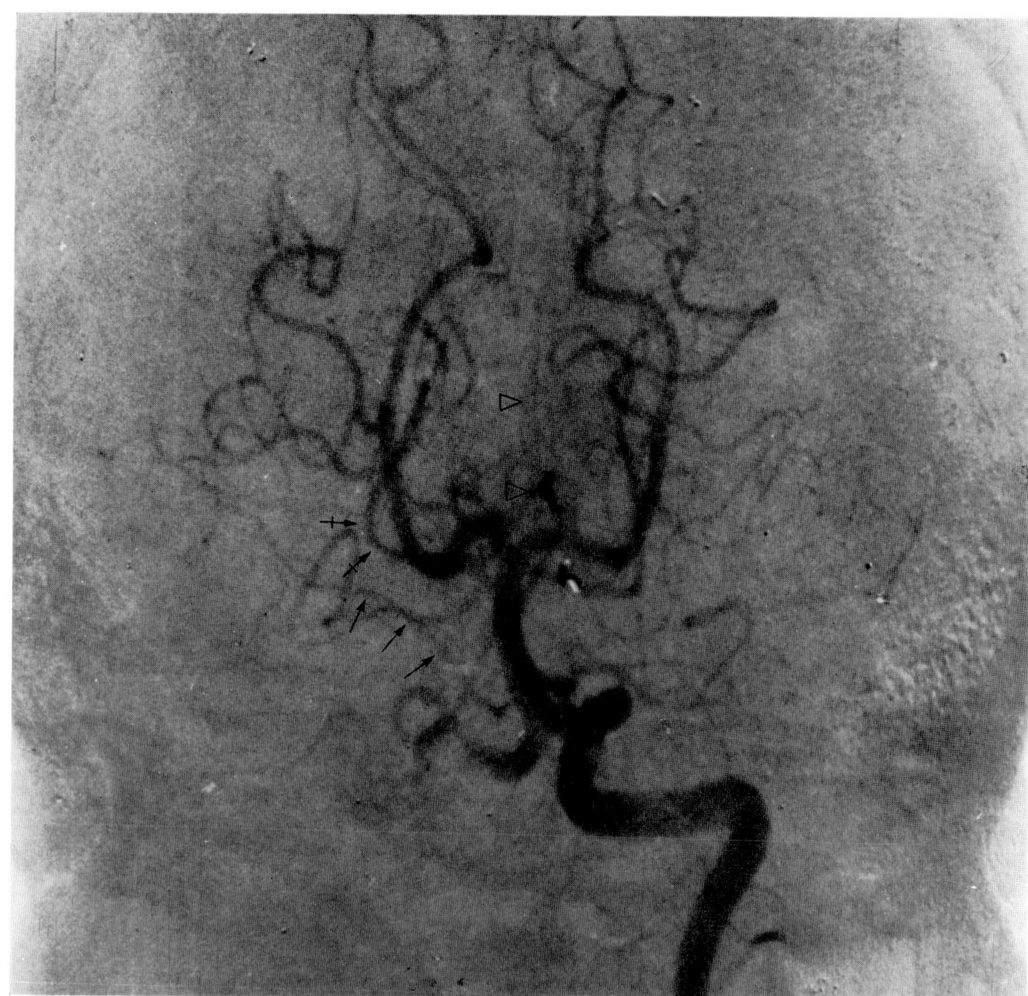

Fig. 213

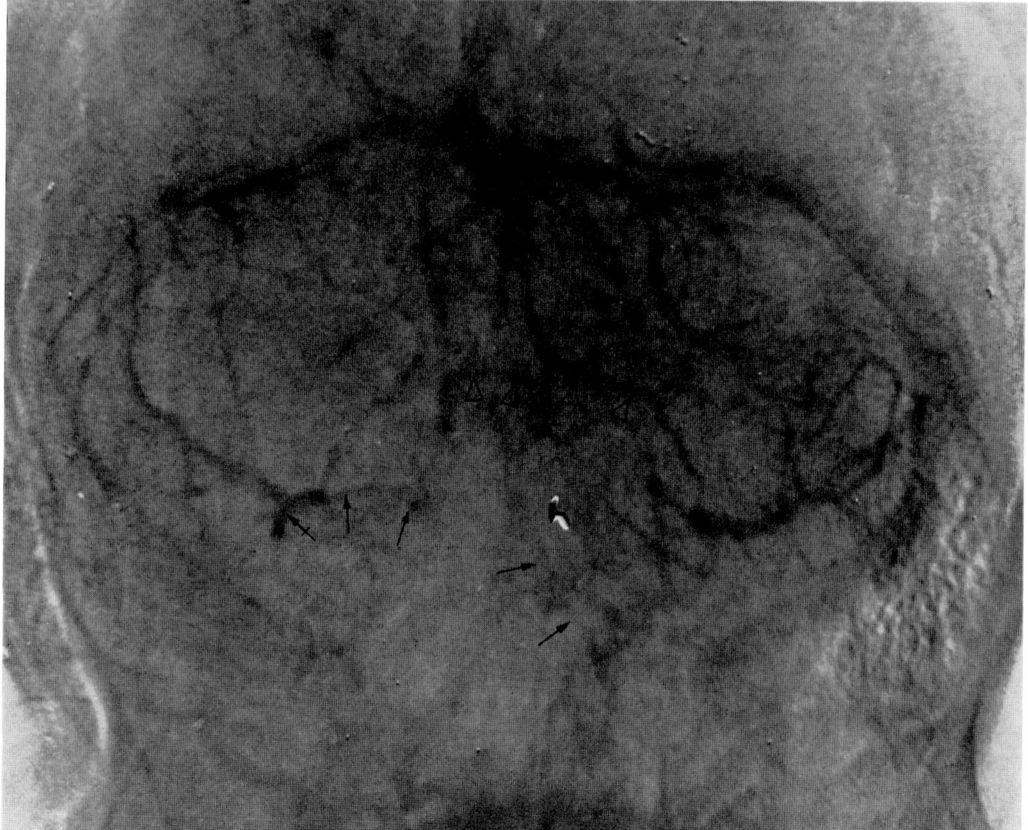

Fig. 214

Chordoma over the Clivus Extending into the Right Cerebellopontine Angle

A 20-year-old male: Figs. 215 and 216

Fig. 215 Arterial phase in the lateral projection. The proximal portion of the basilar artery and the intracranial segments of both vertebral arteries are displaced posteriorly (3 arrows). The lateral medullary and posterior medullary segments of the posterior inferior cerebellar artery are stretched in the anteroposterior direction (3 crossed arrows) with posterior displacement and angulation of the supratonsillar segment (an arrowhead).

Fig. 216 Arterial phase in the anteroposterior projection. There is common origin of the anterior inferior and posterior inferior cerebellar arteries bilaterally. On the right there is elevation of both the anterior inferior (2 arrows) and the posterior inferior (2 crossed arrows) cerebellar arteries. There is an accessory posterior inferior cerebellar artery from the basilar artery (an open arrowhead). These findings indicate tumor extension into the right cerebellopontine angle. The right superior cerebellar and posterior cerebral arteries are elevated (2 open arrowheads).

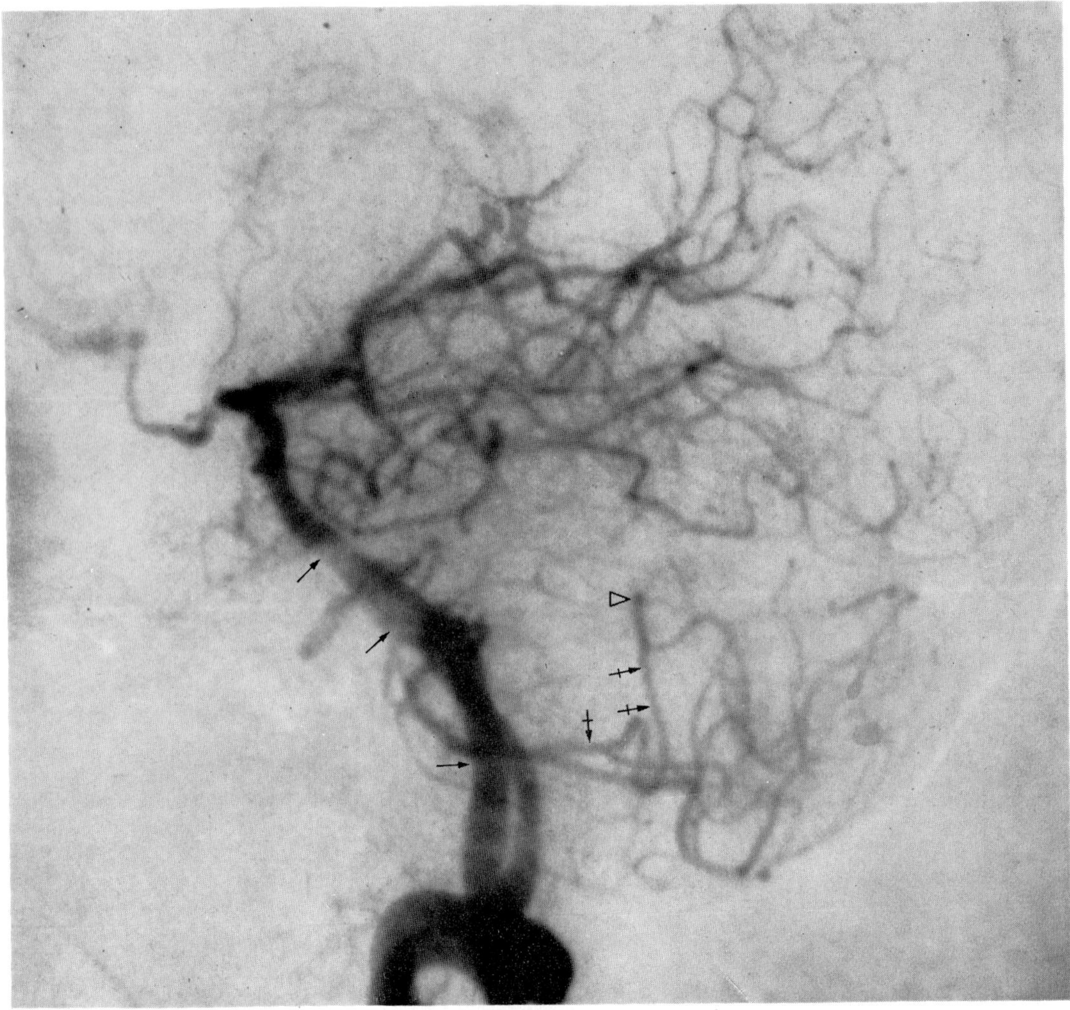

Fig. 215

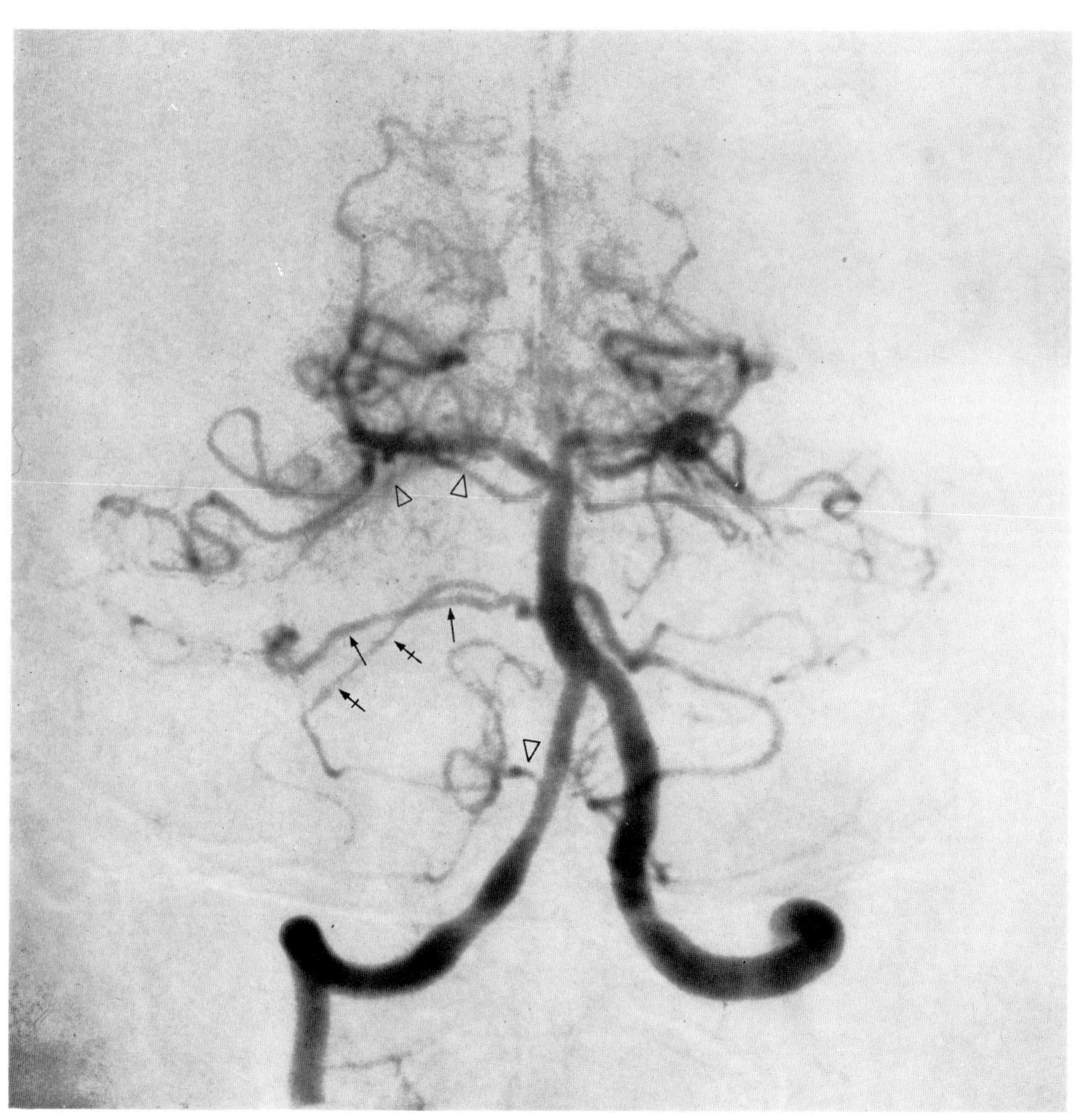

Fig. 216

Multiple Myeloma of the Skull Base Destroying the Right Petrous Apex and the Clivus

A 44-year-old female: Figs. 217–219

Fig. 217 Arterial phase in the lateral projection. The basilar artery is bowed posteriorly with increased distance between the clivus and the basilar artery (3 arrows). The posterior meningeal artery is well shown, but has no clinical significance (2 crossed arrows). The posterior inferior cerebellar arteries are visualized faintly.

Fig. 218 Arterial phase in the Towne projection. The distal vertebral and proximal basilar arteries are displaced to the left (3 arrows). The superior cerebellar artery is diffusely elevated on the right (2 crossed arrows). There is an avascular area in the right cerebellopontine angle.

Fig. 219 Right carotid angiogram in the lateral projection. Extensive tumor stains are noted at the base of the skull. Blood supply is from the external carotid artery.

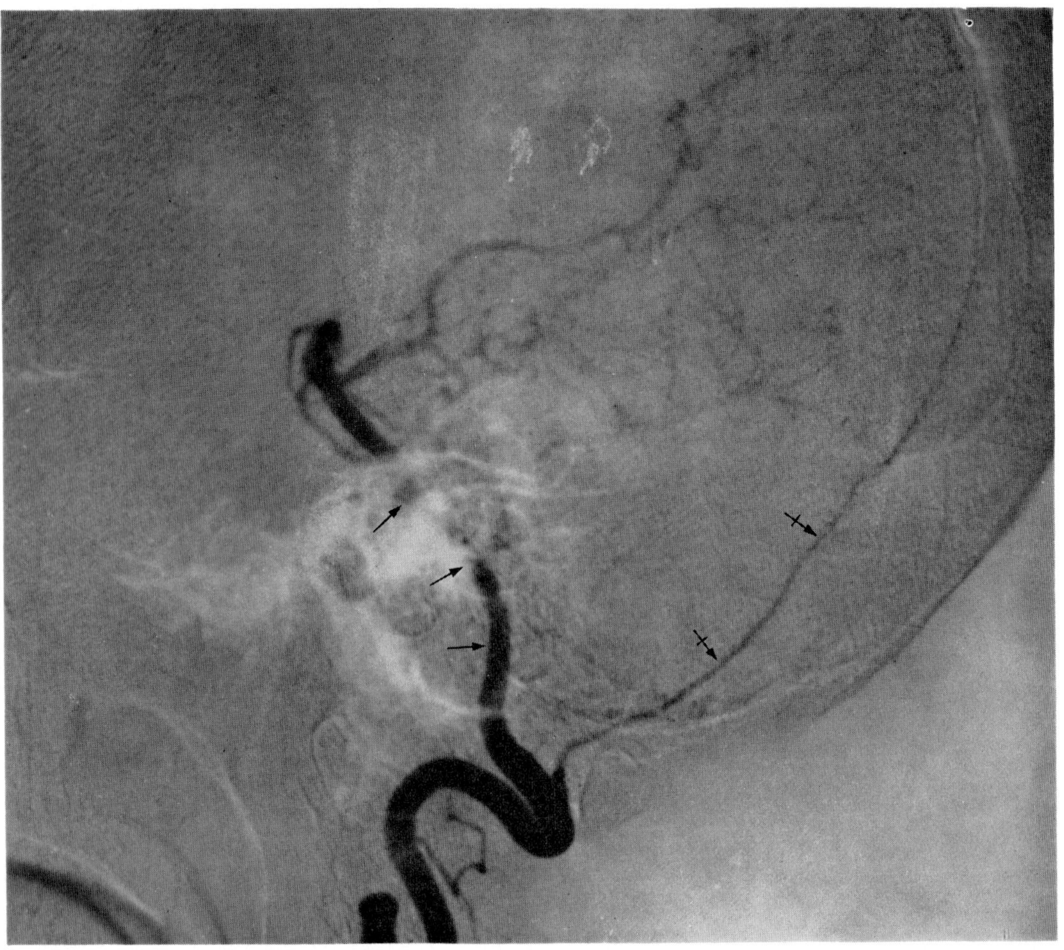

Fig. 217

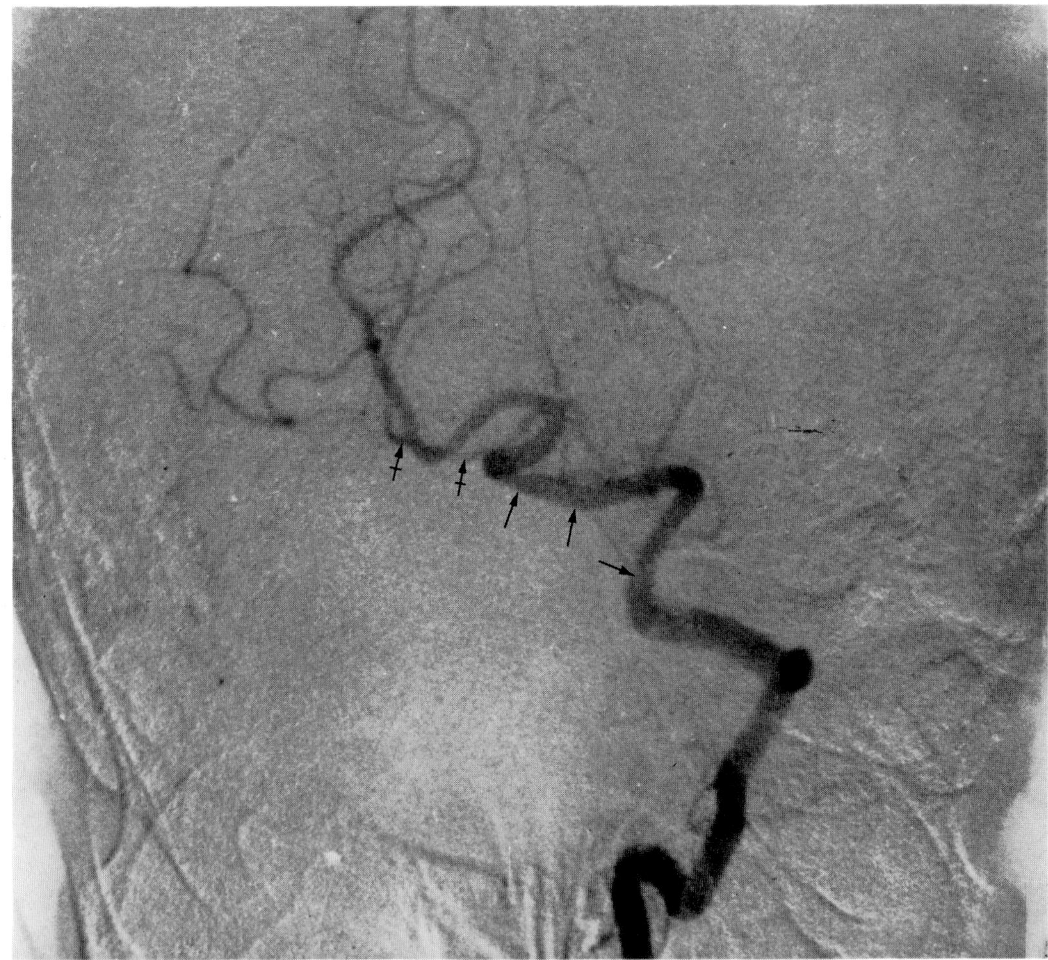

Fig. 218

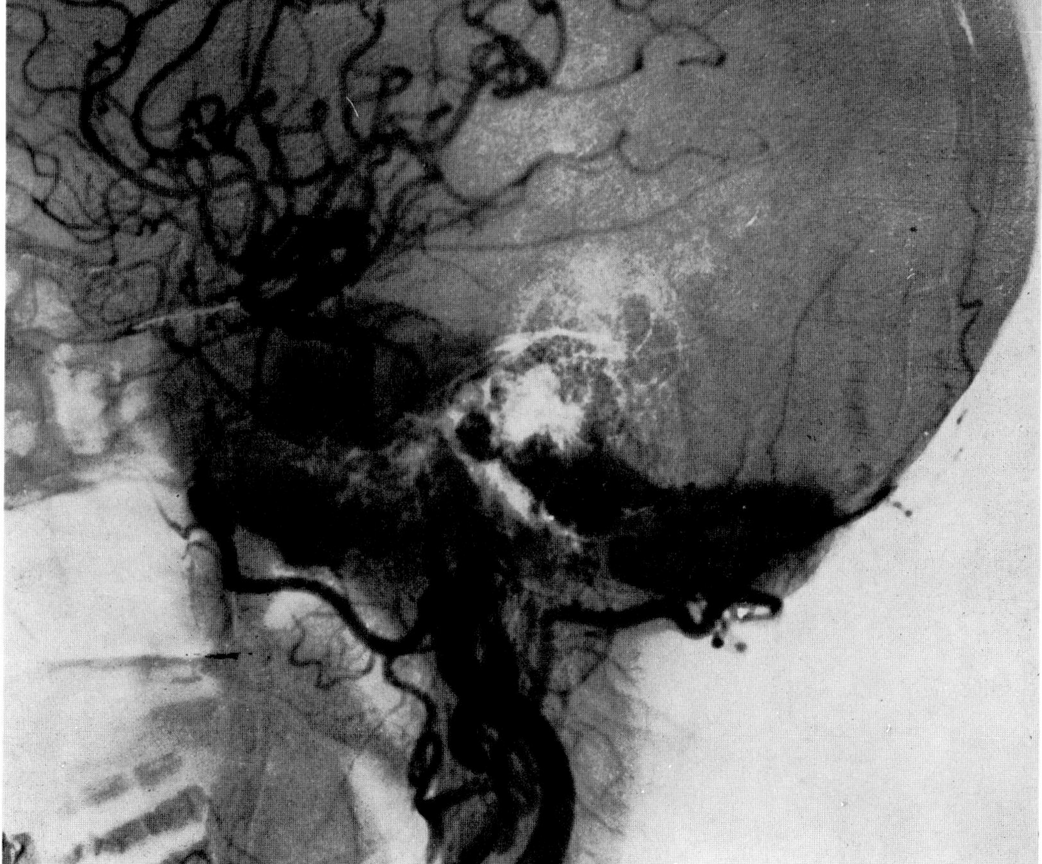

Fig. 219

Malignant Lymphoma of the Nasopharynx Extending into the Posterior Fossa by Destruction of the Clivus

A 31-year-old male: Figs. 220 and 221

Fig. 220. Arterial phase in the lateral projection. The basilar artery is displaced backward with straightening (3 arrows). The supratonsillar segment of the posterior inferior cerebellar artery (a crossed arrow) and the marginal artery from the superior cerebellar artery (3 open arrowheads) are displaced in the posterior direction. Note good visualization of the anterior spinal artery (2 closed arrowheads).

Fig. 221 Venous phase in the lateral projection. The pontine segment of the anterior pontomesencephalic vein is displaced posteriorly (2 arrows), so is the petrosal vein (3 crossed arrows). The precentral cerebellar vein is displaced backward as well (3 arrowheads).

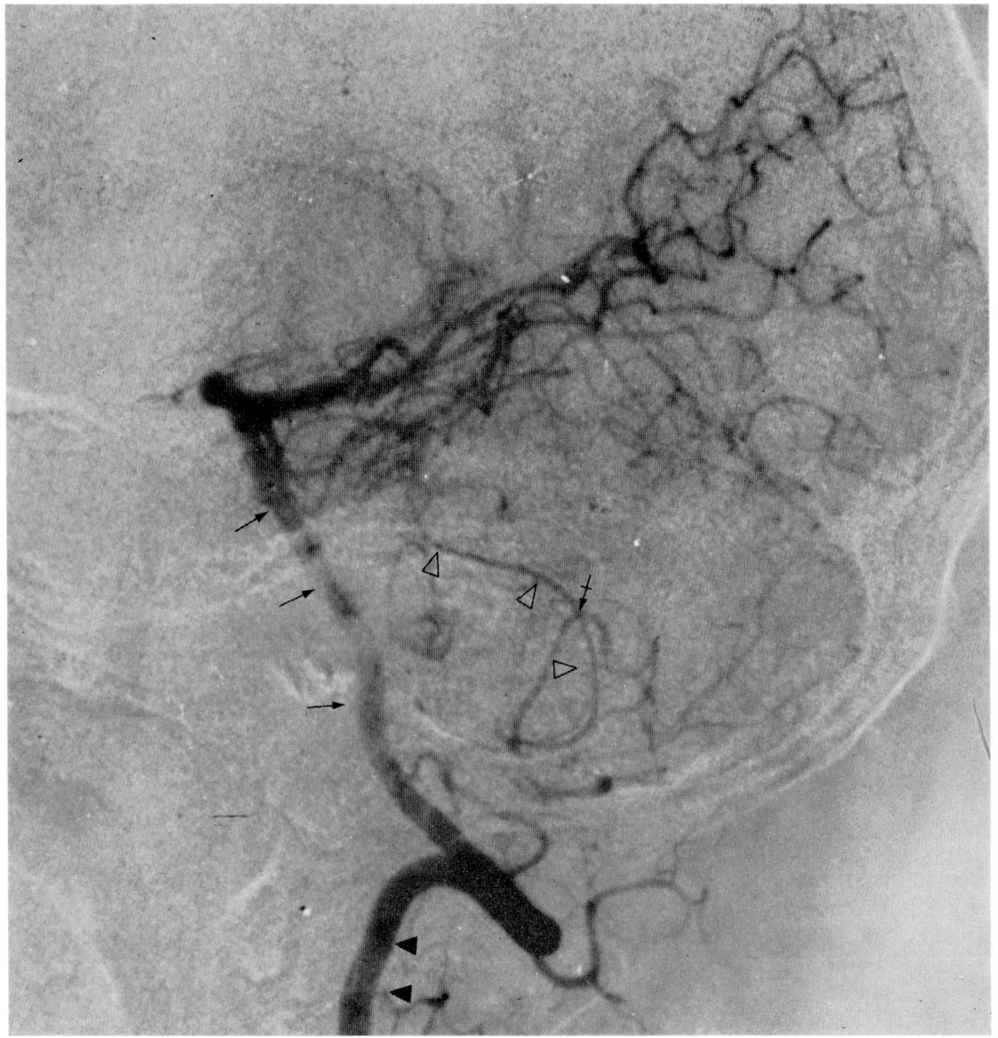

Fig. 220

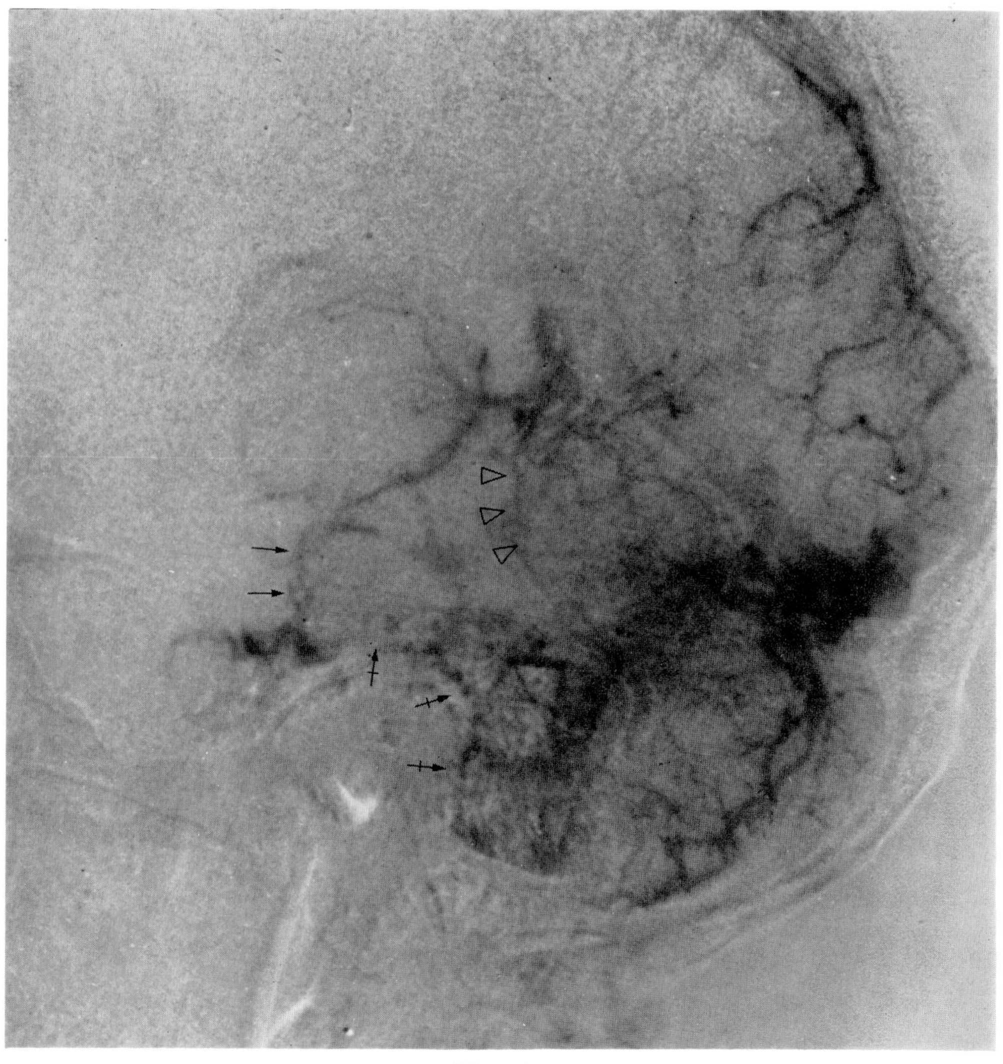

Fig. 221

Large Recurrent Pituitary Tumor with Extention into the Posterior Fossa

A 48-year-old female: Figs. 222 and 223

Fig. 222 Arterial phase in the lateral projection. The left middle cerebral artery is filled via the posterior communicating artery. The sylvian vessels are elevated with marked superior displacement of the posterior communicating artery (2 arrows). The basilar artery is markedly displaced posteriorly (3 crossed arrows). The supratonsillar segment of the posterior inferior cerebellar artery is dislocated posteriorly (a crossed arrow).

Fig. 223 Venous phase in the lateral projection. The petrosal vein and its tributary are displaced backwards (2 arrows). The vein of the lateral recess of the fourth ventricle is also displaced posteriorly (2 arrowheads). The posterior mesencephalic vein is elevated (2 crossed arrows).

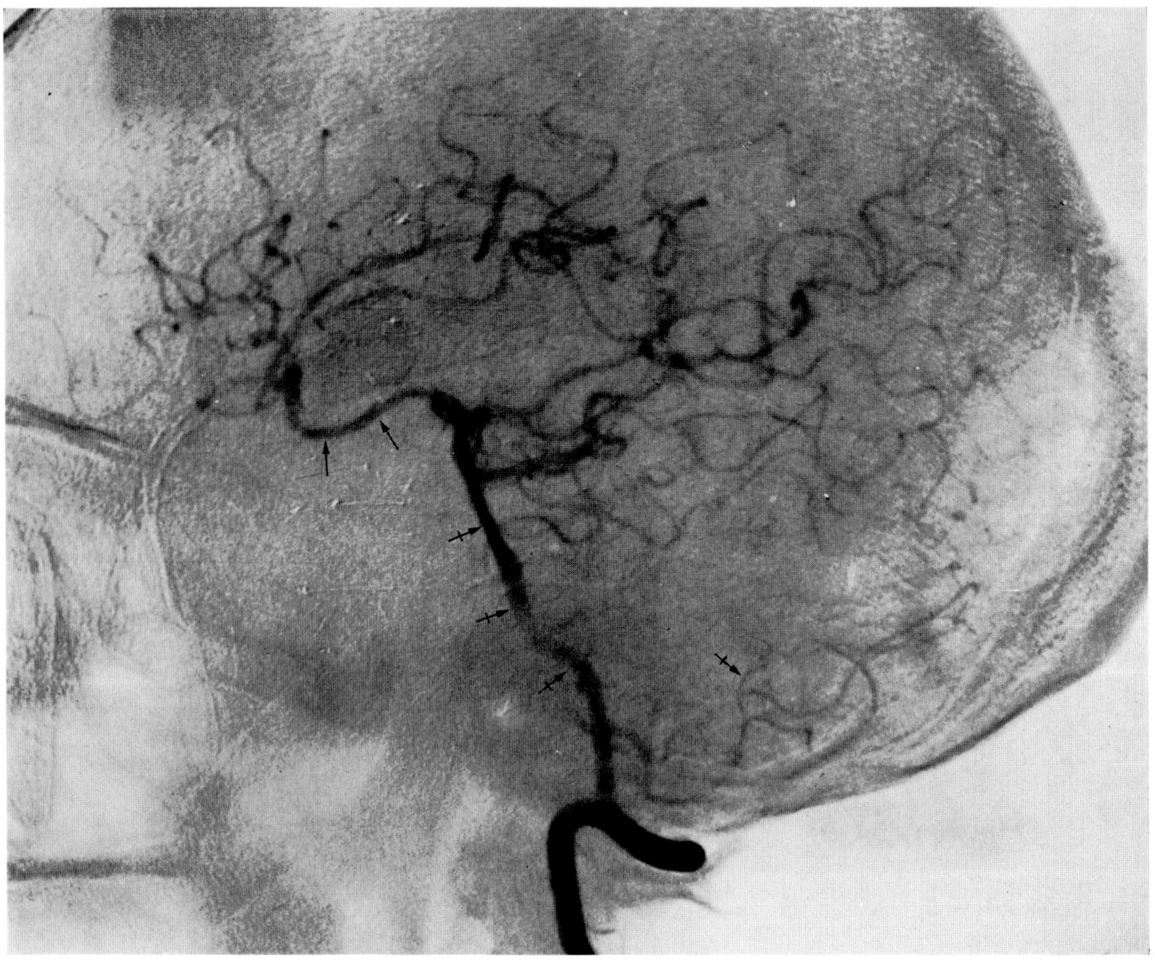

Fig. 222

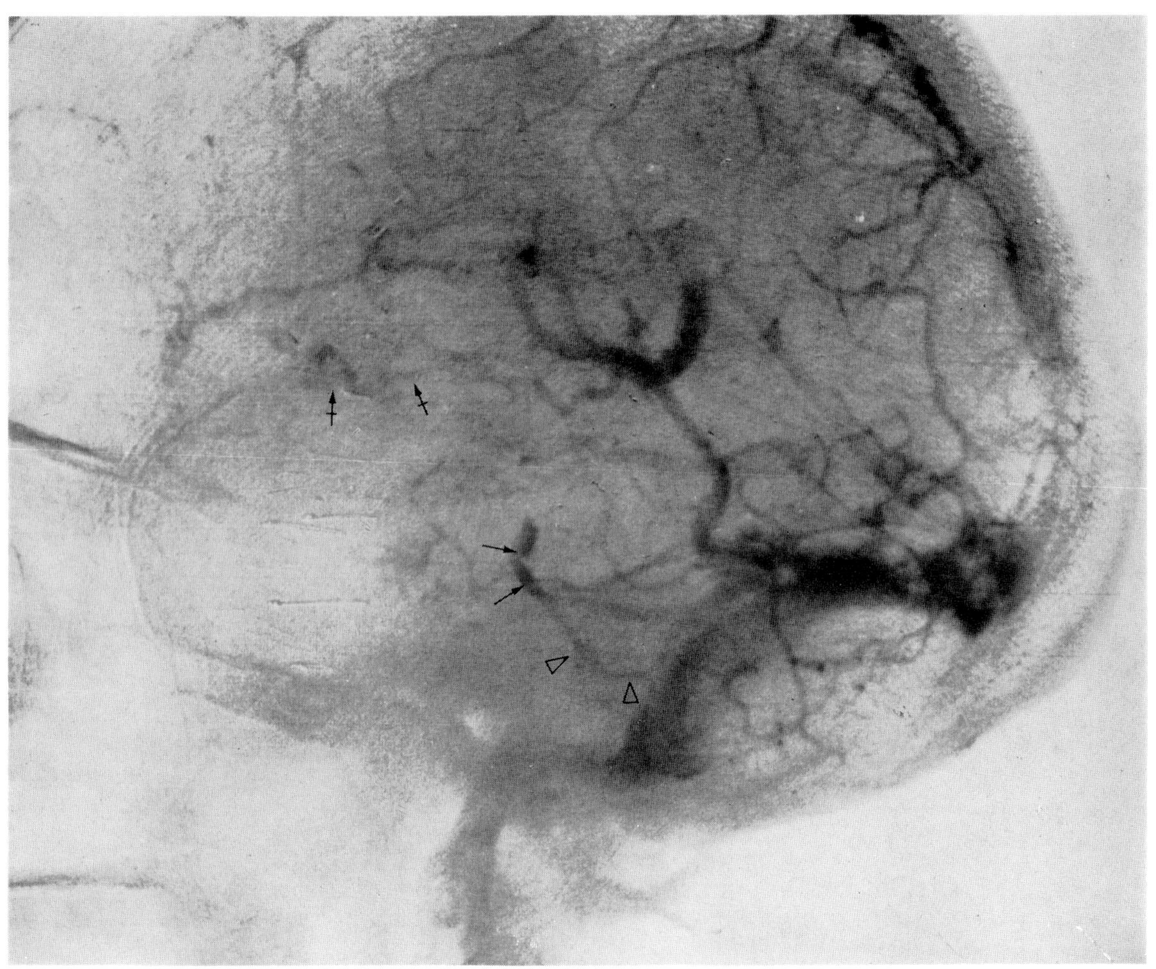

Fig. 223

Large Vascular Tumor over the Inferior Clivus

A 5-year-old male: Figs. 224 and 225

Fig. 224 Arterial phase in the Towne projection. The junction of the vertebral arteries are markedly elevated with foreshortening of the basilar artery. The intracranial vertebral arteries are elongated and displaced laterally (2 arrows). Fenestration of the right intracranial vertebral artery is demonstrated (2 open arrowheads). The right posterior inferior cerebellar artery is marked with a closed arrowhead. There is a small area with tumor vessels superimposed over the left vertebral artery (3 crossed arrows). The feeding arteries are probably the muscular branches of the left vertebral artery (3 double-crossed arrows).

Fig. 225 Arterial phase in the lateral projection. The intracranial vertebral arteries and the basilar artery are markedly displaced backwards (2 arrows), indicating a large clival tumor. The cranial loop of the posterior inferior cerebellar artery is displaced backwards (an arrowhead). The tumor vessels are again demonstrated in the inferior portion of the tumor (3 crossed arrows).

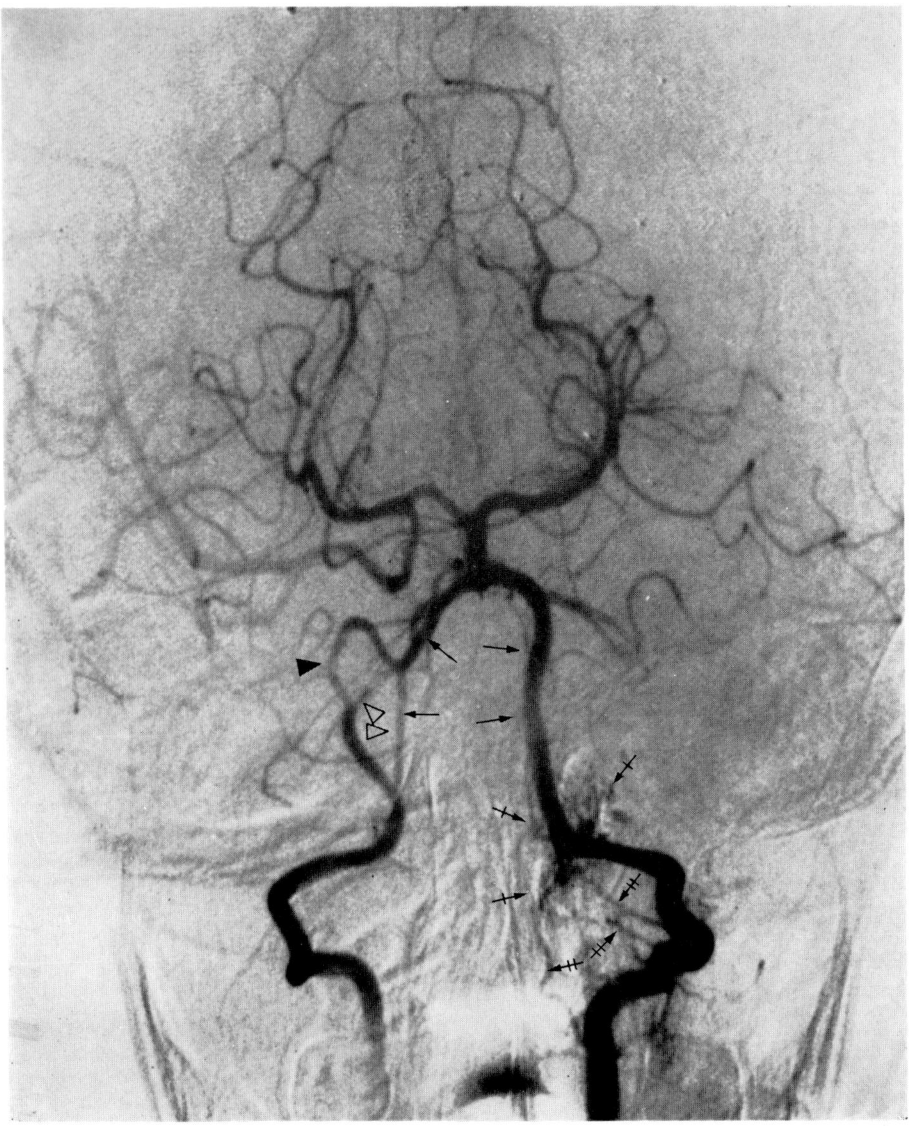

Fig. 224

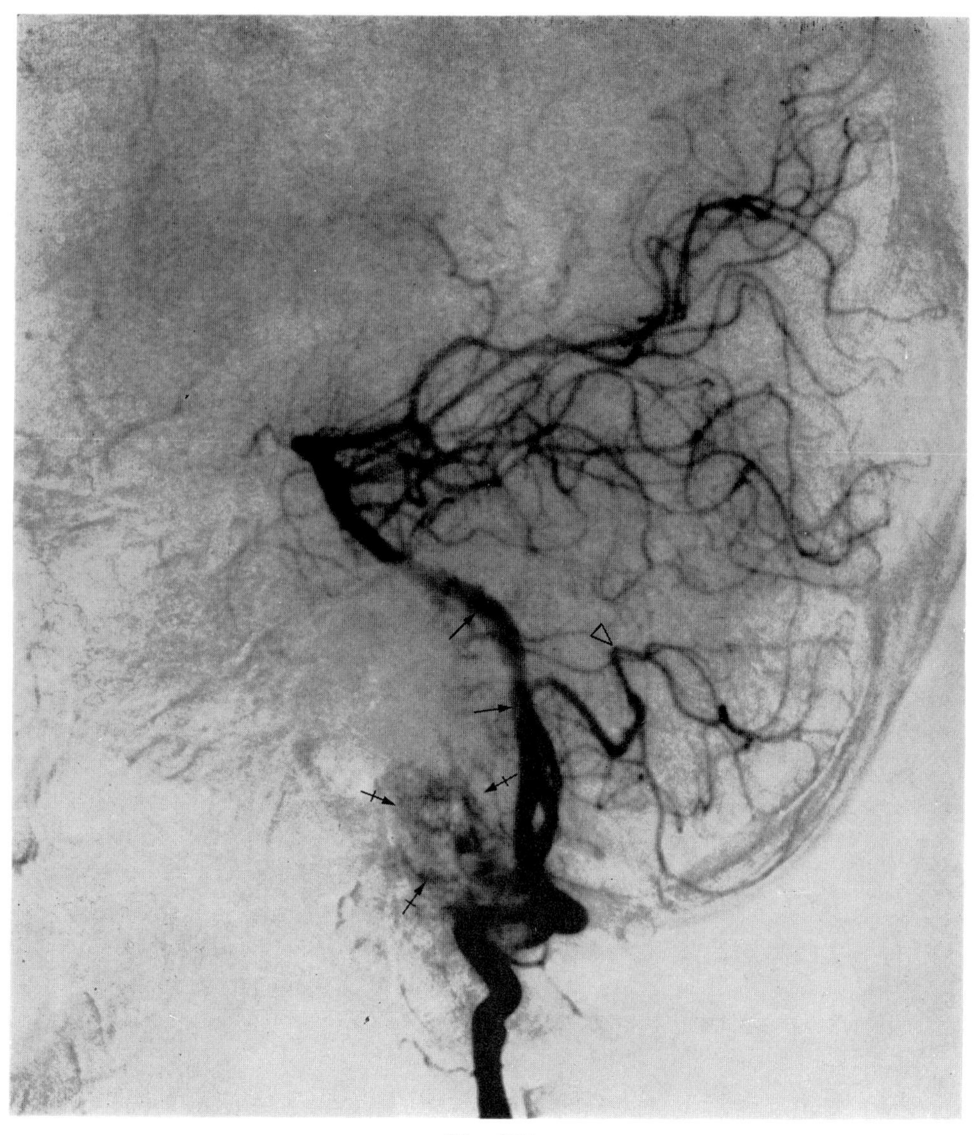

Fig. 225

EXTRACEREBRAL EXPANSIVE PROCESSES

Extradural and intradural tumors are included in this group. Tumors in this group are very uncommon. Meningeal cyst, meningioma, metastatic carcinoma, epidermoid, hematoma and occipital meningocele may present as expansive processes in this location.

Arteriographic features

These tumors usually show arterial displacements similar to cerebellar hemispheric tumors. The only difference is that the arterial branches adjacent to the tumor are all displaced away from the dura and calvarium.

Venographic features

The posterior fossa veins are all displaced away from the dura or calvarium. The torcular, the straight sinus and the transverse sinus may be displaced away from the calvarium.

Infratentorial Arachnoid Cyst

A 3-month-old female: Figs. 226–229

The right tentorium was markedly elevated and a large multicystic lesion was present between the tentorium and the cerebellum on the right.

Fig. 226 Arterial phase in the lateral projection. There is marked elevation of the posterior cerebral arteries (3 arrows). The superior cerebellar artery, probably the right, is elevated and displaced anteriorly (3 crossed arrows). The left superior cerebellar artery takes almost normal course (3 arrowheads). The findings are suggestive of a large infratentorial, extracerebral mass. There is faint visualization of the left posterior cerebral artery (3 double-crossed arrows).

Fig. 227 Venous phase in the lateral projection. There is elevation of the basal vein of Rosenthal (3 arrows). The straight sinus is markedly elevated and elongated (4 crossed arrows). The lateral sinus is normal in position (2 arrowheads). The cerebral cortical vein is marked with 2 open arrowheads.

Fig. 228 Arterial phase in the Towne projection. There is anterior and medial displacement of the right superior cerebellar artery (3 arrows). The left superior cerebellar artery is normal (2 crossed arrows). The right posterior cerebral artery is elongated and displaced laterally (3 arrowheads).

Fig. 229 Arterial phase of the right carotid angiogram in the lateral projection. There is marked unrolling of the anterior cerebral artery, indicating extensive hydrocephalus. The middle cerebral artery and its branches are displaced anteriorly and superiorly, indicating presence of a mass lesion in the posterior portion of the cranial cavity. The lenticulostriate arteries are all stretched (2 arrows).

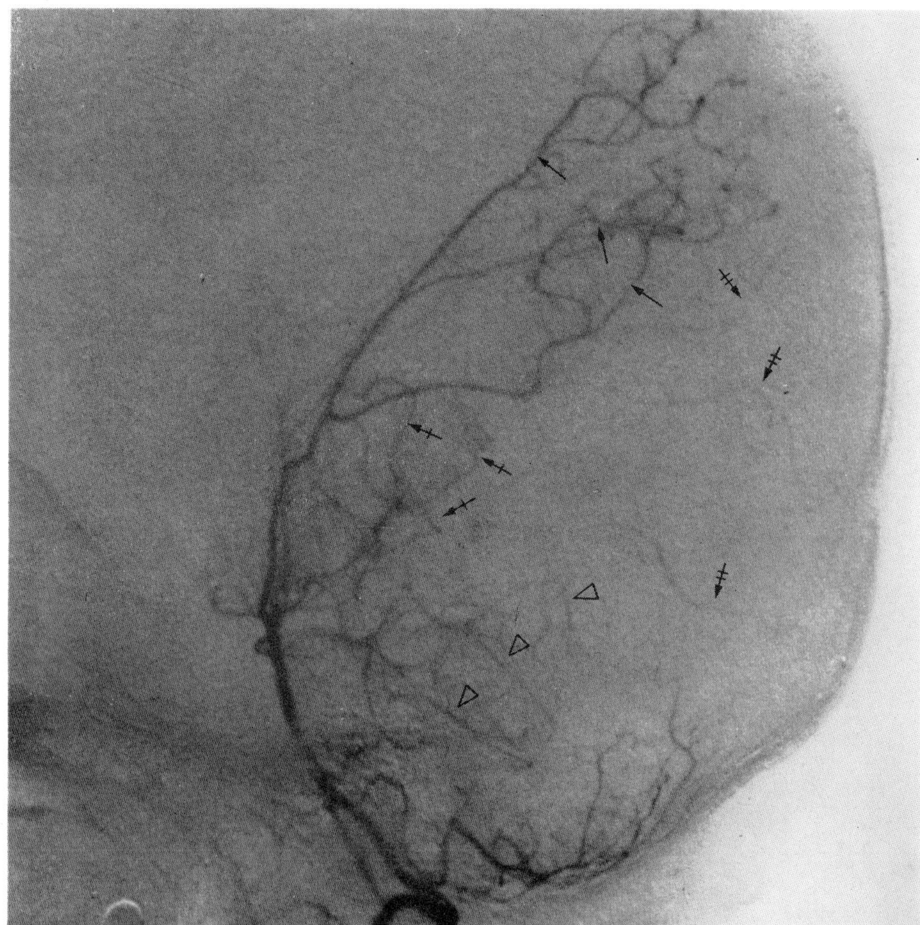

Fig. 226

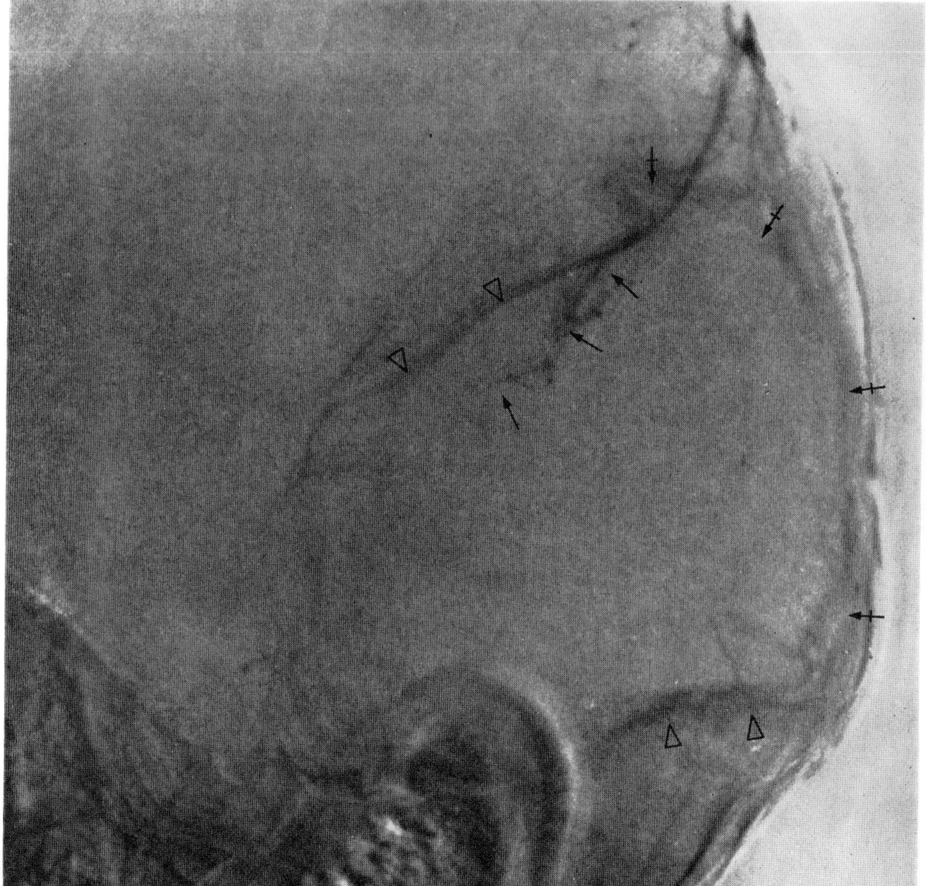

Fig. 227

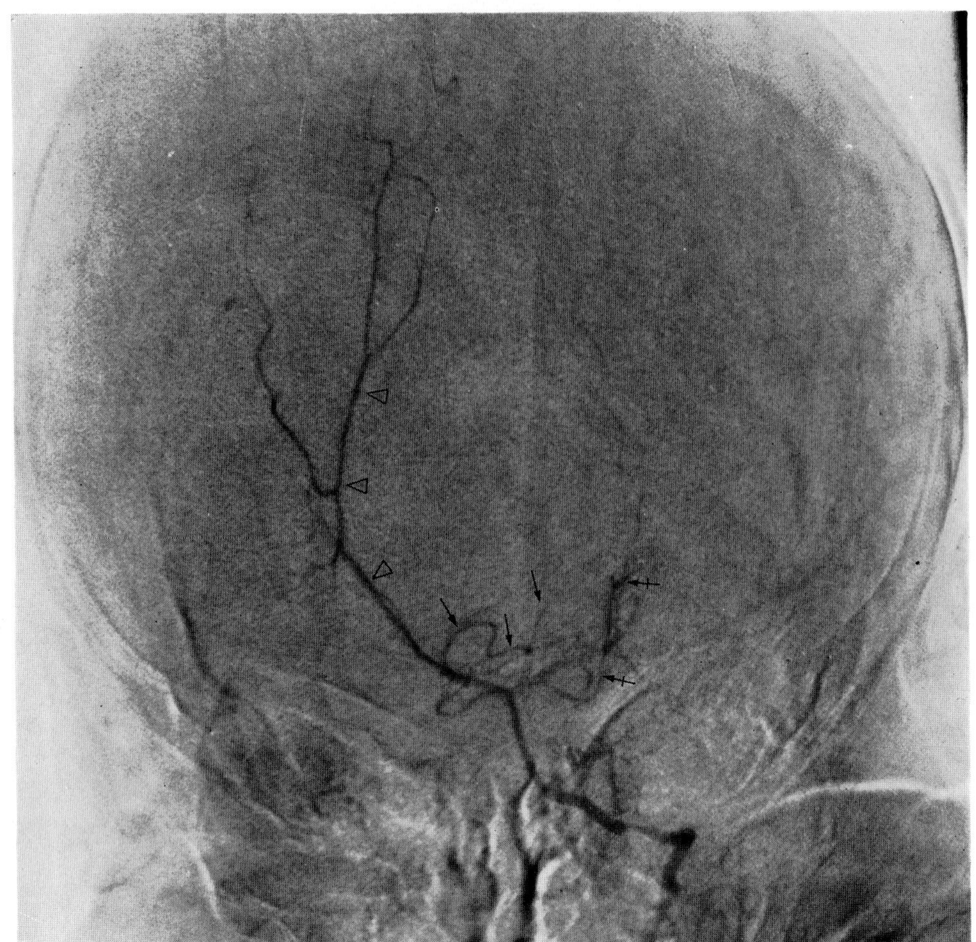

Fig. 228

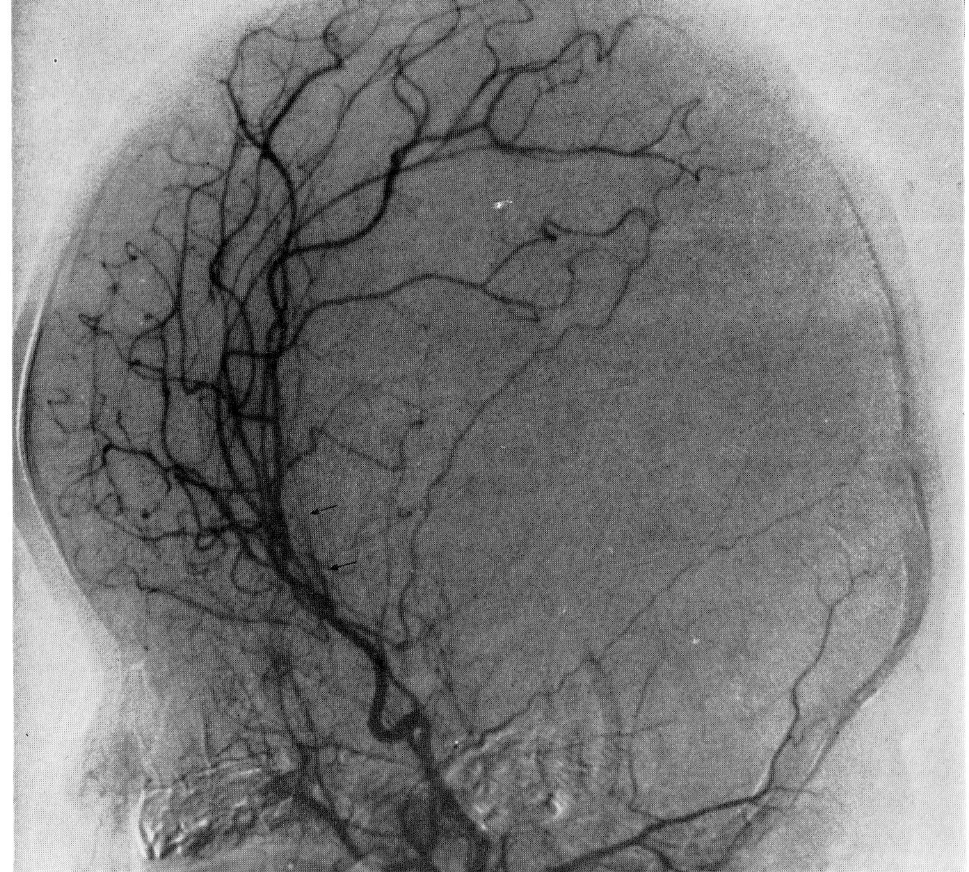

Fig. 229

Large Meningioma Arising from the Junction of the Left Lateral and Sigmoid Sinuses and Compressing the Left Cerebellar Hemisphere

A 48-year-old female: Figs. 230–233

Fig. 230 Arterial phase in the lateral projection. There are arterial changes due to increased intracranial pressure in the posterior fossa: compression of the basilar artery against the clivus, depression of the posterior inferior cerebellar artery (3 arrowheads) and increased distance between the posterior choroidal and posterior pericallosal arteries (2 double-crossed arrows). The marginal artery of the superior cerebellar artery is markedly displaced backwards (3 arrows), suggesting extracerebellar location of the tumor. Another branch of the superior cerebellar artery is also displaced superiorly (3 crossed arrows).

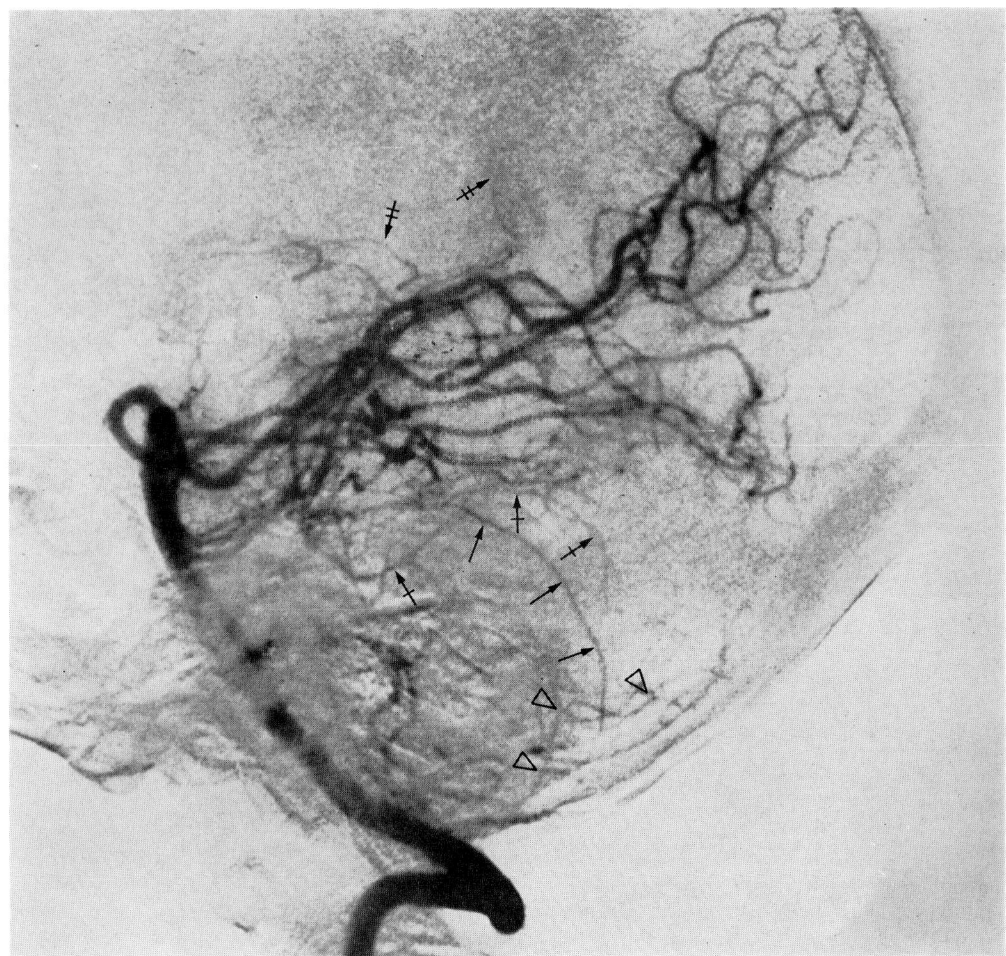

Fig. 230

Fig. 231 Venous phase in the lateral projection. The pontine segment of the anterior pontomesencephalic vein is displaced anteriorly (2 arrows). The copular point of the inferior vermian vein is displaced posteriorly and inferiorly (a crossed arrow). There is decreased distance between the choroid plexus of the lateral ventricle and the internal cerebral vein (2 opposing arrows), due to hydrocephalus.

Fig. 232 Arterial phase in the Towne projection. The posterior inferior cerebellar artery is shifted to the right of the midline (3 arrows). The quadrigeminal and ambient segments of the left superior cerebellar artery is displaced medially (4 arrowheads). These findings indicate a mass lesion in the left posterior fossa. The marginal artery and its branches are stretched and displaced posteriorly (2 medial crossed arrows), indicating an extracerebellar hemispheric tumor. No tumor vessels are demonstrated. The hemispheric branches of the left superior cerebellar artery are stretched (4 lateral crossed arrows).

Fig. 233 Venous phase in the Towne projection. Venous filling of the left posterior fossa is poor due to venous compression by the tumor. Nonvisualization of the unilateral petrosal vein strongly suggests extracerebellar location of the tumor.

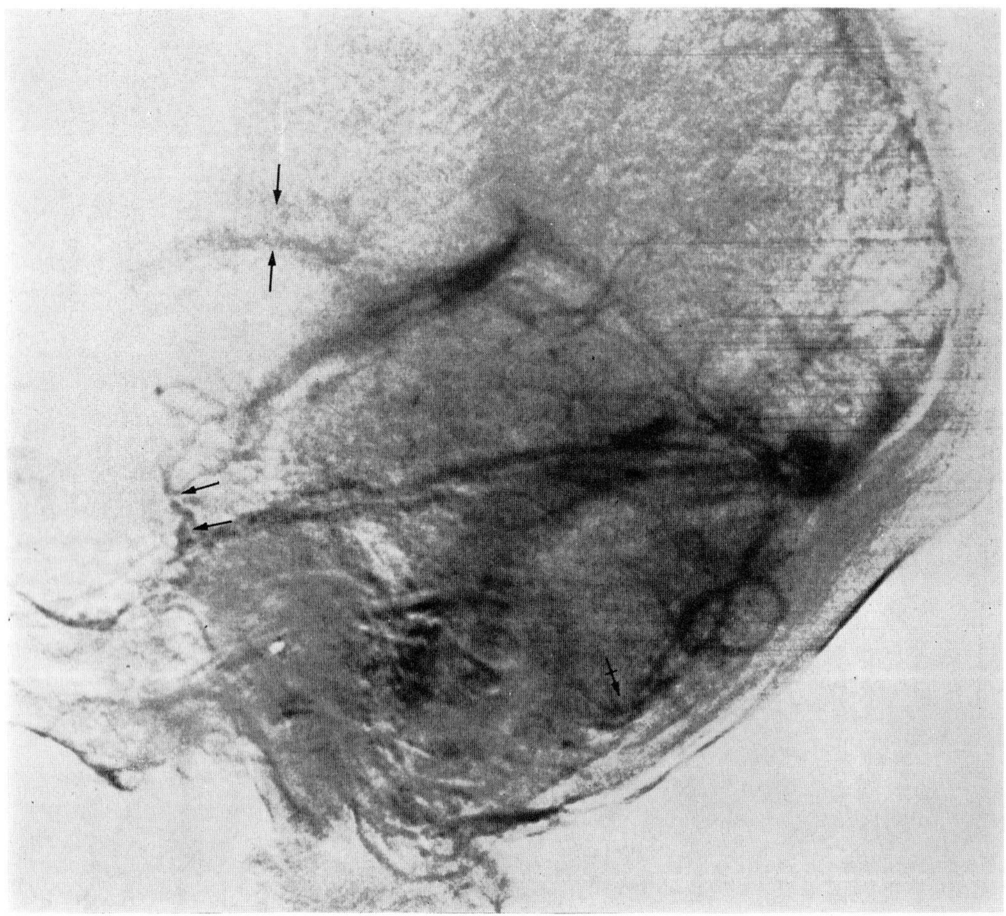

Fig. 231

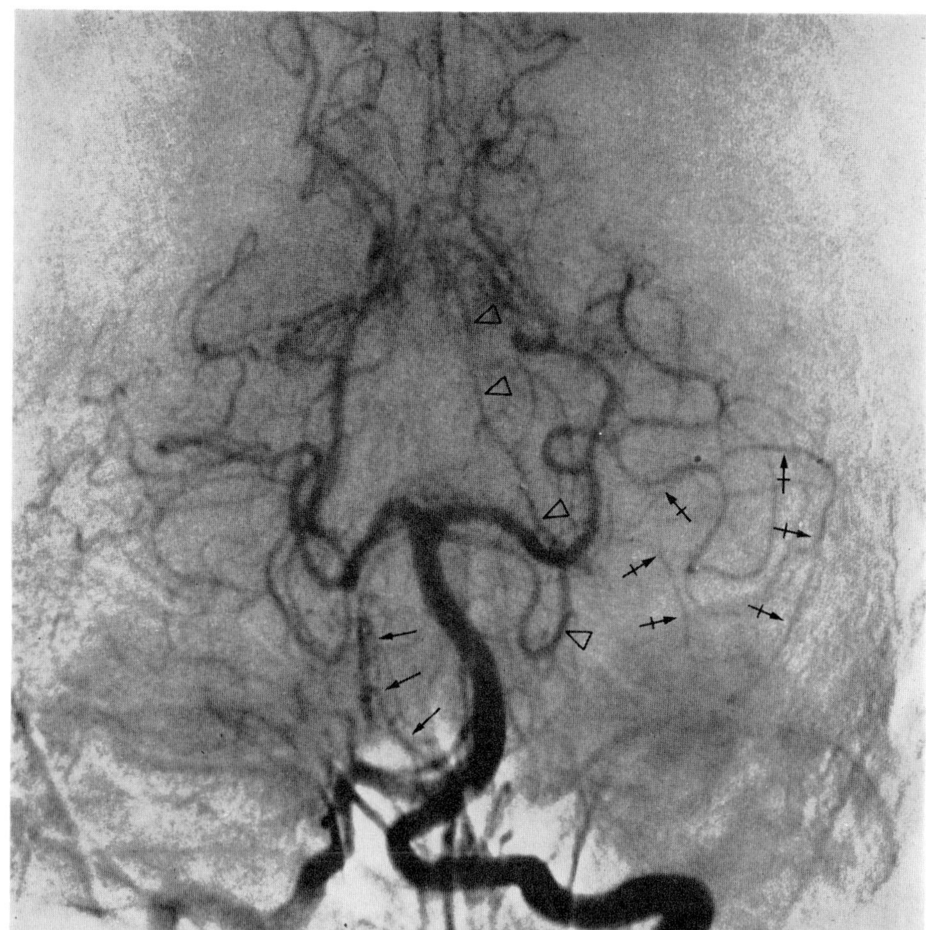

Fig. 232

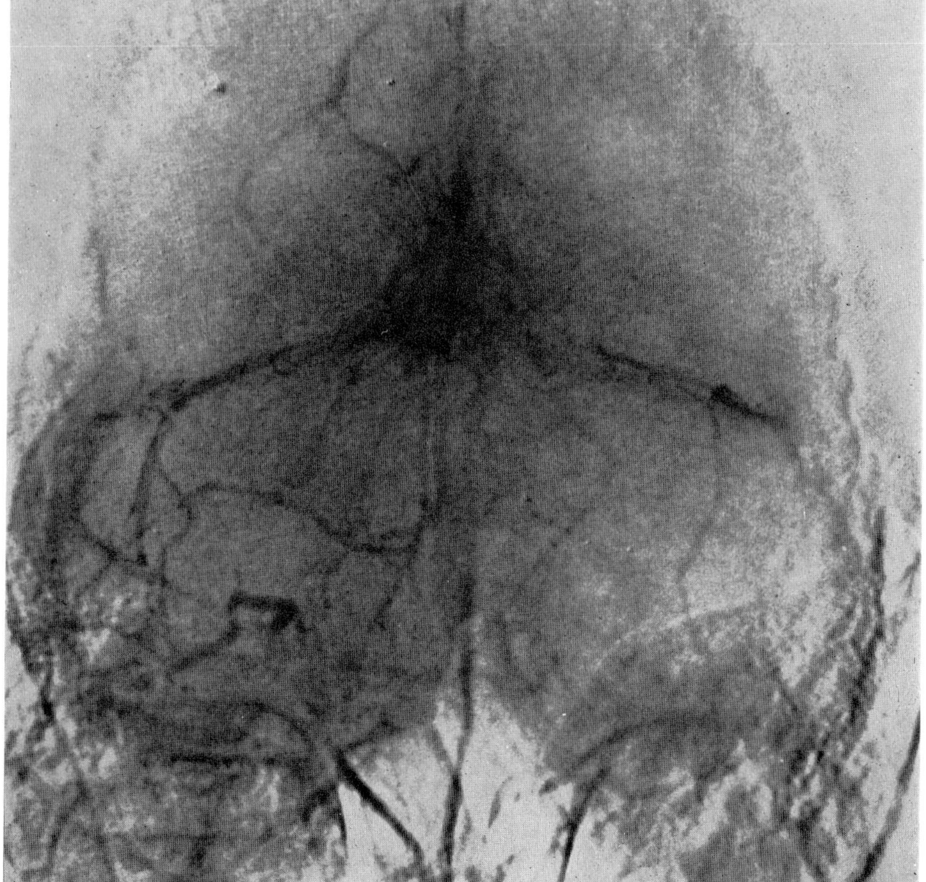

Fig. 233

INCISURAL TUMORS

Tumors which arise from the tentorial incisura are mostly meningiomas. Incisural meningiomas grow supratentorially as well as infratentorially, displacing the brain stem, temporal lobes and the superior cerebellum.

Arteriographic features

The posterior cerebral artery is elevated and displaced laterally by a midline tumor, while the superior cerebellar artery is displaced inferiorly and laterally. Therefore, there is dissociation of the posterior cerebral artery and the superior cerebellar artery in both the anteroposterior and lateral projections. When this tumor arises from the posterior edge of the incisura, the quadrigeminal segment of the superior cerebellar artery is anteriorly displaced with arched configuration. A forward displacement of the posterior pericallosal and posterior choroidal arteries is frequently noted. However, a lateral incisural mass may displace the posterior cerebral artery and superior cerebeller artery medially.

The tentorial branches of the meningohypophyseal arteries from the internal carotid artery are usually enlarged and participate in the blood supply of meningiomas. Characteristically, tumor stains in the meningiomas are homogeneous and remain to the venous phase of angiograms.

Venographic features

The precentral cerebellar vein is usually displaced anteriorly and to the opposite side. The lateral anastomotic mesencephalic vein is also displaced in the lateral, anterior or posterior direction, depending upon the origin of meningiomas. The pontine and interpeduncular segments of the anterior pontomesencephalic vein are dislocated superiorly and anteriorly.

The basal vein of Rosenthal may be elevated and the posterior mesencephalic vein is usually depressed if visualized.

Incisural Meningioma with Major Bulk of Tumor in the Posterior Fossa

A 23-year-old female: Figs. 234–238

Fig. 234 Arterial phase in the lateral projection. The quadrigeminal and vermian segments of the superior cerebellar artery are depressed downwards (3 arrows), while there is elevation and straightening of the quadrigeminal segments of the posterior cerebral artery (2 crossed arrows), suggesting a large tumor at the posterior portion of the tentorial incisura or in the quadrigeminal cistern. The posterior pericallosal (2 open arrowheads) and posterior choroidal arteries (2 closed arrowheads) are dislocated anteriorly. There is minimal depression of the cranial and caudal loops of the posterior inferior cerebellar arteries (a double-crossed arrow) with anterior displacement of the basilar artery, indicating increased intracranial pressure in the posterior fossa.

Fig. 235 Venous phase in the lateral projection. There is marked anterior displacement of the precentral cerebellar vein (3 arrows) and a vein draining into the basal vein, probably the superior vermian vein, is stretched (2 arrows). The basal vein of Rosenthal is pushed anteriorly (2 crossed arrows). The vein of Galen and the straight sinus circumvent the tumor with formation of an arc (3 open arrowheads). The internal cerebral vein is elevated (2 open arrowheads). The copular points, formed by the inferior vermian veins, are depressed downwards (double-crossed arrows). The findings indicate a large mass displacing the tentorium superiorly and the Galenic venous system anteriorly.

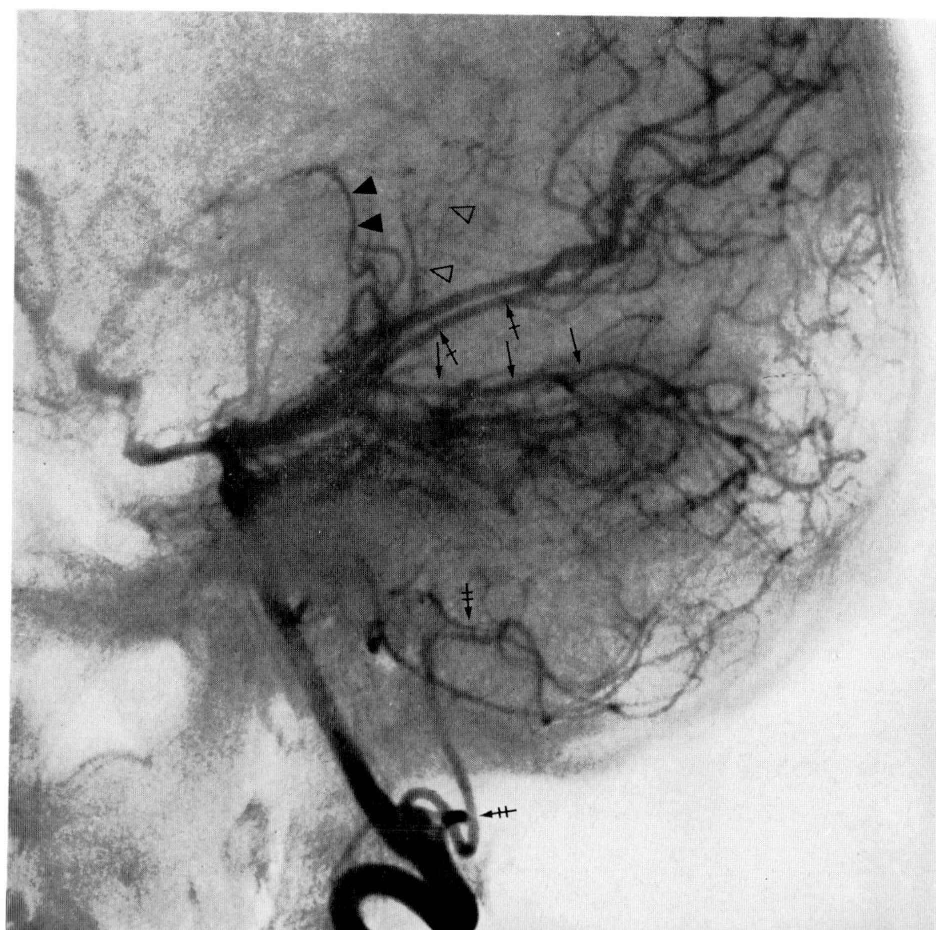

Fig. 234

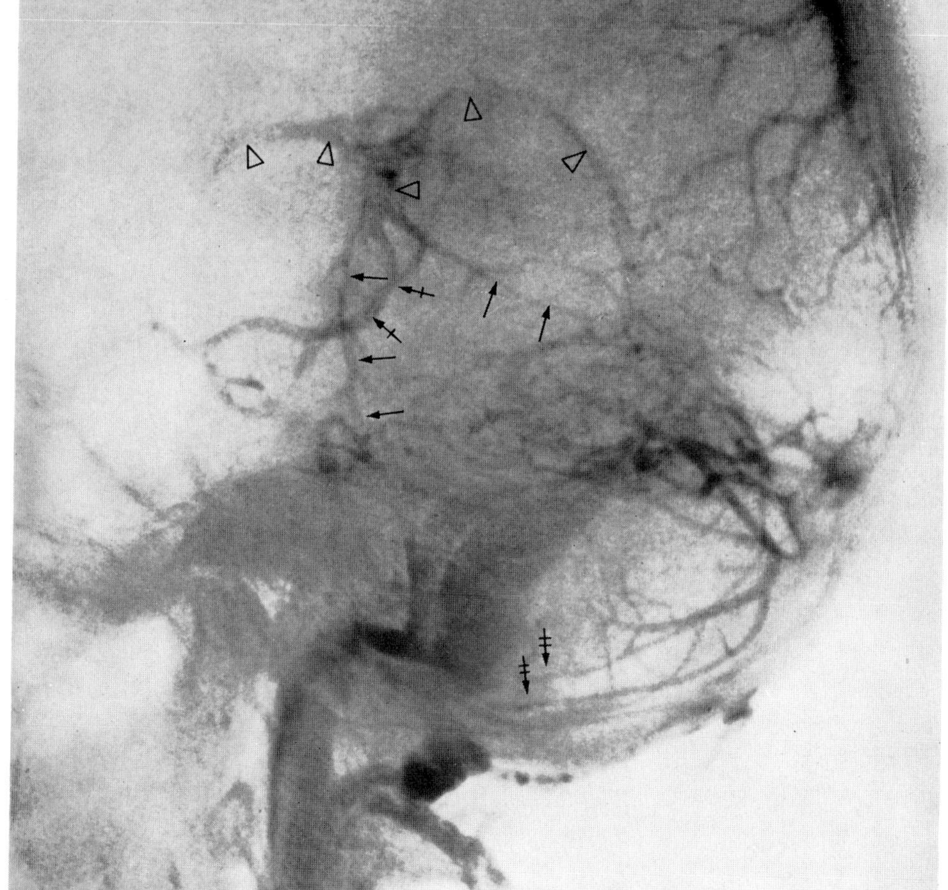

Fig. 235

Fig. 236 Arterial phase in the Towne projection. The quadrigemina land anterior culminate segments of the superior cerebellar artery are displaced laterally and anteriorly in an arcuate fashion (5 arrows), demonstrating a decreased anteroposterior diameter of the midbrain. There is marked separation of the posterior cerebral arteries (2 crossed arrows).

Fig. 237 Arterial phase of the right internal carotid angiogram. The tentorial branch of the meningohypophyseal artery is enlarged and supplies the tumor at the tentorial incisura (4 arrows). Blood supply from this artery usually indicate that the tumor is a meningioma. There is no appreciable arterial displacement except for straightening and minimal elevation of the posterior cerebral artery (2 crossed arrows). There is ventricular dilatation as shown by unrolling of the anterior cerebral artery.

Fig. 238 Venous phase of the right internal carotid angiogram. The proximal portion of the straight sinus is elevated (3 arrows), while the vein of Galen is displaced anteriorly (a crossed arrow). The basal vein is displaced anteriorly (3 open arrowheads) and the internal cerebral vein is moderately elevated (2 closed arrowheads).

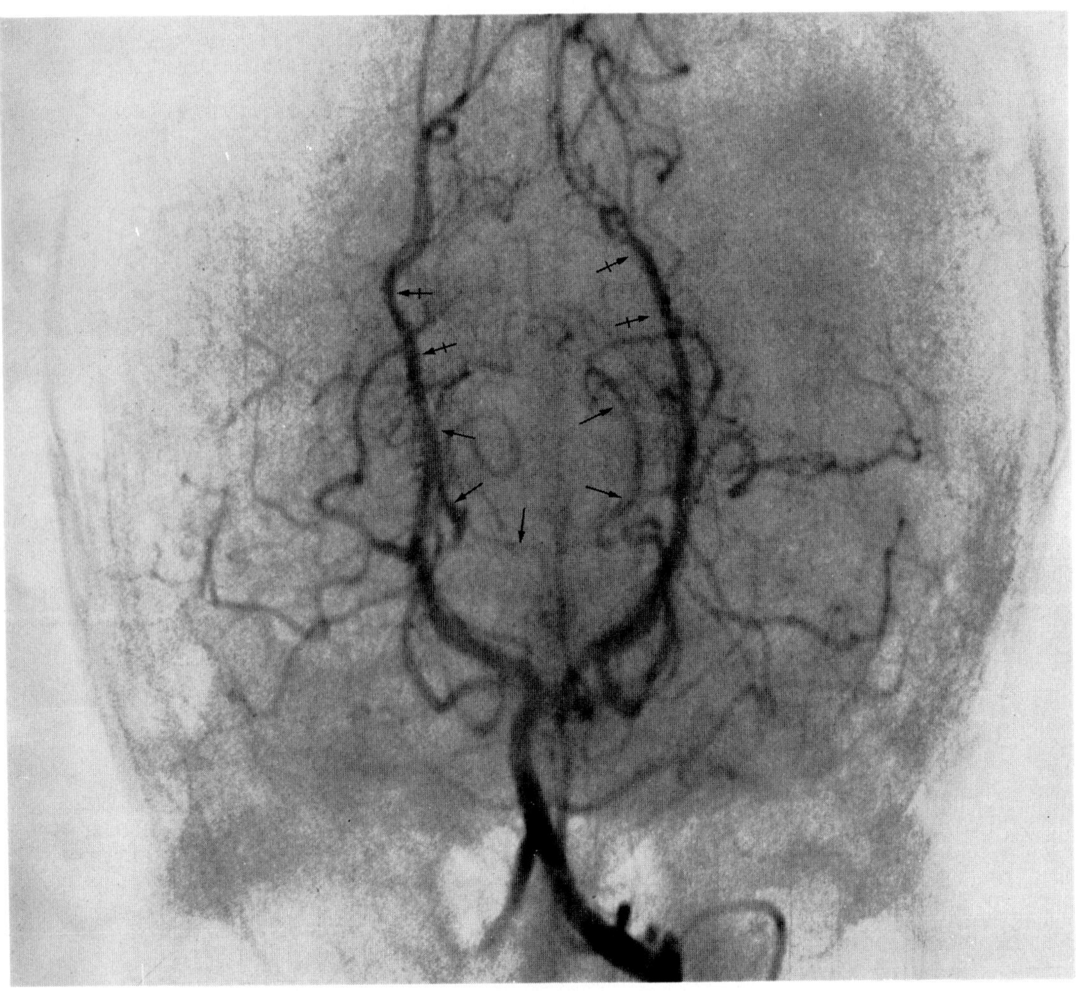

Fig. 236

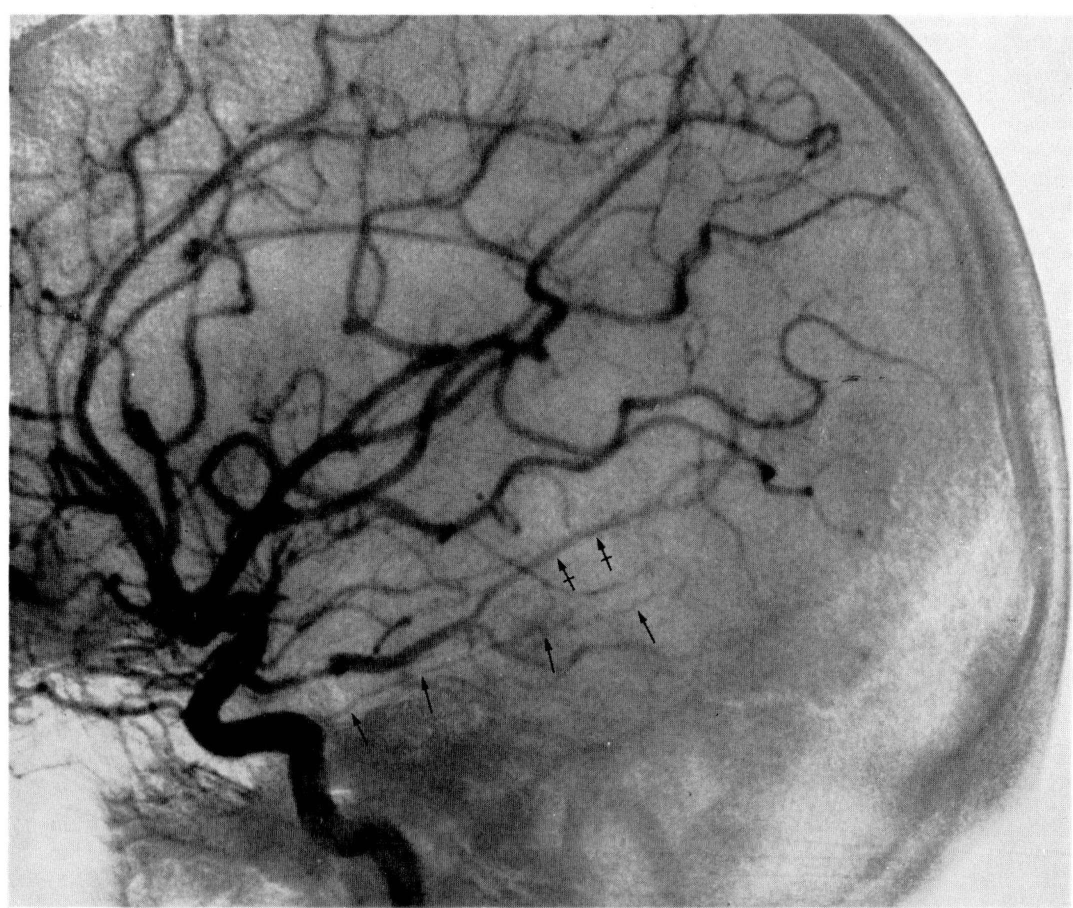

Fig. 237

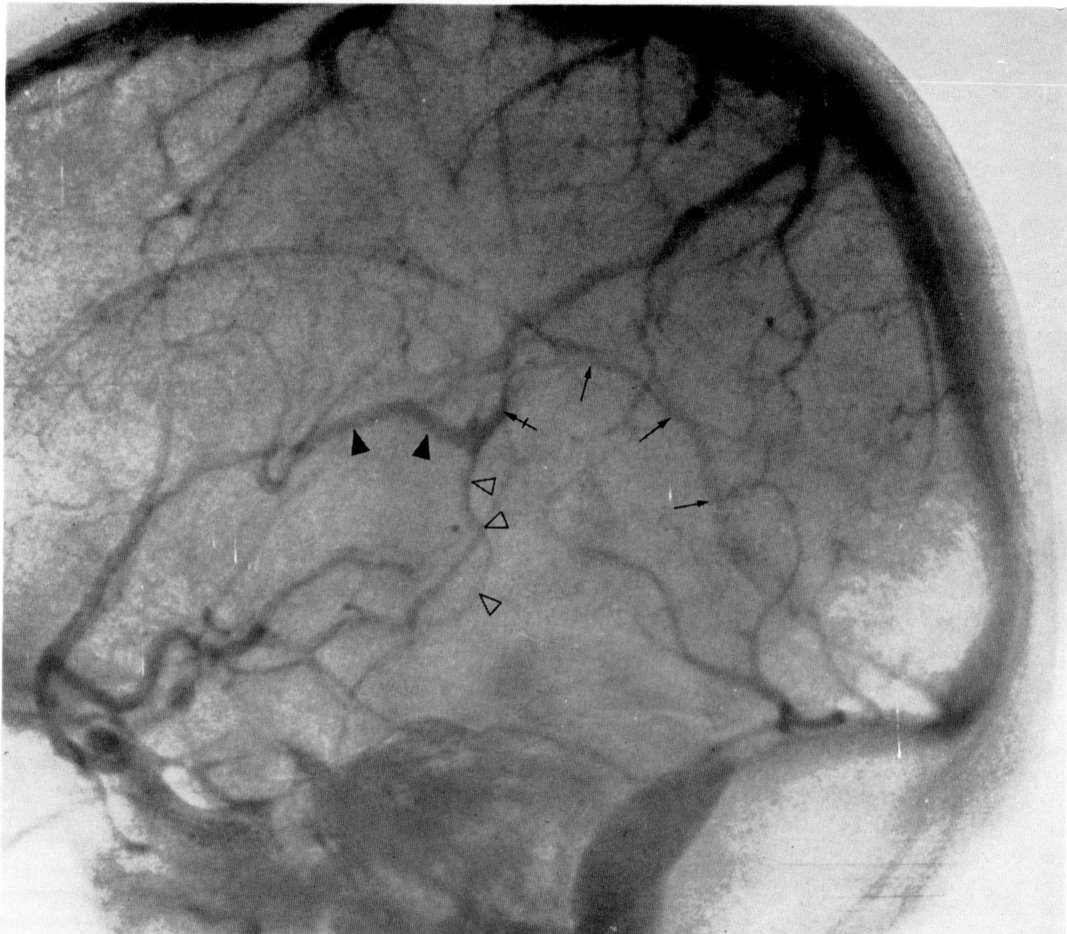

Fig. 238

Recurrent Meningioma of the Tentorial Incisura

A 39-year-old male: Figs. 239–244

This patient had undergone a subtotal removal of a meningioma 5 years previously. The tumor extended supratentorially along the falx on both sides.

Fig. 239 Arterial phase of the left vertebral angiogram in the lateral projection. There is a large vascular tumor with superior displacement of the calcarine (3 arrows) and parieto-occipital (3 crossed arrows) branches of the right posterior cerebral artery. Irregular tumor vessels are noted above the tentorium. In addition, there are tumor vessels in the area of the tentorial incisura, being supplied by the superior cerebellar artery (4 arrowheads). This artery may be slightly displaced downwards with increased distance from the posterior cerebral artery (2 opposing arrows).

Fig. 240 Capillary phase in the lateral projection. There is diffuse, homogeneous tumor stain supratentorially (4 arrowheads) as well as infratentorially (4 arrows).

Fig. 241 Arterial phase in the Towne projection. The right posterior cerebral artery is displaced laterally with minimal tumor stain (3 arrows). There is also flush filling of the left posterior cerebral artery with slight stretching (2 closed arrowheads). The quadrigeminal segment of the superior cerebellar artery is displaced anteriorly and laterally in arcuate fashion, suggesting infratentorial extension of the tumor (7 crossed arrows). There are minimal tumor vessels at the posterior tentorial incisura (2 open arrowheads).

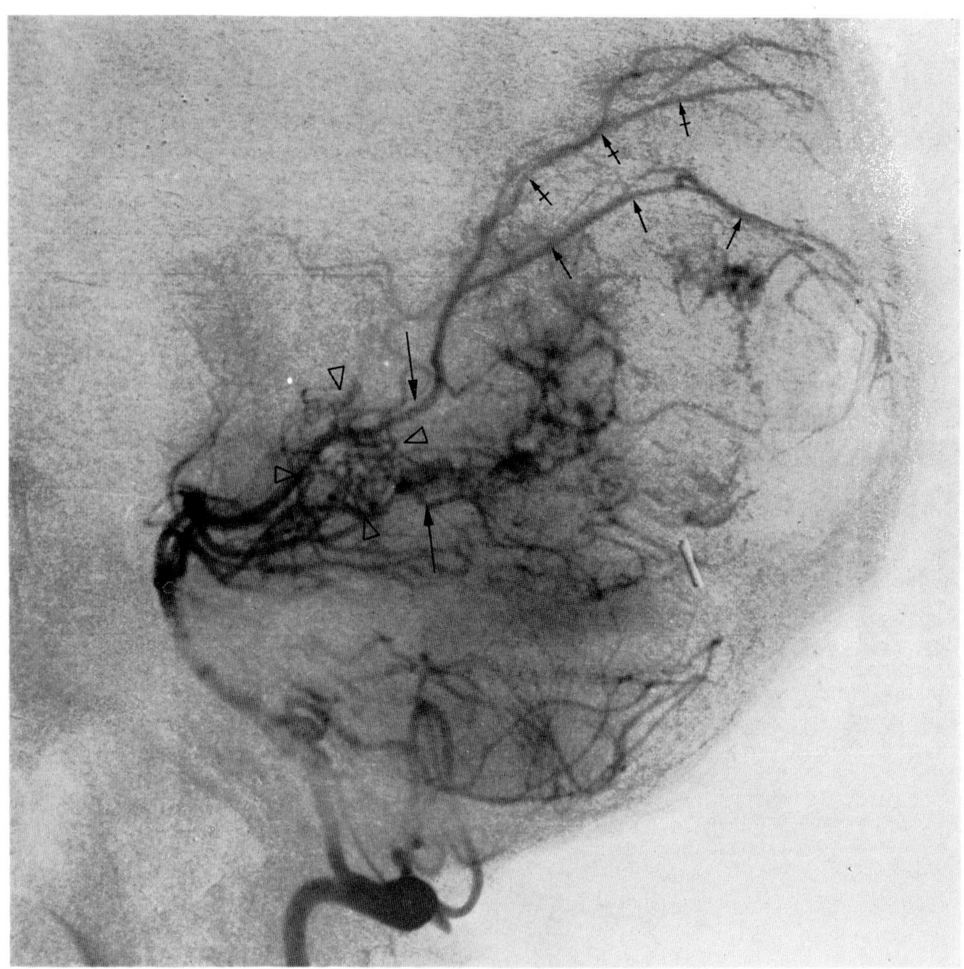

Fig. 239

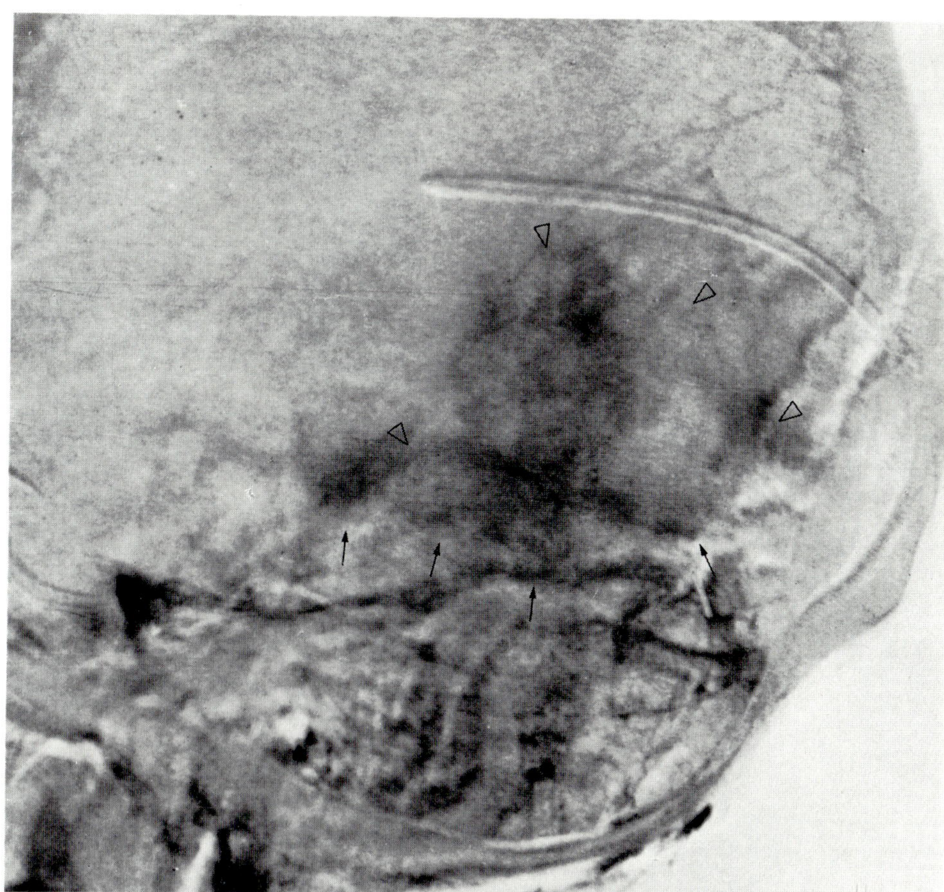

Fig. 240

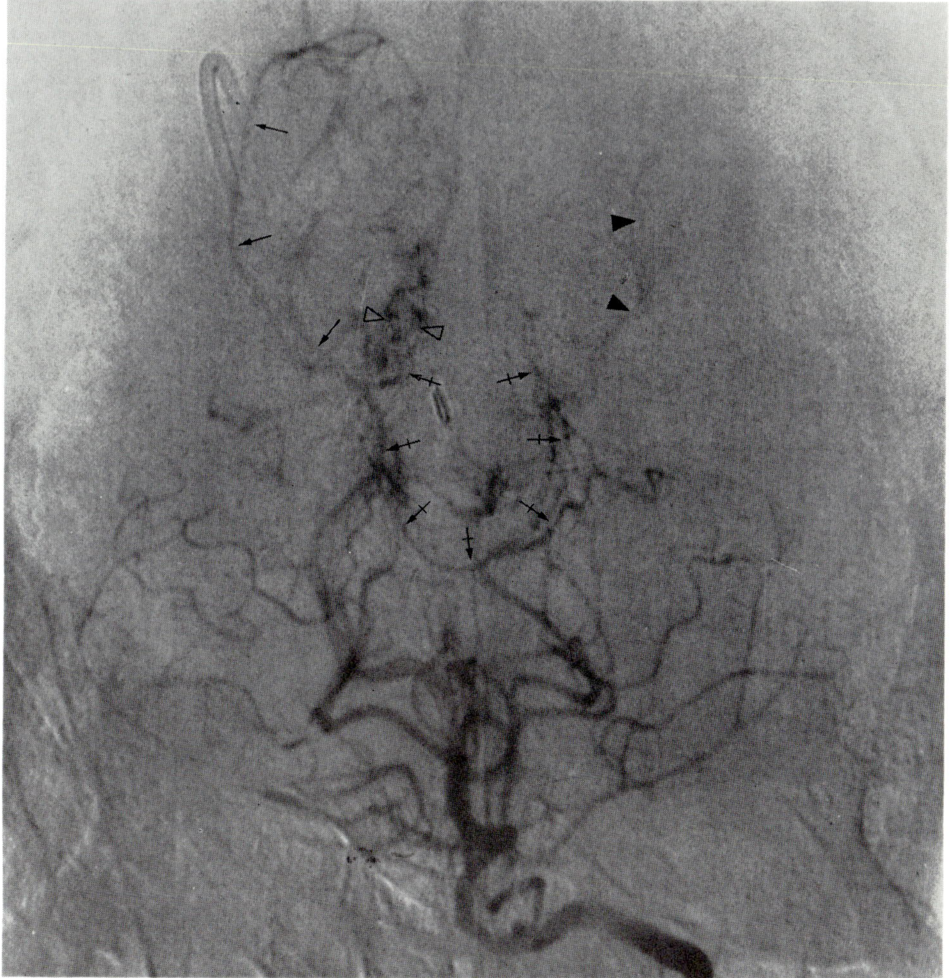

Fig. 241

Fig. 242 Venous phase in the Towne projection. Tumor stains are noted in both occipital regions (2 crossed arrows) and in the posterior fossa below the tentorial incisura (5 arrows).

Fig. 243 Arterial phase of the left internal carotid angiogram. There is a 6 × 5 cm vascular tumor supplied by the enlarged posterior cerebral artery. The calcarine branch of the posterior cerebral artery is depressed downward (4 arrows), while the parieto-occipital branch is elevated (3 crossed arrows). The sylvian point is displaced anteriorly and superiorly (an arrowhead).

Fig. 244 Venous phase of the left internal carotid angiogram. Diffuse, homogeneous tumor stain is noted above the tentorium (5 arrows). The basal vein of Rosenthal is displaced anteriorly (a crossed arrow) and the internal cerebral vein is compressed in an accordion fasion (2 arrowheads). The cortical veins in the posterior parietal area are stretched due to cerebral edema.

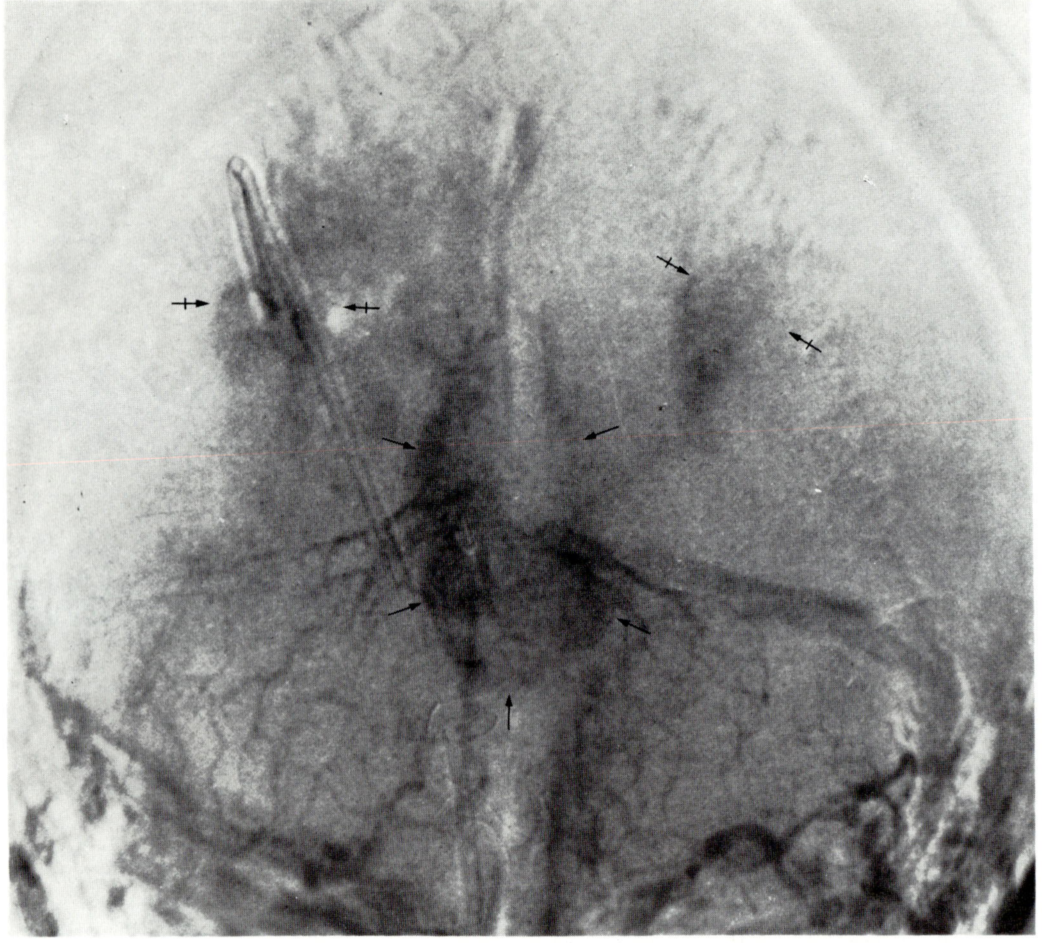

Fig. 242

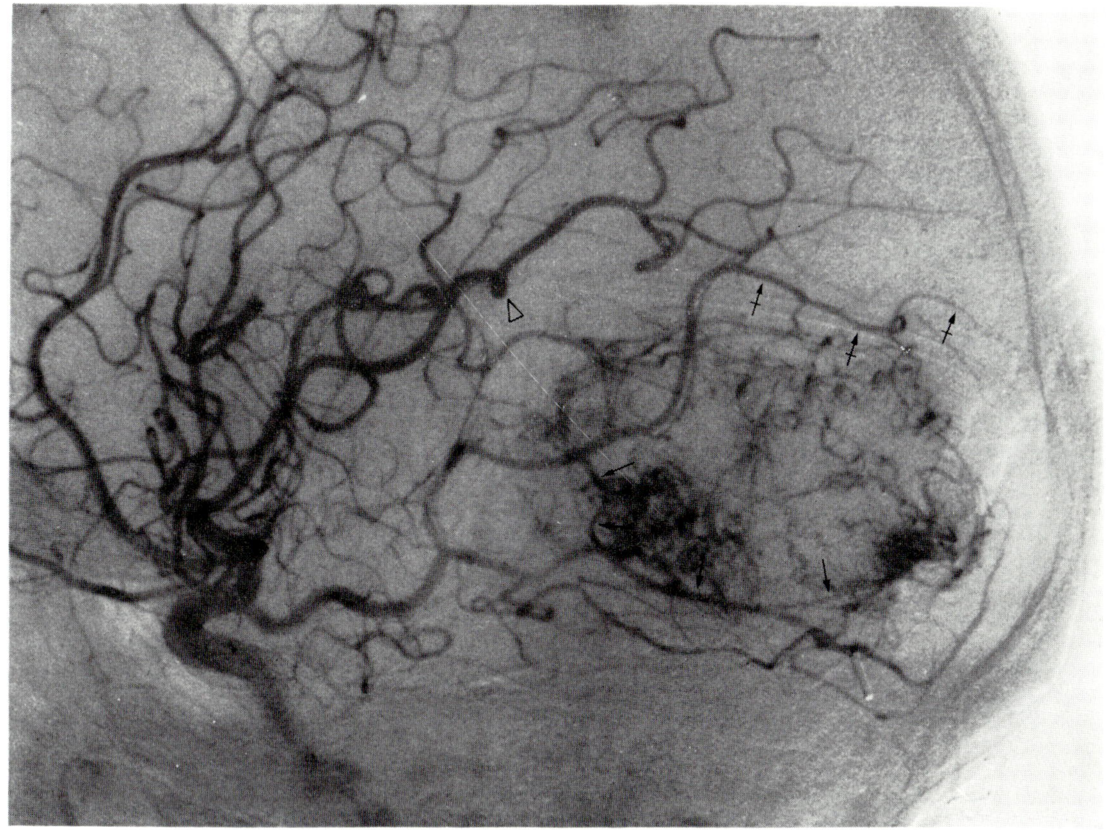

Fig. 243

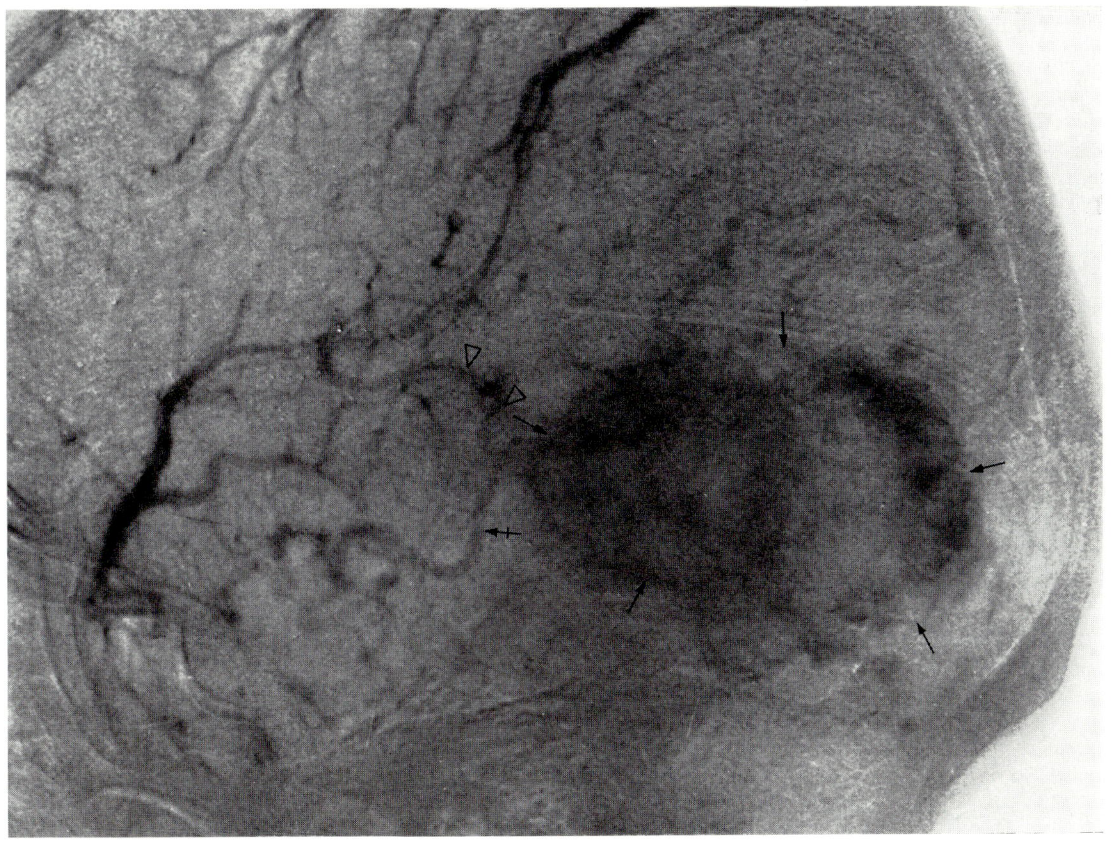

Fig. 244

7

Supratentorial Tumors

OCCIPITAL TUMORS

It is unusual to encounter a tumor localized in the occipital lobe. Tumors in this area easily extend and invade the posterior temporal and posterior parietal lobes. The occipital lobe may be involved as a result of extension of tumors originating in the adjacent areas. The lesions of frequent occurrence in the occipital lobe are glioma, metastatic tumor, meningioma and brain abscess. Epidermoid tumor and hemorrhage due to arterio-venous malformation or ruptured aneurysm are infrequently observed in the occipital lobes.

Arteriographic features

The posterior cerebral artery shows the most marked changes. The calcarine branch of this artery is displaced upward or downward. The parieto-occipital branch is displaced upward in an arcuate fashion, while the posterior temporal branch is depressed inferiorly. Therefore, there is usually separation of the parieto-occipital branch and the posterior temporal branch. These findings are observed not only in the lateral projection, but also in the anteroposterior projection.

The posterior choroidal arteries, especially the lateral posterior choroidal artery, is anteriorly displaced in the lateral projection.

On carotid angiograms, the sylvian point is displaced anteriorly and superiorly and the anterior choroidal artery is accordioned anteriorly. There may be a midline shift of the anterior cerebral artery to the opposite side.

Venographic features

The superficial veins and capillaries of the occipital lobe may be stretched, showing curvilinear distribution. These findings are produced by compression of the capillaries and veins within the cerebral sulci secondary to cerebral edema. This appearance of vessels is called "onion skinning" or "onion peeling".

The direct atrial vein and the vein of the occipital horn are distorted and displaced anteriorly. The midline shift of the internal cerebral vein is greater than the shift of the anterior cerebral artery. Occlusion of the superior sagittal sinus may occur with tumors invading the dura such as meningiomas.

Large Cystic Astrocytoma in the Right Occipital, Parietal and Temporal Lobes

A 10-year-old female: Figs. 245 and 246

Fig. 245 Arterial phase in the lateral projection. The parieto-occipital branch (3 arrows) of the right posterior cerebral artery is markedly displaced superiorly with moderate superior dislocation of the calcarine branch (3 crossed arrows). The posterior temporal branch is dislocated downwards (3 closed arrowheads). The posterior choroidal artery is displaced anteriorly (2 open arrowheads).

Fig. 246 Arterial phase in the Towne projection. The parieto-occipital branch is straightened (4 arrows). There is accordioning of the calcarine branch (3 crossed arrows). The posterior temporal branch is anteriorly displaced (2 arrowheads), indicating tumor extension into the posterior temporal lobe.

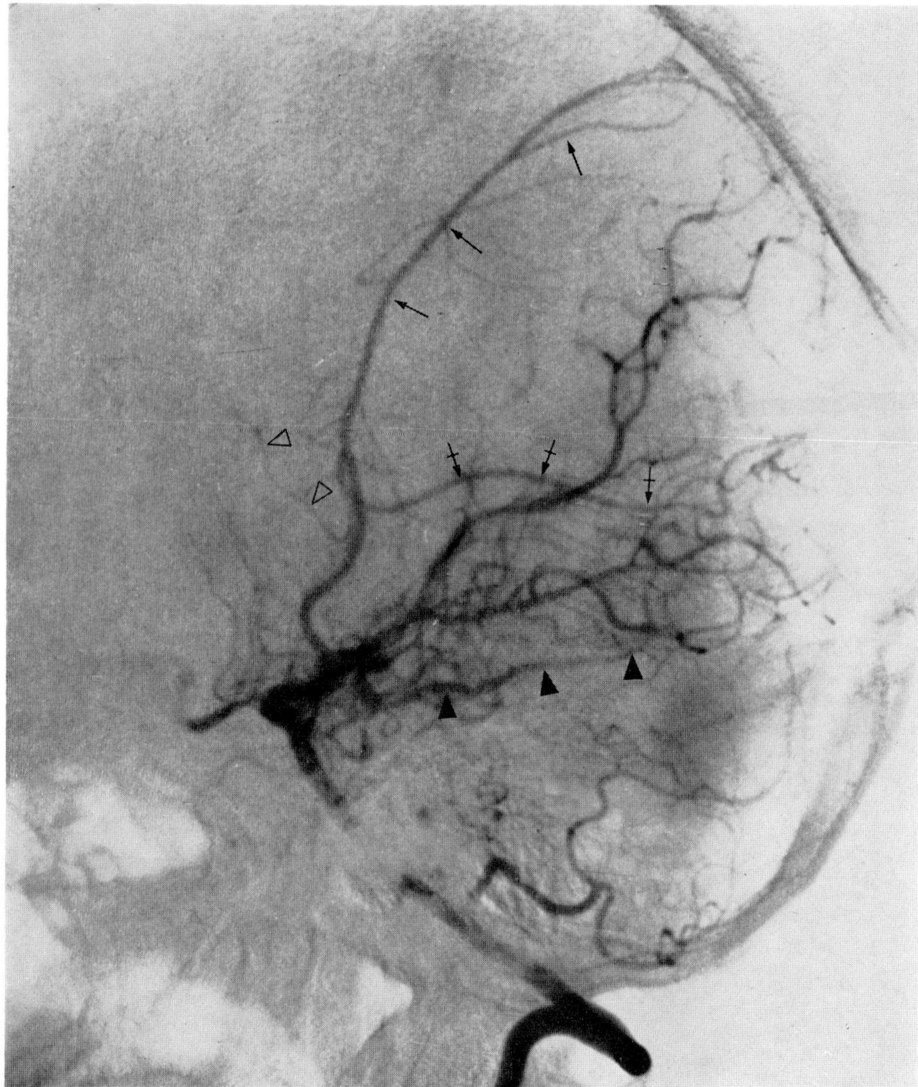

Fig. 245

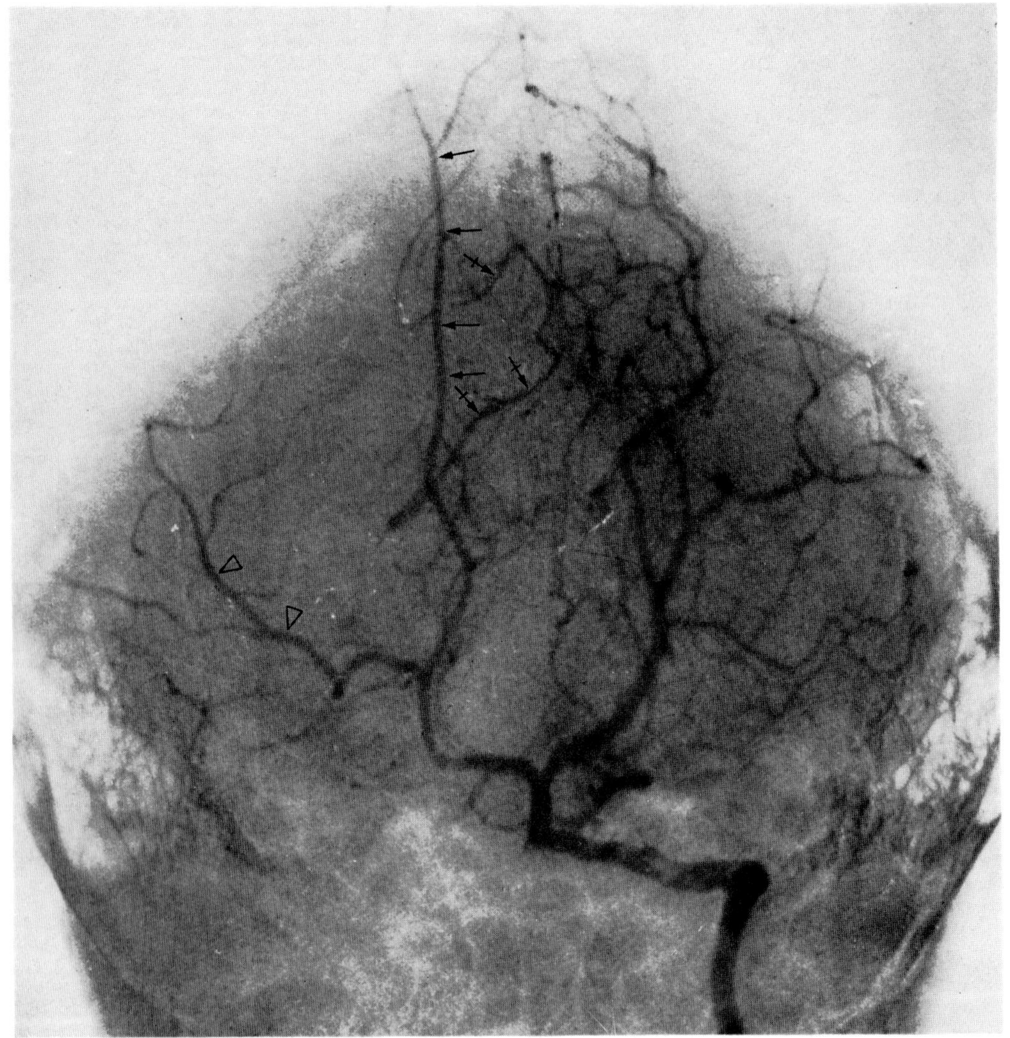

Fig. 246

Metastatic Tumor in the Right Occipital Lobe Secondary to Carcinoma of the Lung

A 60-year-old male: Figs. 247 and 248

Fig. 247 Arterial phase in the lateral projection. The quadrigeminal segment of the posterior cerebral artery is diffusely elevated on the right (a closed arrowhead). The parieto-occipital branch (3 arrows) and the calcarine branch (4 crossed arrows) are stretched in an arcuate fashion. The posterior choroidal arteries are dislocated anteriorly (2 open arrowheads). The findings suggest a large mass in the occipital lobe. The basilar artery is displaced anteriorly and the posterior inferior cerebellar artery is depressed (3 open arrowheads), probably indicating increased intracranial pressure with tendency of tonsillar herniation.

Fig. 248 Arterial phase in the Towne projection. The quadrigeminal segment of the right posterior cerebral artery is displaced anteriorly (2 arrowheads). The calcarine (2 crossed arrows) and parieto-occipital branches (2 arrows) are displaced laterally.

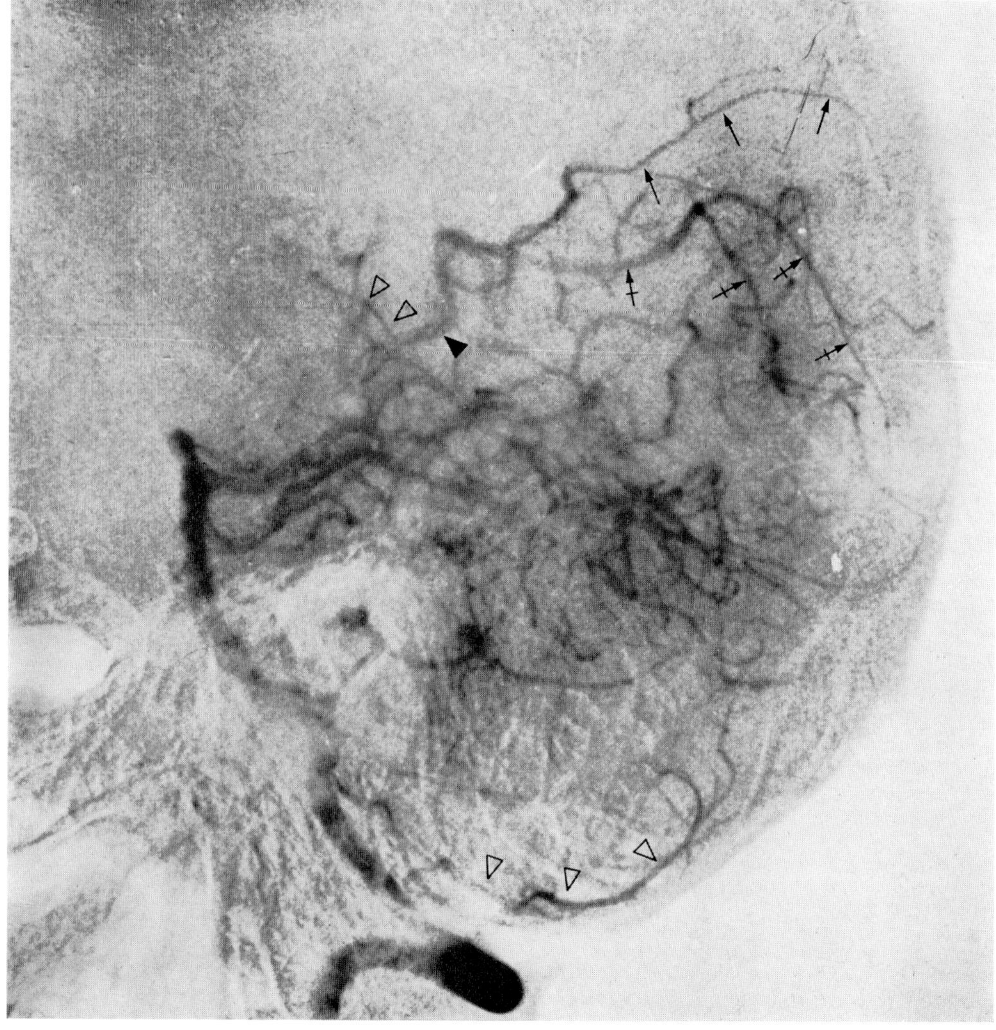

Fig. 247

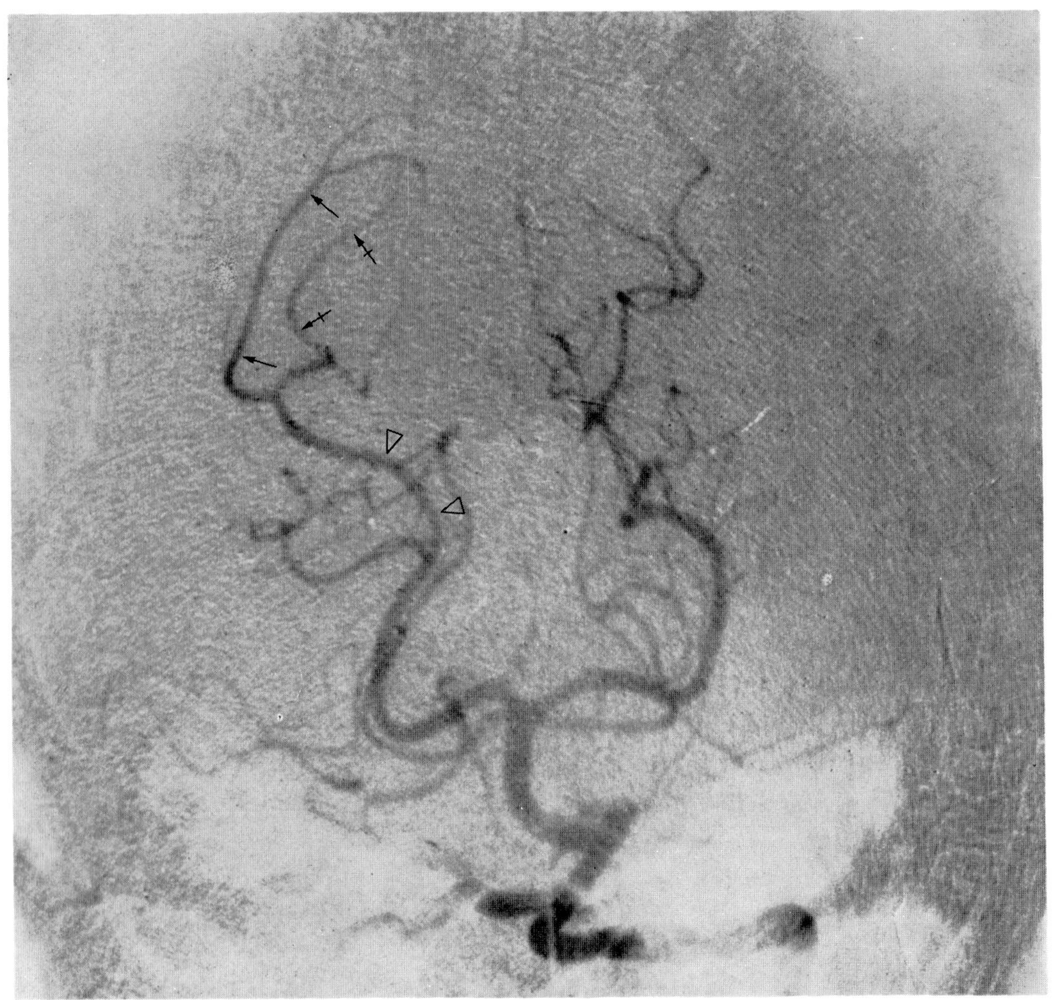

Fig. 248

Large Bilateral Occipital Meningioma with Attachment to the Posterior Portion of the Falx

A 54-year-old male: Figs. 249–254

Fig. 249 Arterial phase in the lateral projection. A 4 × 5 cm occipital tumor is present with arcuate displacement of the parieto-occipital and calcarine branches of the right posterior cerebral artery (6 arrows). A branch of the right posterior cerebral artery is also elevated (2 arrowheads). The parieto-occipital and calcarine branches of the left posterior cerebral artery are separated and displaced anteriorly by a left occipital tumor (4 crossed arrows). The posterior meningeal artery is enlarged and supplies the tumor by two terminal branches (5 double-crossed arrows). The posterior choroidal and the thalamoperforate arteries are displaced anteriorly (2 long arrows). Main blood supply comes from the posterior meningeal artery, left calcarine artery and the right parieto-occipital artery. Findings were supplemented with the use of bilateral carotid angiograms with good demonstration of individual posterior cerebralar teries.

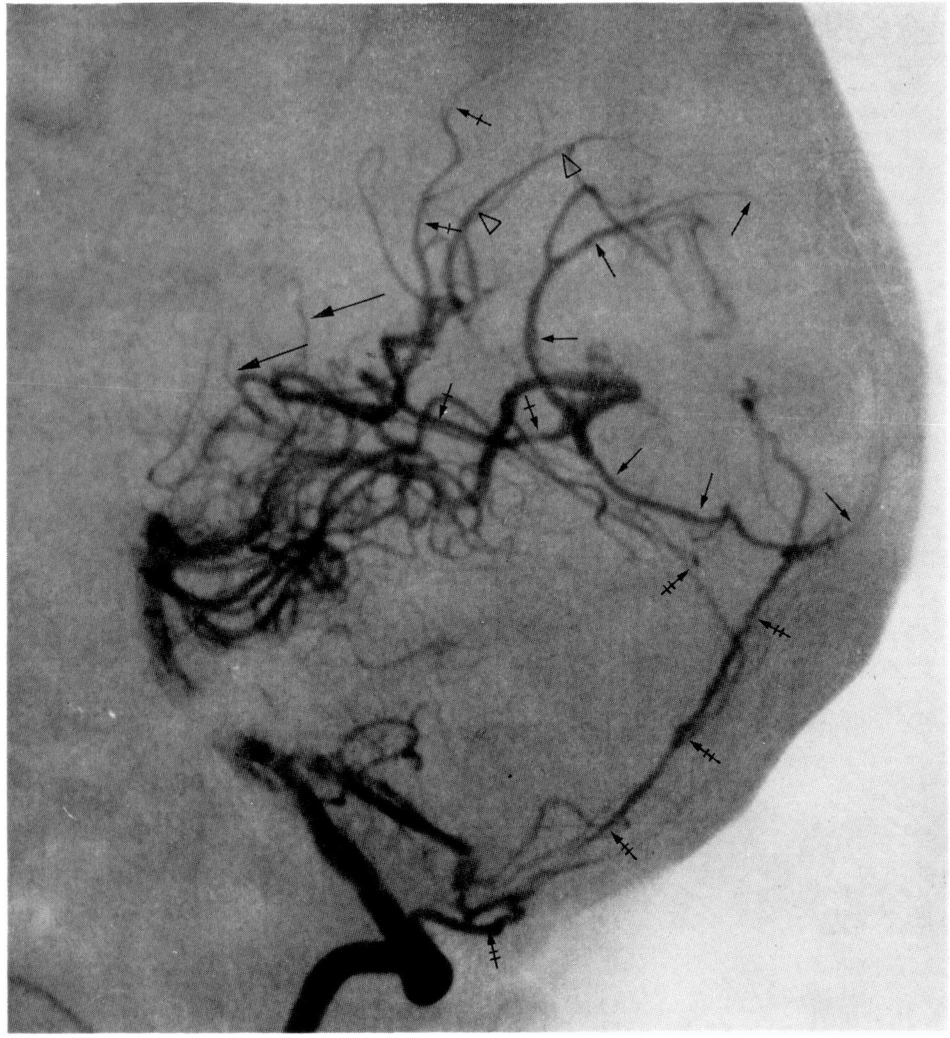

Fig. 249

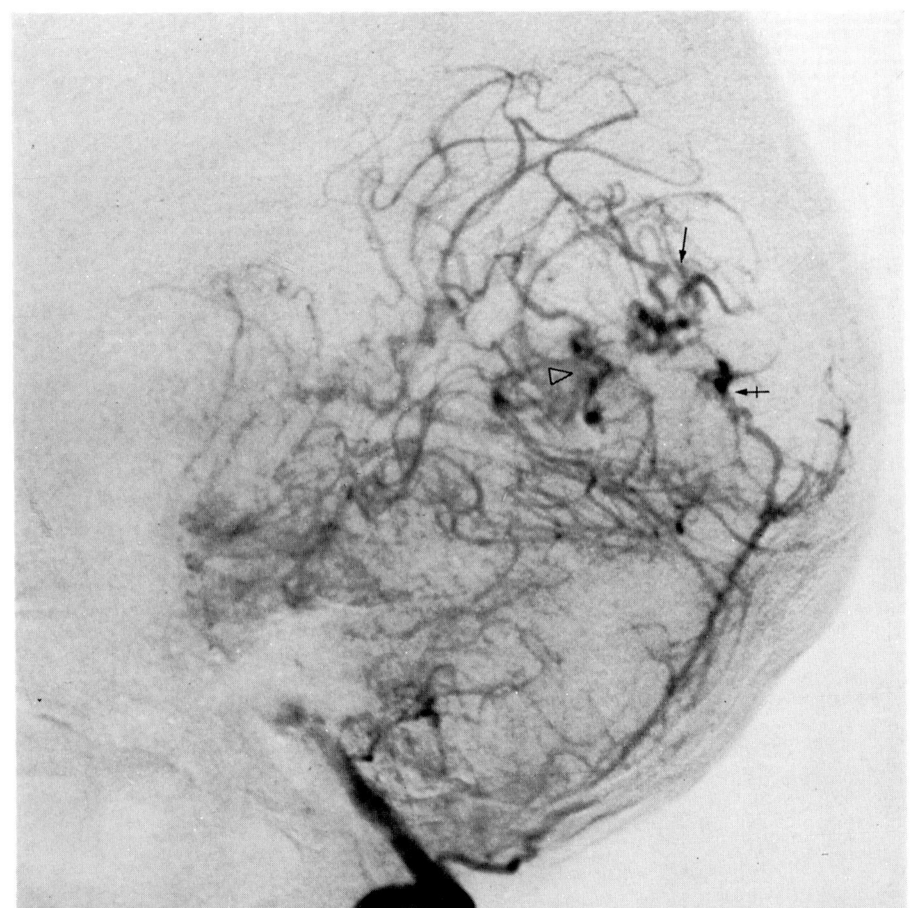

Fig. 250

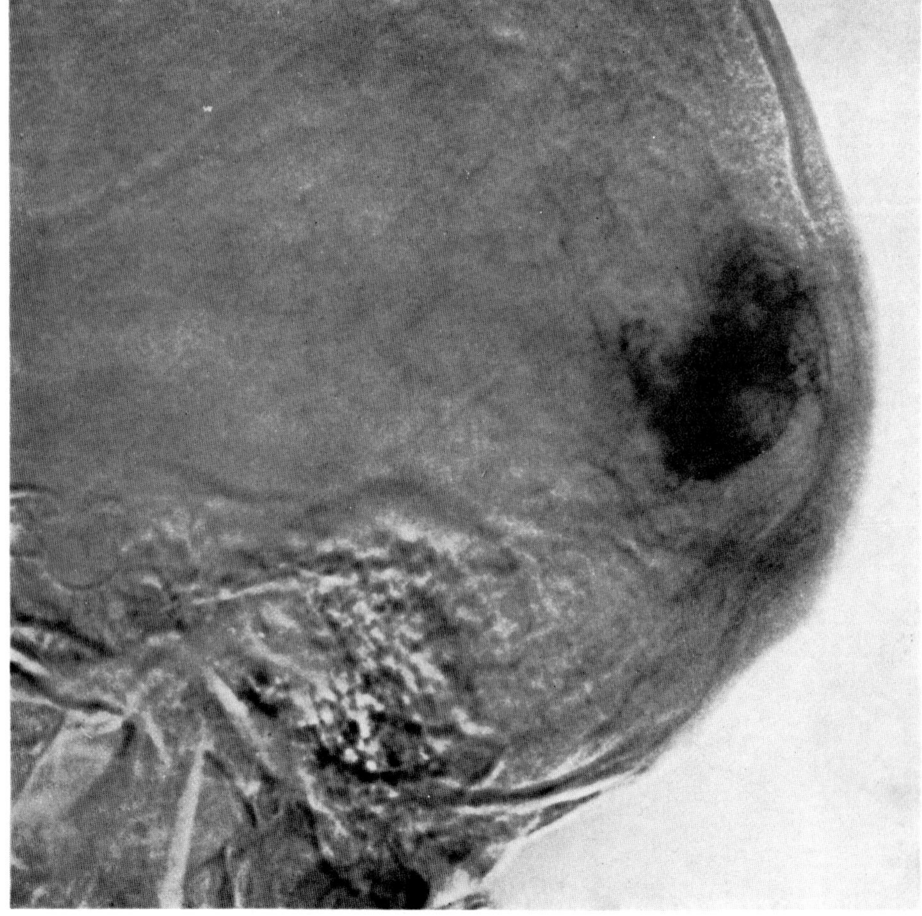

Fig. 251

Fig. 250 Late arterial phase in the lateral projection. Tumor vessels and blood supply are well shown. There are tumor vessels supplied by the posterior meningeal artery (a crossed arrow), right parieto-occipital artery (an arrow) and left calcarine artery (an arrowhead).

Fig. 251 Capillary phase in the lateral projection. Dense tumor stains are noted in the posterior aspect of the tumors. These appear to be supplied mostly by the posterior meningeal artery, probably indicating the tumor attachment to the falx.

Fig. 252 Arterial phase in the Towne projection. The left calcarine branch is enlarged and angulated anteriorly (2 arrows). The left parieto-occipital branch is compressed against the falx (2 crossed arrows). The right parieto-occipital (2 arrows)and the calcarine (2 crossed arrows) arteries are displaced anteriorly and laterally. The posterior meningeal artery arises from the terminal vertebral artery, courses upwards in the midline and reaches the posterior falx (4 arrowheads).

Fig. 253 Late arterial phase in the Towne projection. The findings described above are well shown. The markers are same as Fig. 252.

Fig. 254 Capillary phase in the Towne projection. The posterior meningeal artery is shown to good advantage. There appear to be two parallel branches (2 opposing arrows) which supply tumor vessels on each side. The meningeal artery enters the tumors via a small area (a crossed arrow), which probably indicates the tumor attachment to the falx. The tumor vessels are well shown on each side of the tumor.

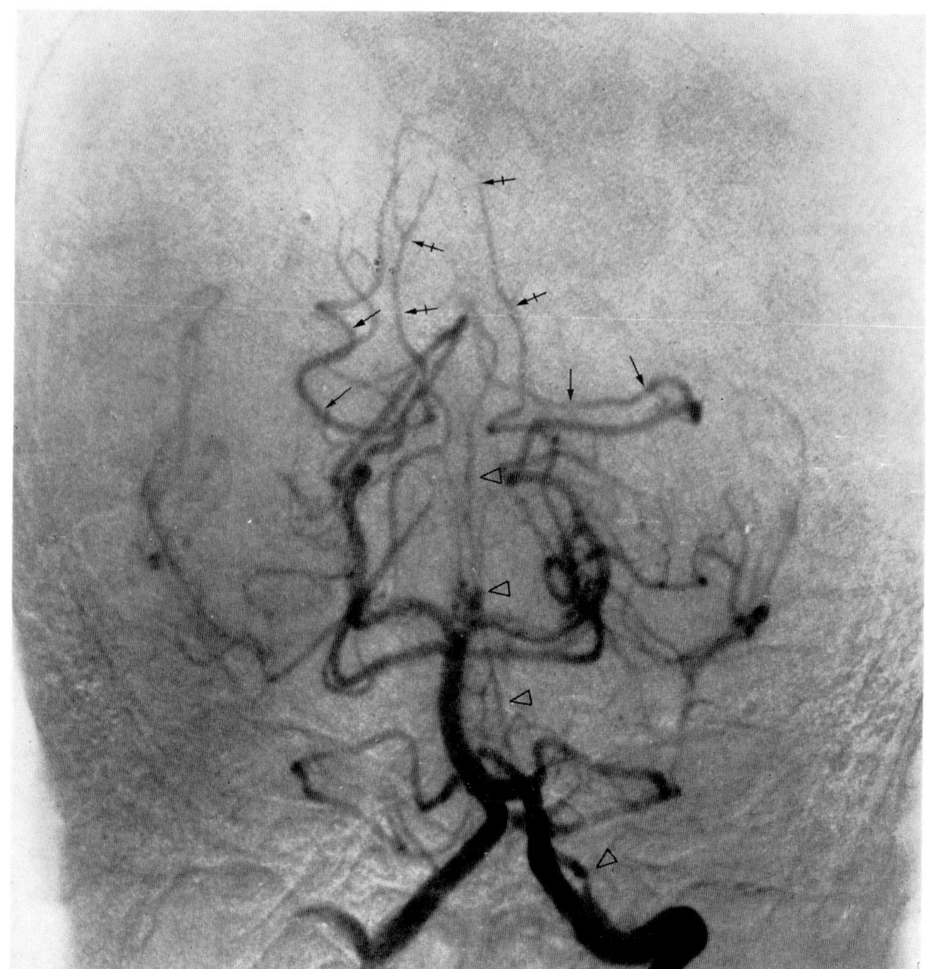

Fig. 252

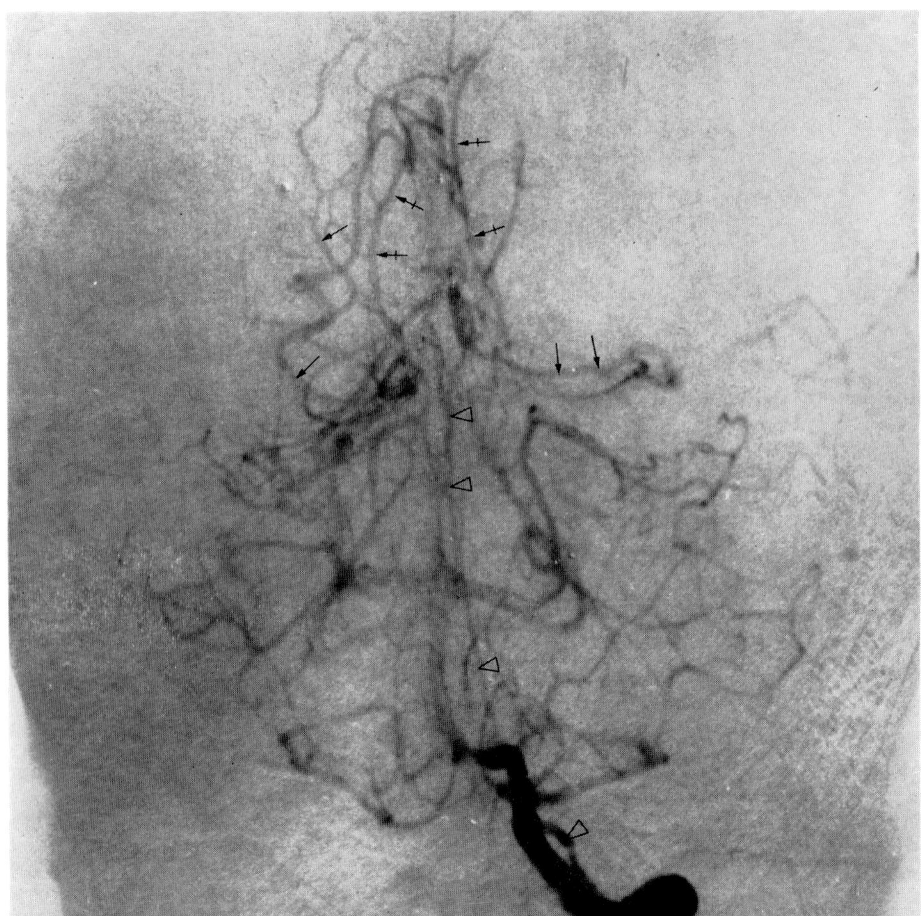

Fig. 253

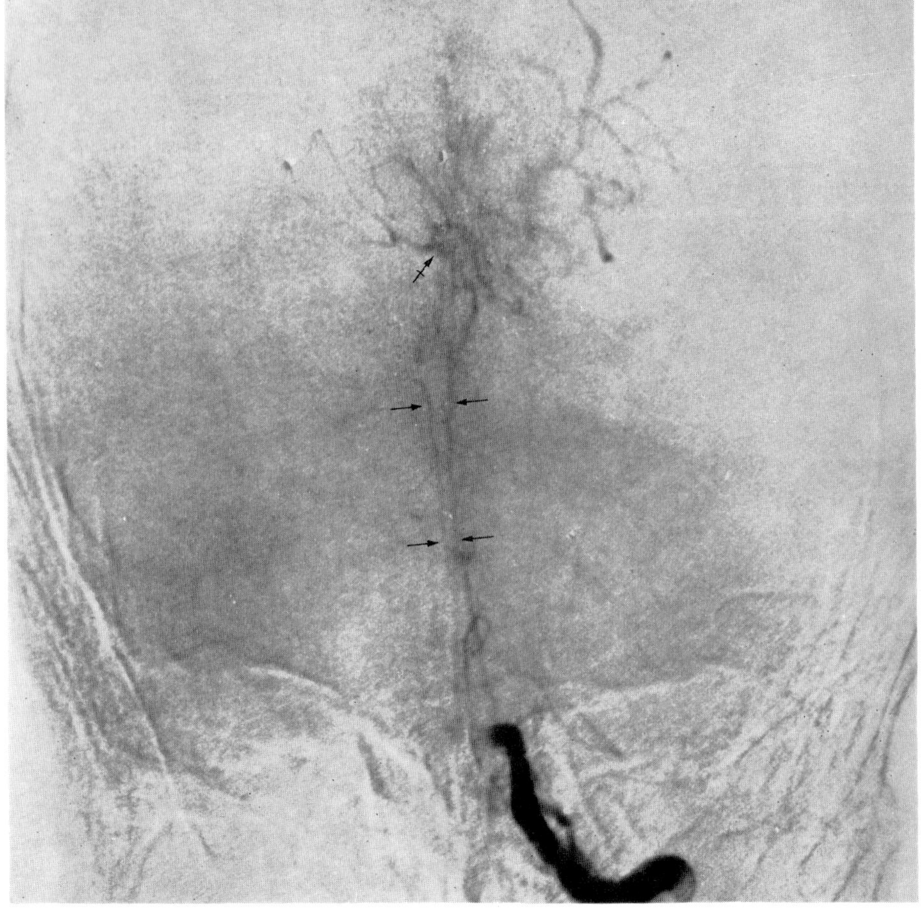

Fig. 254

TEMPORAL TUMORS

Histologically similar tumors are encountered in this location as in the occipital lobe tumors. An incisural tumor may present as a temporal tumor, and this latter entity was discussed in the preceding section.

Arteriographic features

The main portion of the posterior cerebral artery may be displaced in various directions, depending upon the origin of tumors. The anterior temporal and posterior temporal arteries of the posterior cerebral artery are displaced in either anterior, posterior or superior direction. Tumor vessels or tumor stains are supplied by small arterial branches of the posterior cerebral artery. The thalamoperforate arteries may be displaced to the opposite side in the anteroposterior projection. When there is tumor invasion into the thalamus, the lateral posterior choroidal artery may be displaced posteriorly.

Carotid angiograms show superior and anterior displacement of the sylvian point with draping of temporal branches of the middle cerebral artery. The meningohypophyseal artery may be enlarged when there is a tentorial meningioma.

Venographic features

The basal vein of Rosenthal and the posterior mesencephalic vein may be displaced medially and posteriorly. The internal cerebral vein is displaced to the opposite side.

Ependymoma of the Left Temporal Lobe with Transtentorial Herniation

A 3-year-old male: Figs. 255–258

Fig. 255 Arterial phase in the Towne projection. The crural segment and the anterior ambient segment of the left posterior cerebral artery is medially displaced (3 arrows) and the anterior temporal artery is stretched and elongated (3 crossed arrows), suggesting an expanding lesion in the anterior and middle temporal lobe. There is medial displacement of the left posterior communicating artery (2 long arrows). The thalamoperforate arteries are deviated to the right (an arrowhead).

Fig. 256 Arterial phase in the lateral projection. There is increased distance between the clivus and the basilar artery (arrowheads). The proximal segments of the posterior cerebral artery are depressed downwards (3 arrows), suggesting a transtentorial herniation. The thalamoperforate arteries are displaced posteriorly (2 crossed arrows).

Fig. 257 Venous phase in the lateral projection. The pontine segment of the anterior pontomesencephalic vein is displaced posteriorly with increased distance from the clivus (3 arrows). The superior thalamic veins are depressed due to hydrocephalus (3 crossed arrows).

Fig. 258 Left internal carotid angiogram. There are tumor vessels in the middle portion of the temporal lobe. The supraclinoid portion of the internal carotid artery is anteriorly displaced. The anterior choroidal artery is enlarged and displaced superiorly (3 arrows). There is anterior and superior displacement of the sylvian segment of the middle cerebral artery (3 crossed arrows). Unrolling of the anterior cerebral artery is noted.

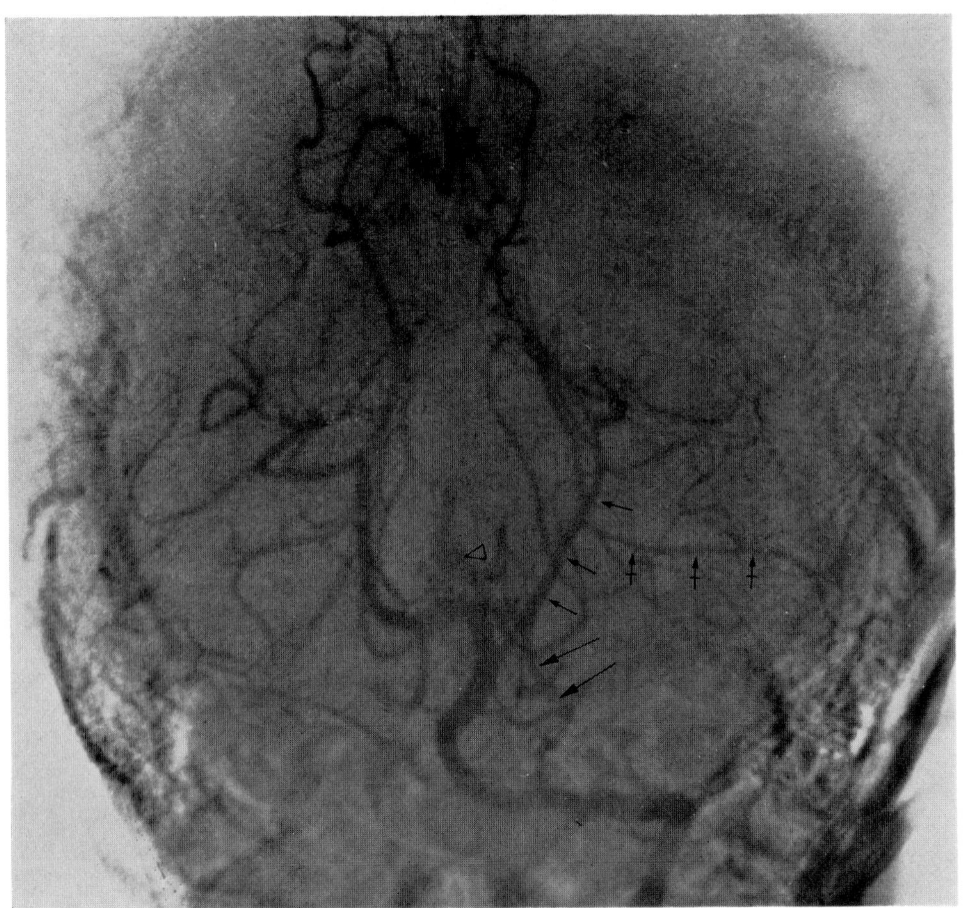

Fig. 255

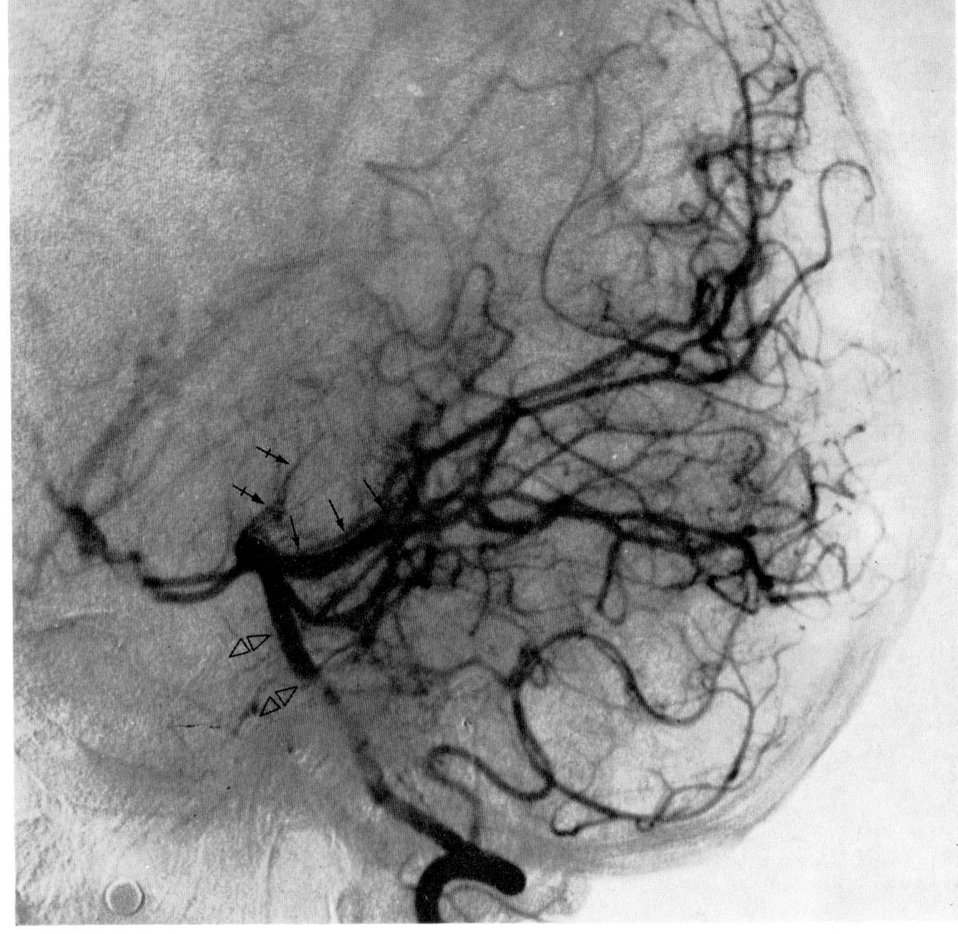

Fig. 256

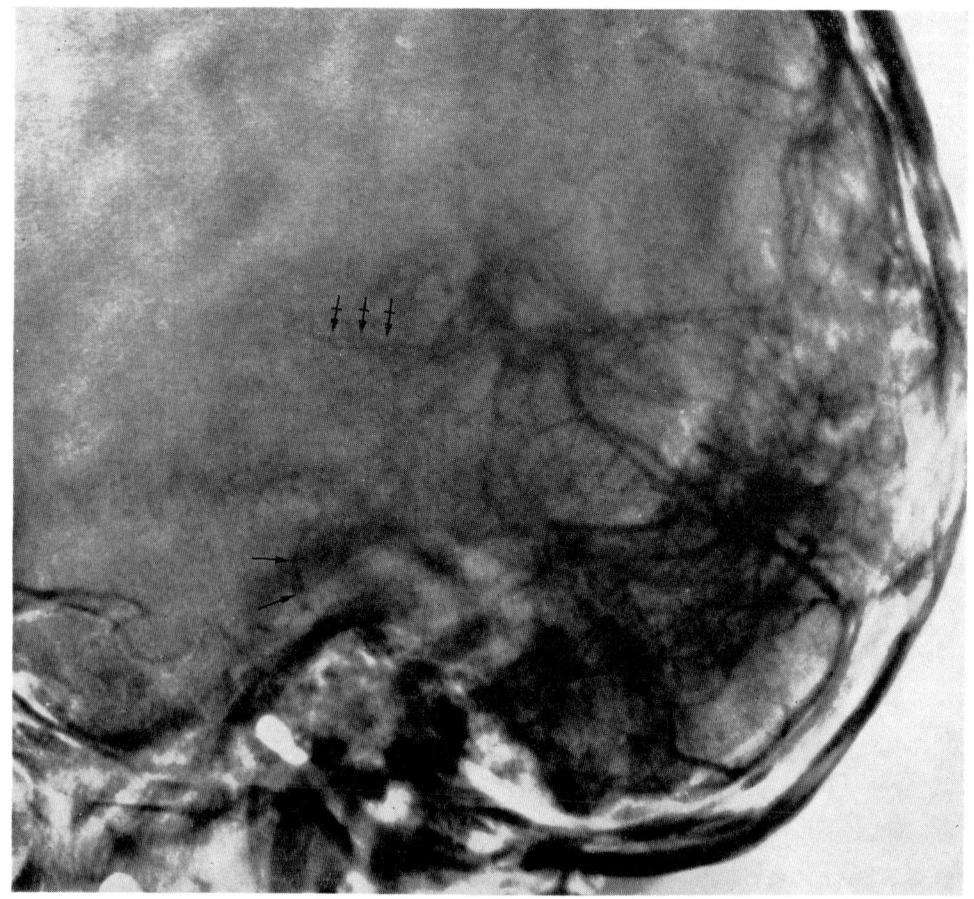

Fig. 257

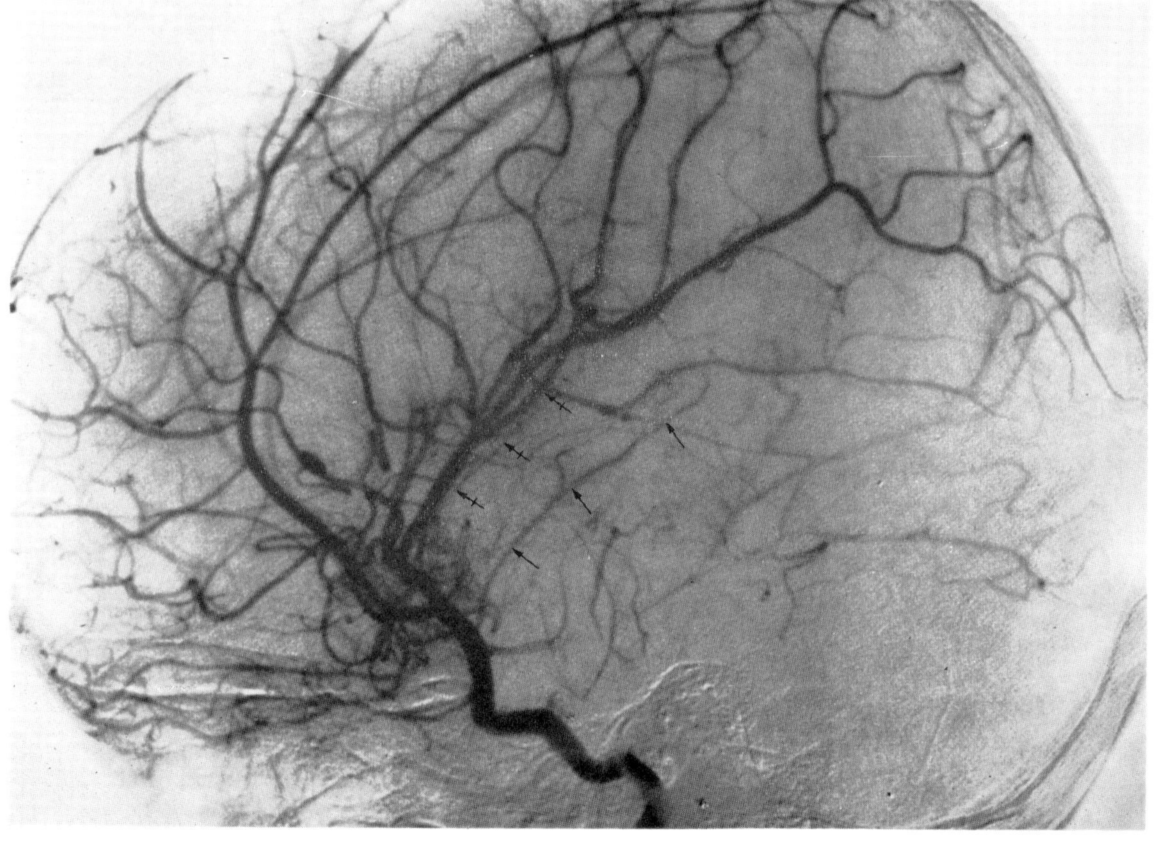

Fig. 258

Large Neurinoma Arising from the Right Gasselian Ganglion and Extending into the Right Cerebellopontine Angle

A 28-year-old female: Figs. 259–263

Fig. 259 Arterial phase in the Towne projection. The right posterior cerebral artery and its anterior temporal artery are displaced posteriorly in an arcuate fashion (3 arrows), indicating a large mass in the area of the anterior temporal lobe. The posterior displacement of the superior cerebellar artery and its marginal branch represents tumor extention into the cerebellopontine angle (3 crossed arrows). The anterior inferior cerebellar artery is depressed downwards (2 arrowheads).

Fig. 260 Venous phase in the Towne projection. The right petrosal vein and the transverse pontine vein are displaced laterally and inferiorly (3 arrows).

Fig. 261 Arterial phase in the lateral projection. The posterior cerebral artery is elevated and the anterior temporal artery is pushed backwards (5 arrows). There is also superior and posterior displacement of the superior cerebellar artery and its marginal artery (5 crossed arrows), outlining the posterior extent of the tumor. The posterior choroidal arteries are dislocated posteriorly (3 arrowheads).

Fig. 262 Right internal carotid angiogram. The carotid siphon is opened with marked elevation of the anterior choroidal artery (3 arrows) and the sylvian point (a crossed arrow). The anterior temporal branch of the middle cerebral artery is also elevated (2 arrowheads). The findings suggest a large extracerebral tumor in the middle fossa.

Fig. 263 Right external carotid angiogram. The anterior branch of the middle meningeal artery is well shown (3 arrowheads), while its posterior branches supply tumor vessels in the middle fossa (3 arrows). The posterior meningeal artery from the ascending pharyngeal artery also supplies the tumor (4 crossed arrows). Because of blood supply from the meningeal arteries, differentiation from a meningioma was not possible.

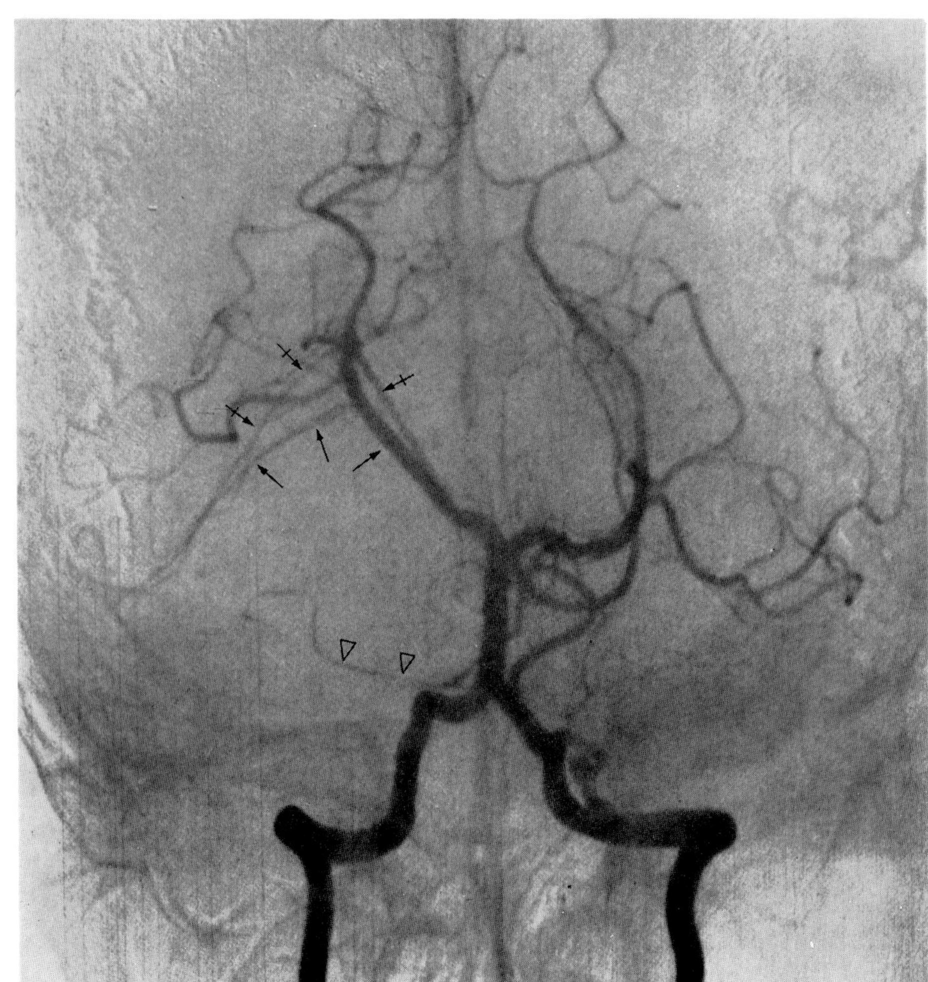

Fig. 259

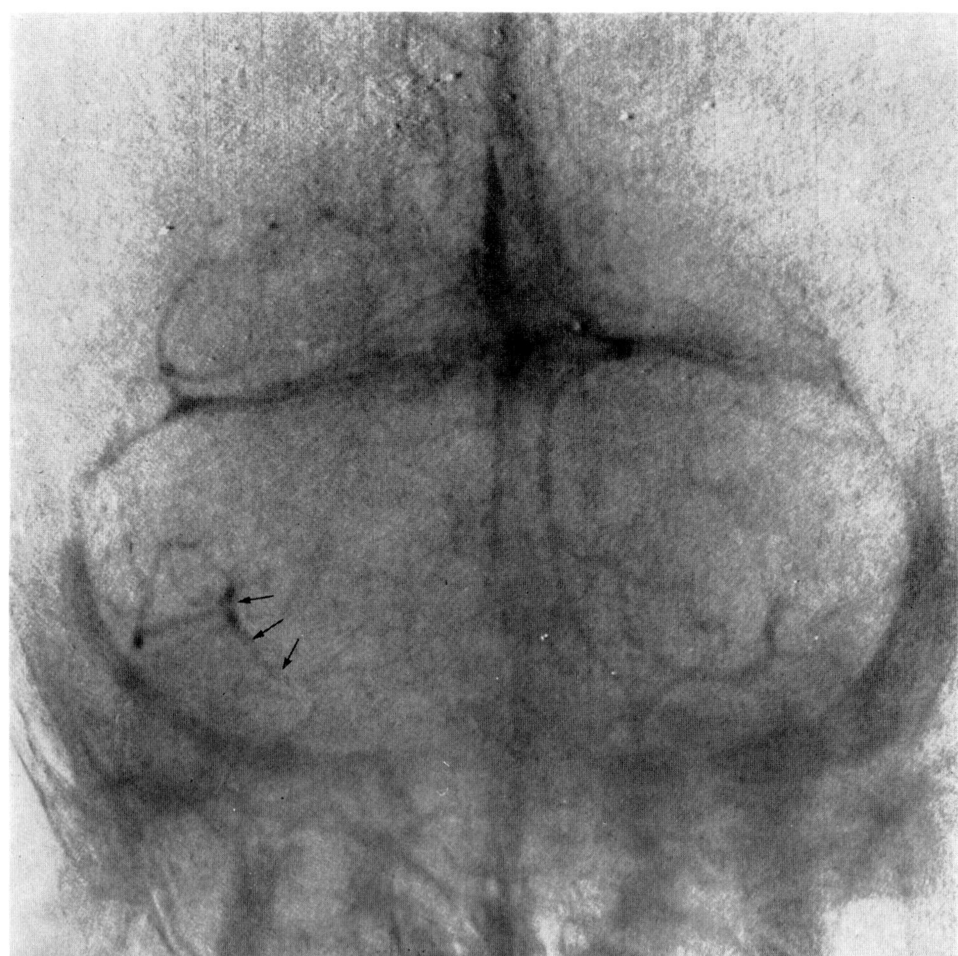

Fig. 260

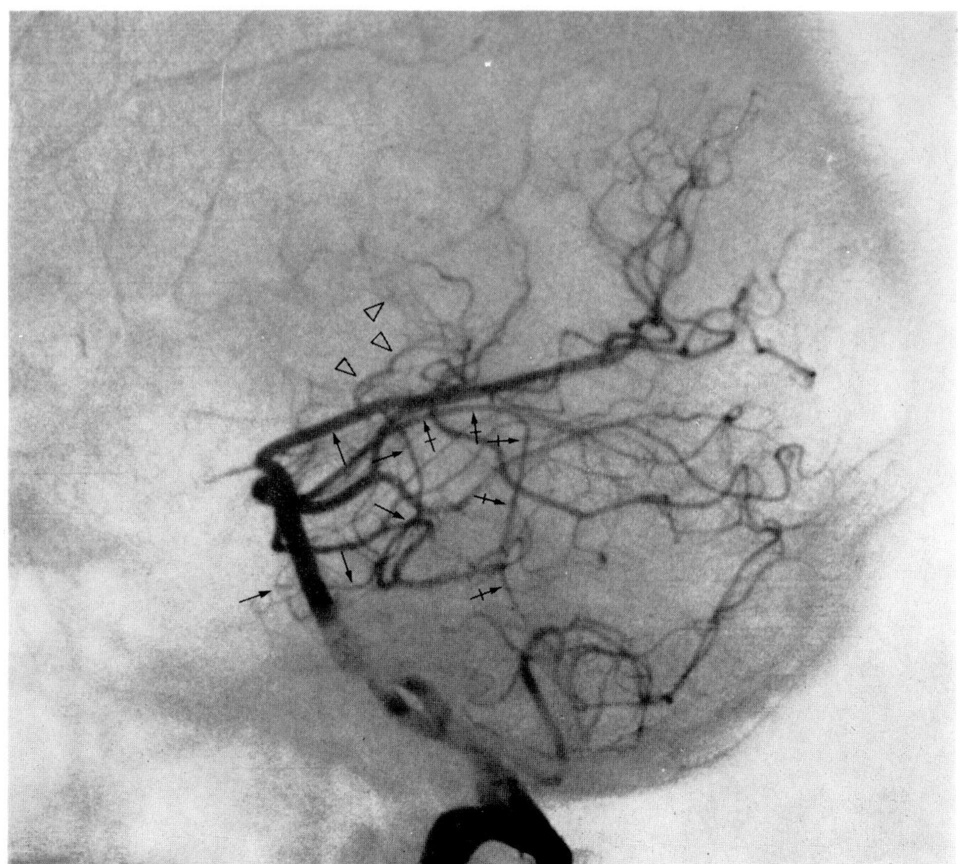

Fig. 261

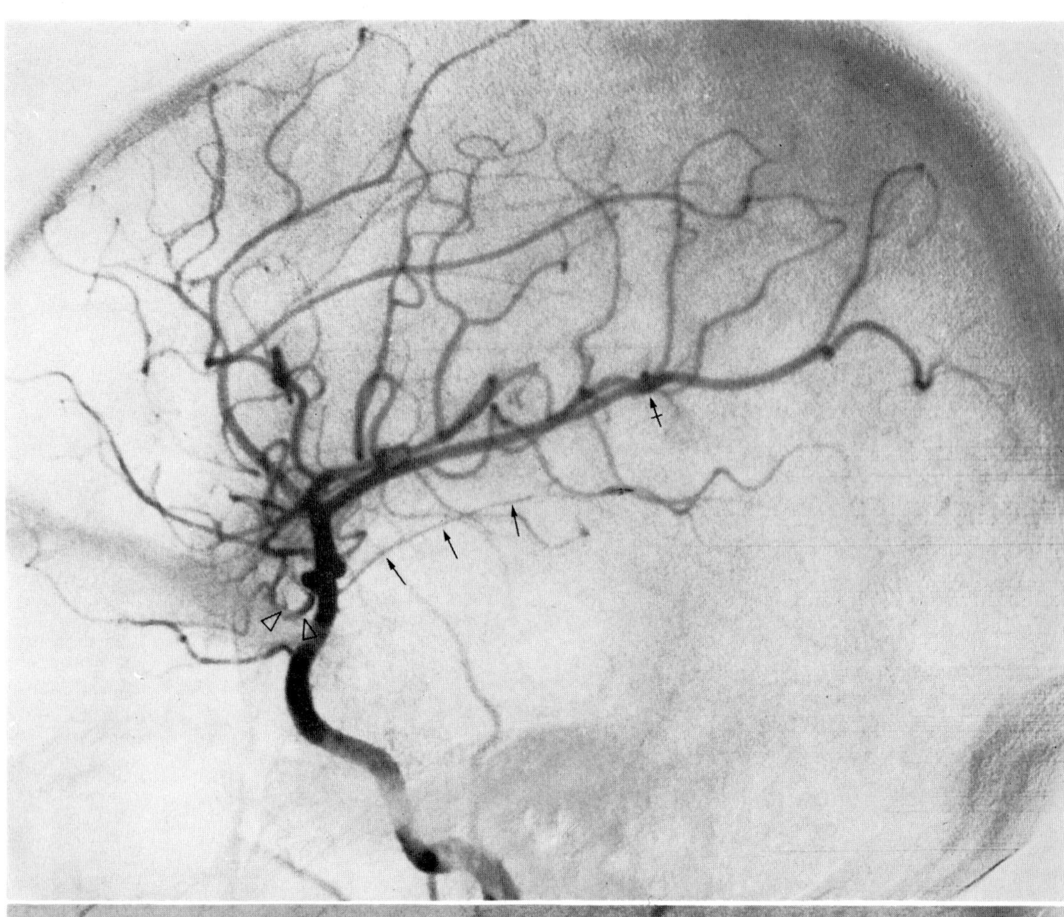

Fig. 262

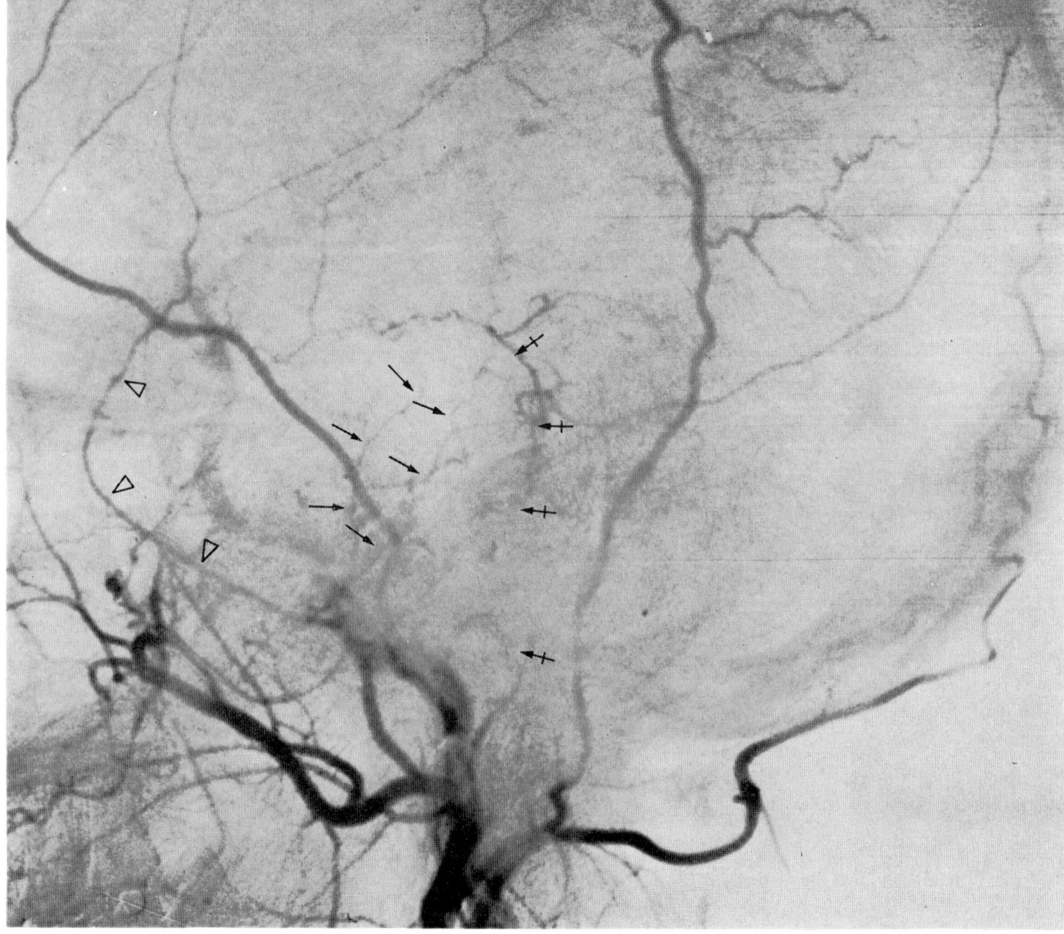

Fig. 263

THALAMIC TUMORS (TUMORS OF THE POSTERIOR THALAMUS)

Arteriographic features

Posterior choroidal artery

The lateral posterior choroidal artery is displaced posteriorly in an arcuate fashion with increased radius of its curvature. The artery outlines the posterior surface of the tumor. Only rarely is lateral displacement of this artery observed. When the tumor encases this artery, there may be anterior displacement of the artery.

The medial choroidal artery is usually normal in position at the early stage of the disease, but posterior displacement of this artery is observed when the tumor becomes larger or infiltrates the brain stem.

Colliculi quadrigemini and corpori geniculati arteries

These arteries may participate in the blood supply of the tumor. They become enlarged with anterior or posterior displacement.

Thalamoperforate arteries

These arteries are usually hypertrophied and displaced anteriorly. The arteries, embedded in the tumor, may show rigidity and displacement to various directions depending upon the growth of the tumor. In the frontal projection these arteries may be displaced to the opposite side.

Tumor vessels and tumor stains

Irregular tumor vessels may be supplied by the arteries described above. Tumor stains are frequently demonstrated on the capillary phase and the extent of the tumor can be evaluated.

Venographic features

The internal cerebral vein is elevated and displaced to the opposite side. The superior choroid vein, running on the floor of the lateral ventricle, is frequently displaced superiorly and posteriorly. The distance between the superior choroid vein and the internal cerebral vein is increased, since the superior choroid vein is more markedly elevated than the internal cerebral vein.

The basal vein of Rosenthal is displaced downwards and posteriorly. The superior and anterior thalamic veins are poorly visualized in the presence of thalamic tumors, but these thalamic veins may be displaced upwards when visualized.

Large Thalamic Tumor on the Right

A 43-year-old male: Figs. 264–267

Fig. 264 Arterial phase in the lateral projection. The right lateral posterior choroidal artery is markedly displaced posteriorly in an arcuate fashion (3 arrows). The left lateral and bilateral medial posterior choroidal arteries are depressed due to hydrocephalus (4 crossed arrows). There is straightening of the posterior thalamoperforate arteries (2 arrowheads). In addition, there are multiple small arterial branches supplying the tumor (not properly reproduced). Some of these arterial branches are probably the colliculi quadrigemini and corpori geniculati arteries arising from the ambient segment of the posterior cerebral artery. The posterior pericallosal artery is well demonstrated (2 long arrows).

Fig. 265 Venous phase in the lateral projection. The superior choroid vein is enlarged and displaced superiorly and posteriorly (4 arrows) with elongated connecting vein (a crossed arrow). The internal cerebral vein is displaced superiorly on the side of tumor (4 open arrowheads). The internal cerebral vein (2 double-crossed arrows), and the anterior and superior thalamic veins (3 closed arrowheads) are well demonstrated on the nomal side.

Fig. 266 Arterial phase in the Towne projection. The posterior choroid artery, presumably the right medial branch, is stretched and displaced medially (2 arrows). The lateral posterior choroidal arteries are displaced laterally (4 crossed arrows).

Fig. 267 Venous phase in the Towne projection. The superior choroid vein and choroid blush are displaced laterally and posteriorly on the right (4 arrows), while the choroid plexus is normal on the left (2 crossed arrows).

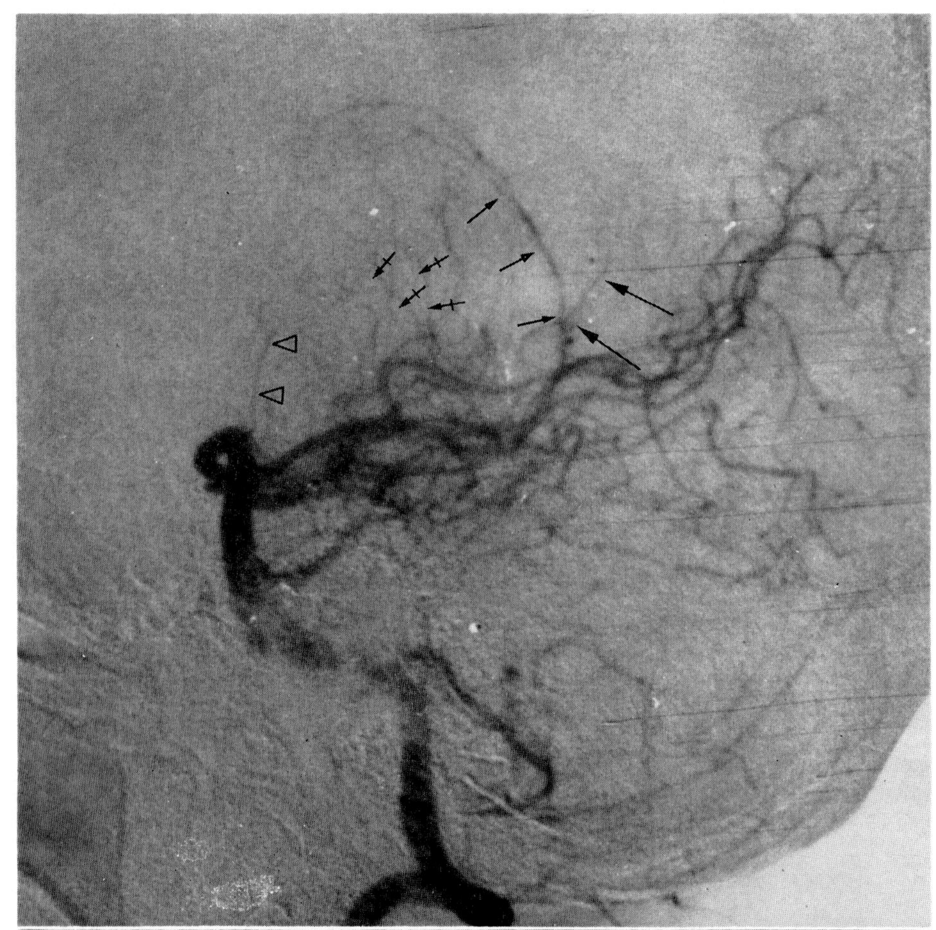

Fig. 264

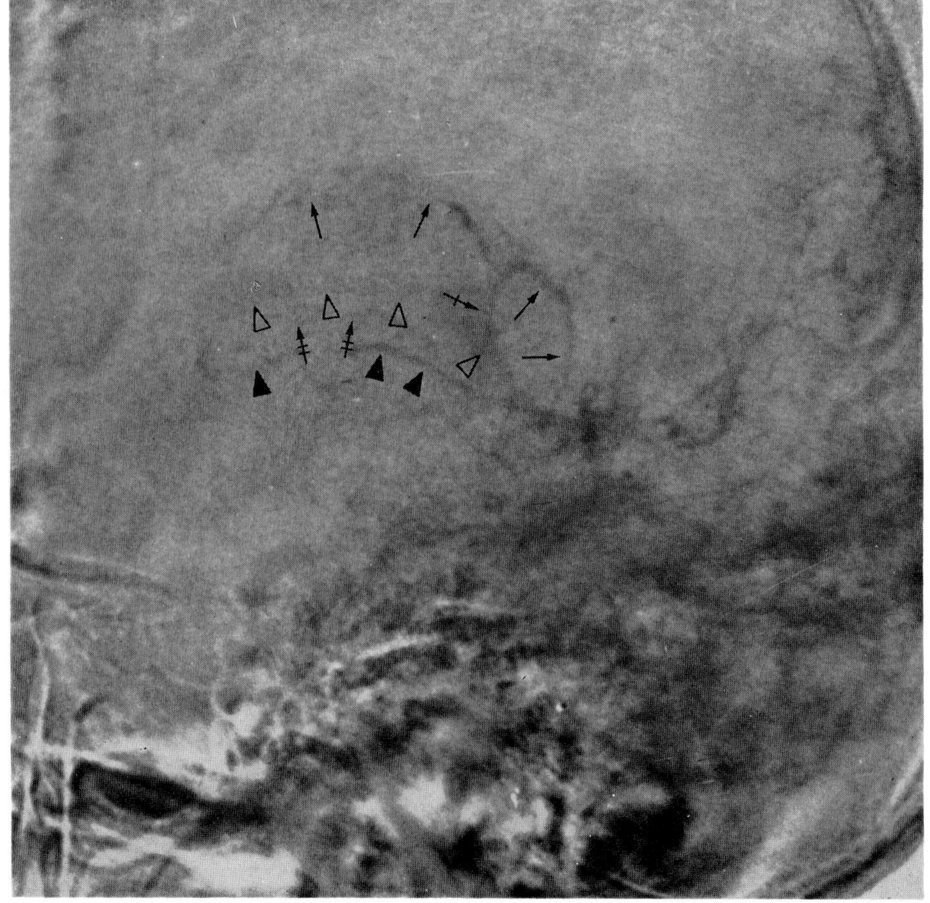

Fig. 265

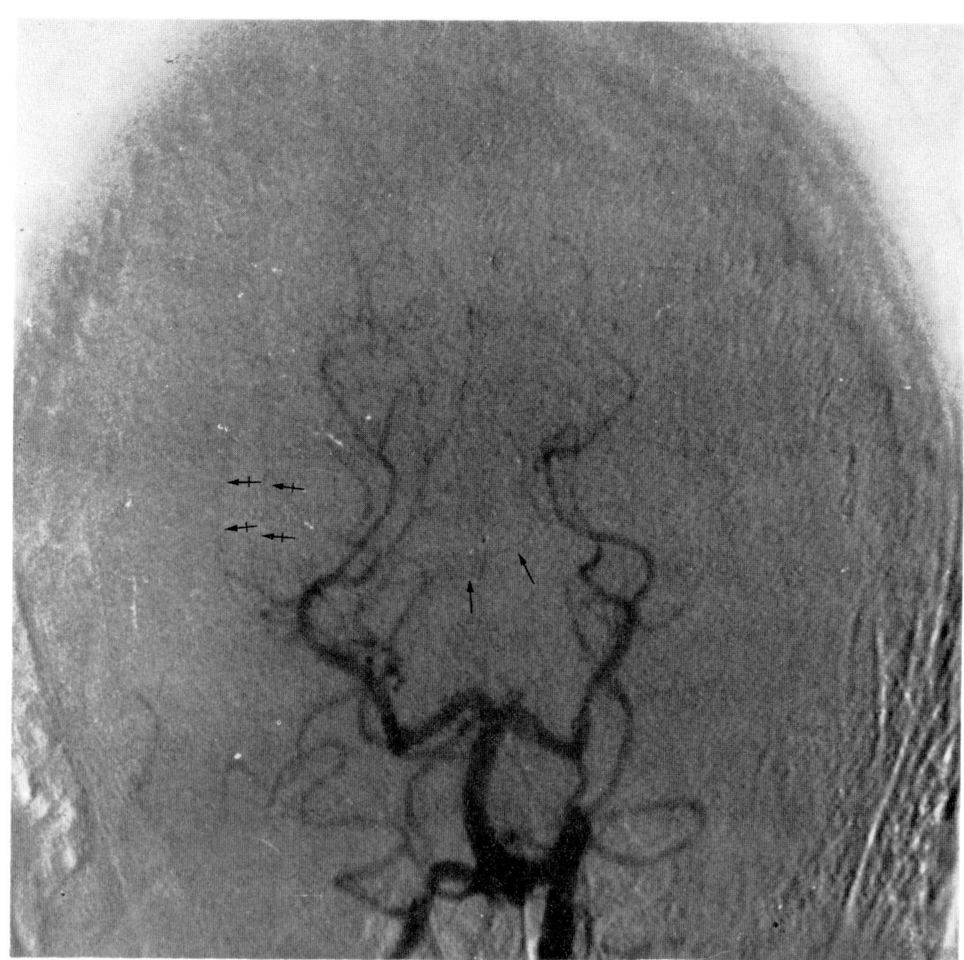

Fig. 266

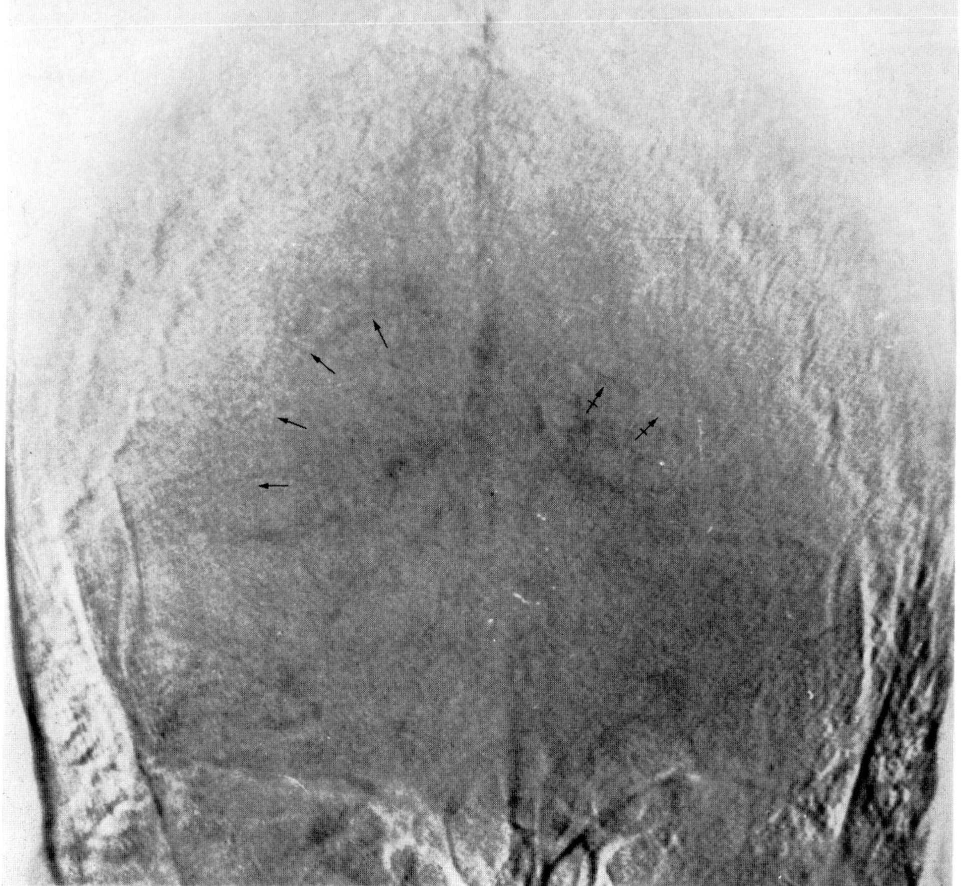

Fig. 267

Right Thalamic Tumor Extending into the Caudate Nucleus and Anterior and Middle Portion of the Right Temporal Lobe

A 44-year-old female: Figs. 268–272

Fig. 268 Arterial phase in the lateral projection. The posterior thalamoperforate arteries are bowed posteriorly (2 arrows). The posterior choroidal arteries are also elevated and displaced posteriorly (3 crossed arrows). The sylvian segments, filled via the posterior communicating artery, are elevated (3 arrowheads), suggesting extension into the temporal lobe.

Fig. 269 Venous phase in the lateral projection. The right superior choroid vein is markedly displaced superiorly in an arcuate fashion (3 closed arrowheads). The internal cerebral vein on the right is also displaced superiorly (2 short arrows). The internal cerebral vein is also slightly elevated on the normal side (3 crossed arrows). The anterior thalamic vein is normal (a double-crossed arrow). The basal vein of Rosenthal is depressed downwards (3 open arrowheads).

Fig. 270 Arterial phase in the Towne projection. The posterior choroidal artery, presumably the right medial branch, is stretched and displaced medially (3 arrows).

Fig. 271 Capillary phase in the Towne projection. The choroid blush on the right is displaced superiorly (3 arrows), while there is normal position of the choroid plexus on the left (3 crossed arrows).

Fig. 272 Venous phase in the Towne projection. Superiorly displaced choroid vein is well seen on the right (3 arrows) with normal choroid vein on the left (3 crossed arrows).

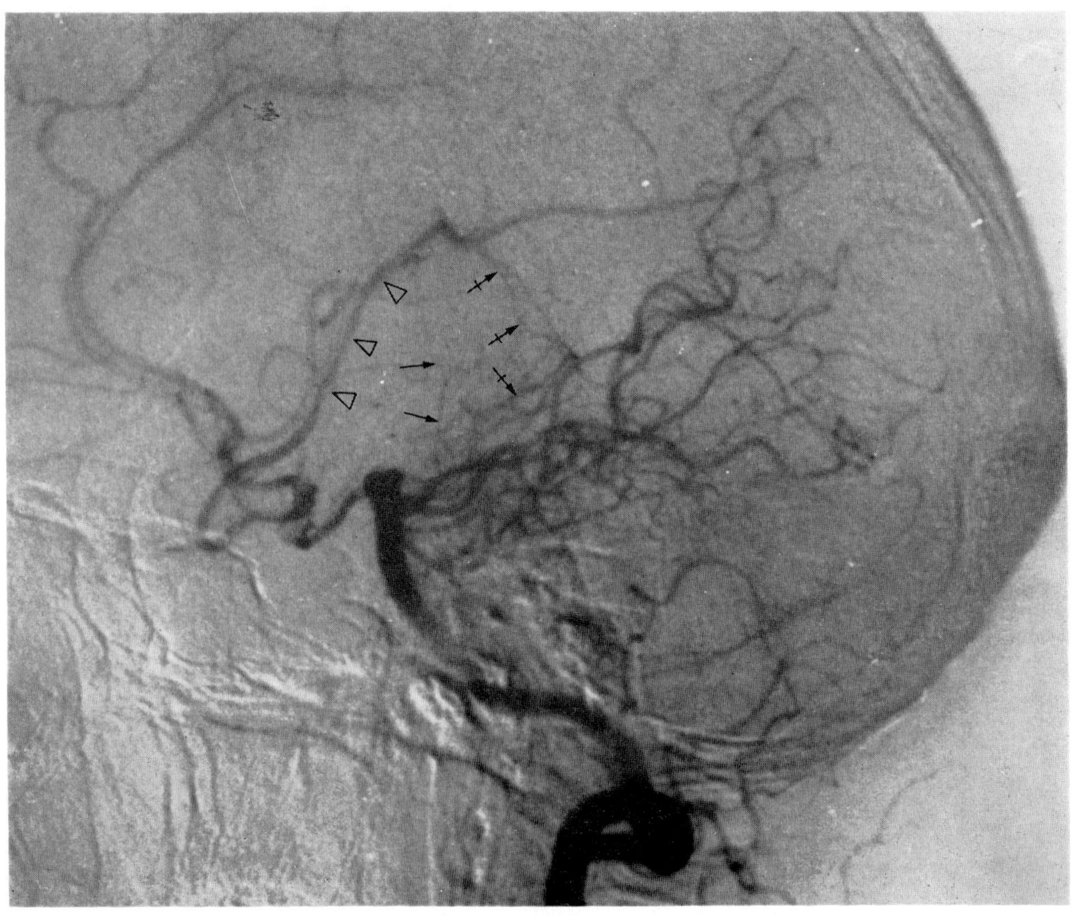

Fig. 268

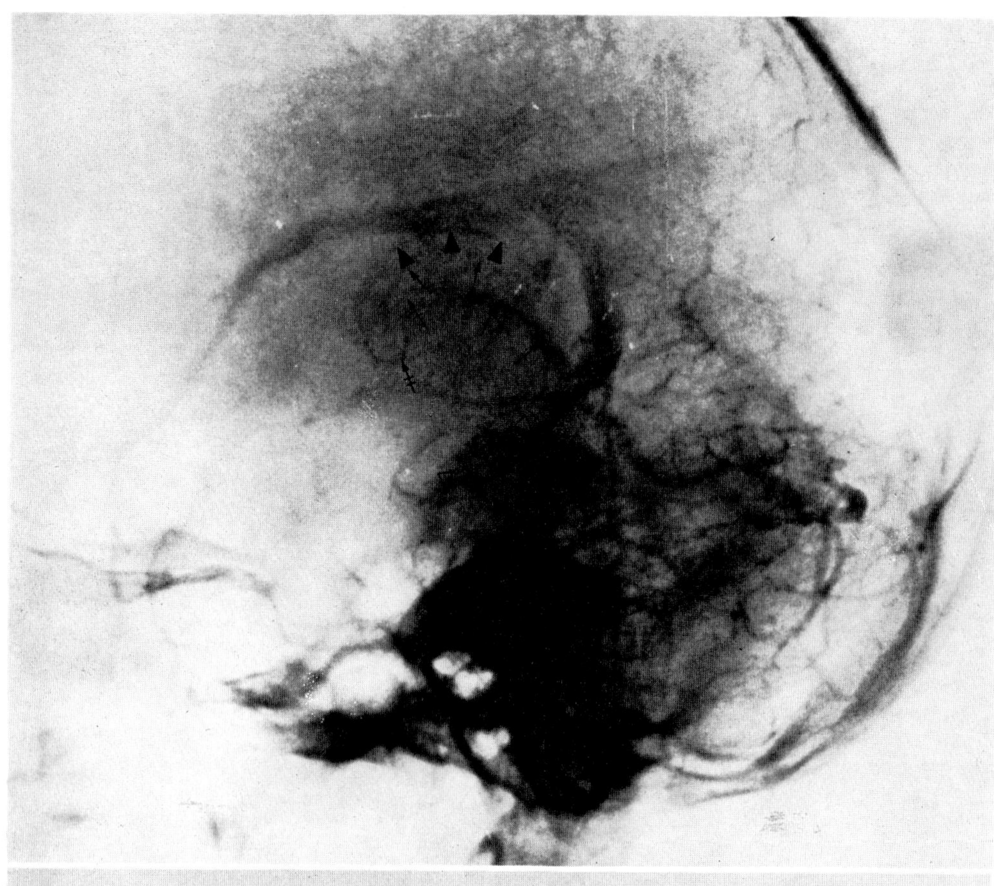

Fig. 269

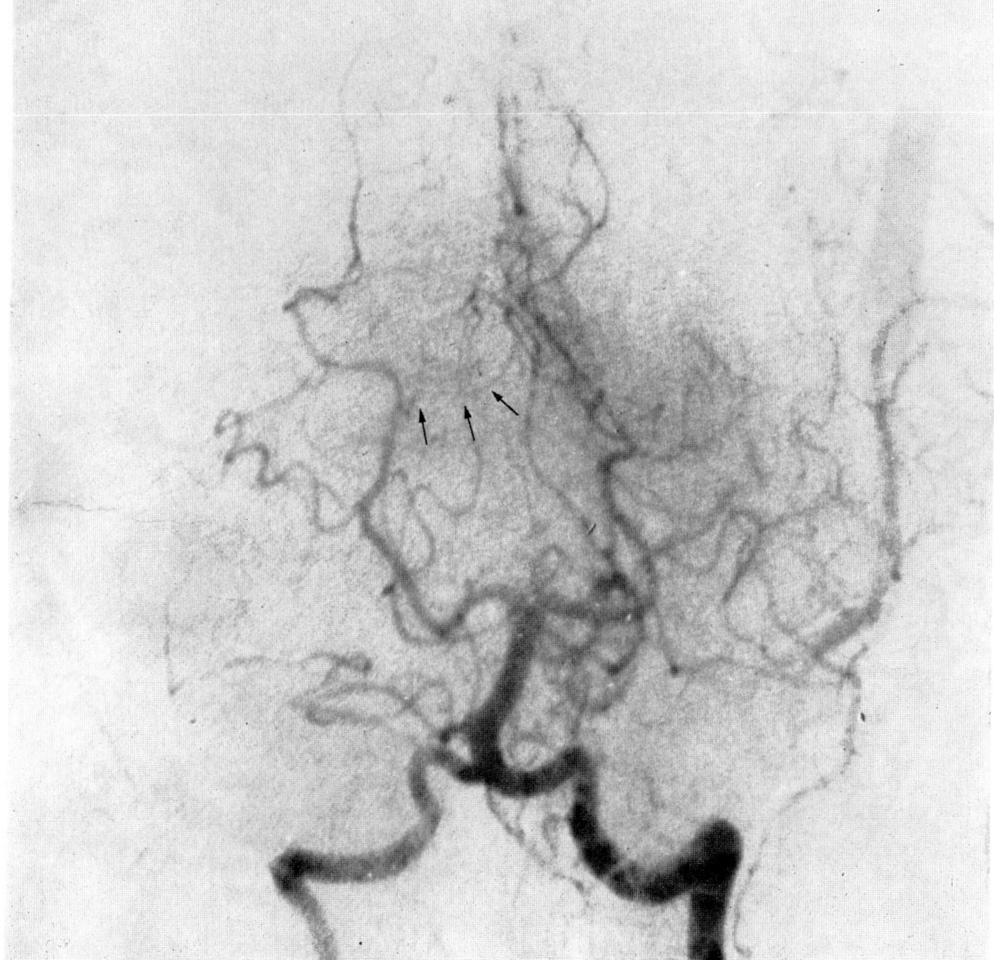

Fig. 270

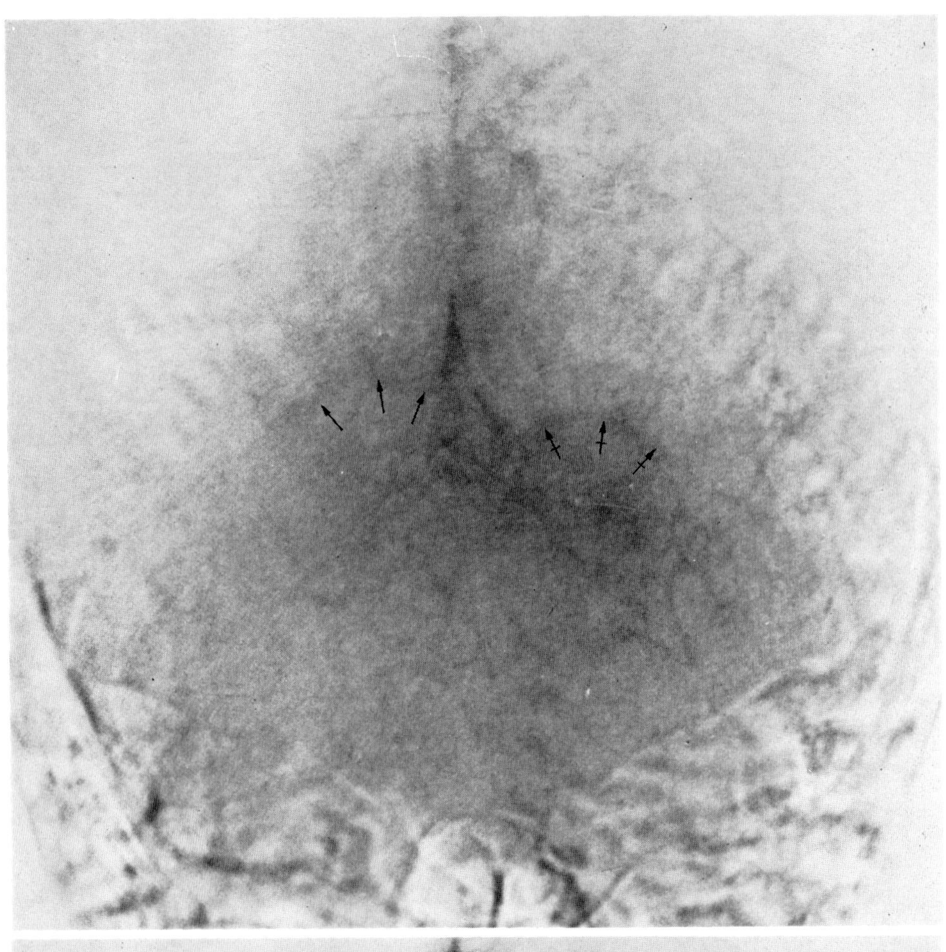

Fig. 271

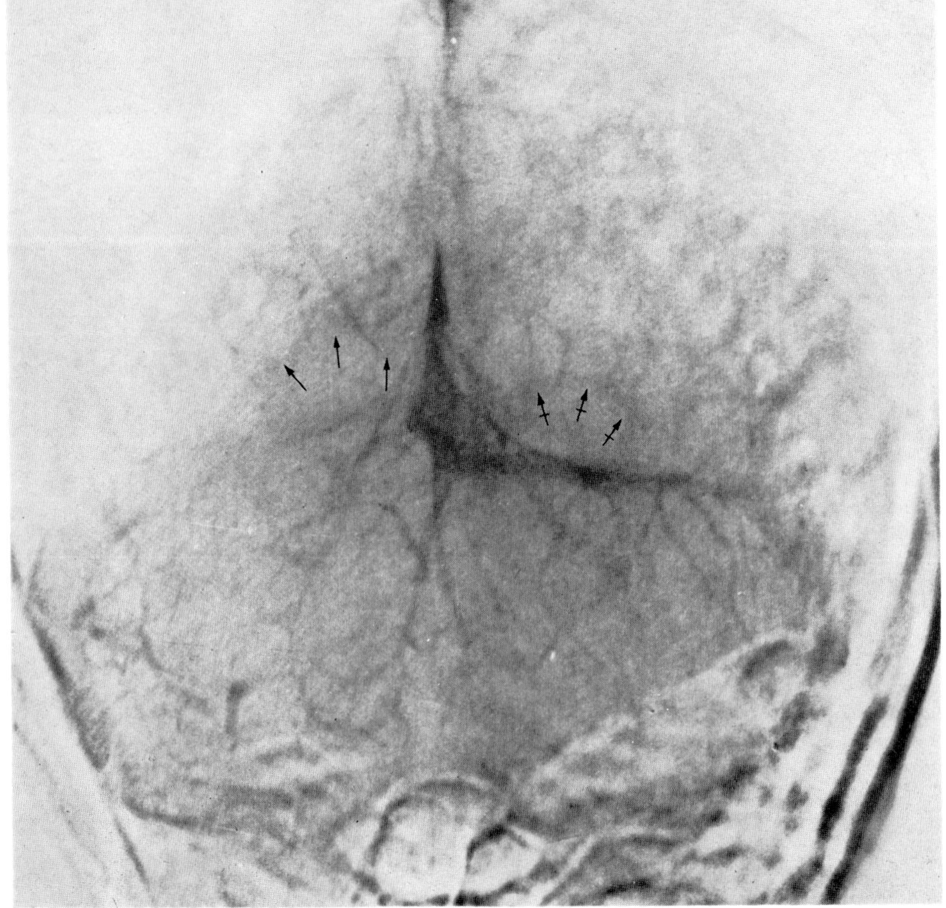

Fig. 272

PINEAL TUMORS

Arteriographic features

Posterior choroidal artery

The medial posterior choroidal artery is displaced posteriorly in an arcuate fashion with loss of its characteristic figure "3". The lateral posterior choroidal artery is also displaced posteriorly when the tumor becomes large. When a pineal tumor extends laterally, the most significant displacement is seen in the lateral posterior choroidal artery.

Thalamoperforate arteries

These arteries may be pushed forwards with anterior convexity when a pineal tumor is large or there is extension into the thalamus.

Colliculi quadrigemini and corpori geniculati arteries

They may be enlarged when they supply tumors. These arteries are not visible on angiograms without hypertrophy of the vessels or with use of fine detail magnification techniques.

Posterior cerebral artery

The quadrigeminal segment may be separated in the presence of large tumors.

Venographic features

The terminal portion of the internal cerebral vein is elevated and separated laterally in the presence of large tumors. No change is observed in small tumors. The basal vein of Rosenthal may be displaced downwards with inferior convexity.

The superior choroid vein may be elevated when the tumor extends laterally with elevation of the floor of the lateral ventricle. The cisternal portion of the precentral cerebellar vein, near the junction with the basilar vein of Rosenthal, is frequently displaced backwards with straightening or posterior convexity.

Large Pineal Tumor

A 13-year-old male: Figs. 273–275

Fig. 273 Arterial phase in the lateral projection. The medial posterior choroidal artery is markedly displaced posteriorly in an arcuate fashion bilaterally (3 arrows). The lateral posterior choroidal arteries are also stretched and displaced posteriorly (3 crossed arrows). The thalamoperforate arteries are bowed anteriorly (3 arrowheads). Findings are those of a huge mass in the pineal region. The proximal portion of the posterior cerebral arteries are depressed and the basilar artery is compressed against the clivus, secondary to increased intracranial pressure.

Fig. 274 Venous phase in the lateral projection. The internal cerebral veins (4 arrowheads) are displaced superiorly above the superior choroid veins (3 upper arrows). This finding was obtained by superimposition of venous phases of bilateral carotid and vertebral angiograms. The superior choroid vein on the other side is displaced superiorly (a crossed arrow), while the internal cerebral vein on the same side is visualized faintly (2 crossed arrows). The basal veins of Rosenthal on both sides are displaced inferiorly together with the inferior and posterior thalamic veins (3 lower arrows).

Fig. 275 Arterial phase in the Towne projection. The quadrigeminal portion of the posterior cerebral arteries are separated. The medial posterior choroidal arteries are stretched laterally and separated (3 arrows). The arteries, presumably the lateral posterior choroidal arteries, are displaced laterally (4 crossed arrows). The course of the superior cerebellar artery is normal.

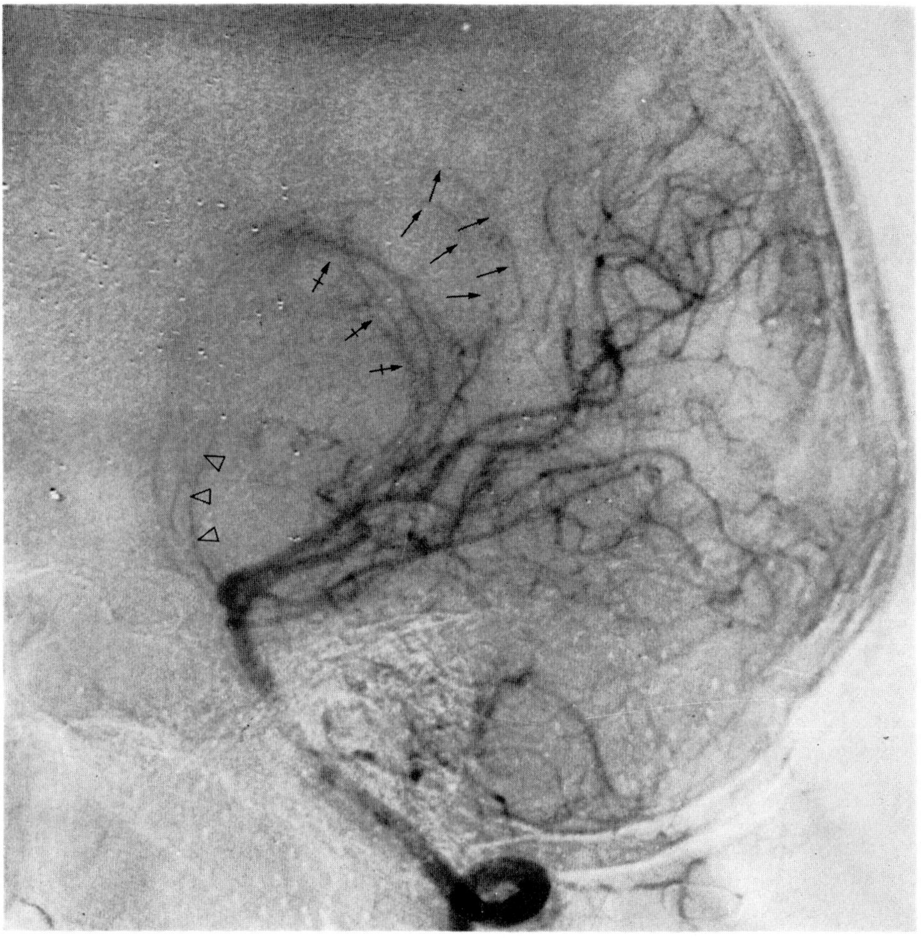

Fig. 273

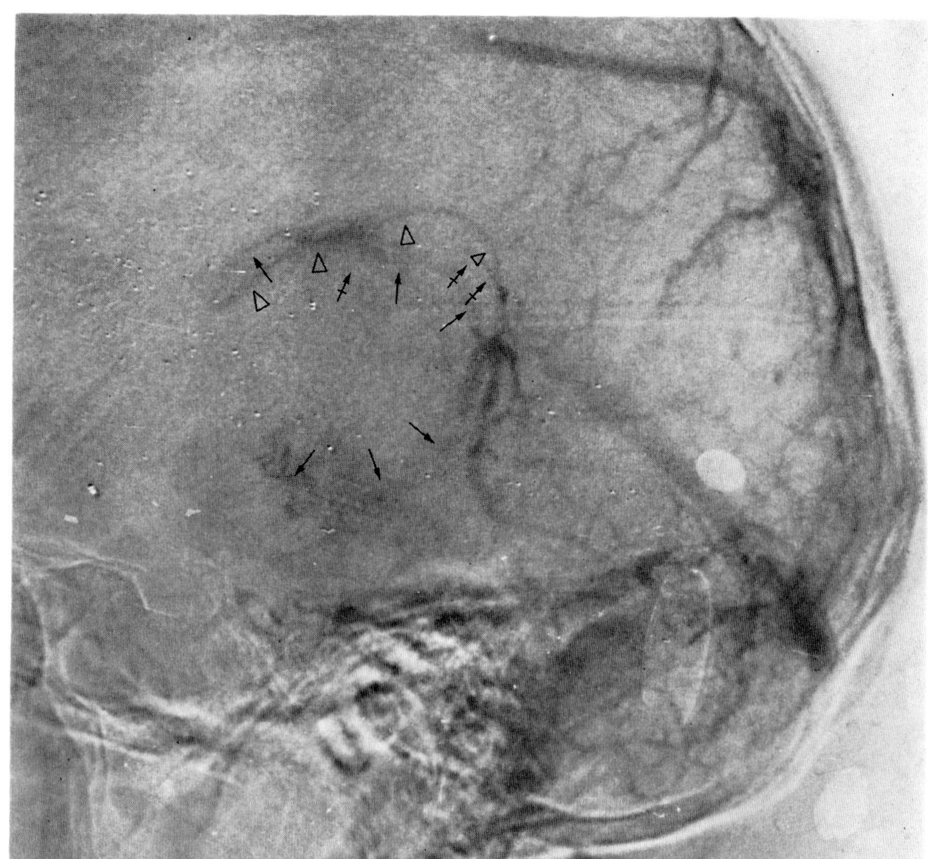

Fig. 274

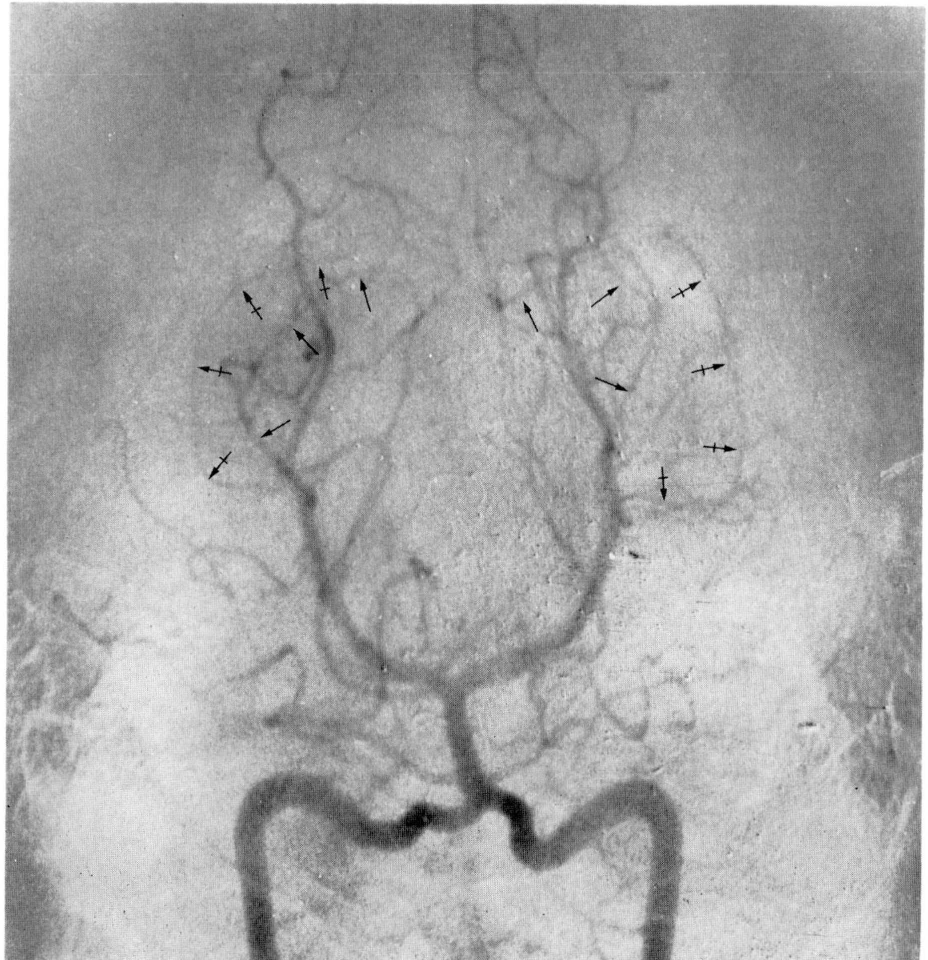

Fig. 275

Pinealoma

A 20-year-old male: Figs. 276 and 277

Fig. 276 Arterial phase in the lateral projection. There is a 2.0 × 2.0 cm round, homogeneous tumor stain in the pineal region. The medial and lateral posterior choroidal arteries are superimposed, but they are both displaced posteriorly (4 arrows). The distal segment of the thalamoperforate arteries are bowed anteriorly (2 crossed arrows). The proximal portion of the posterior cerebral arteries are depressed downwards.

Fig. 277 Venous phase in the lateral projection. The distal portion of the internal cerebral vein and the venous plexus over the pineal region are displaced superiorly and posteriorly with sharp margins (3 arrows). The cisternal portion of the precentral cerebellar vein is slightly displaced posteriorly.

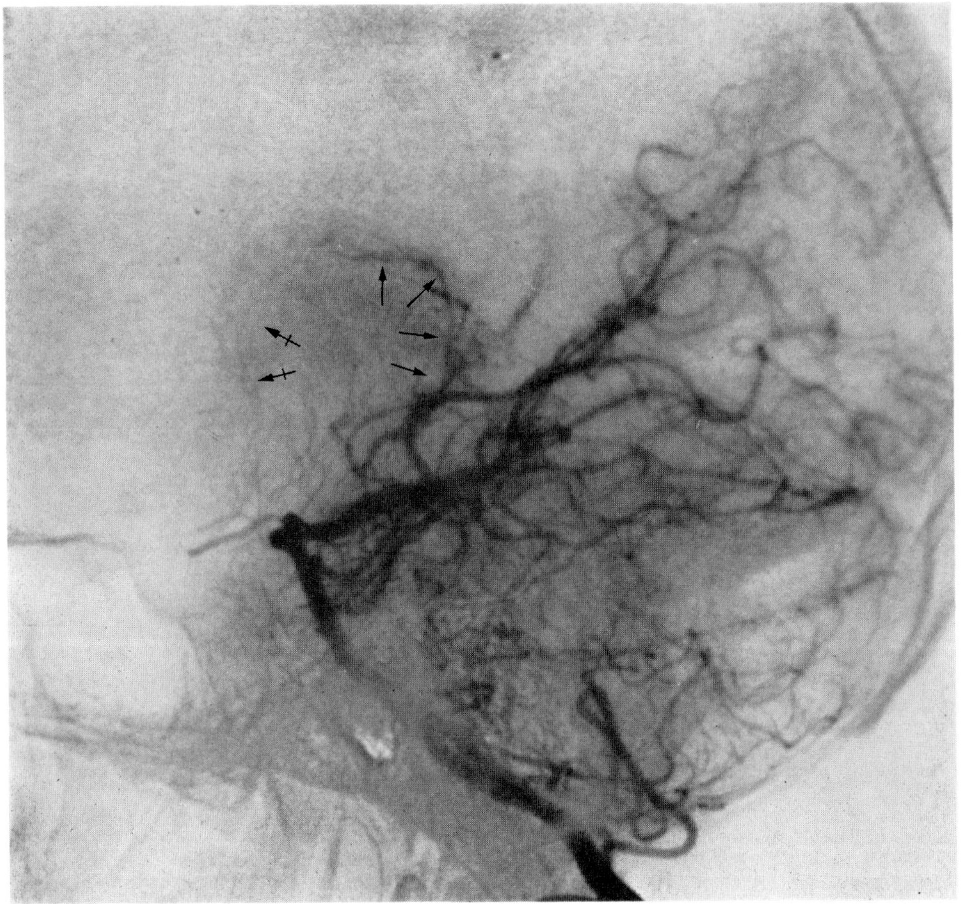

Fig. 276

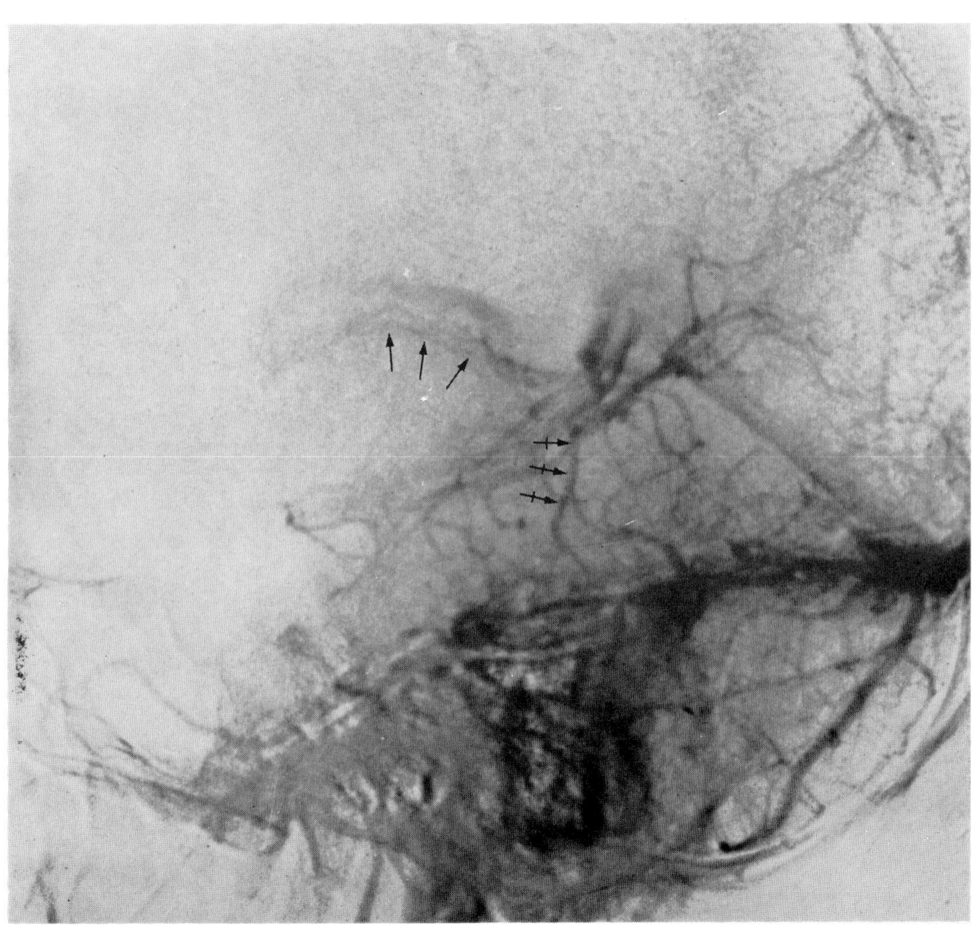

Fig. 277

Pinealoma

An 11-year-old male: Figs. 278 and 279

Fig. 278 Arterial phase in the lateral projection. Both medial posterior choroidal arteries are displaced posteriorly in an arcuate fashion (2 opposing arrows). The lateral posterior choroidal arteries are minimally stretched (2 opposing crossed arrows). The colliculi quadrigemini and corpori geniculati arteries are enlarged (2 opposing arrowheads).

Fig. 279 Venous phase in the lateral projection. The cisternal portion of the precentral cerebellar vein is displaced posteriorly (2 arrows). There are no other venous changes.

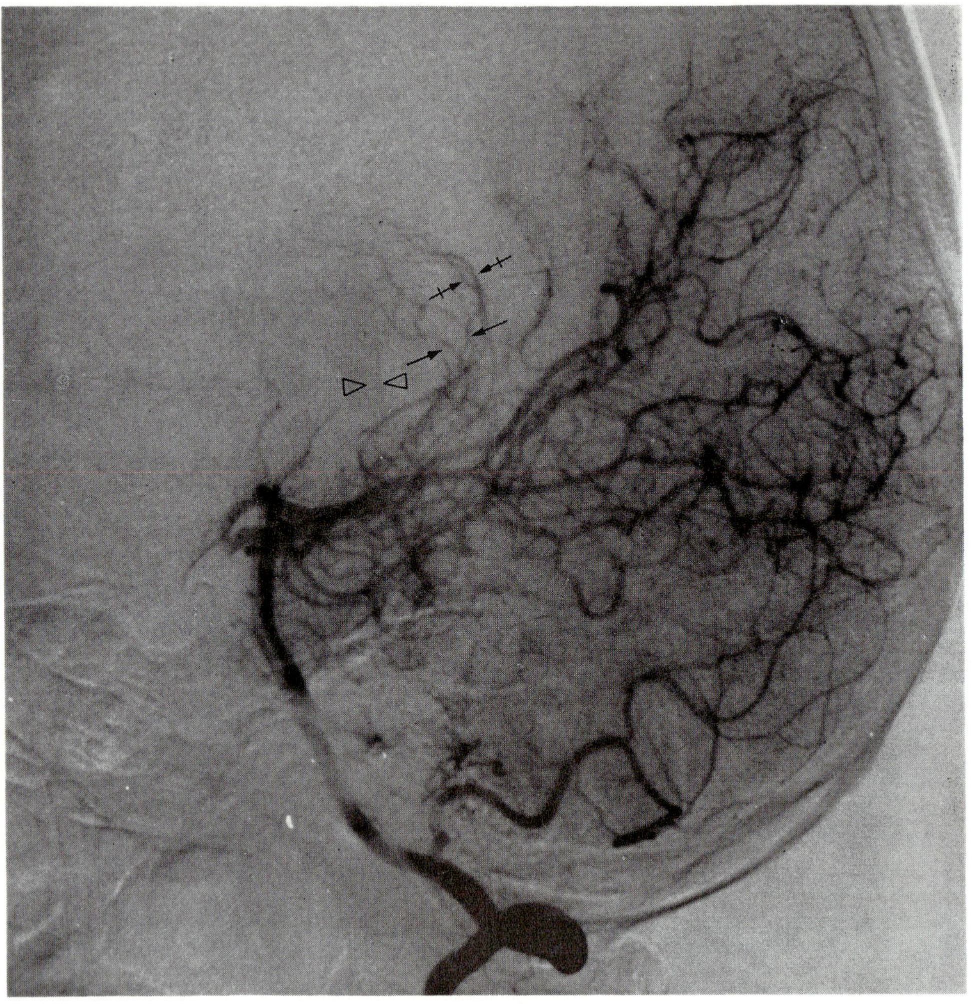

Fig. 278

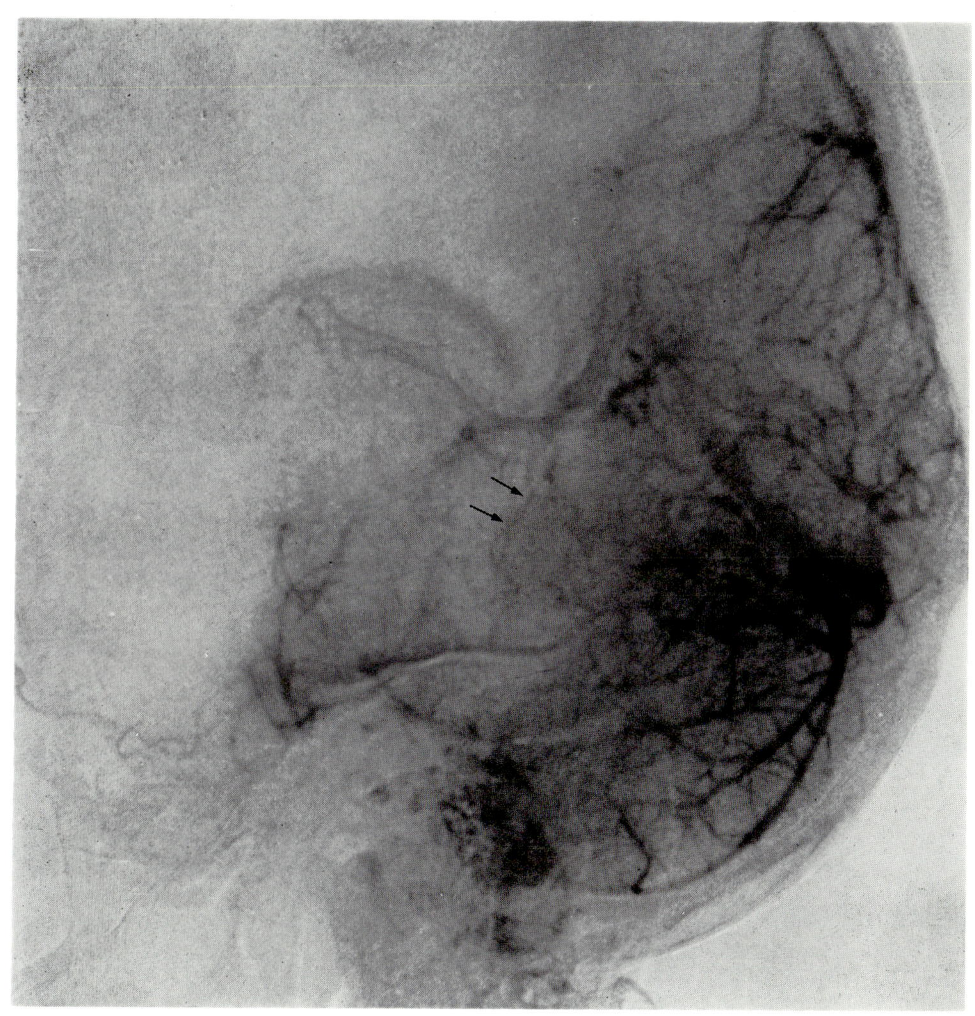

Fig. 279

Large Glioblastoma in the Pineal Region

A 7-year-old male: Figs. 280 and 281

Fig. 280 Arterial phase in the lateral projection. The medial (3 arrows) and lateral (3 crossed arrows) posterior choroidal arteries are both displaced posteriorly in an arcuate fashion. The thalamoperforate arteries are stretched (2 arrowheads). The ambient segment of the posterior cerebral arteries is depressed downwards. These vessels outline the tumor in the pineal region. The basilar artery is compressed against the clivus.

Fig. 281 Capillary phase in the lateral projection. There is a large round tumor stain in the pineal region corresponding to the arterial phase. The superior choroid vein is displaced superiorly and posteriorly (4 arrows). There is superior displacement of the internal cerebral (2 crossed arrows) and the superior thalam ic vein (2 arrowheads).

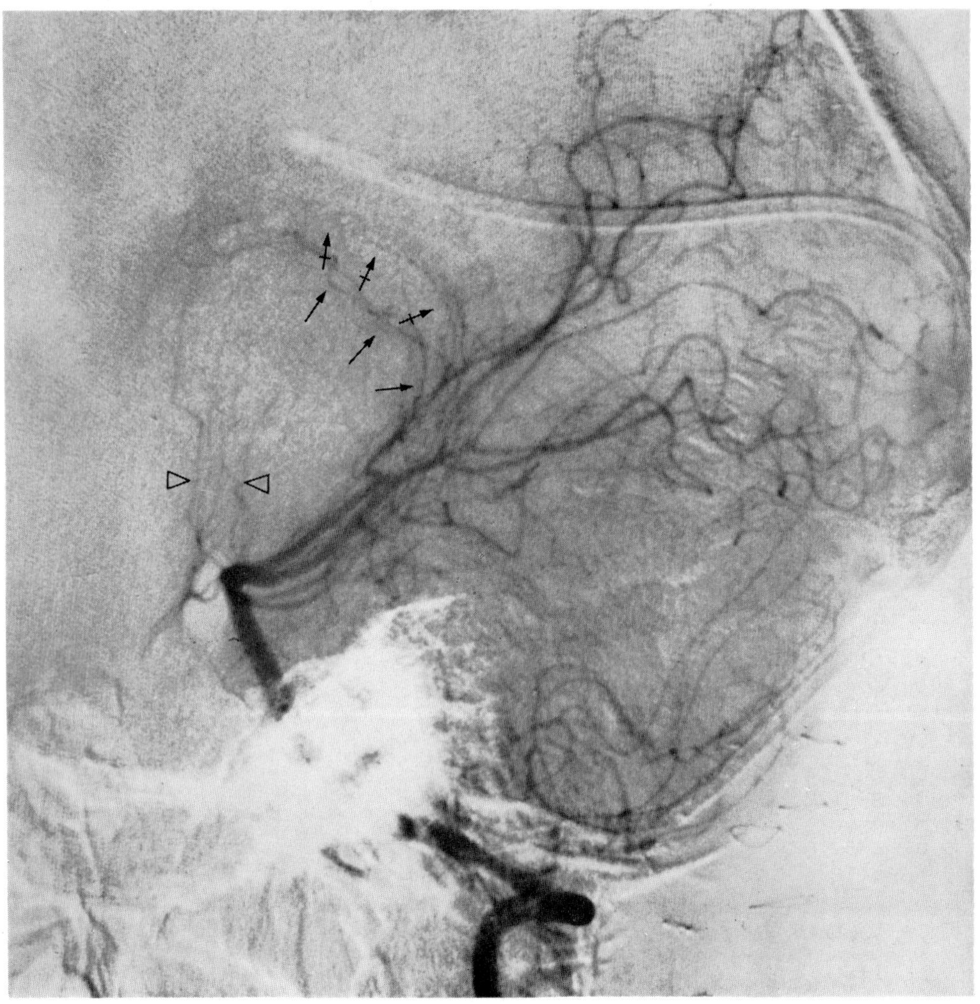

Fig. 280

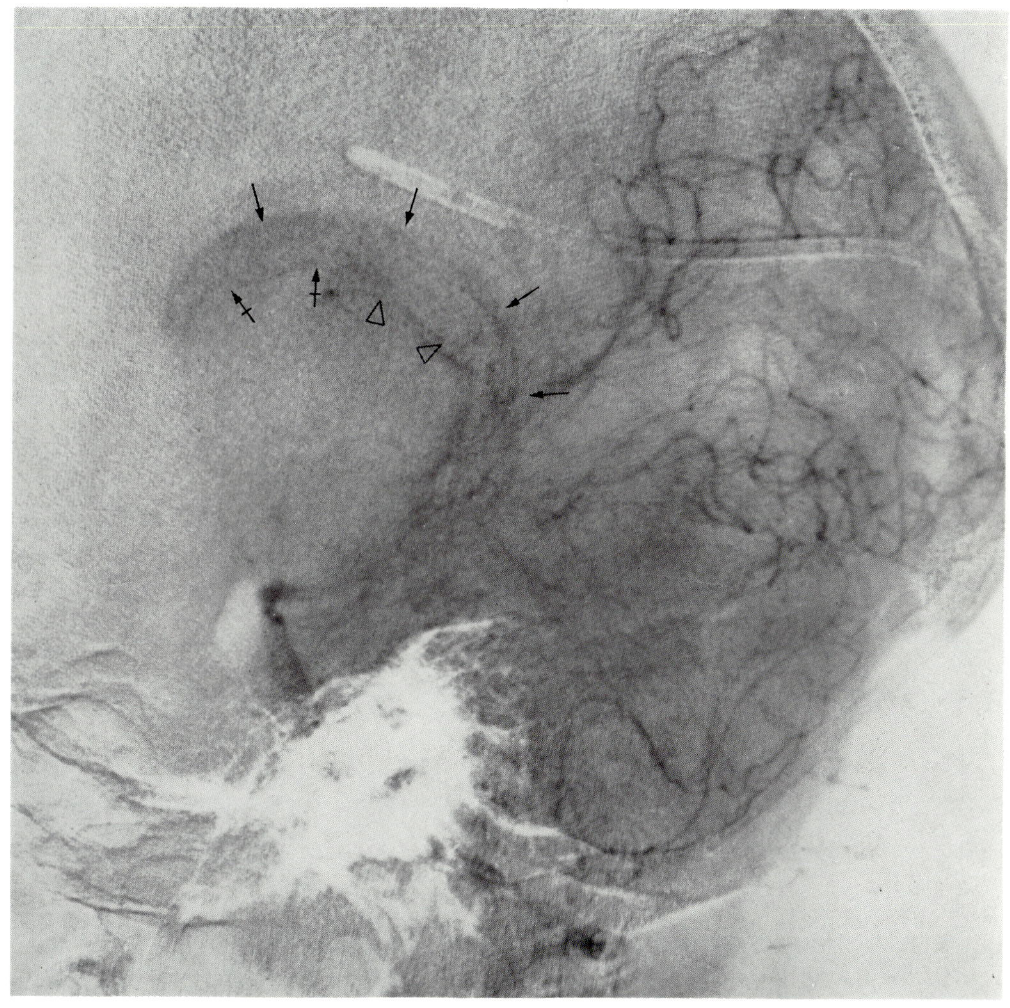

Fig. 281

PARASELLAR AND SUPRASELLAR TUMORS

Tumors included in this group mainly consist of large pituitary tumors, craniopharyngiomas, parasellar epidermoid, meningiomas and suprasellar pinealomas. Hypothalamic gliomas present similar angiographic findings. These tumors extend posteriorly by displacing the midbrain backwards and elevating the temporal lobe. There is frequent extension of tumors into the posterior fossa, usually into the prepontine cistern and the cerebellopontine angle.

Arteriographic features

The distal portion of the basilar artery is displaced posteriorly by extension of the tumor into the interpeduncular cistern. This segment may be buckled. When the tumor extends posteriorly under the temporal lobe, the posterior cerebral artery is elevated or displaced posteriorly. The anterior temporal and posterior temporal arteries may be elevated. With extension into the prepontine and cerebellopontine angle cistern, the basilar artery is dislocated away from the clivus and the anterior inferior cerebellar artery is depressed downwards. The superior cerebellar artery is elevated.

Venographic features

The pontine and interpeduncular segments of the anterior pontomesencephalic vein are displaced inferiorly and posteriorly with backward dislocation of the precentral cerebellar vein. The basal vein of Rosenthal may be pushed upwards and backwards, while the posterior mesencephalic vein is depressed.

Large Craniopharyngioma Displacing the Midbrain Posteriorly

A 10-year-old male: Figs. 282–284

Fig. 282 Arterial phase in the lateral projection. The distal segment of the basilar artery is markedly displaced posteriorly with the proximal segment of the posterior cerebral artery (3 arrows). The thalamoperforate (2 opposing arrows), medial posterior choroidal (3 crossed arrows) and the lateral posterior choroidal (3 open arrowheads) are pushed backwards in arcuate configuration. There is minimal posterior dislocation of the posterior pericallosal artery (3 closed arrowheads).

Fig. 283 Venous phase in the lateral projection. The internal cerebral vein and the superior thalamic vein are superimposed and pushed superiorly (3 arrows), while the posterior mesencephalic vein is amputated and displaced downwards (2 crossed arrows). The interpeduncular segment of the anterior pontomesencephalic vein is markedly displaced downwards (3 closed arrowheads), suggesting tumor encroachment upon the interpeduncular fossa. The precentral cerebellar vein is displaced posteriorly (2 open arrowheads). All these findings indicate a large suprasellar mass displacing the midbrain posteriorly.

Fig. 284 Arterial phase in the Towne projection. The basilar artery is elongated with rigid appearance. The interpeduncular segment of the posterior cerebral artery is bowed posteriorly and superiorly (4 arrows), indicating the presence of a large mass in the interpeduncular fossa.

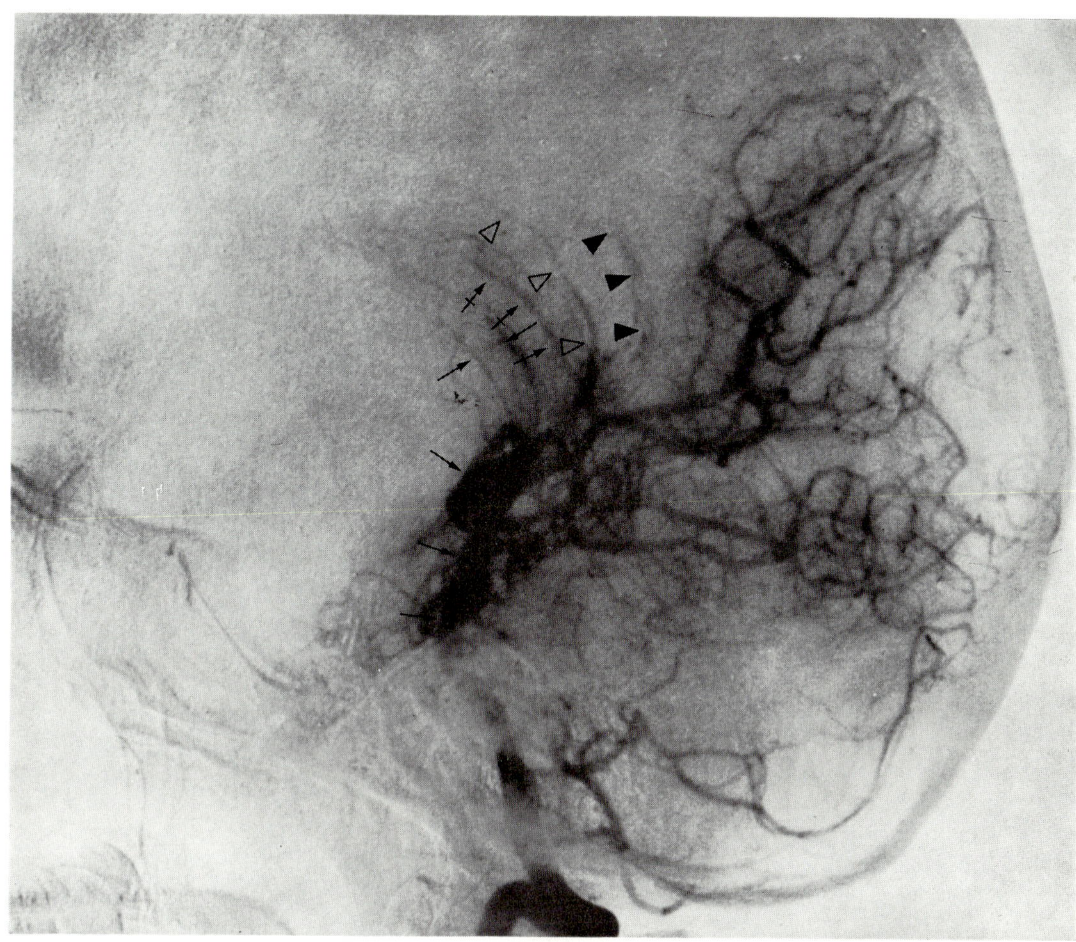

Fig. 282

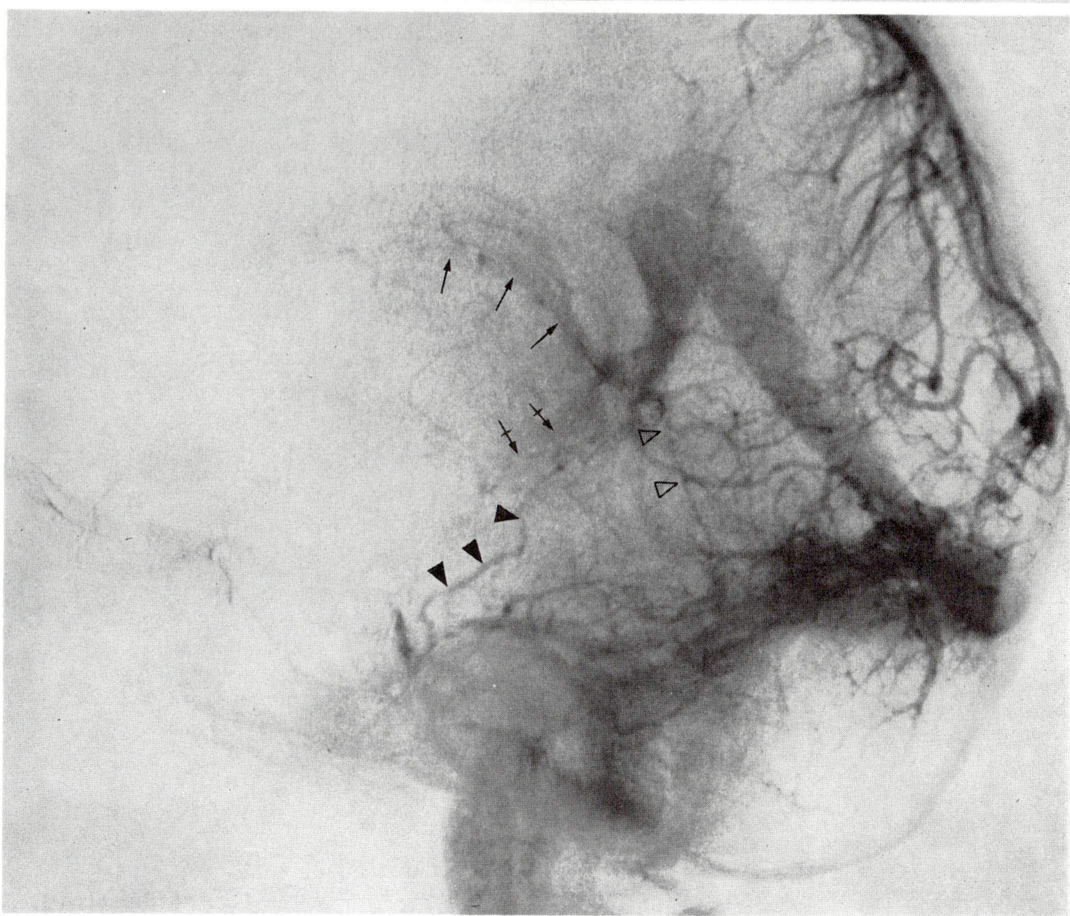

Fig. 283

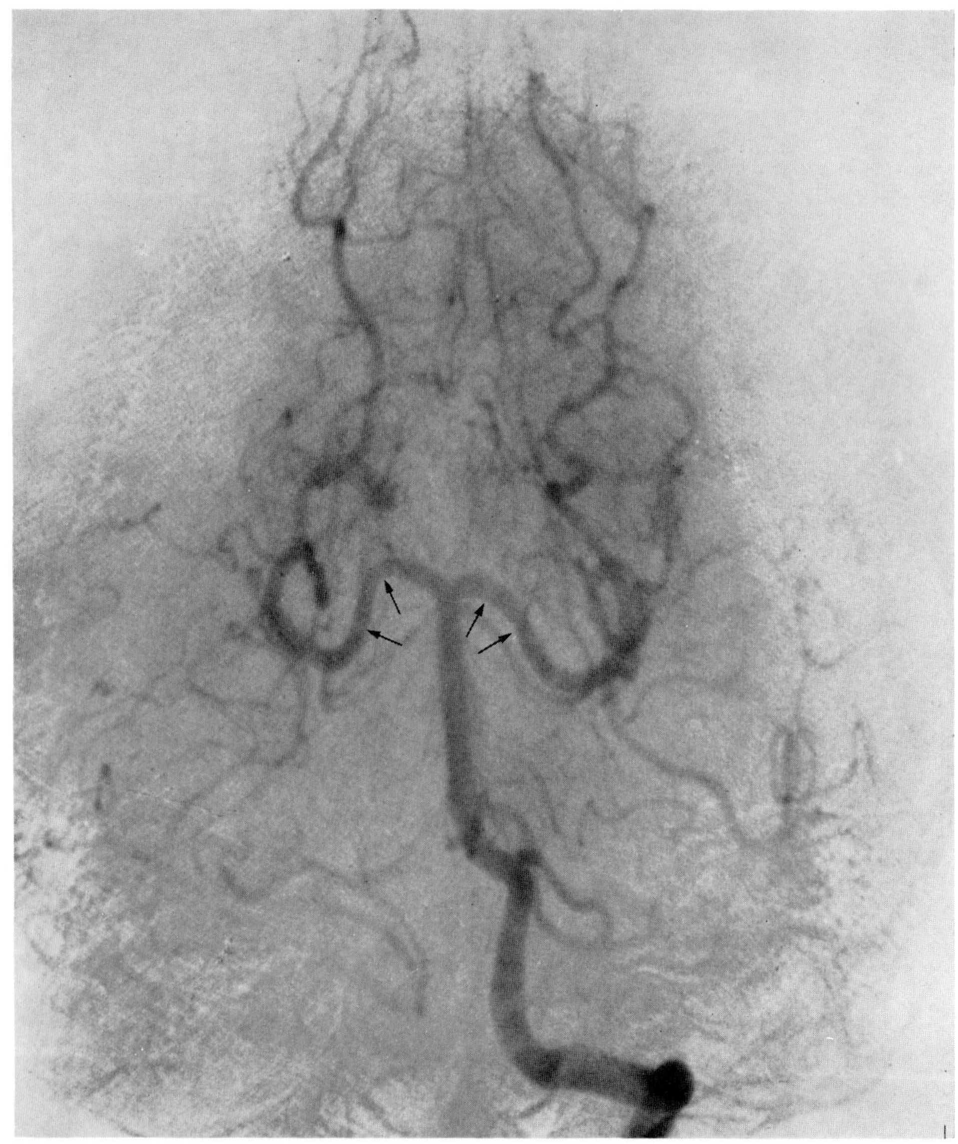

Fig. 284

Craniopharyngioma with Posterior Extention

A 9-year-old male: Figs. 285–288

Fig. 285 Arterial phase in the lateral projection. The distal segment of the basilar artery is buckled with posterior displacement (the posterior clinoid is shown with a double-crossed arrow). The posterior communicating artery (2 open arrowheads) and the most proximal posterior cerebral artery are pushed downwards by a suprasellar tumor extending posteriorly. The posterior thalamoperforate arteries and colliculi quadrigemini arteries are displaced posteriorly (4 arrows), while the posterior choroidal arteries are dislocated posteriorly and superiorly (3 crossed arrows). The anterior thalamoperforate artery is stretched and displaced posteriorly (2 closed arrowheads).

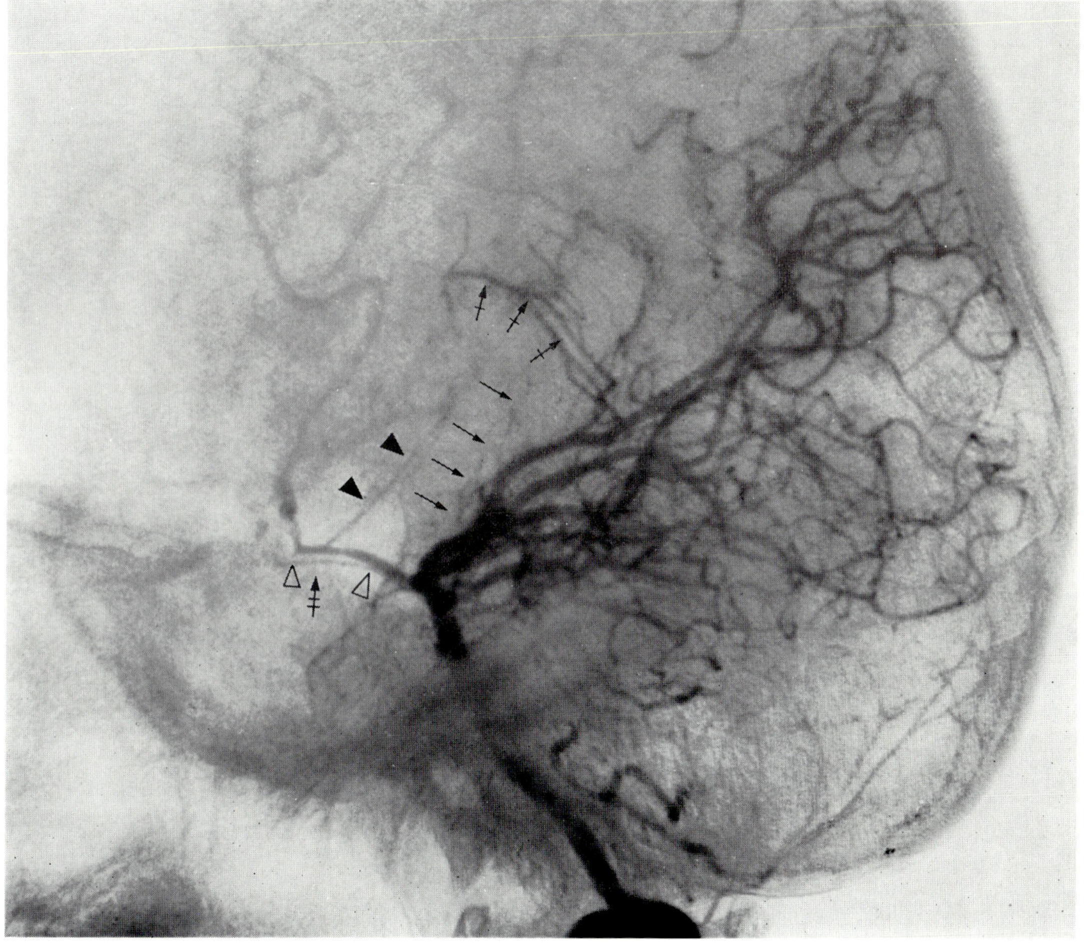

Fig. 285

Fig. 286 Venous phase in the lateral projection. The interpeduncular and pontine segments of the anterior pontomesencephalic vein and the posterior mesencephalic vein are markedly displaced infero-posteriorly (3 arrows). The internal cerebral vein is displaced supero-posteriorly (3 crossed arrows). The posterior clinoid is shown with a double-crossed arrow.

Fig. 287 Arterial phase in the Towne projection. The short segments of the posterior communicating arteries are both visualized with lateral displacement (2 arrows on each side), secondary to a midline suprasellar tumor extending posteriorly.

Fig. 288 Venous phase in the Towne projection. The posterior mesencephalic vein is pushed backwards at its anterior portion (3 arrows).

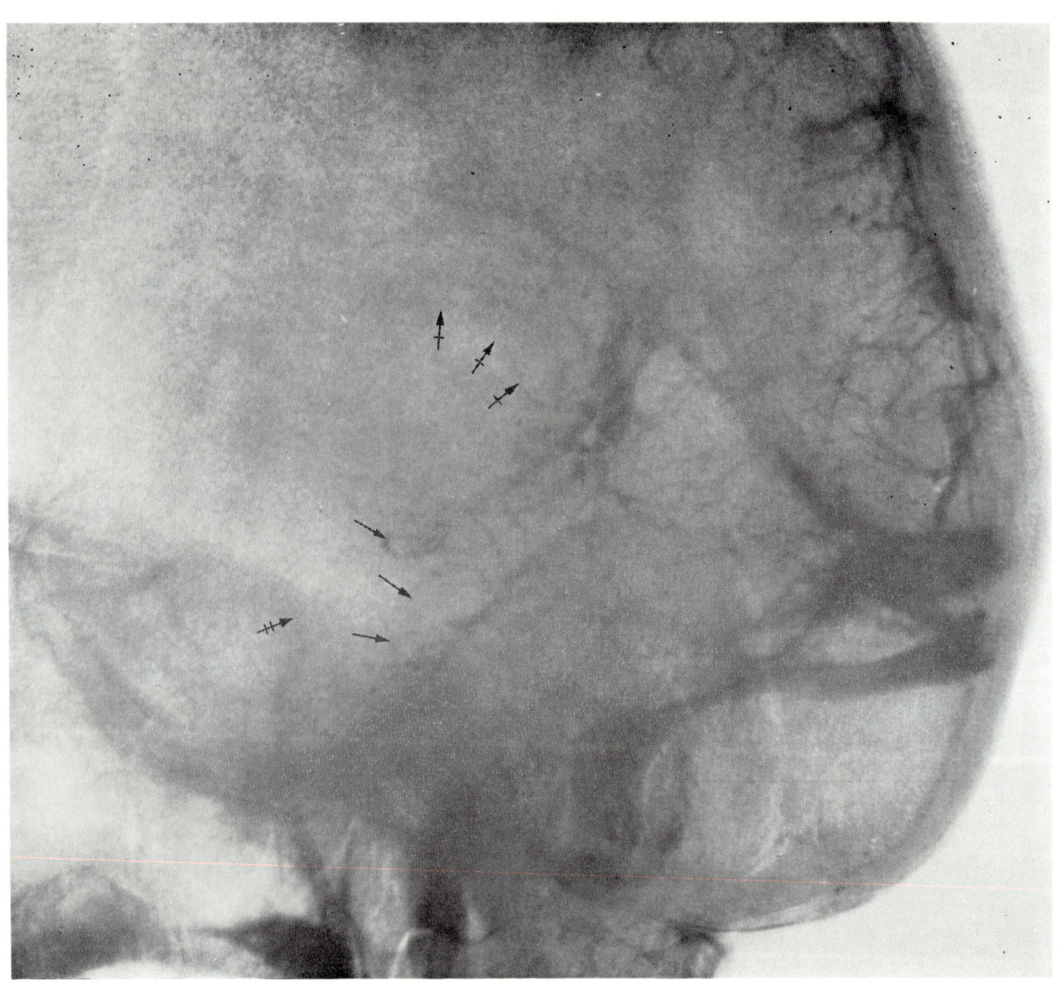

Fig. 286

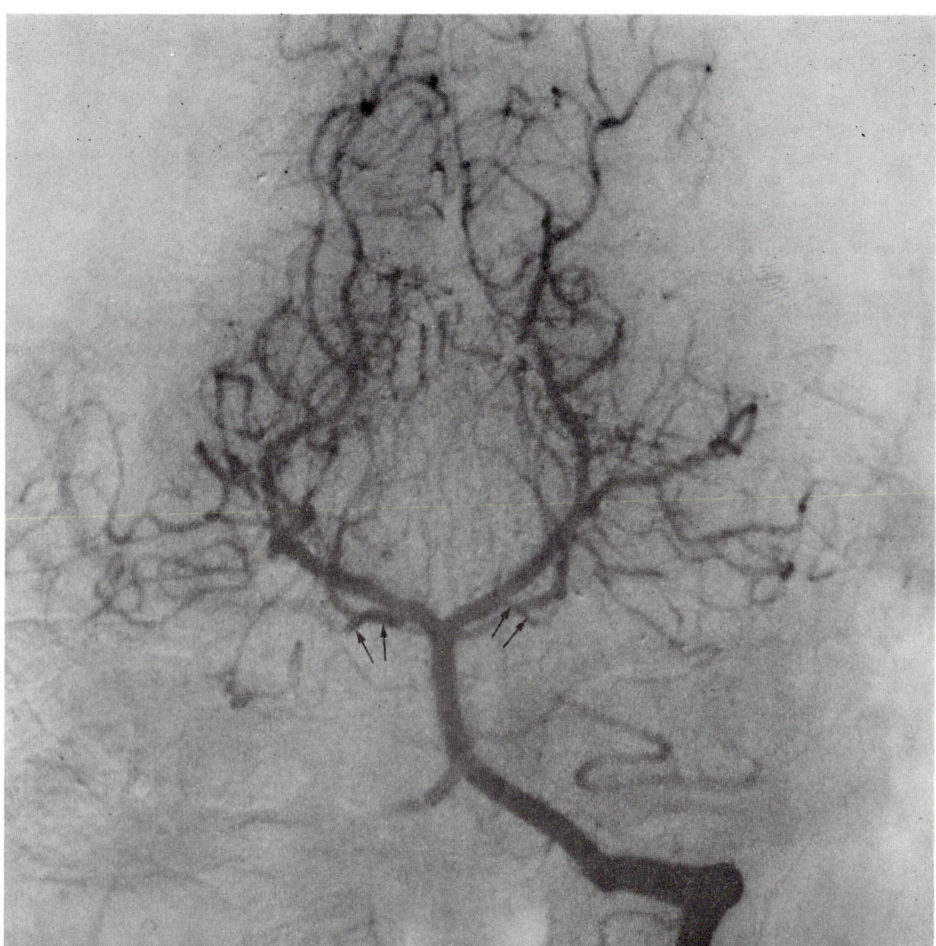

Fig. 287

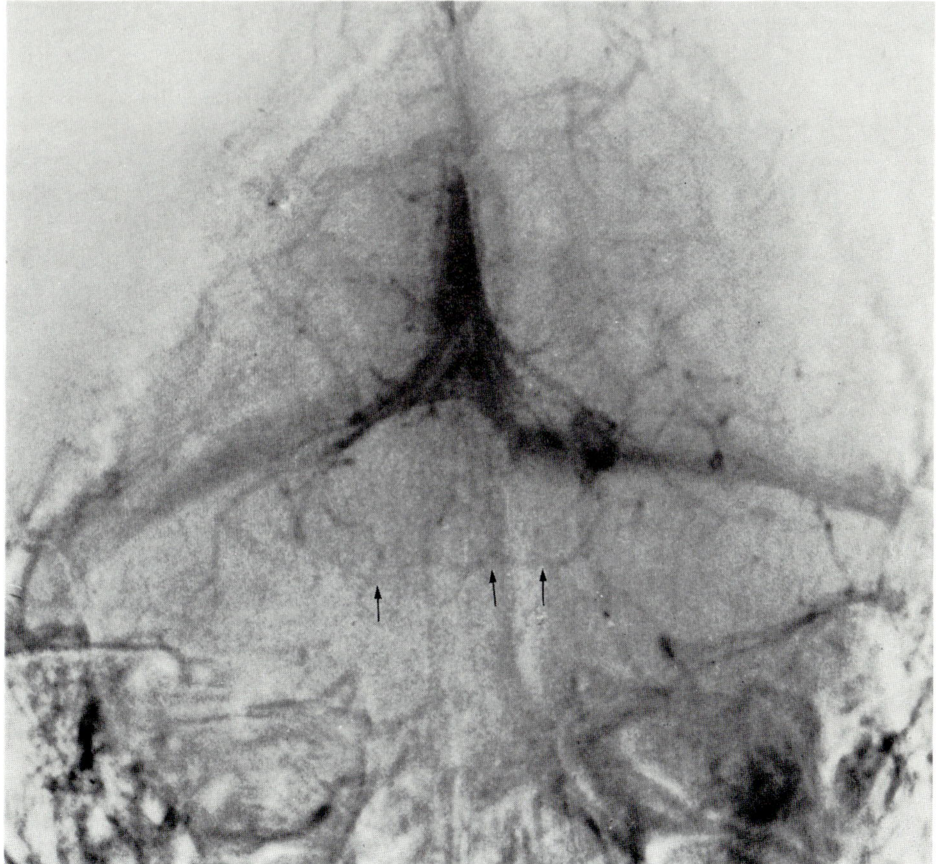

Fig. 288

Craniopharyngioma Extending into the Prepontine and Right Cerebellopontine Angle Cisterns

A 17-year-old male: Figs. 289–292

Fig. 289 Arterial phase in the lateral projection. The basilar artery is pushed backwards by a tumor over the clivus (3 arrows). The terminal segment of this artery is slightly elevated. The posterior clinoid process is marked with a crossed arrow.

Fig. 290 Venous phase in the lateral projection. The interpeduncular and pontine segments of the anterior pontomesencephalic vein are displaced posteriorly (3 arrows). The precentral cerebellar vein is displaced posteriorly (2 arrowheads). A crossed arrow indicates the posterior clinoid process.

Fig. 291 Arterial phase in the Towne projection. The crural and anterior ambient segments of the posterior cerebral and superior cerebellar arteries are elevated (3 arrows), indicating tumor extension into the right cerebellopontine angle. The basilar artery is shifted to the left of the midline.

Fig. 292 Venous phase in the Towne projection. The right petrosal vein and the vein of the lateral recess of the fourth ventricle are displaced laterally and inferiorly in an arcuate fashion (4 crossed arrows).

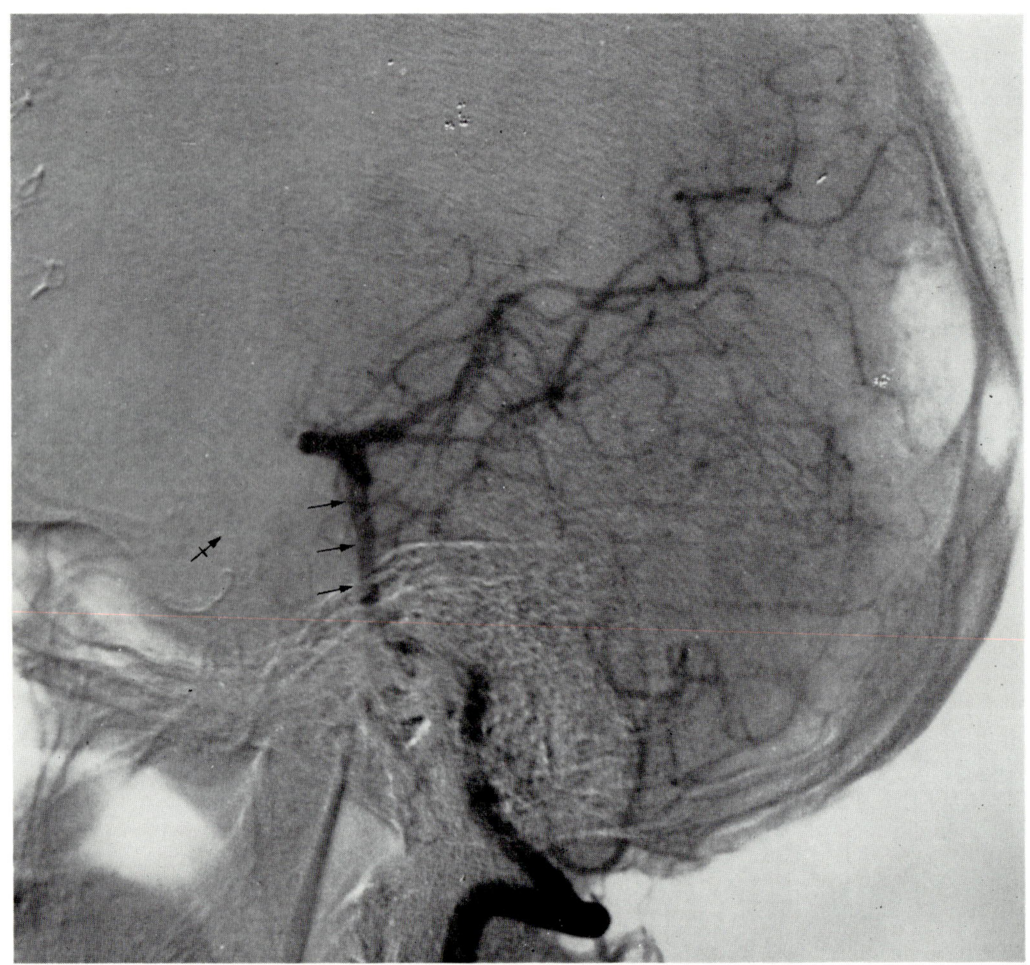

Fig. 289

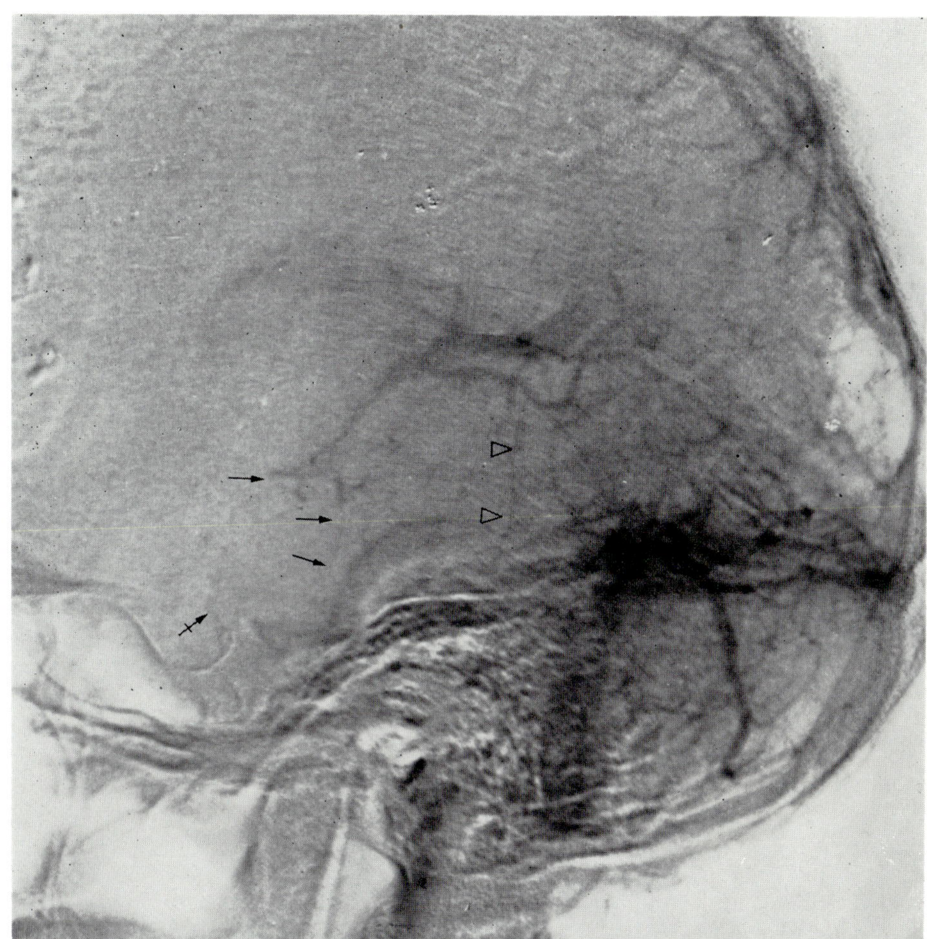

Fig. 290

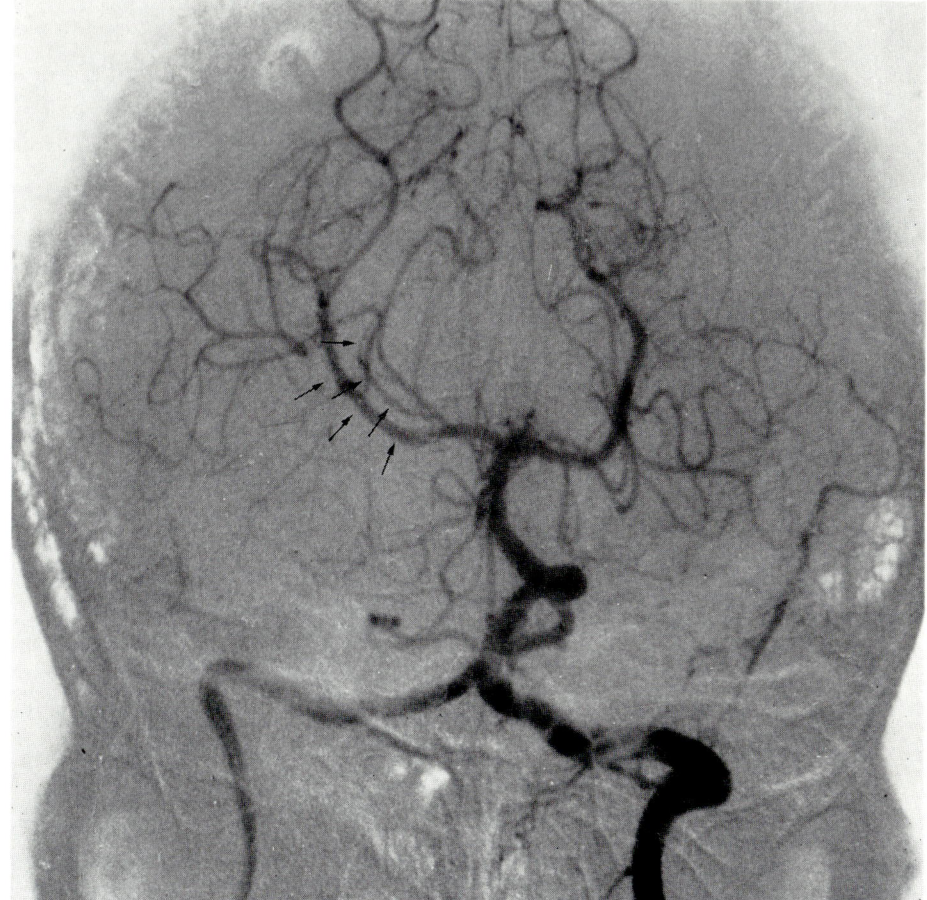

Fig. 291

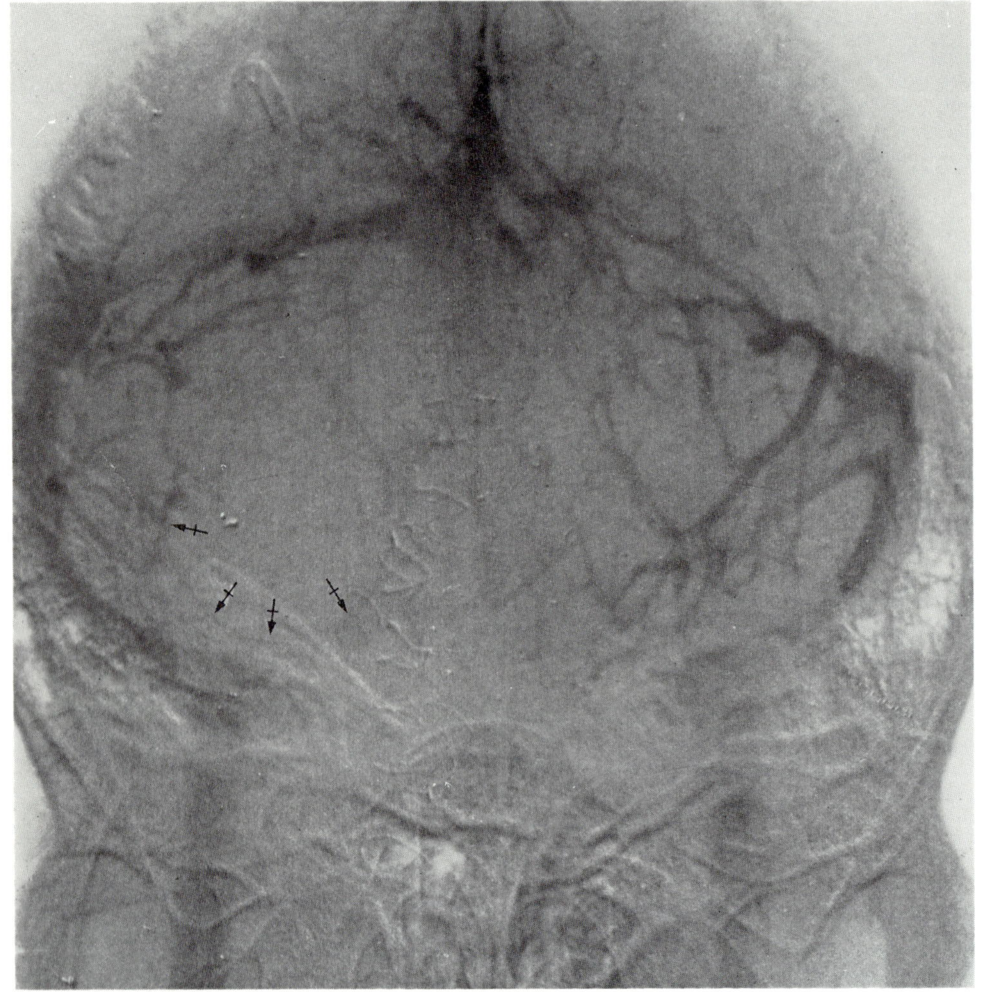

Fig. 292

Large Chromophobe Adenoma Extending Posteriorly along the Right Tentorial Incisura

A 39-year-old male: Figs. 293 and 294

Fig. 293 Arterial phase in the Towne projection. The crural and anterior ambient segments of the posterior cerebral artery are markedly elevated with posterior displacement of the anterior temporal artery (4 arrows), suggesting tumor extension under the temporal lobe. The same segment of the superior cerebellar artery is markedly depressed (2 crossed arrows). The findings indicate that the tumor extends posteriorly along the tentorial incisura. The right posterior communicating artery is laterally displaced (2 arrowheads).

Fig. 294 Arterial phase in the lateral projection. The basilar artery is slightly pushed away from the clivus (3 open arrowheads). There is increased distance between the right posterior cerebral artery (2 arrows) and the right superior cerebellar artery (3 crossed arrows), probably outlining the superior and lower surface of the tumor. The posterior communicating artery is stretched with marked elevation (2 closed arrowheads). The posterior clinoid process is marked with a crossed arrow.

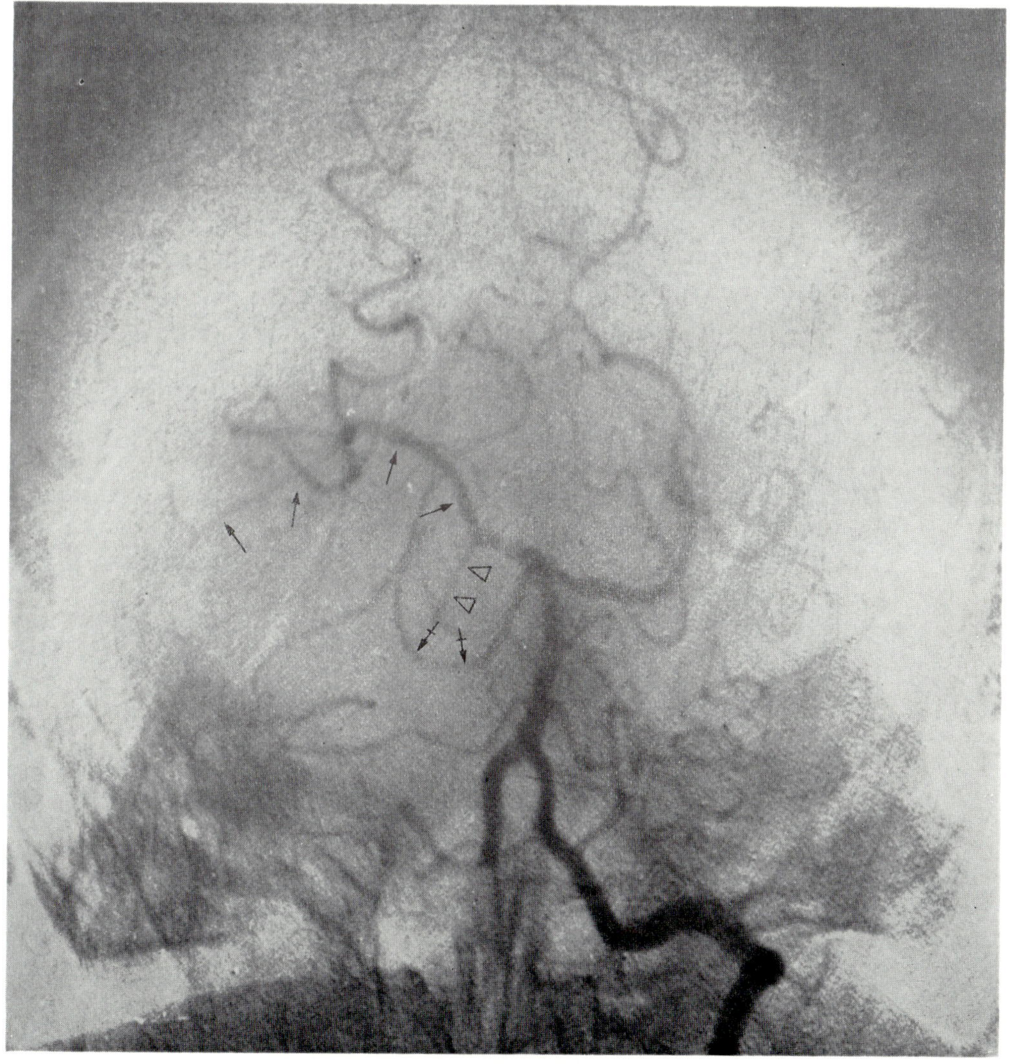

Fig. 293

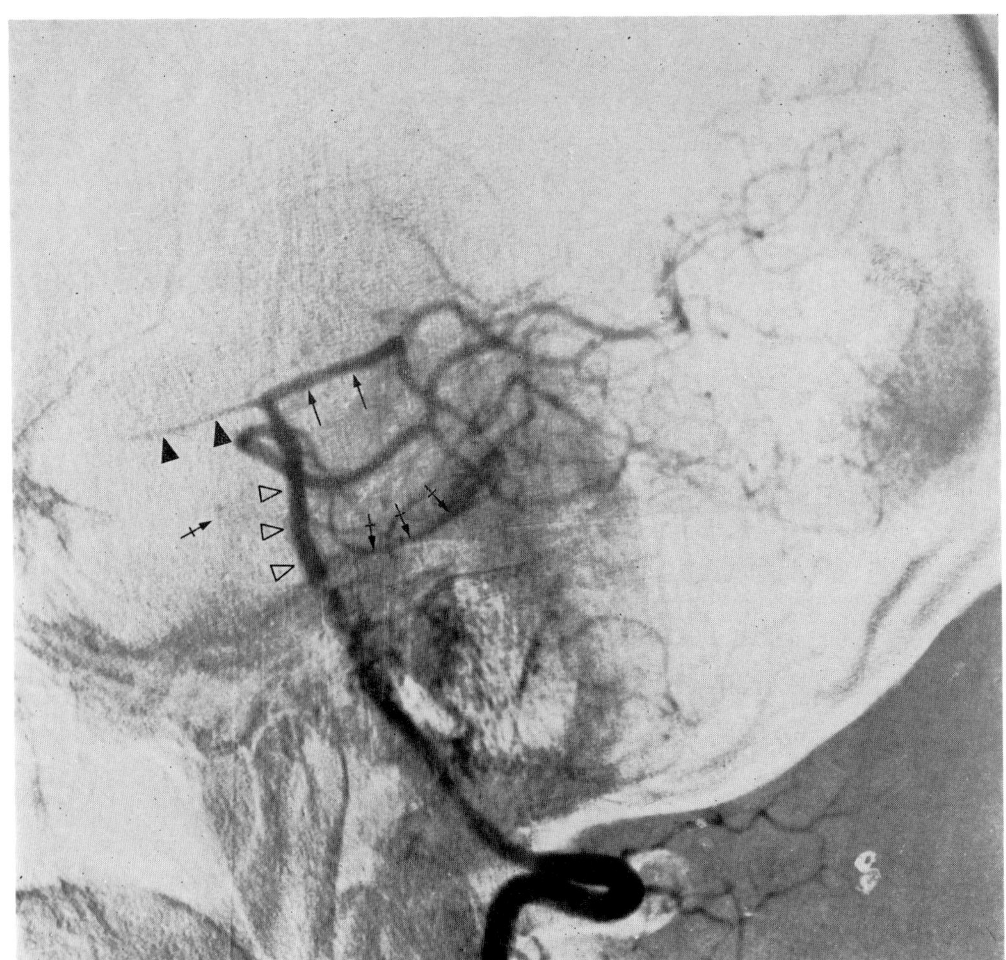

Fig. 294

TUMORS OF THE SPLENIUM OF THE CORPUS CALLOSUM

Vertebral angiography is useful in the diagnosis of the tumors in the posterior portion of the corpus callosum. The tumors in the anterior portion of the corpus callosum are usually diagnosed by carotid angiography. Glioblastomas and astrocytomas are the most common tumors in this location. Oligodendrogliomas may also be encountered.

Arteriographic features

In the presence of tumors in the posterior portion, the posterior pericallosal artery is displaced posteriorly, while the posterior choroidal arteries are depressed downwards. The pericallosal artery of the anterior cerebral artery may be elevated by these tumors. If the tumor is located laterally, the pericallosal and callosomarginal arteries are displaced laterally, although the arterial midline shift is infrequently seen. Tumor vessels are supplied by the pericallosal artery and the posterior pericallosal arteries.

Venographic features

The venous phase, is very important for the diagnosis of these tumors. The internal cerebral vein and the thalamostriate vein are depressed downwards with increased distance to the inferior sagittal sinus. The vein of Galen may be displaced posteriorly. The posterior cerebral vein may be enlarged and drain the tumor.

Glioblastoma in the Splenium of the Corpus Callosum with Invasion of the Right Temporal Lobe and the Lateral Ventricle

A 43-year-old male: Figs. 295–298

Fig. 295 Arterial phase in the lateral projection. The posterior pericallosal artery is displaced posteriorly in an arcuate fashion (3 arrows), while the posterior choroidal arteries are depressed downwards (3 crossed arrows). Irregular tumor vessels are noted between these two arteries. Several enlarged arteries (2 arrowheads) are probably the colliculi quadrigemini and corpori geniculati arteries.

Fig. 296 Venous phase in the lateral projection. The internal cerebral vein (2 arrows) and the superior choroid vein (2 crossed arrows) are markedly depressed.

Fig. 297 Arterial phase in the Towne projection. The quadrigeminal segment of the right posterior cerebral artery, calcarine artery (2 arrows) and the parieto-occipital artery (2 crossed arrows) are displaced laterally due to invasion of the temporal lobe. An unnamed arterial branch, probably a medial branch of the posterior cerebral artery, is displaced laterally (3 open arrowheads). There are tumor vessels medial to these arterial branches (4 closed arrowheads). The medial posterior choroidal artery is seen bilaterally (2 double-crossed arrows).

Fig. 298 Right internal carotid angiogram. There are tumor vessels (5 arrowheads) in the splenium of the corpus callosum, being supplied by the enlarged pericallosal artery (2 arrows). The great vein of Galen and the straight sinus are opacified early (crossed arrows).

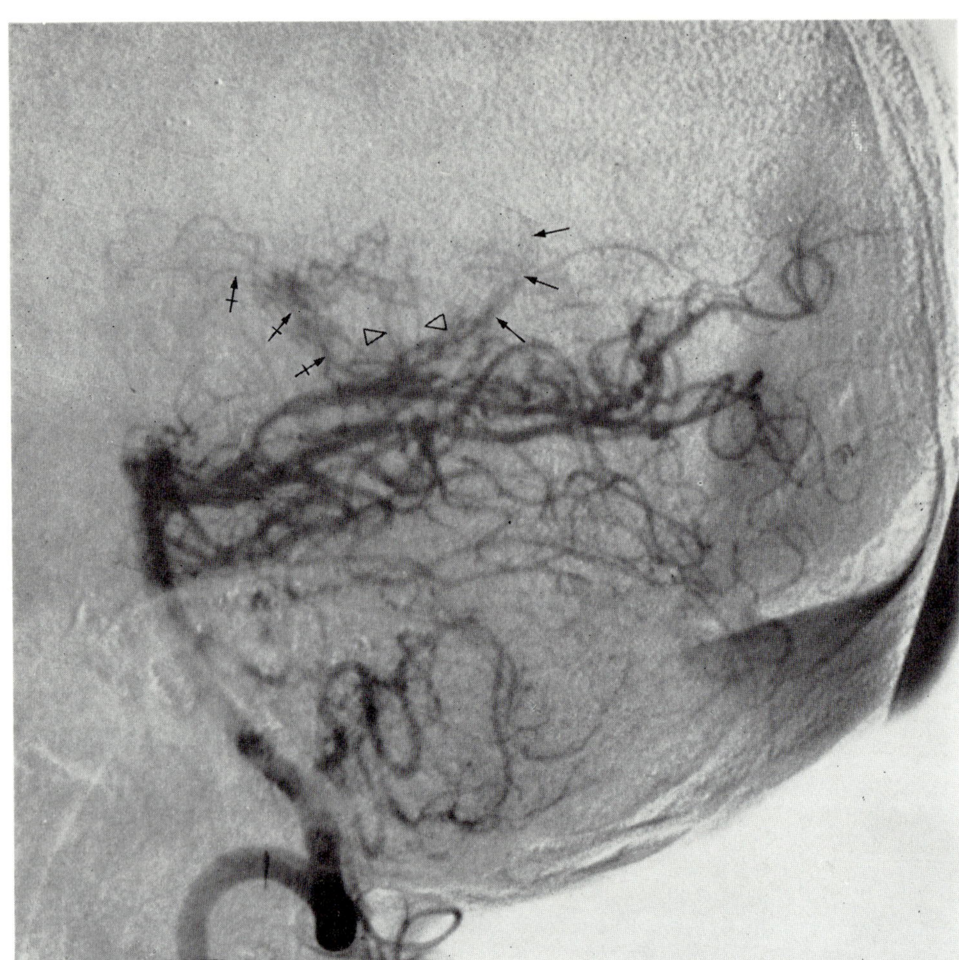

Fig. 295

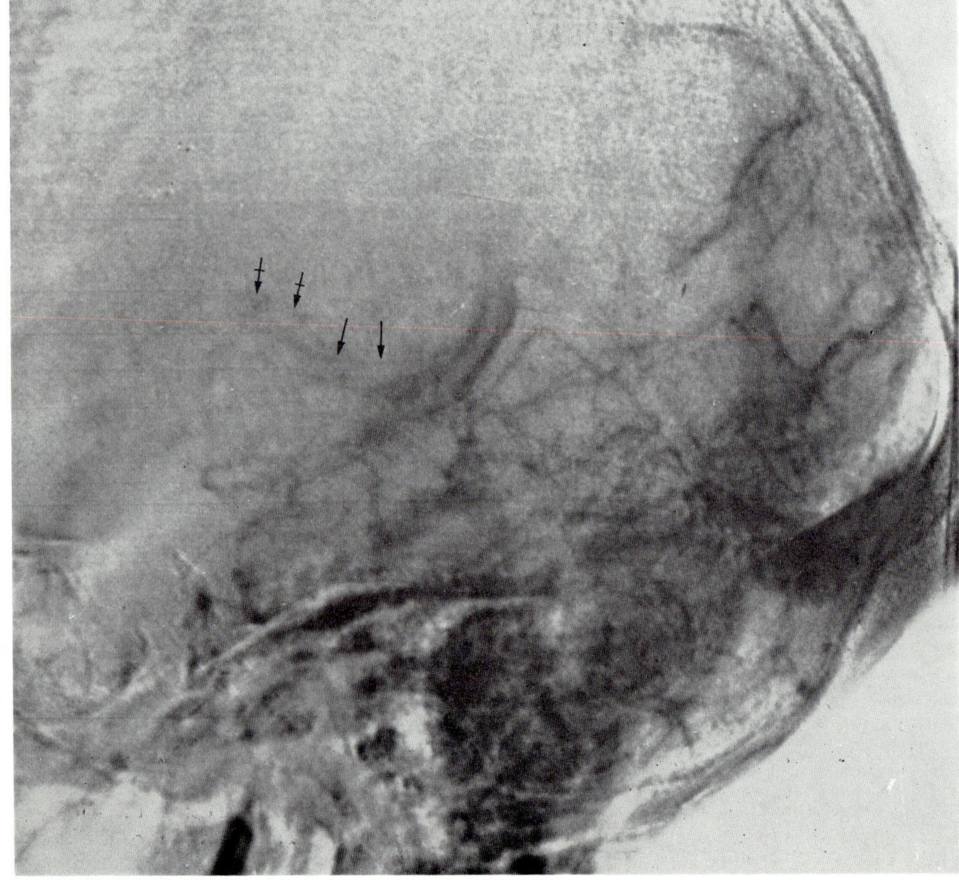

Fig. 296

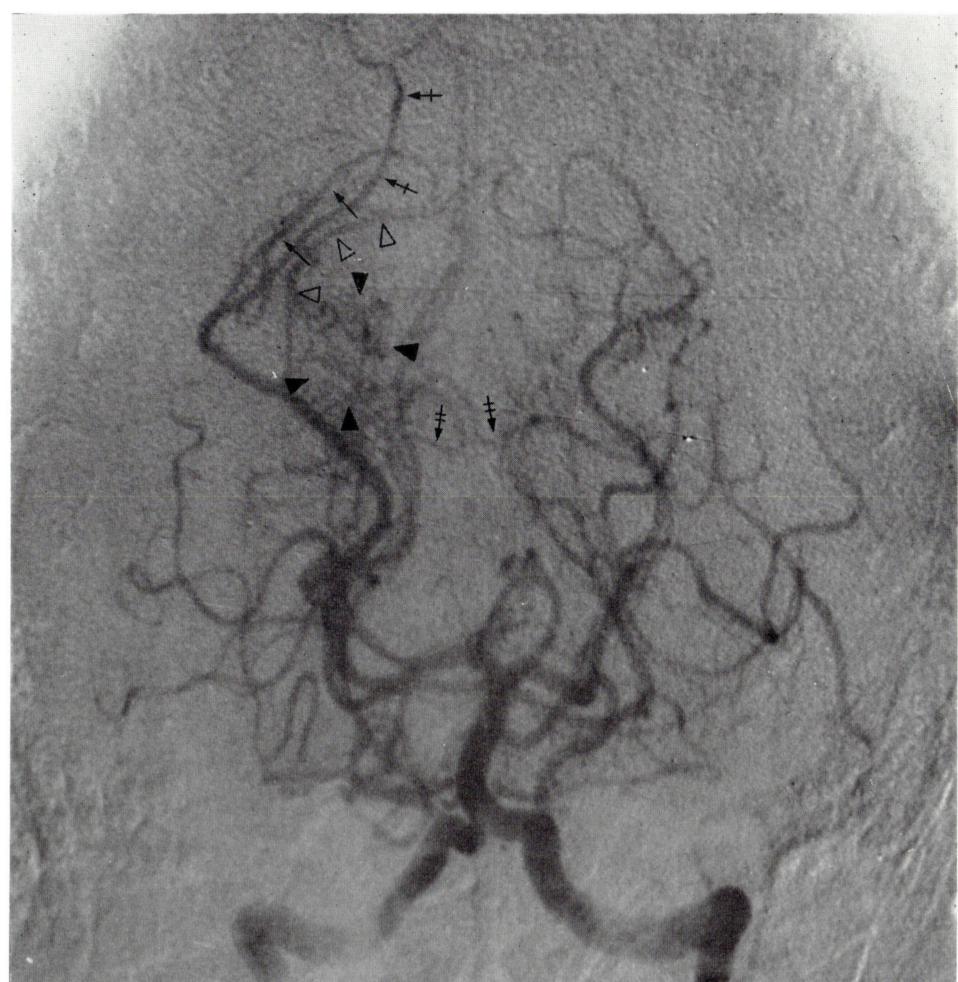

Fig. 297

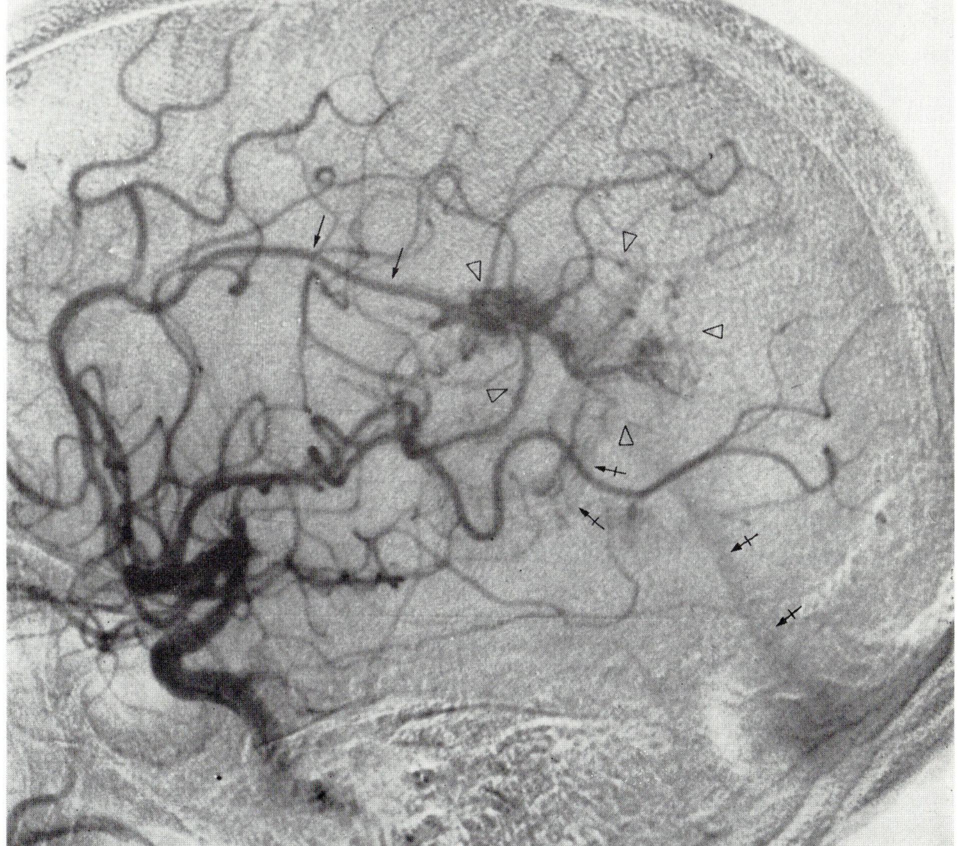

Fig. 298

INTRAVENTRICULAR TUMORS

The tumors in the lateral ventricle are ependymomas, oligodendrogliomas, choroid plexus papillomas, meningiomas and epidermoid tumors. A mixed glioma, usually oligodendroglioma and astrocytoma, may also be observed. Some intracerebral tumors may extend into the lateral ventricle, presenting as intraventricular tumors.

In the third ventricle, colloid cysts arise from the anterior portion while the pinealomas are the most common tumors arising from the posterior portion of the third ventricle. Choroid plexus papillomas, ependymomas and epidermoid tumors may occur in this location.

Arteriographic features

When these tumors are vascular, the blood supply is derived from the posterior choroidal arteries as well as the anterior choroidal arteries. The posterior choroidal arteries may be depressed and the posterior pericallosal artery is dislocated backwards. There is contralateral shift of the anterior cerebral artery as well as lateral and superior displacement of the sylvian group of the middle cerebral arteries.

Additional arterial changes develop when the tumor invades the adjacent structures.

Venographic features

The choroid plexus and the superior choroid vein are depressed and there are changes due to ventricular dilatation. The internal cerebral vein is displaced to the opposite side.

With vascular tumors, large draining veins may be demonstrated, draining into the internal cerebral vein directly or indirectly via the thalamostriate vein.

Oligodendroglioma of the Right Lateral Ventricle Involving the Third Ventricle and the Thalamus

A 24-year-old female: Figs. 299–303

Fig. 299 Early arterial phase in the lateral projection. The distal basilar artery is buckled and displaced downwards. The thalamoperforate arteries are accordioned inferiorly (2 opposing arrows). The posterior communicating artery is depressed downwards. The posterior clinoid process is marked with a crossed arrow.

Fig. 300 Arterial phase in the lateral projection. There are multiple irregular tumor vessels between the depressed posterior choroidal artery (3 crossed arrows) and the posteriorly arched posterior pericallosal artery (3 arrows). Blood supply partly comes from the colliculi quadrigemini and corpori geniculati arteries as well as the posterior choroidal arteries. The parieto-occipital branch of the posterior cerebral artery is displaced posteriorly (3 open arrowheads).

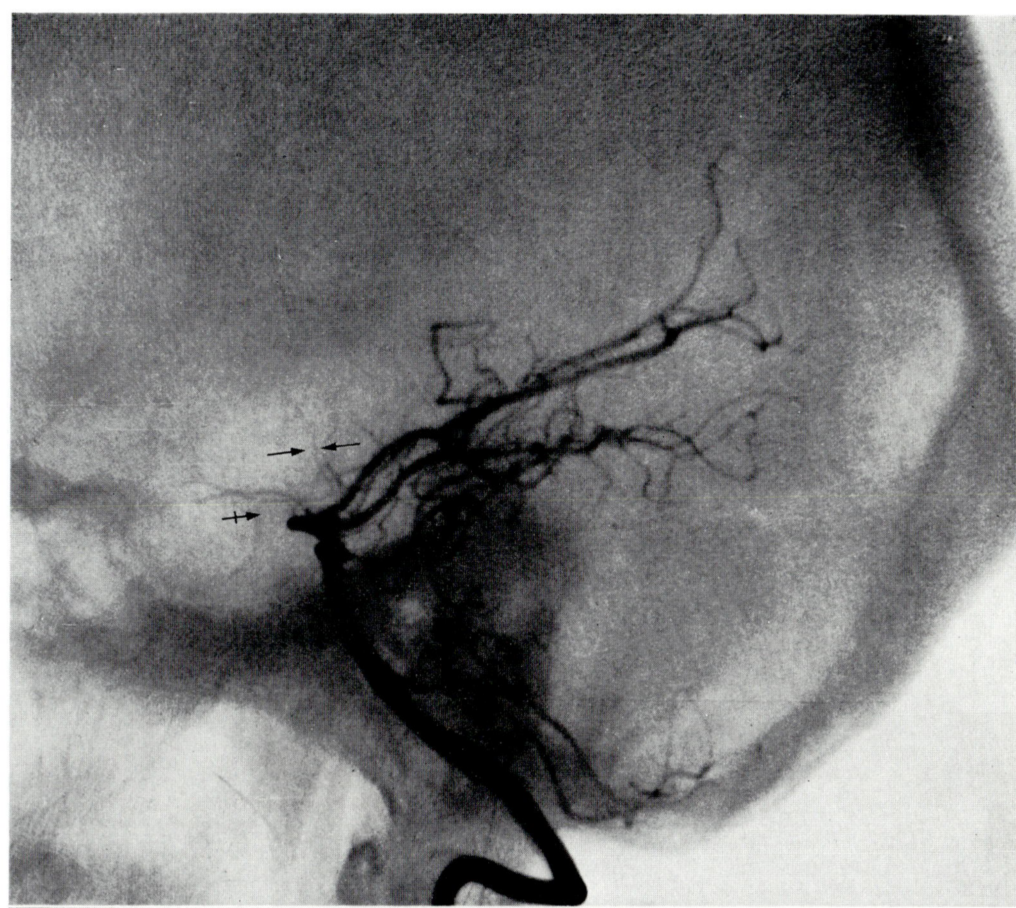

Fig. 299

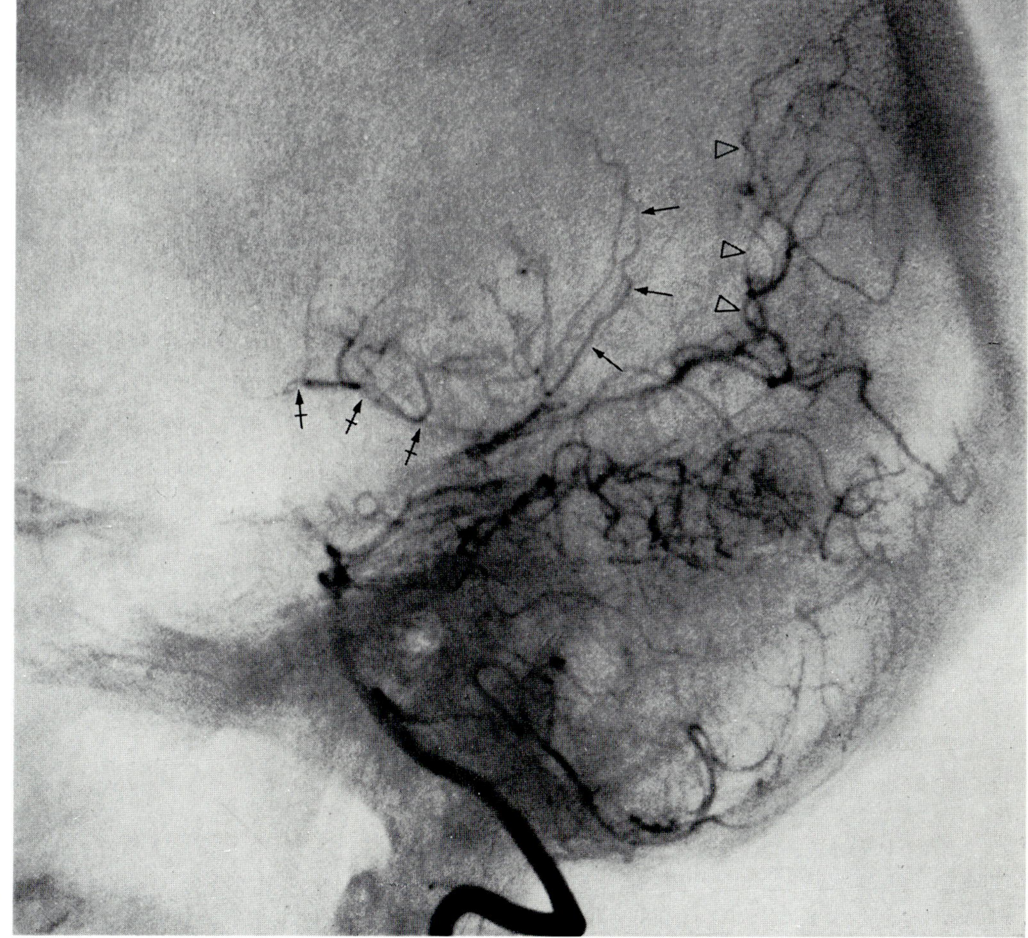

Fig. 300

Fig. 301 Venous phase in the lateral projection. The internal cerebral vein and the vein of Galen are moderately depressed downwards (4 arrows). There appears to be homogeneous tumor stain above these veins (3 arrowheads).

Fig. 302 Venous phase of the right internal carotid angiogram in the lateral projection. There is marked depression of the internal cerebral vein as well as posterior displacement of the vein of Galen (5 arrows). The thalamostriate vein is anteriorly displaced (2 arrowheads). An abnormal vein, arising from the tumor, drains into the proximal portion of the vein of Galen (2 crossed arrows). This abnormal vein is superimposed over the vein of Labbe.

Fig. 303 Venous phase of the right internal carotid angiogram in the anteroposterior projection. The tumor fills the entire lateral ventricle, displacing the veins on the ventricular floor, one of which probably represents the thalamostriate vein (3 arrows). The abnormal vein, probably on the medial surface of the tumor, is displaced to the left across the midline by the large tumor projecting into the left lateral ventricle (3 crossed arrows). This abnormal vein drains downwards. The basal vein of Rosenthal is shown (2 arrowheads).

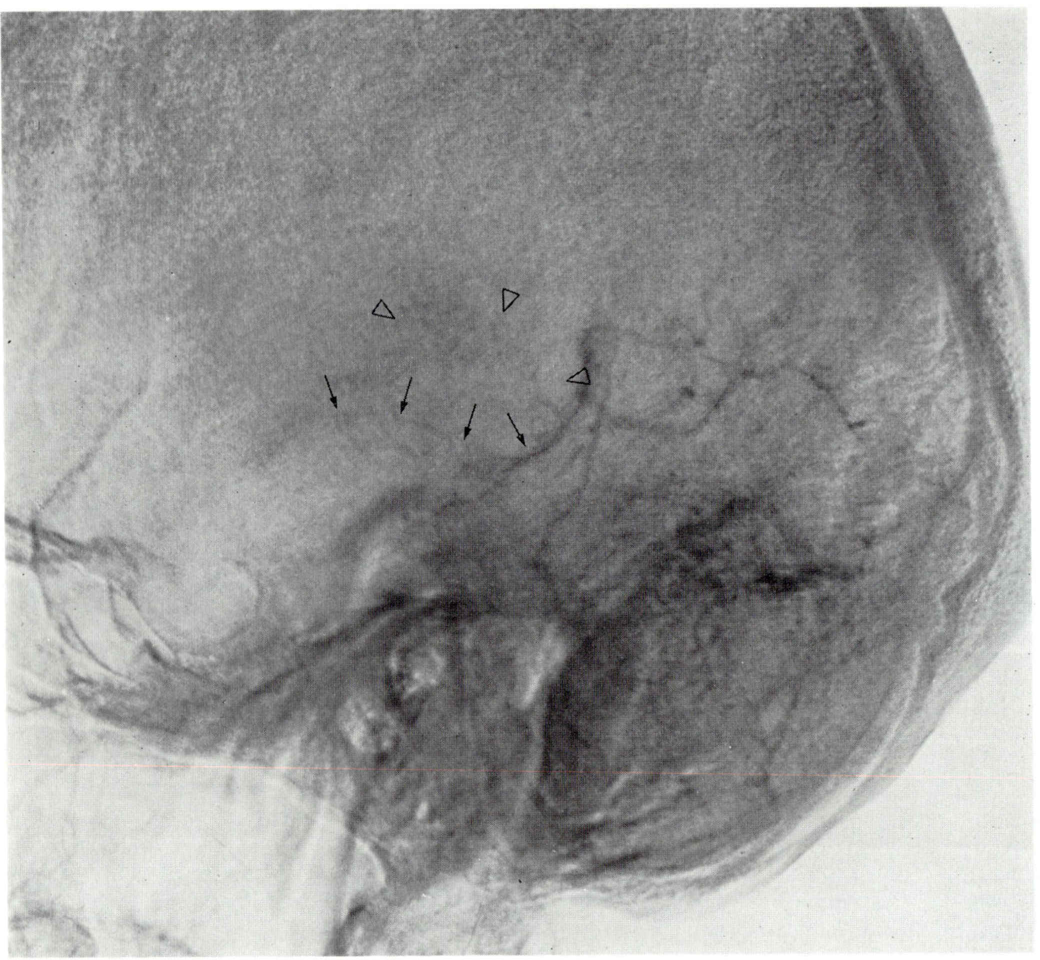

Fig. 301

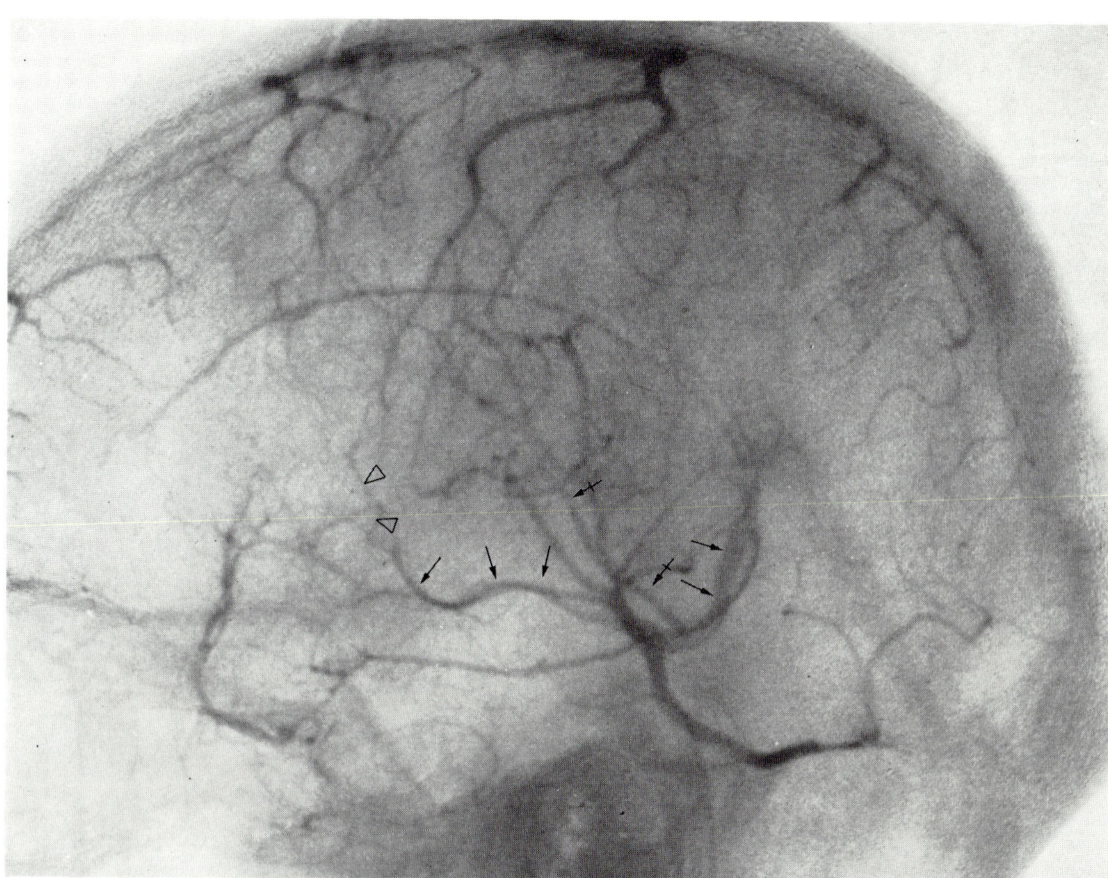

Fig. 302

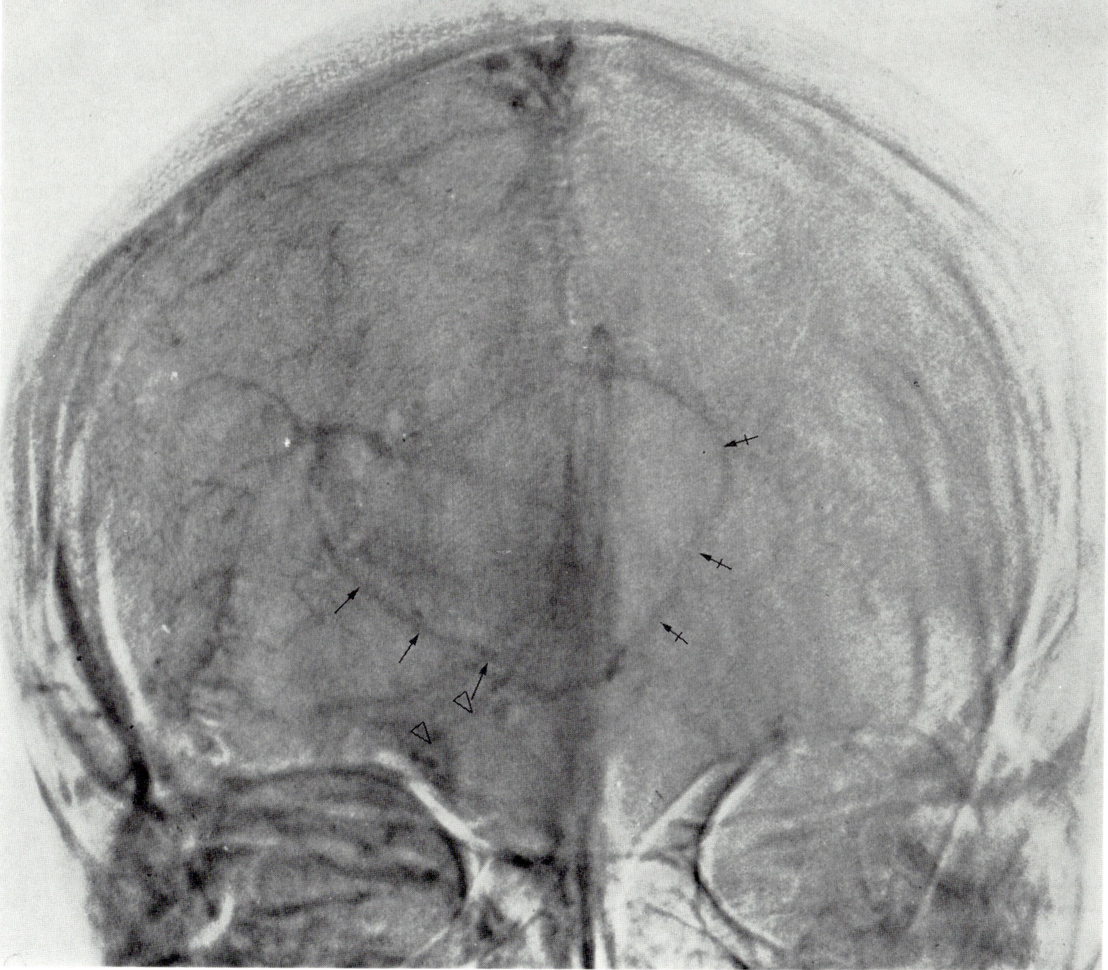

Fig. 303

Right Intraventricular Oligodendroglioma Involving the Posterior Parietal Lobe and the Posterior Thalamus

A 34-year-old male: Figs. 304–307

Fig. 304 Arterial phase in the lateral projection. The distal basilar artery is pushed downwards (the tip of the dorsum sellae is marked with a crossed arrow). The posterior choroidal arteries (3 arrows) and the posterior pericallosal artery (3 crossed arrows) are markedly separated with tumor vessels being supplied by the posterior choroidal arteries (3 closed arrowheads). The parieto-occipital artery is displaced posteriorly (2 open arrowheads).

Fig. 305 Venous phase in the lateral projection. The internal cerebral vein and the vein of Galen are markedly displaced inferiorly and posteriorly (4 arrows), so is the basal vein of Rosenthal (2 crossed arrows). Tumor stains are observed above the internal cerebral vein (2 arrowheads).

Fig. 306 Arterial phase of the right internal carotid angiogram in the lateral projection. The anterior choroidal artery is moderately enlarged because of blood supply to the tumor (2 arrows). There is unrolling of the anterior cerebral artery. The sylvian point is moderately displaced anteriorly (a crossed arrow), secondary to involvement of the posterior parietal lobe.

Fig. 307 Venous phase of the right internal carotid angiogram in the lateral projection. The internal cerebral vein and the vein of Galen are markedly displaced downwards by the intraventricular tumor (3 arrows). The tumor stains are seen within the lateral ventricle (3 arrowheads).

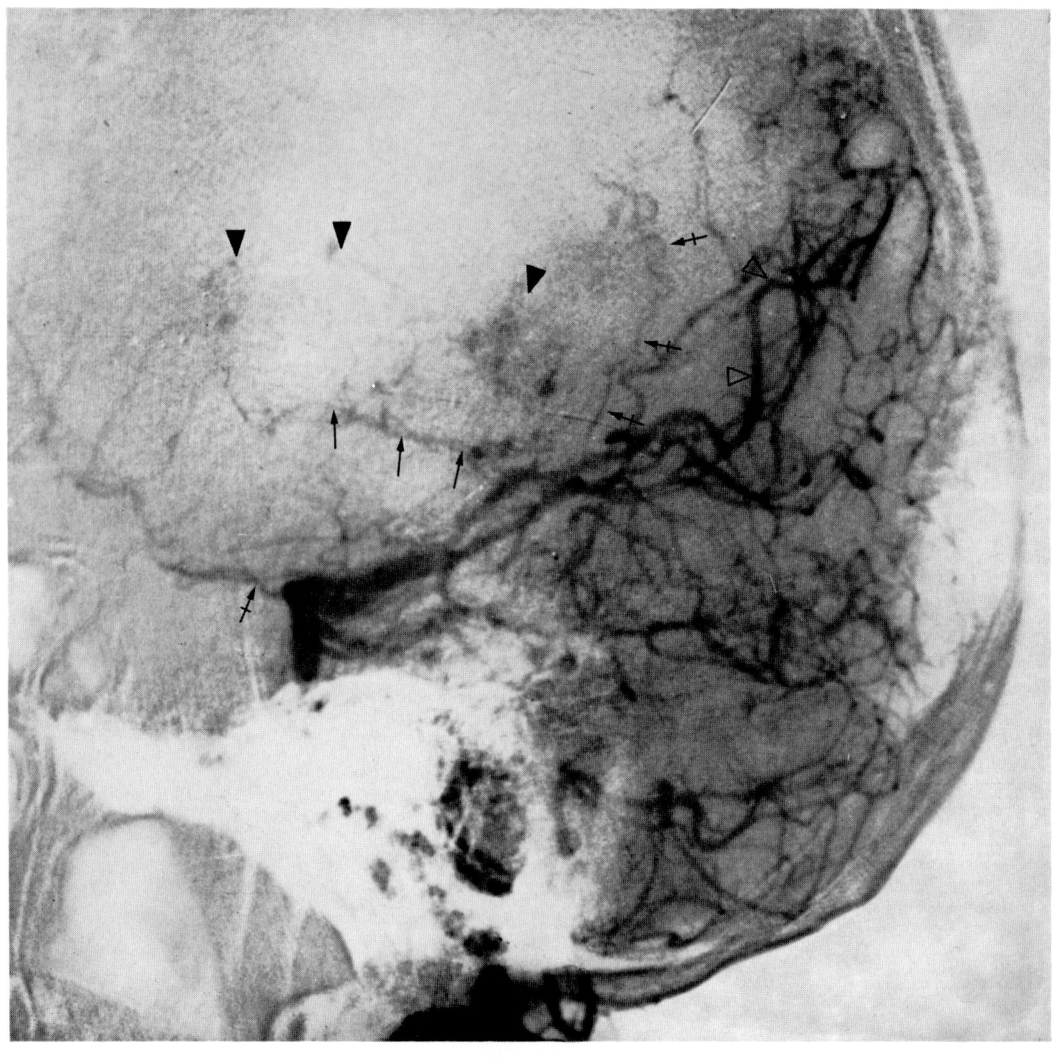

Fig. 304

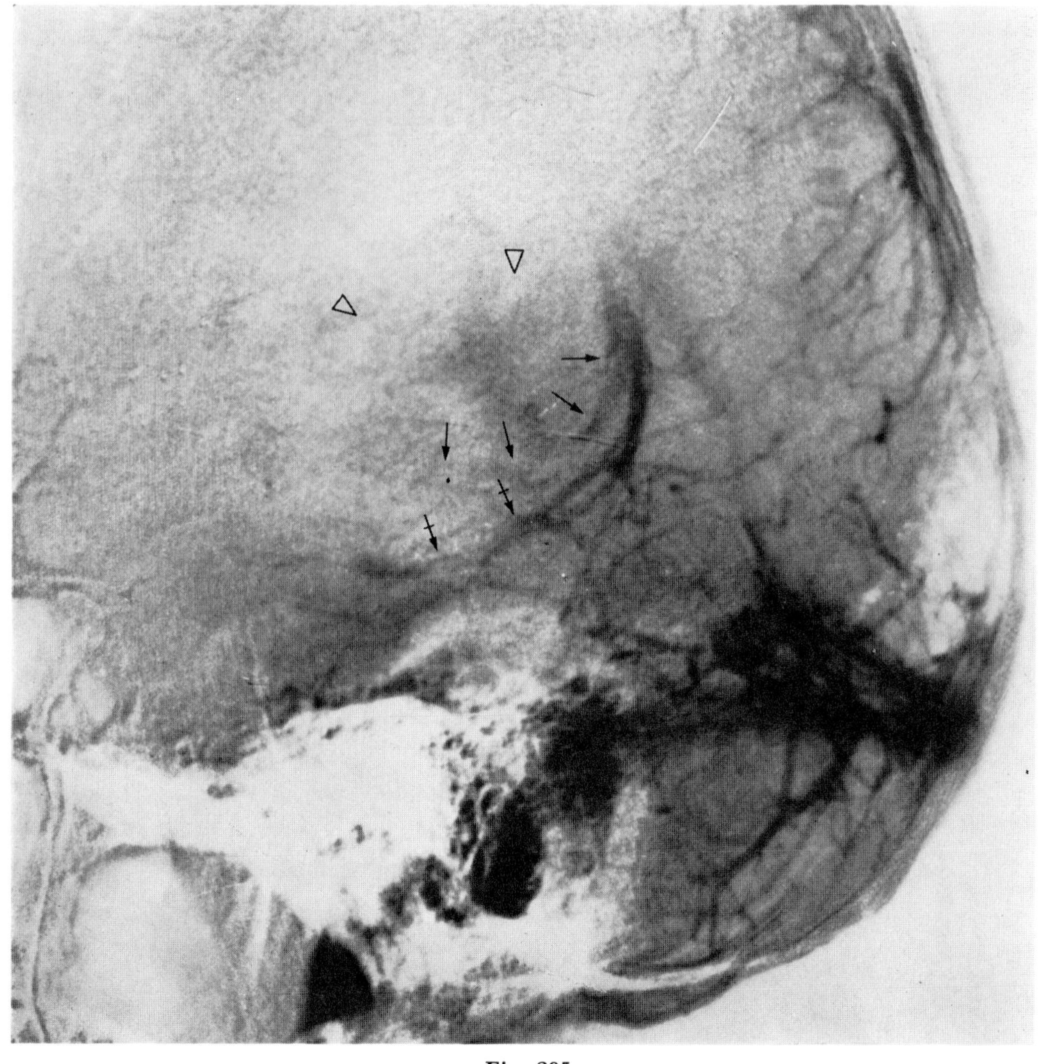

Fig. 305

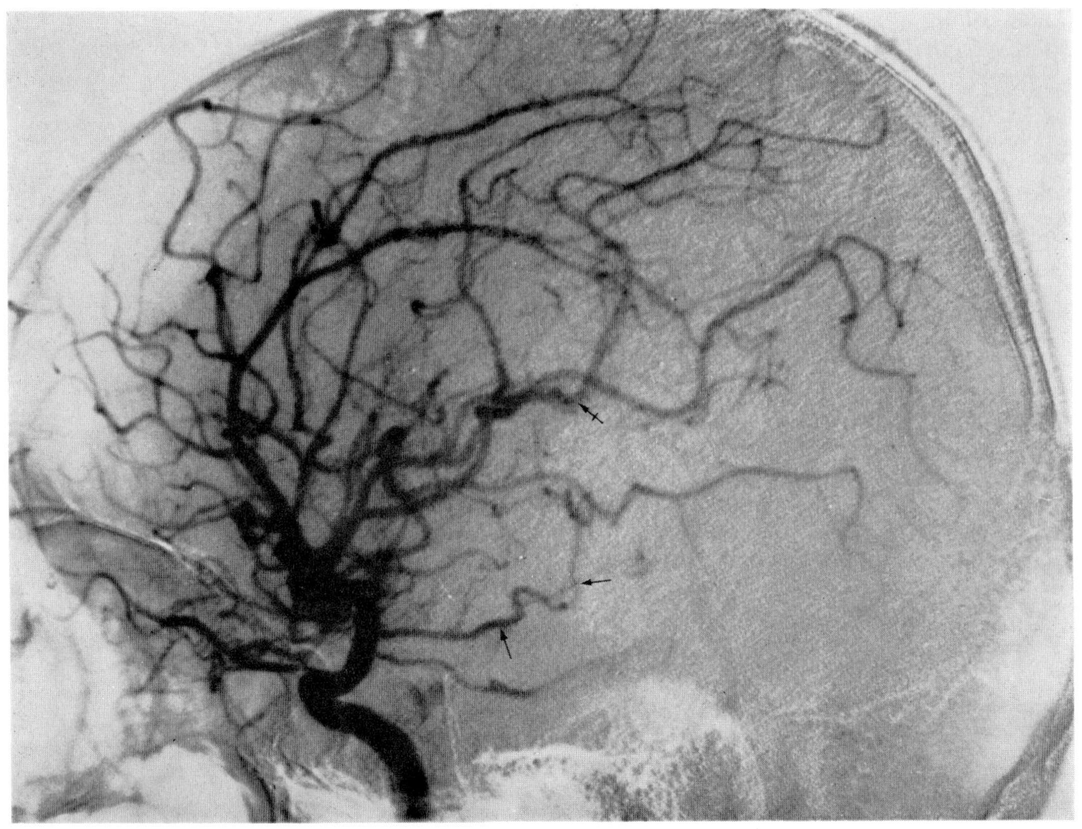

Fig. 306

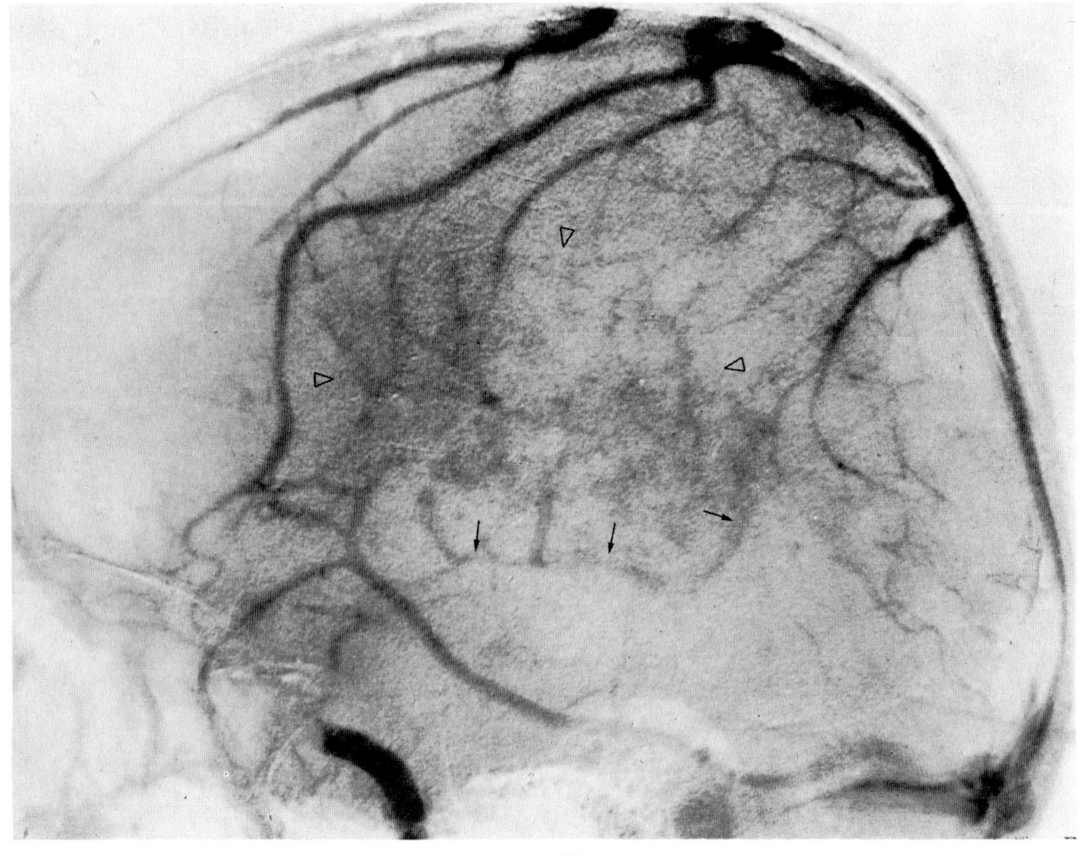

Fig. 307

Ependymoma of the Right Trigone Invading the Temporo-parieto-occipital Region

A 3-year-old female: Figs. 308–312

Fig. 308 Arterial phase in the lateral projection. The posterior choroidal arteries are displaced anteriorly in an arcuate fashion (3 arrows), while the posterior pericallosal artery is pushed backwards (3 crossed arrows). The right parieto-occipital artery is displaced posteriorly (4 closed arrowheads). There is straightening and downward displacement of the right posterior temporal artery (3 open arrowheads). The findings indicate a large tumor in the lateral ventricle involving the temporal lobe.

Fig. 309 Early venous phase in the lateral projection. The internal cerebral vein and the superior thalamic vein are superimposed and markedly depressed (3 arrows). The basal vein of Rosenthal is dislocated inferiorly (3 crossed arrows). There is posterior displacement of the cisternal portion of the precentral cerebellar vein (2 arrowheads).

Fig. 310 Venous phase in the lateral projection. There are at least three abnormal veins draining into the vein of Galen. They are all stretched around the tumor (3 arrows).

Fig. 311 Arterial phase in the Towne projection. The posterior temporal artery is stretched with rigid appearance (3 arrows), probably due to encasement by the tumor. The parieto-occipital arteries on both sides are displaced medially because of marked hydrocephalus.

Fig. 312 Venous phase in the Towne projection. The abnormal veins are stretched around the tumor (2 arrows). The vein of Galen is displaced to the left of the midline (2 crossed arrows).

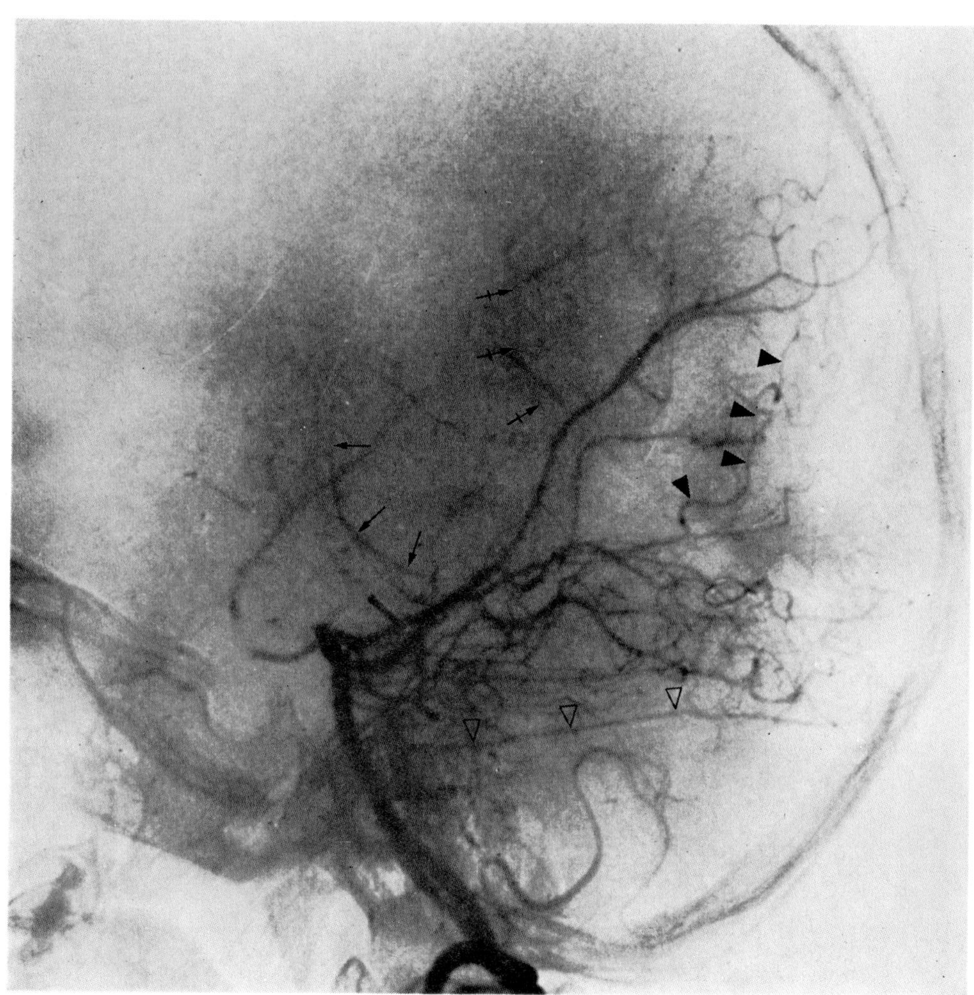

Fig. 308

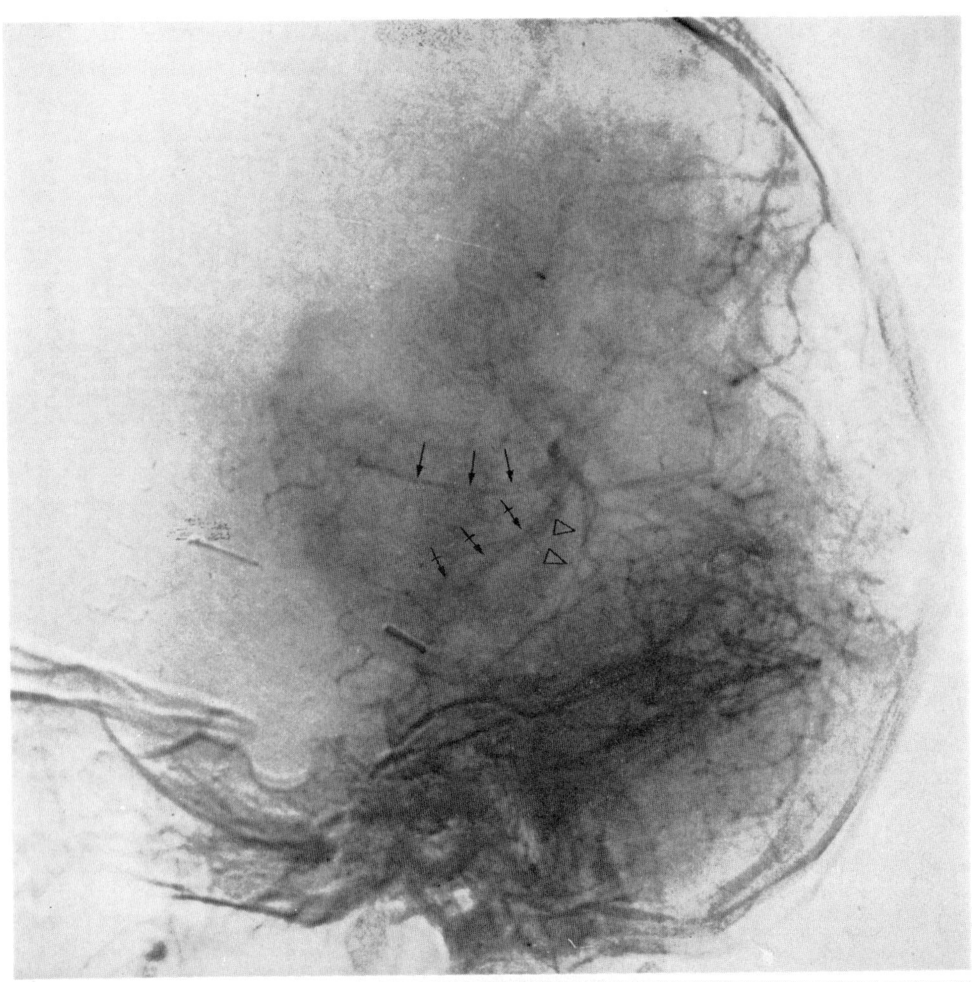

Fig. 309

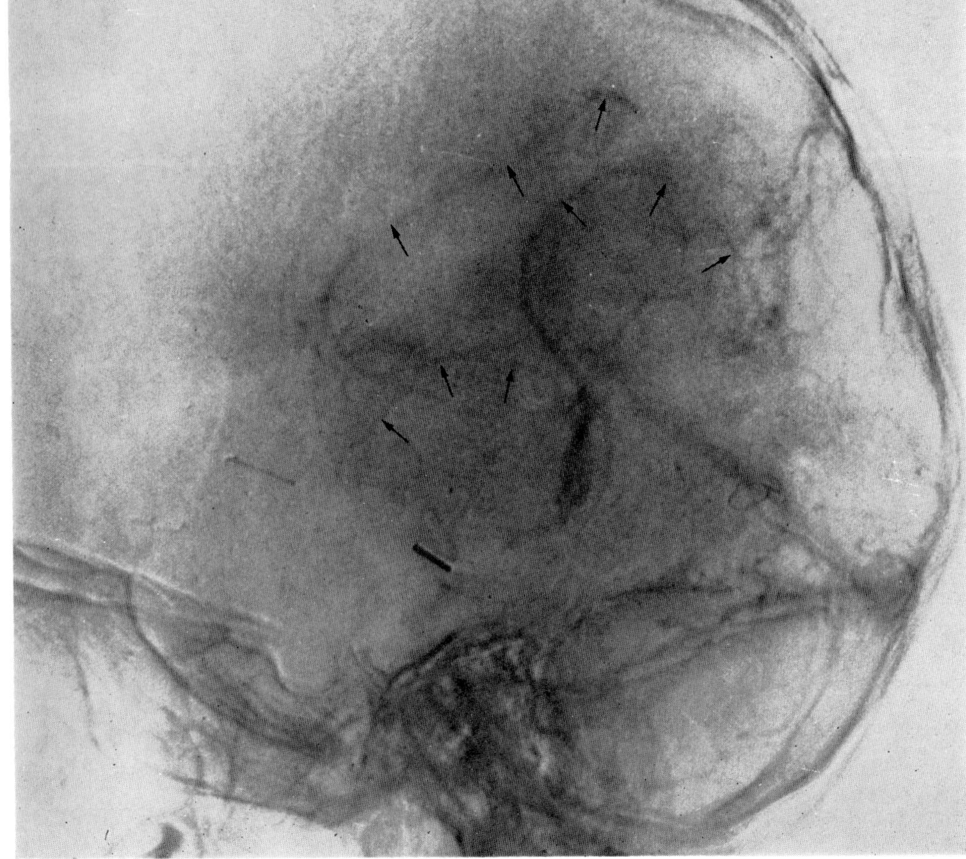

Fig. 310

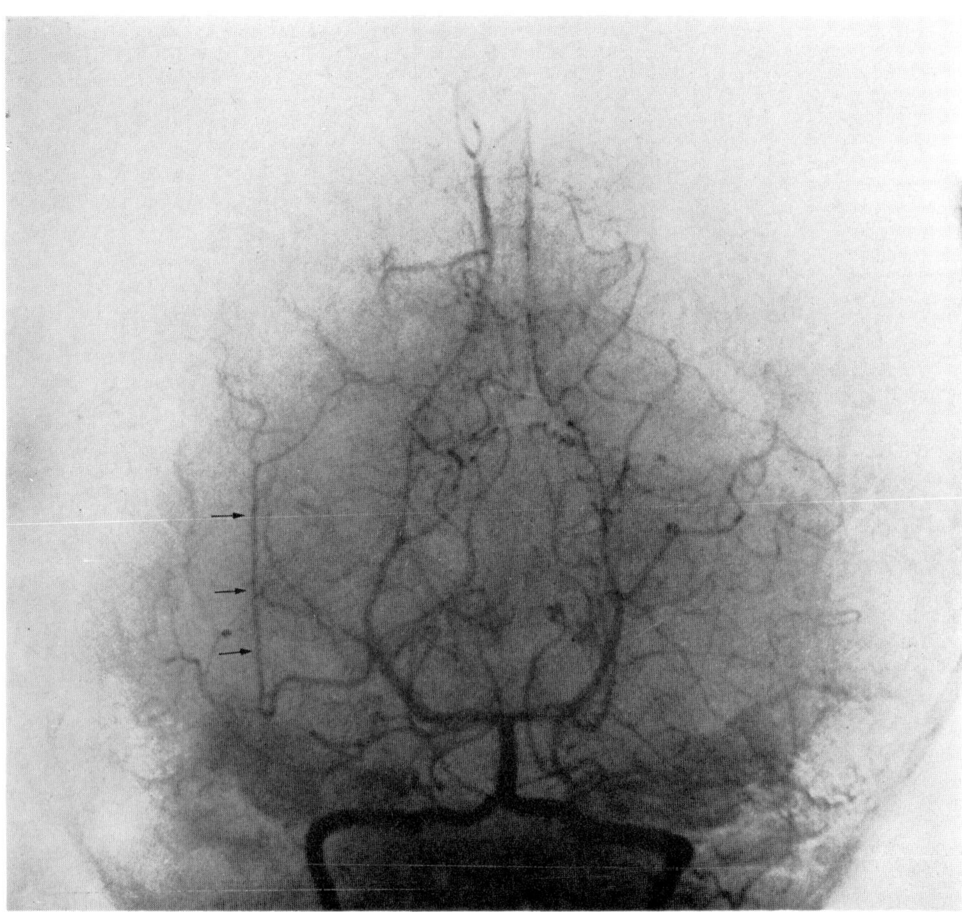

Fig. 311

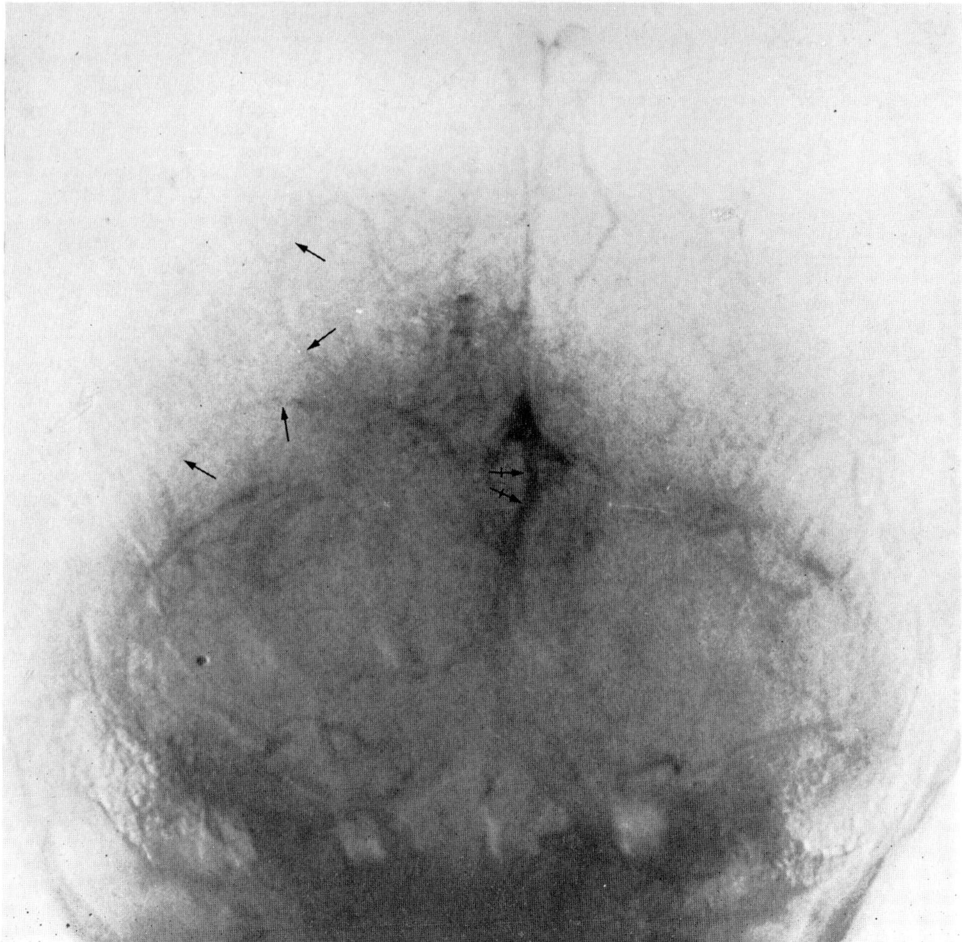

Fig. 312

Intraventricular Teratoma with Extensive Involvement of the Trigone, Temporal Horn and Occipital Horn on the Right

A 43-year-old male: Figs. 313–317

Fig. 313 Arterial phase in the lateral projection. The right posterior choroidal artery is depressed downwards (3 arrows). The left choroidal artery is normal in its course (2 crossed arrows). The course of the posterior thalamoperforate arteries is redundant with buckling of the distal basilar artery (2 arrowheads). The posterior clinoid process is marked with a double-crossed arrow. The findings are suggestive of an intraventricular tumor.

Fig. 314 Early venous phase in the lateral projection. There is marked depression of the internal cerebral vein and the superior thalamic vein on the right (3 arrows). The internal cerebral vein is also depressed on the left (3 crossed arrows). The posterior mesencephalic vein is depressed (3 open arrowheads), while posterior displacement is noted of the anterior pontomesencephalic vein (3 closed arrowheads). The posterior clinoid process is marked with an arrow.

Fig. 315 Venous phase in the lateral projection. Marked depression of the internal cerebral vein (3 arrows) and the choroid plexus (2 crossed arrows) are noted. These findings of the vertebral angiogram strongly suggest presence of a large mass in the lateral ventricle.

Fig. 316 Arterial phase of the internal carotid angiogram on the right. The sylvian point (a crossed arrow) is markedly displaced forwards, so are the other segments of the middle cerebral artery (3 arrows).

Fig. 317 Venous phase of the same angiogram. Tumor stains (2 arrows) are noted just above the internal cerebral vein, which is markedly depressed downwards with straight appearance (3 crossed arrows). The thalamostriate vein is displaced anteriorly (2 arrowheads).

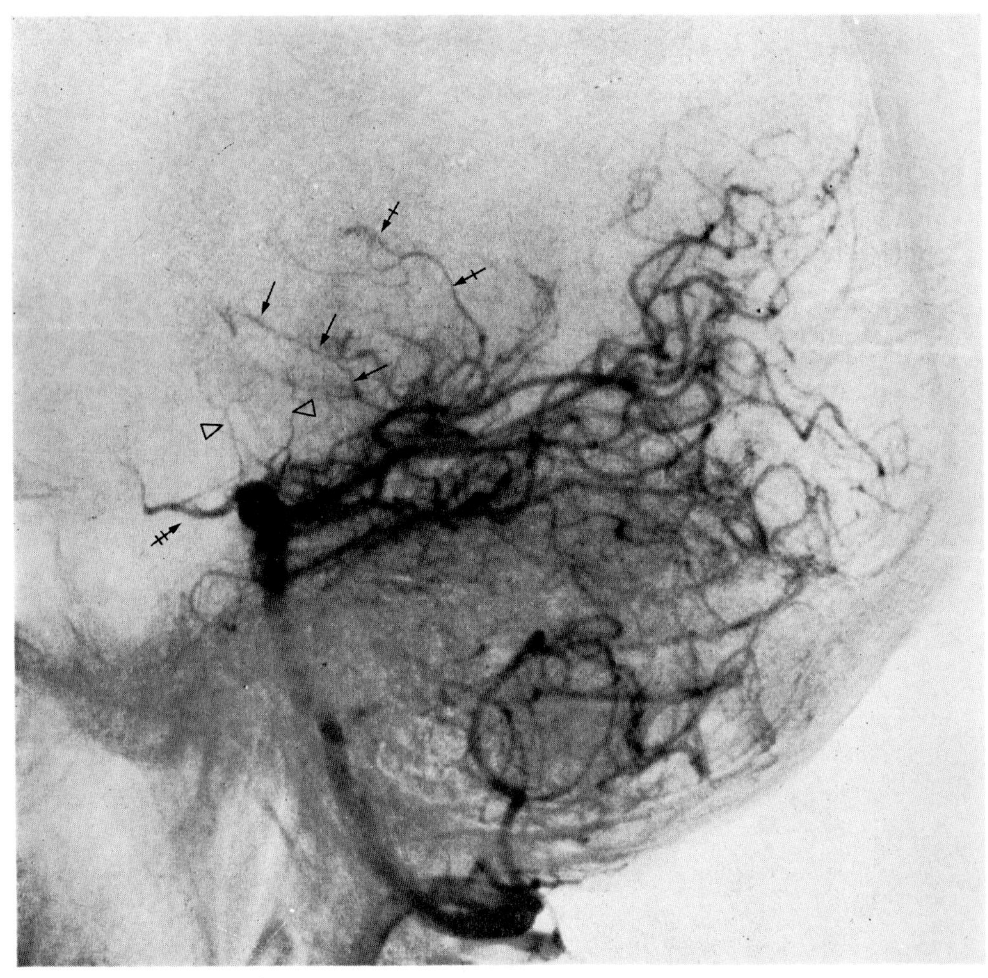

Fig. 313

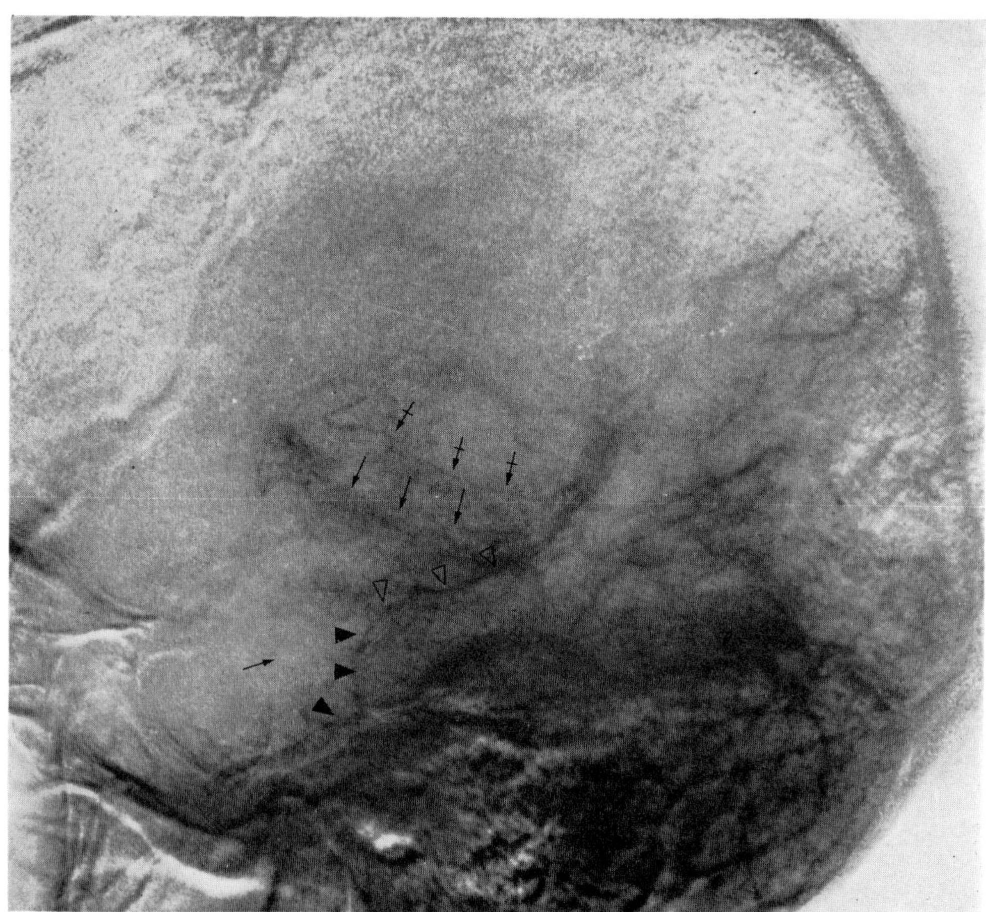

Fig. 314

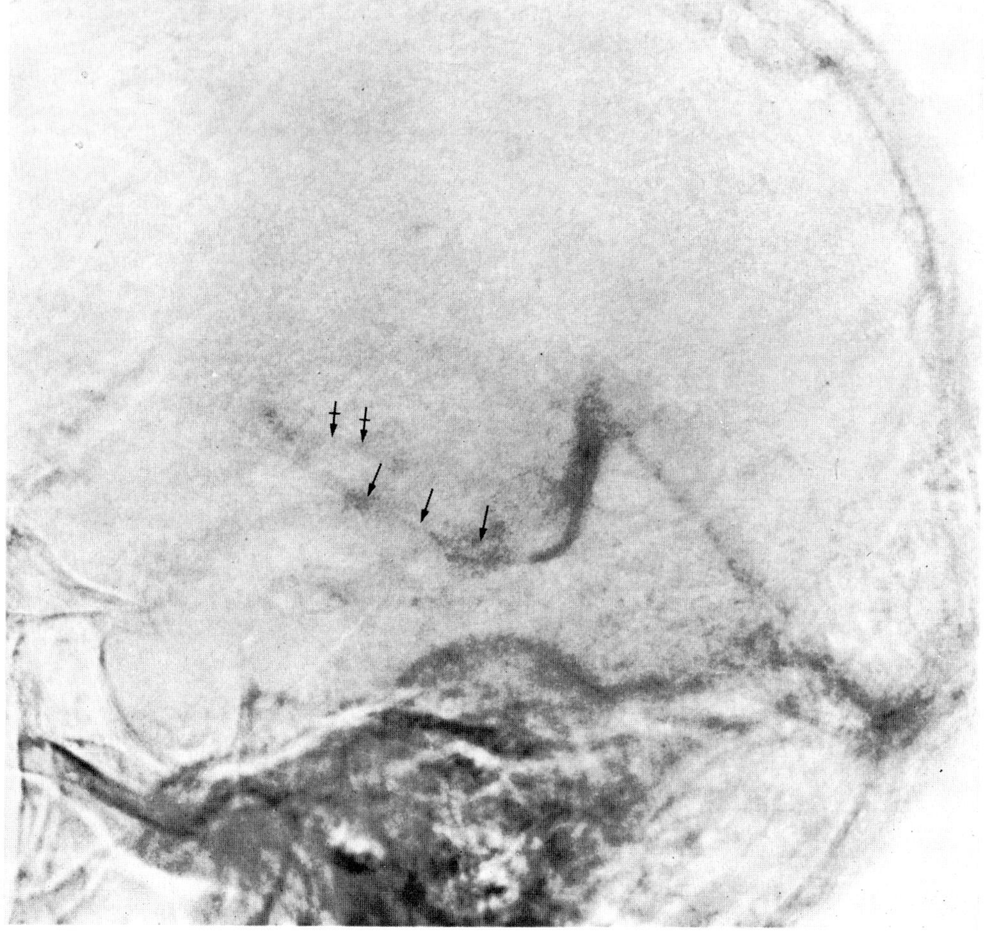

Fig. 315

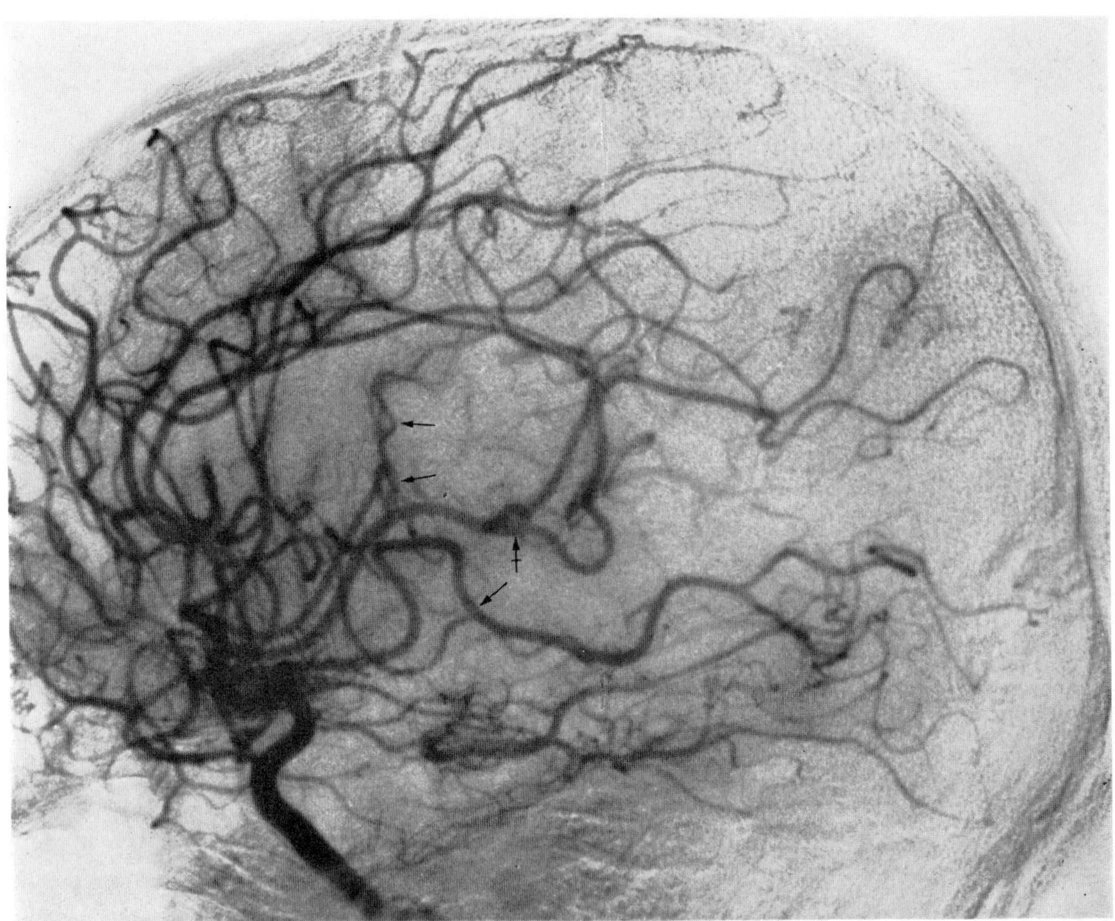

Fig. 316

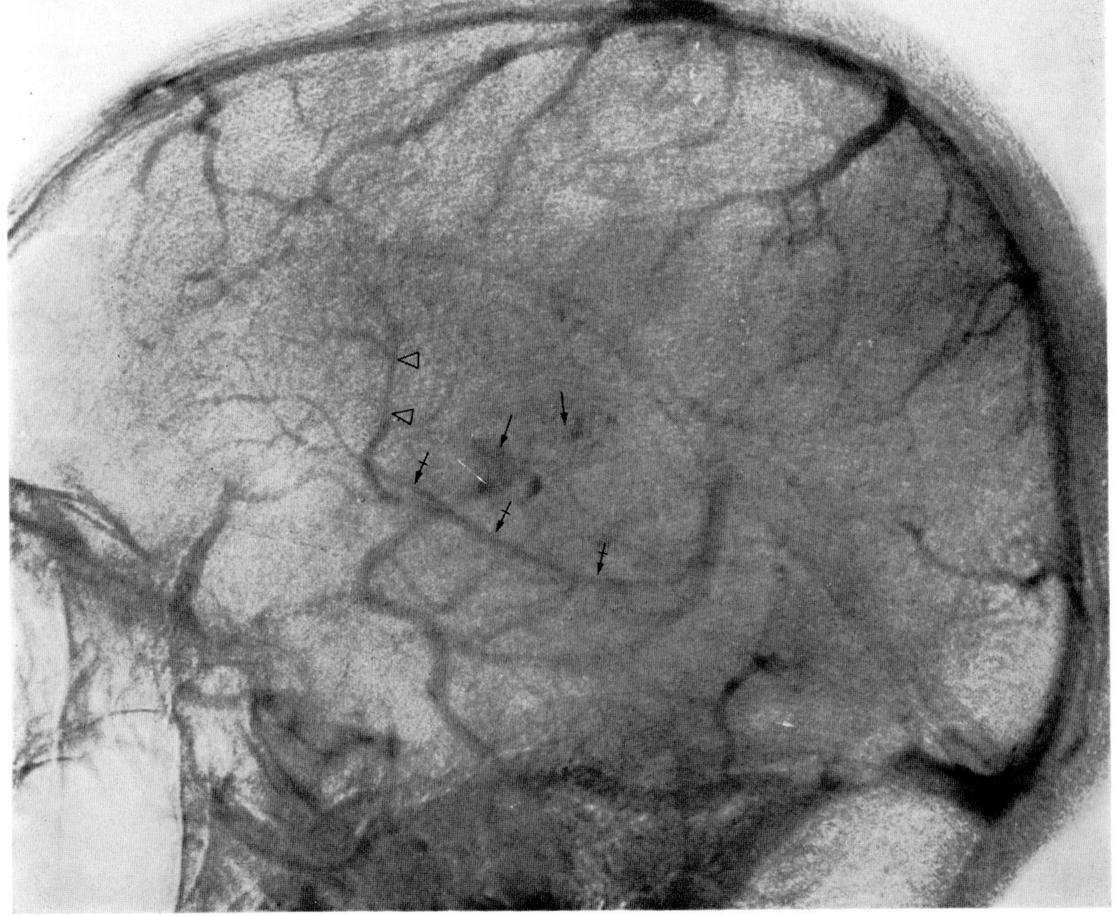

Fig. 317

Meningioma Filling the Trigone, Body and Temporal Horn of the Left Lateral Ventricle

A 38-year-old female: Figs. 318–324

Fig. 318 Arterial phase in the lateral projection. The lateral posterior choroidal artery is enlarged and dislocated anteriorly (3 arrows) with supply of tumor vessels in the superior aspect of the tumor (4 open arrowheads). The posterior pericallosal artery is pushed backwards on the left (3 crossed arrows). The ambient segment of the posterior cerebral artery is depressed downwards (3 double-crossed arrows) with tumor vessels just above this segment (2 closed arrowheads).

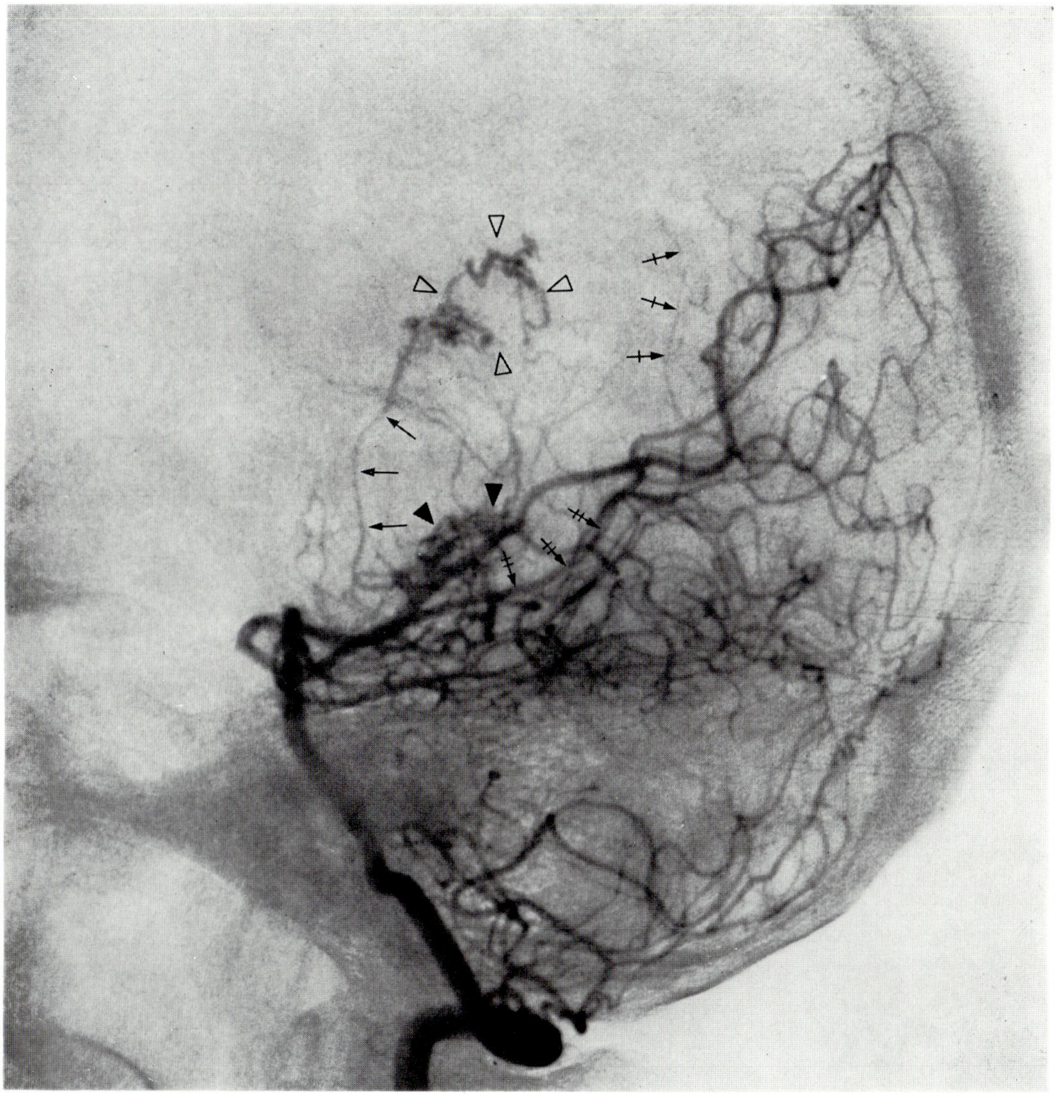

Fig. 318

Fig. 319 Venous phase in the lateral projection. The tumor stain is well demonstrated in the superior aspect of the tumor (4 arrows). The posterior mesencephalic vein is depressed (2 crossed arrows).

Fig. 320 Arterial phase in the Towne projection. The quadrigeminal and posterior ambient segments of the posterior cerebral artery are displaced medially (2 arrows) with arcuate stretching of the parieto-occipital artery (2 crossed arrows). The tumor vessels are again demonstrated (an arrowhead). The left superior cerebellar artery is also displaced medially, probably due to indirect pressure through the tentorium.

Fig. 321 Capillary phase in the Towne projection. The tumor stains are visualized (4 arrows).

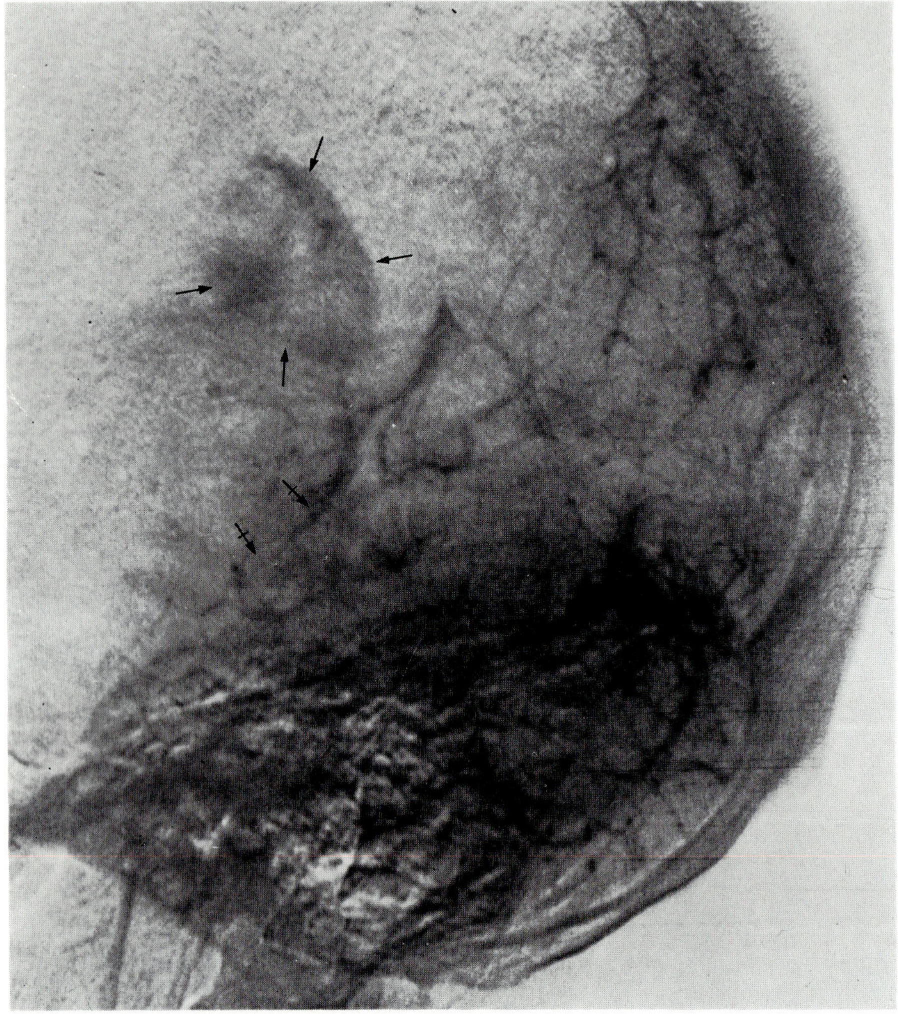

Fig. 319

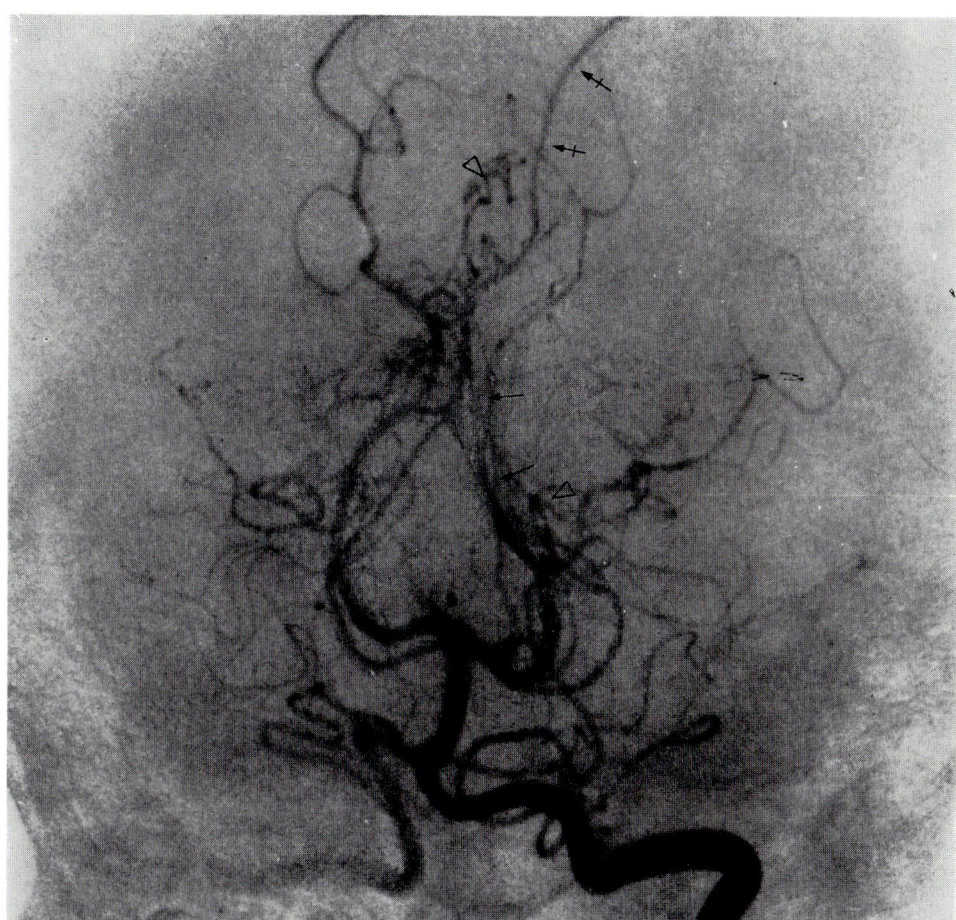

Fig. 320

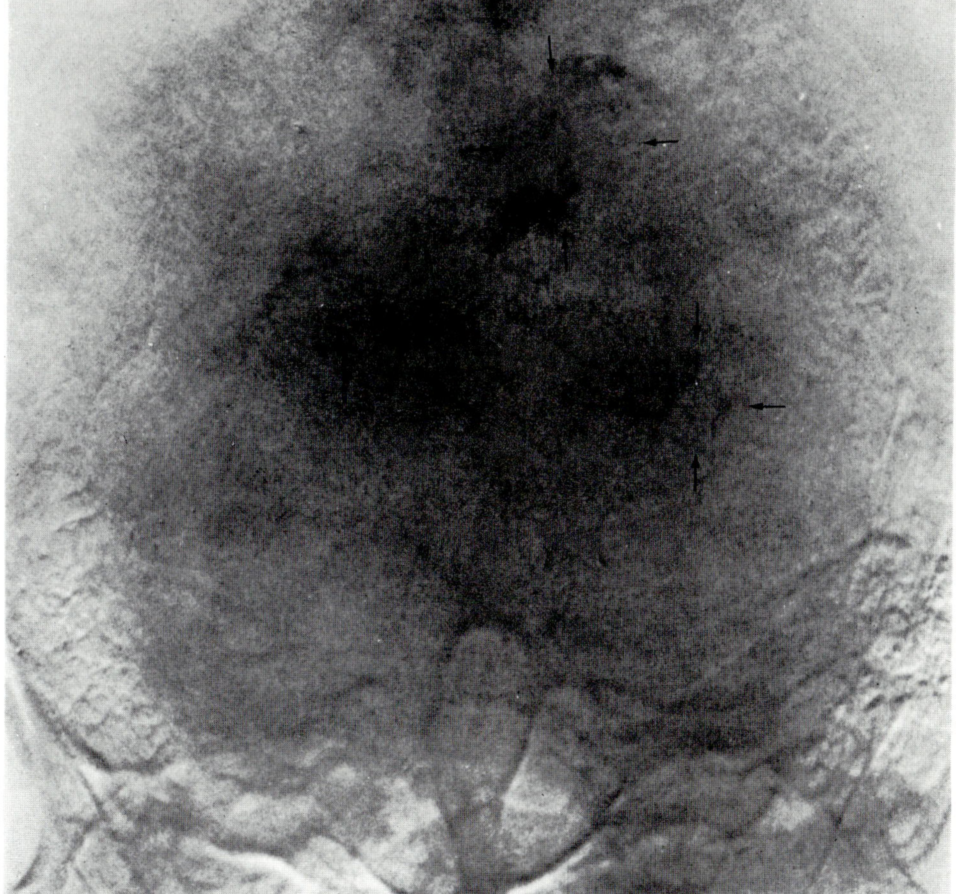

Fig. 321

Fig. 322 Arterial phase of the left internal carotid angiogram. The anterior choroidal artery is enlarged and supplies tumor vessels in the lateral ventricle. The cisternal portion of the anterior choroidal artery is accordioned (3 arrows). The sylvian vessels are displaced anteriorly and superiorly (3 arrowheads).

Fig. 323 Capillary phase of the internal carotid angiogram. There are irregular tumor vessels in the area of the trigone of the lateral ventricle (4 arrows).

Fig. 324 Venous phase of the internal carotid angiogram. Diffuse, homogeneous tumor stain is demonstrated in the entire tumor of the trigone, body and temporal horn (4 arrows). The superior, posterior aspect of the tumor is not stained (3 arrowheads), since this area is supplied by the posterior choroidal artery. The internal cerebral vein appears to be depressed (4 crossed arrows). Homogeneous tumor stains, remaining to the venous phase and having blood supply from the choroidal arteries, strongly suggest an intraventricular meningioma.

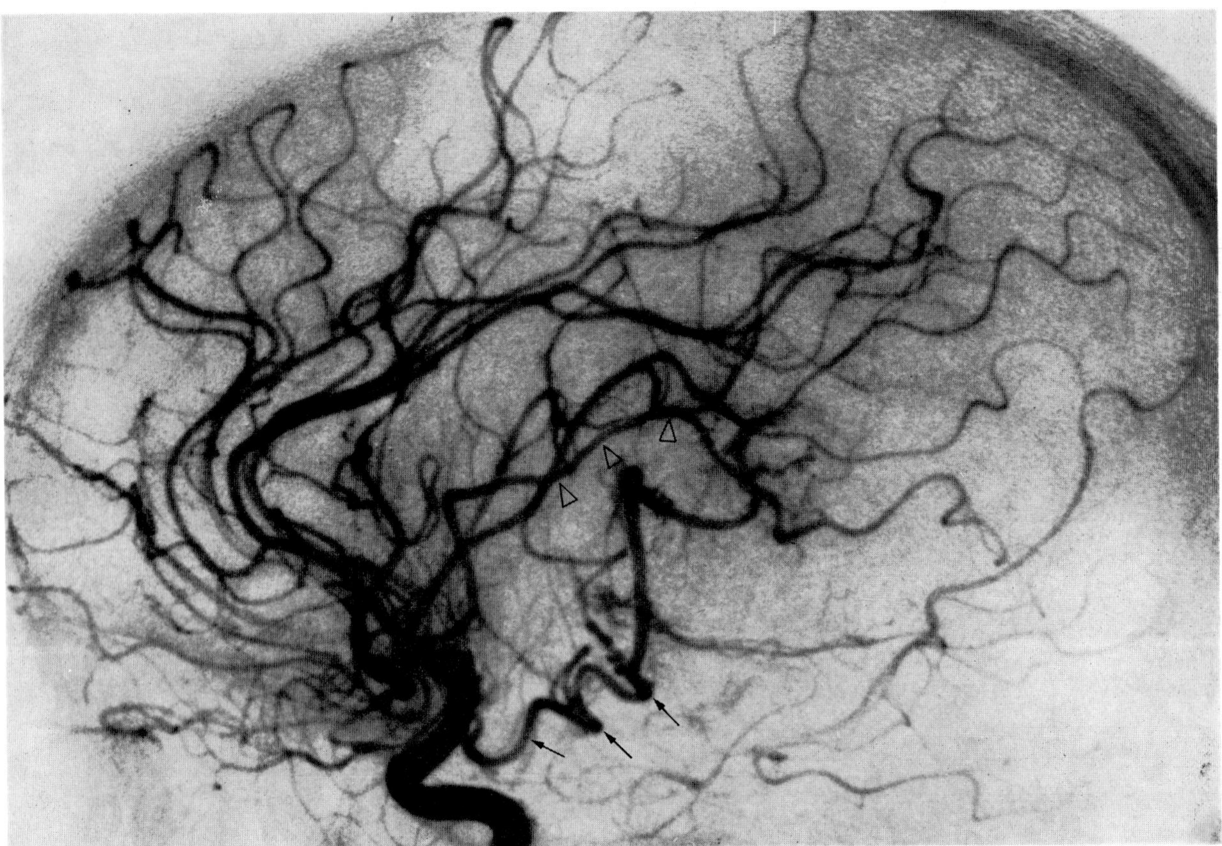

Fig. 322

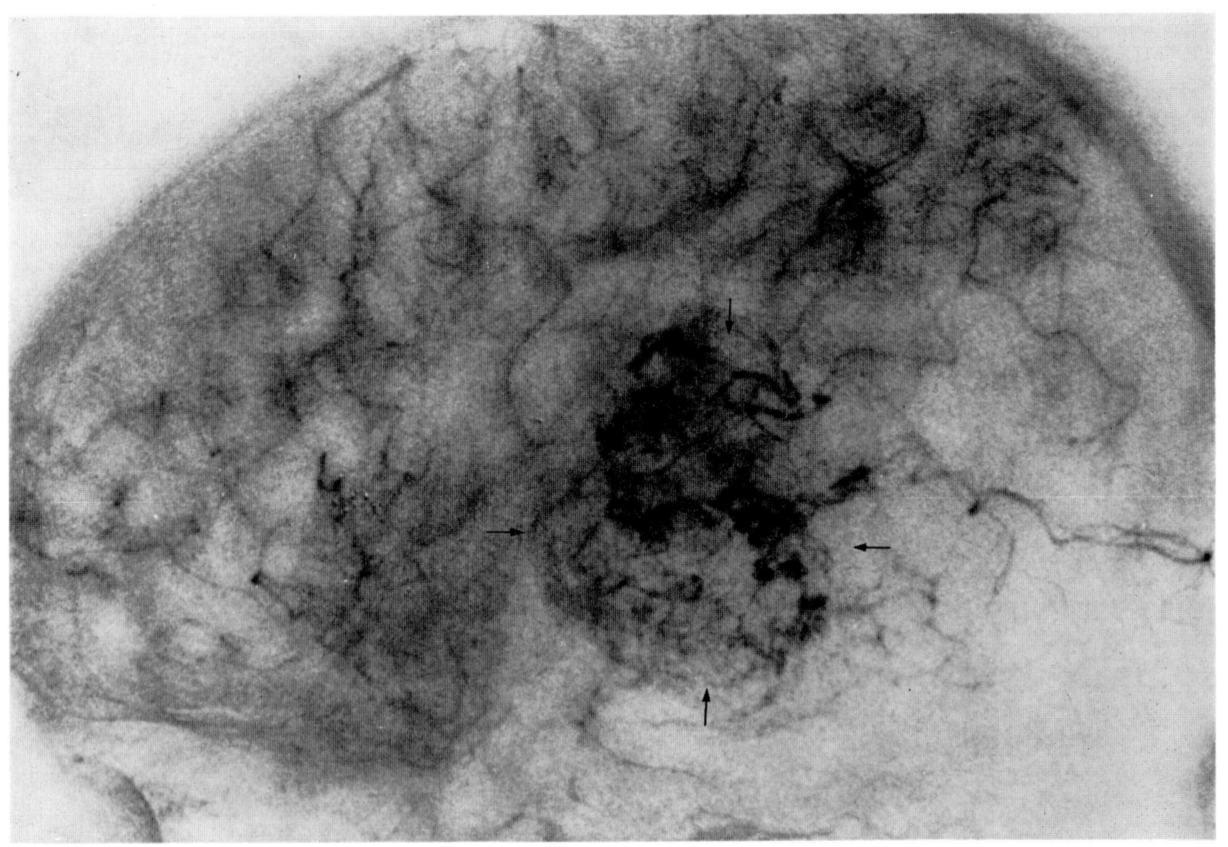

Fig. 323

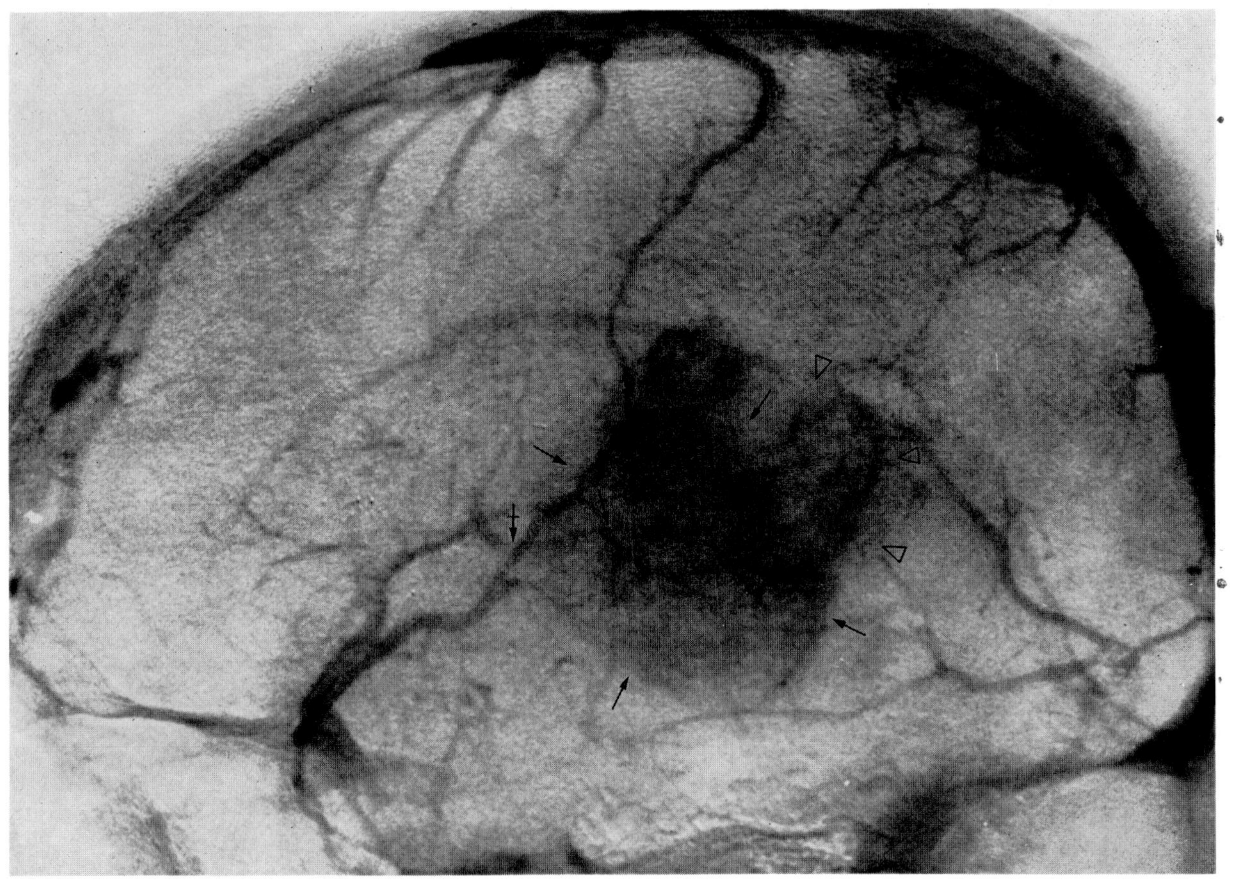

Fig. 324

8

Vascular Diseases

ANEURYSM

Etiologic factors of aneurysms are mostly congenital and atherosclerotic. Basal skull fractures may involve the basilar artery with formation of an aneurysm.

Aneurysms of the vertebrobasilar system comprise 15 to 20% of all intracranial aneurysms of autopsy materials (PASSERINI and TAGLIABUE, 1966). The radiological incidence of these aneurysms is less than 5% in the most reported series (BULL, 1964; PASSERINI and TAGLIABUE, 1966). According to BULL's series (1964) of 64 aneurysms of the vertebrobasilar system (1962), 97% of all aneurysms arose from only 4 major sites, termination of the basilar artery in 63%, junction of the vertebral and posterior inferior cerebellar arteries in 20%, junction of the basilar and superior cerebellar arteries in 11% and junction of the basilar and vertebral arteries in 3%. Aneurysms may develop at the origin of the anterior inferior cerebellar arteries. In another series of 168 vertebrobasilar aneurysms (PASSERINI and TAGLIABUE, 1964), 102 aneurysms (61%) were of the basilar artery, 32 (21%) of the vertebral artery and 30 (18%) of the remaining portions of the vertebrobasilar system.

Vertebrobasilar aneurysms are often a manifestation of multiple aneurysms. JAMIESON (1964) reported that 7 out of 19 patients with posterior fossa aneurysms also had aneurysms in the carotid system. According to McKISSOCK's statistics (1964) there were 231 multiple aneurysms, more than 10% of which invloved the basilar arterial system together with the carotid system. Thus, it is quite important to look for a second or third aneurysm in the vertebrobasilar system in the presence of an aneurysm on the carotid tree and vice versa.

Aneurysms of the vertebrobasilar system may be responsible for subarachnoid hemorrhage. PASSERINI and TAGLIABUE (1966) found 4 aneurysms and 3 angiomas (11.4%) in the posterior fossa as the source of bleeding following 61 negative bilateral carotid angiograms. SPATZ and BULL (1957) also reported similar experience in 8 aneurysms and 8 angiomas (26%) out of 60 vertebral angiograms performed in the similar condition. Thus, complete exploration of the cerebral circulation is necessary in the presence of subarachnoid hemorrhage.

It is now a routine practice at our institution to perform vertebral angiography in patients with subarachnoid hemorrhage or aneurysms of the carotid system. If the two carotid and one vertebral angiograms are negative, we perform angiograms on the other vertebral artery.

Aneurysm Arising from the Junction of both Vertebral Arteries

A 53-year-old female: Figs. 325–327

Fig. 325 Arterial phase in the Towne projection. There is a 1.0×1.0 cm saccular aneurysm arising from the junction of the right and left vertebral arteries (2 opposing arrows).

Fig. 326 Arterial phase in the lateral projection. The aneurysm is seen tangentially (2 opposing arrows). There is minimally increased distance between the clivus and the basilar artery, probably due to posterior displacement of the basilar artery by the anteriorly located aneurysm. The clivus is marked with 3 crossed arrows.

Fig. 327 Half-axial projection with slight rotation of the head to the right. This projection was obtained to demonstrate the neck of the aneurysm, but this was not successful. The aneurysm is marked with 2 opposing arrows.

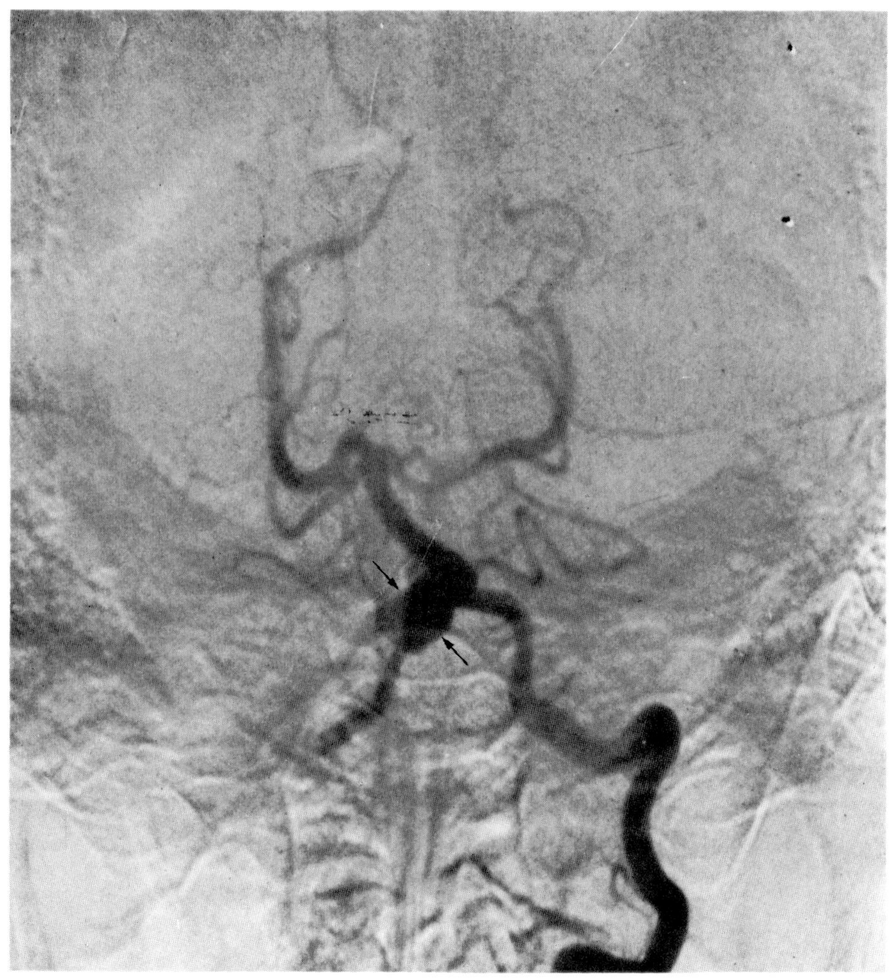

Fig. 325

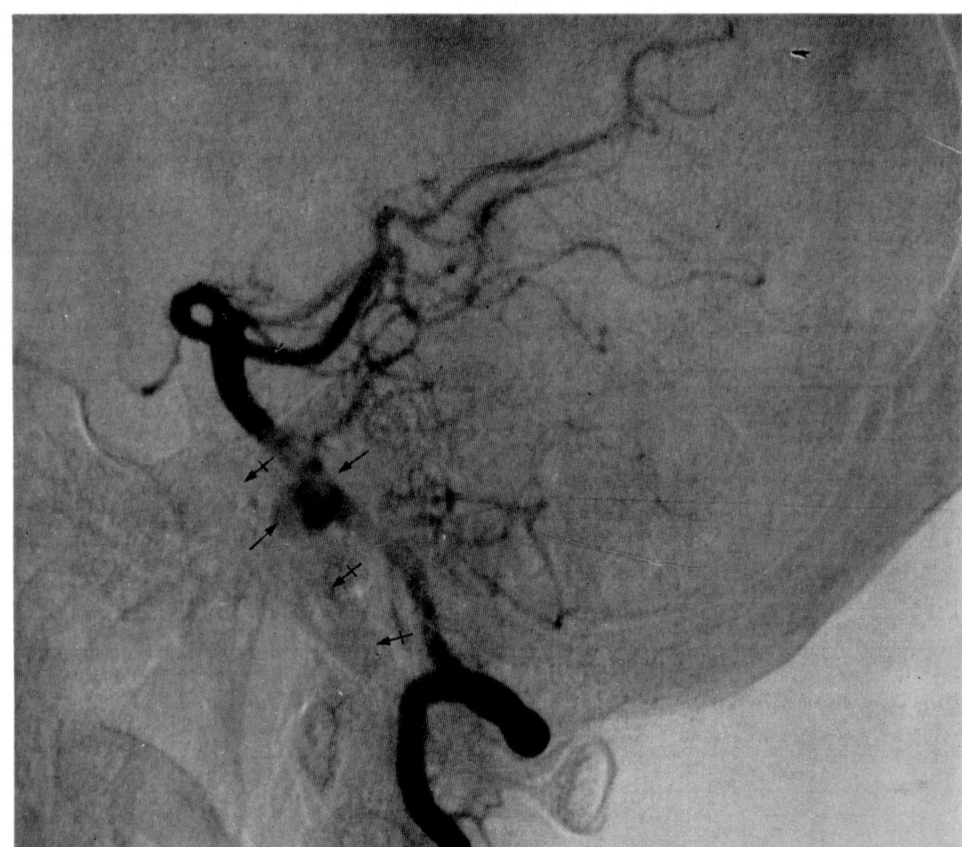

Fig. 326

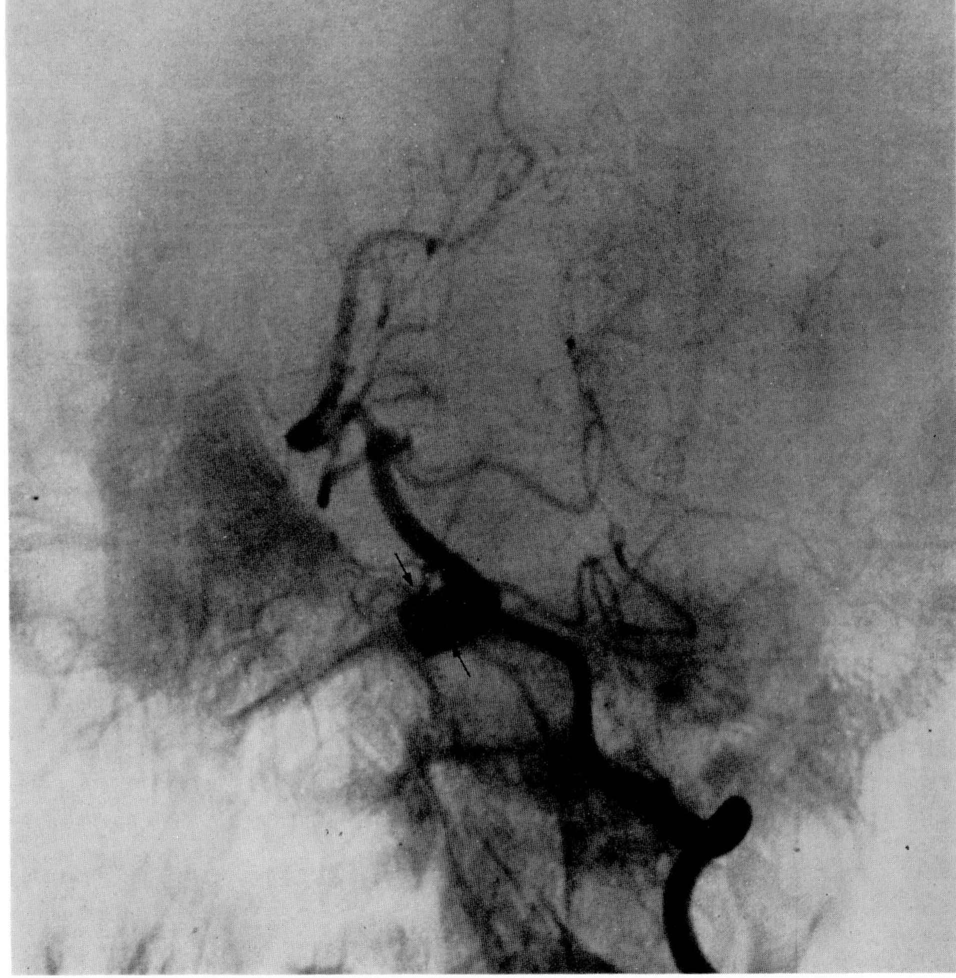

Fig. 327

Saccular Aneurysm Originating from the Junction of both Vertebral Arteries

A 54-year-old female: Figs. 328 and 329

Fig. 328 Arterial phase in the Towne projection. There is a 1.0 × 1.2 cm aneurysm as the junction of both vertebral arteries (2 opposing arrows). The neck of the aneurysm is not demonstrated. The arteries are moderately tortuous.

Fig. 329 Arterial phase in the lateral projection. The aneurysm is not well shown because of superimposition of the mastoids. The basilar artery (3 open arrowheads) is displaced backwards from the clivus (3 crossed arrows), secondary to the mass effect of the aneurysm. The distal basilar artery is projecting into the interpeduncular fossa, probably elevating the floor of the third ventricle (a closed arrowhead).

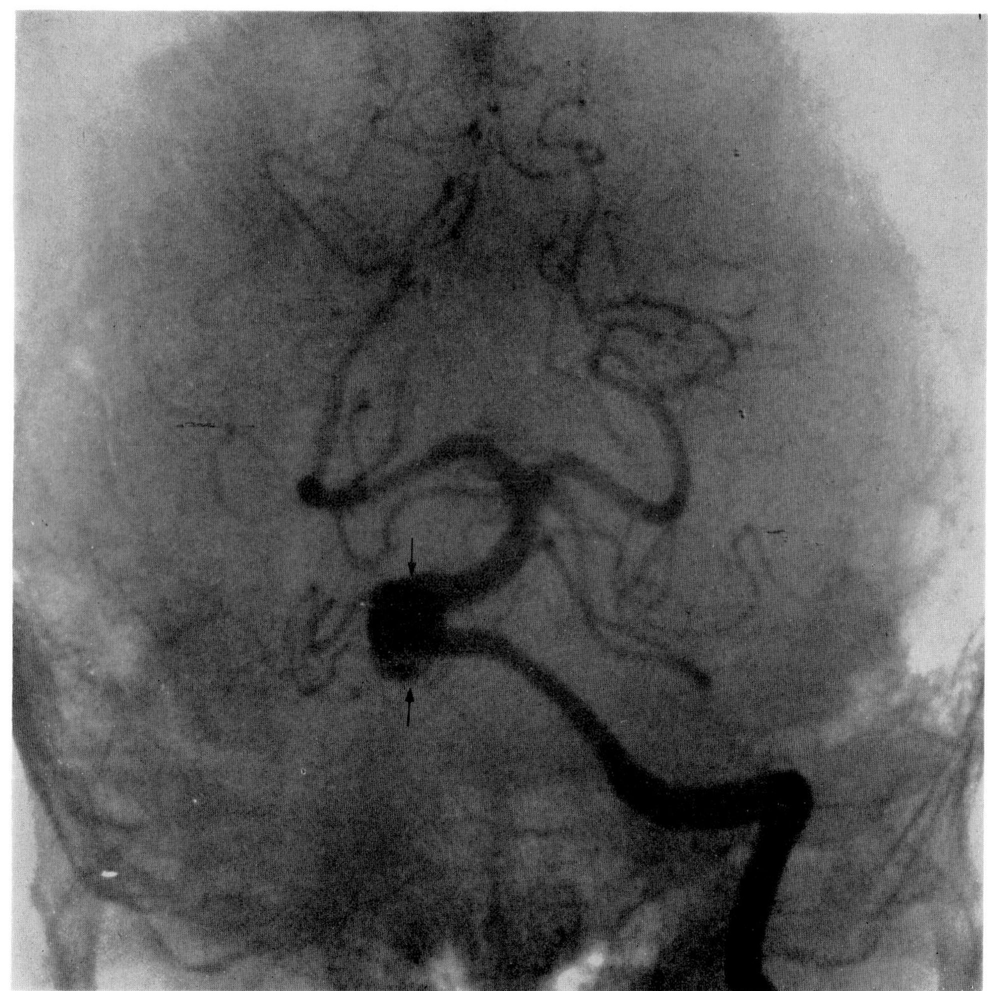

Fig. 328

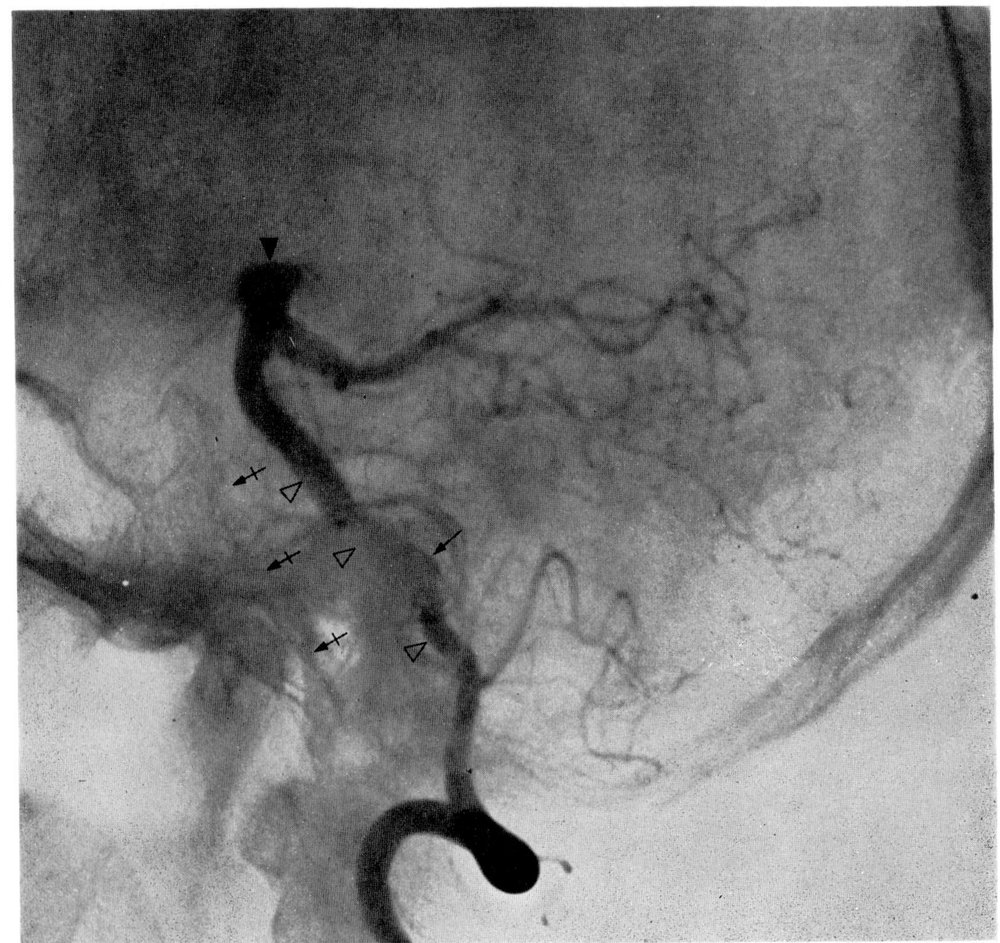

Fig. 329

Saccular Aneurysm Arising from the Right Distal Vertebral Artery at the Origin of the Posterior Inferior Cerebellar Artery

A 39-year-old female: Figs. 330 and 331

Fig. 330 Arterial phase in the Towne projection. There is a 1.5×1.2 cm saccular aneurysm at the origin of the right posterior inferior cerebellar artery (2 opposing arrows).

Fig. 331 Arterial phase in the lateral projection. The saccular aneurysm extends into the upper cervical subarachnoid space (2 arrows). There is a narrow neck at the superior aspect of the aneurysm (a crossed arrow).

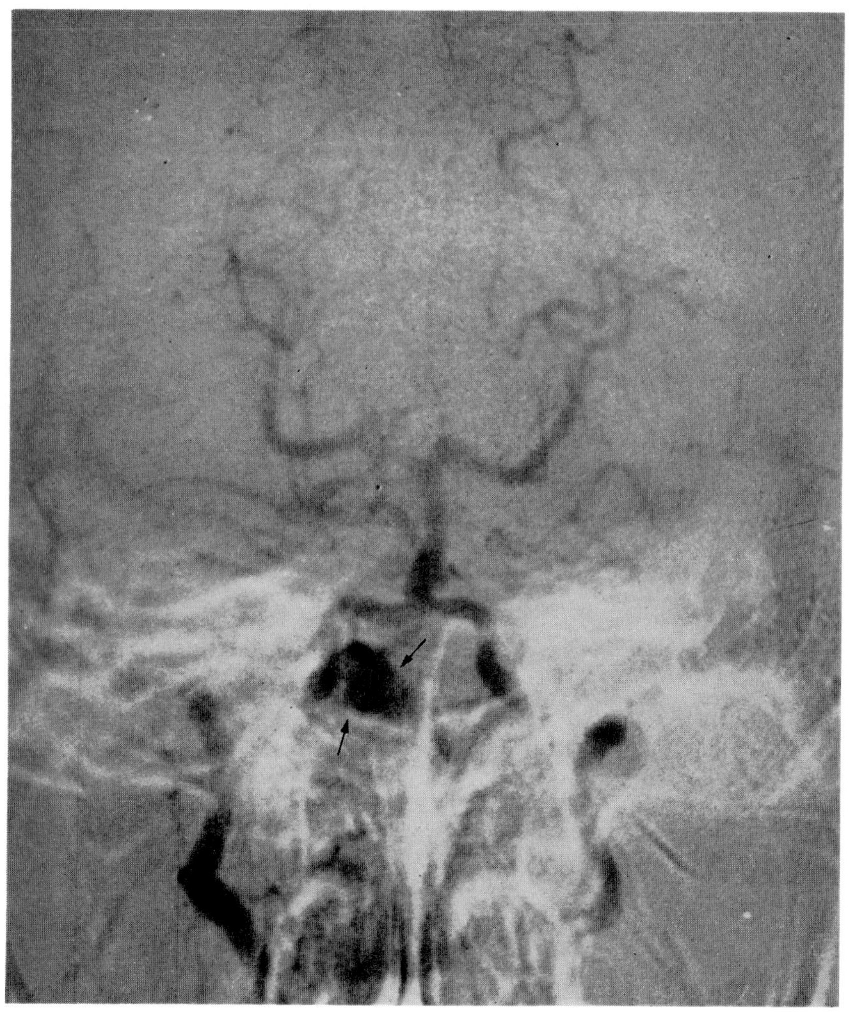

Fig. 330

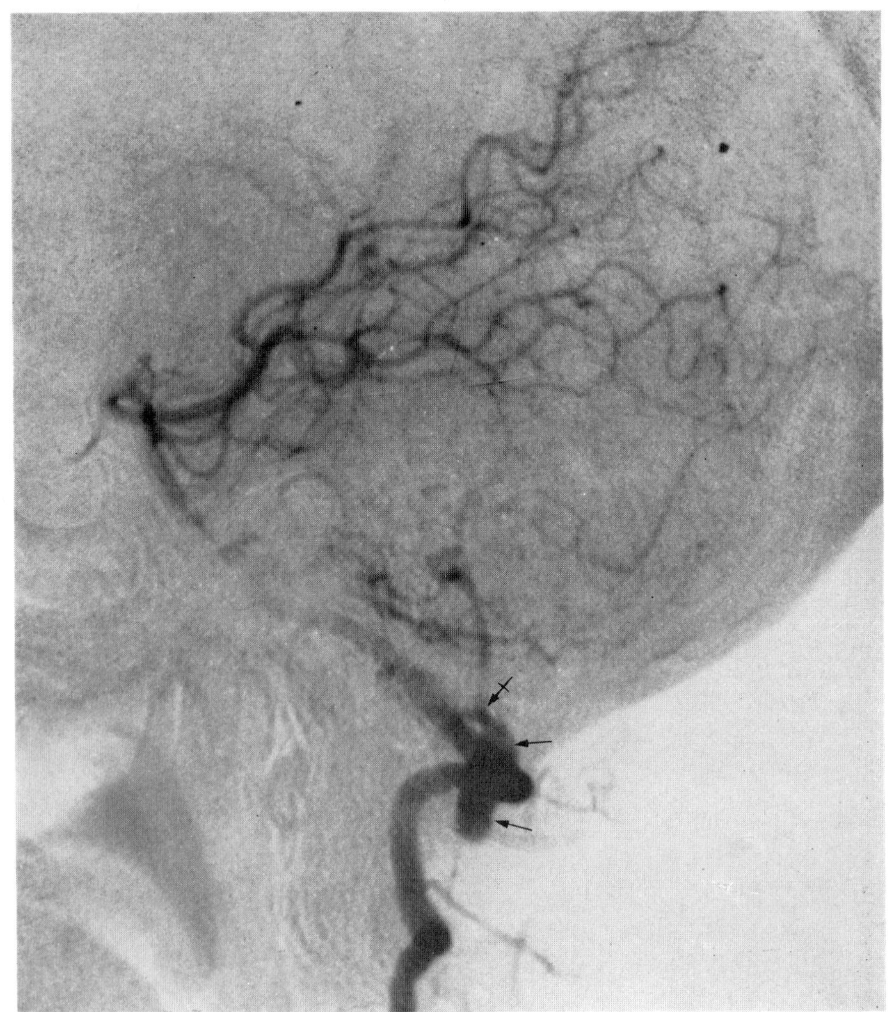

Fig. 331

Aneurysm Originating from the Distal Segment of the Basilar Artery

A 51-year-old female: Figs. 332 and 333

Fig. 332 Arterial phase in the anteroposterior projection. A saccular aneurysm is noted from the terminal segment of the basilar artery, projecting to the left. The left posterior cerebral artery appears to be tortuous and superimposed on the aneurysm (2 crossed arrows). The left superior cerebellar artery courses below the aneurysm. Therefore, the aneurysm appears to arise from the basilar artery between the origins of the posterior cerebral and superior cerebellar arteries. The origin of the left superior cerebeller artery is marked with an arrow.

Fig. 333 Arterial phase in the lateral projection. The aneurysm is superimposed on the distal end of the basilar artery (2 opposing arrows).

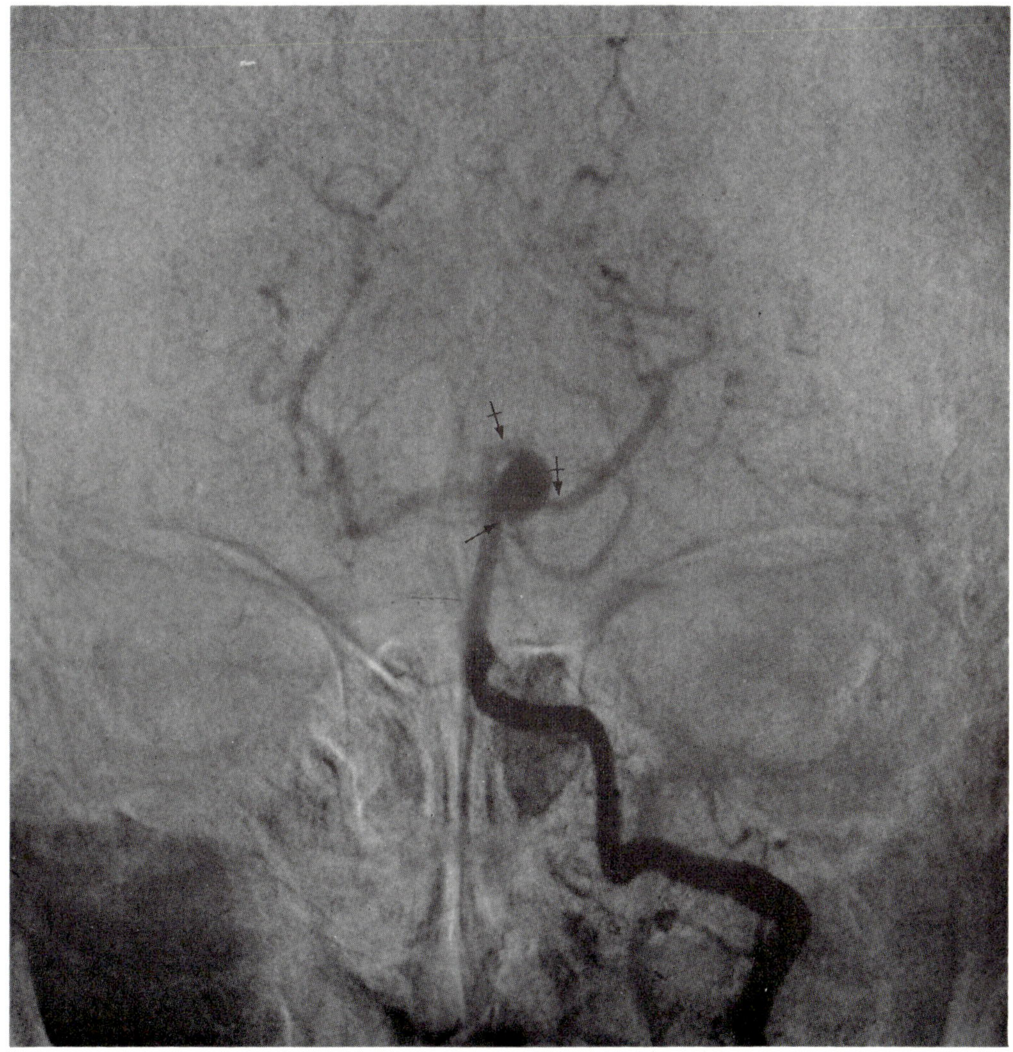

Fig. 332

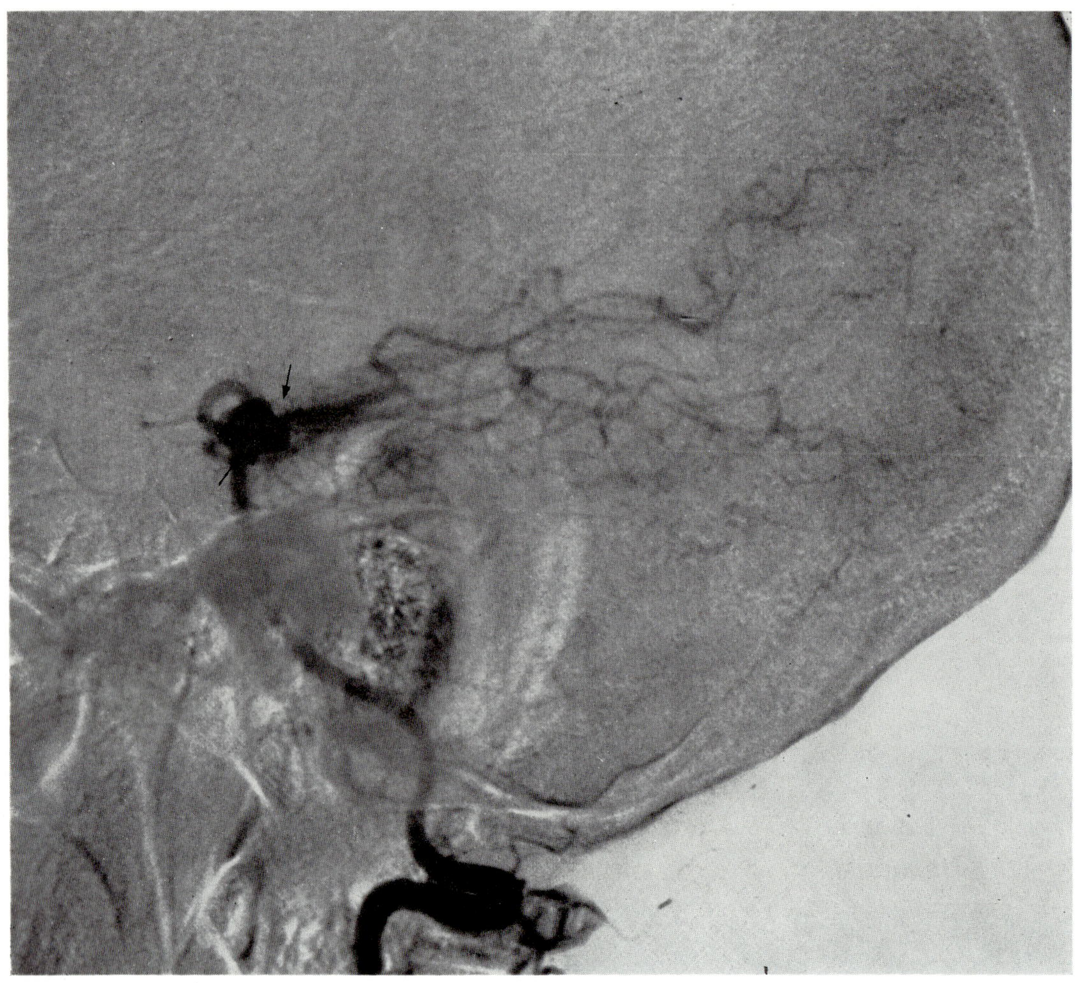

Fig. 333

Aneurysm Arising from the Basilar Artery at the Origin of the Superior Cerebellar Artery

A 35-year-old female: Fig. 334

Fig. 334 Arterial phase in the Towne projection. A 3 mm saccular aneurysm is noted at the origin of the superior cerebellar artery (an arrow). The aneurysm was not demonstrated on the lateral view.

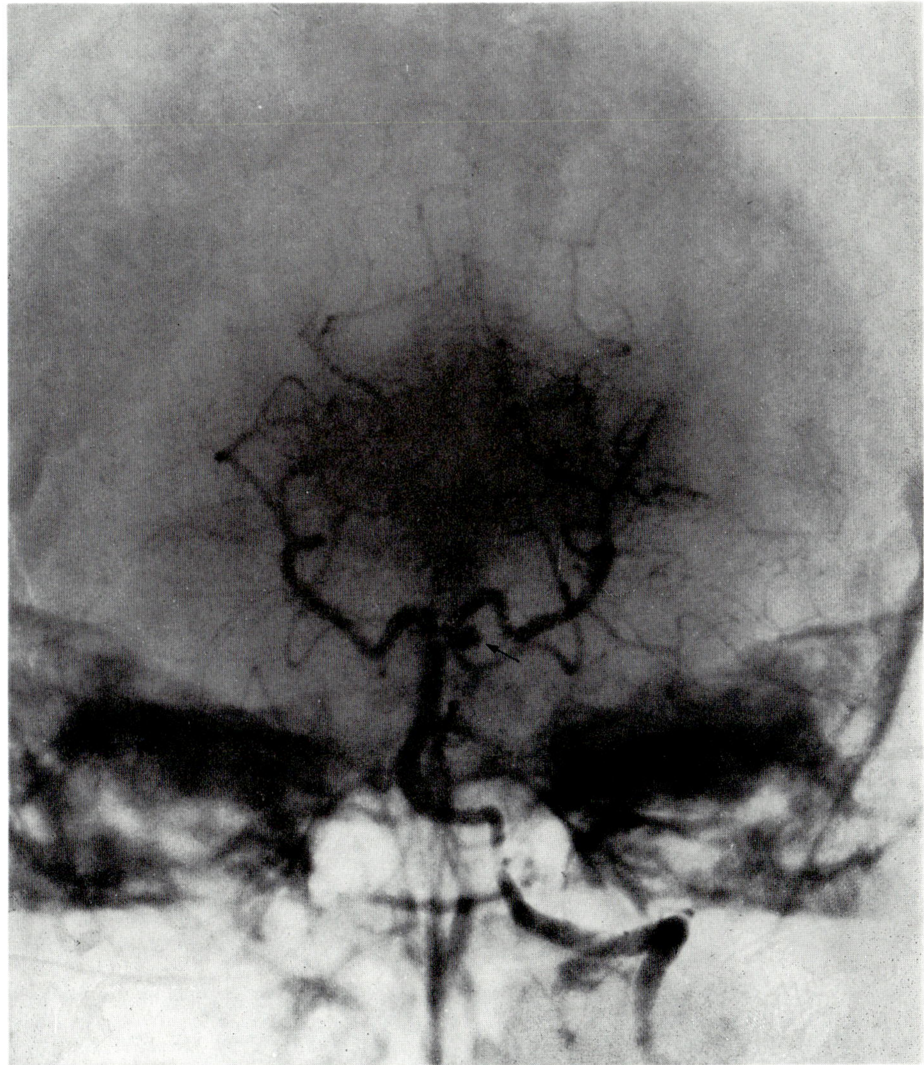

Fig. 334

Aneurysm Arising from the Terminal Segment of the Basilar Artery

A 55-year-old male: Figs. 335 and 336

Fig. 335 Arterial phase in the Towne projection. There is a 1.0×0.6 cm aneurysm at the distal end of the basilar artery (an arrow), projecting superiorly into the interpeduncular fossa. The left posterior cerebral and the posterior temporal arteries are enlarged (4 crossed arrows). These arteries supplied an arteriovenous malformation of the left temporal lobe.

Fig. 336 Arterial phase in the lateral projection. The aneurysm is projecting superiorly from the distal end of the basilar artery (an arrow). There is enlargement of the posterior cerebral artery and the posterior temporal artery (4 crossed arrows).

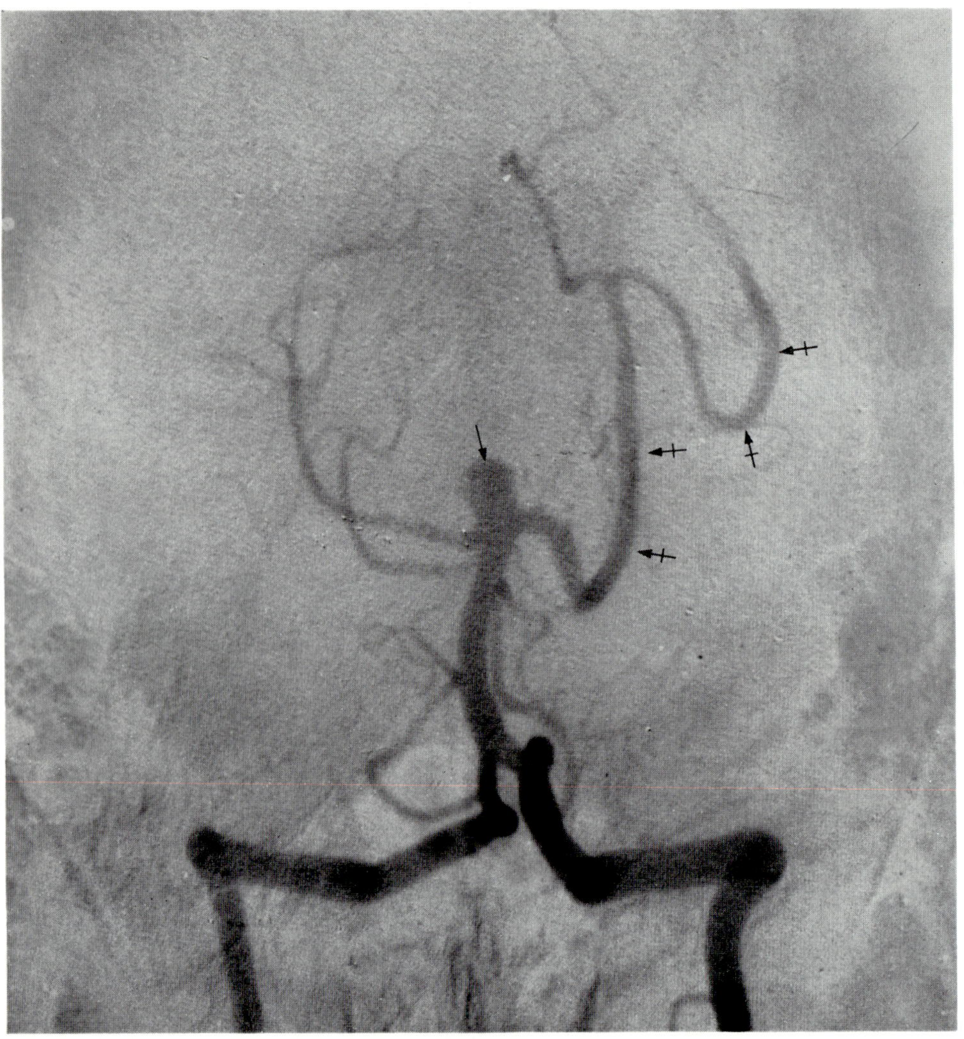

Fig. 335

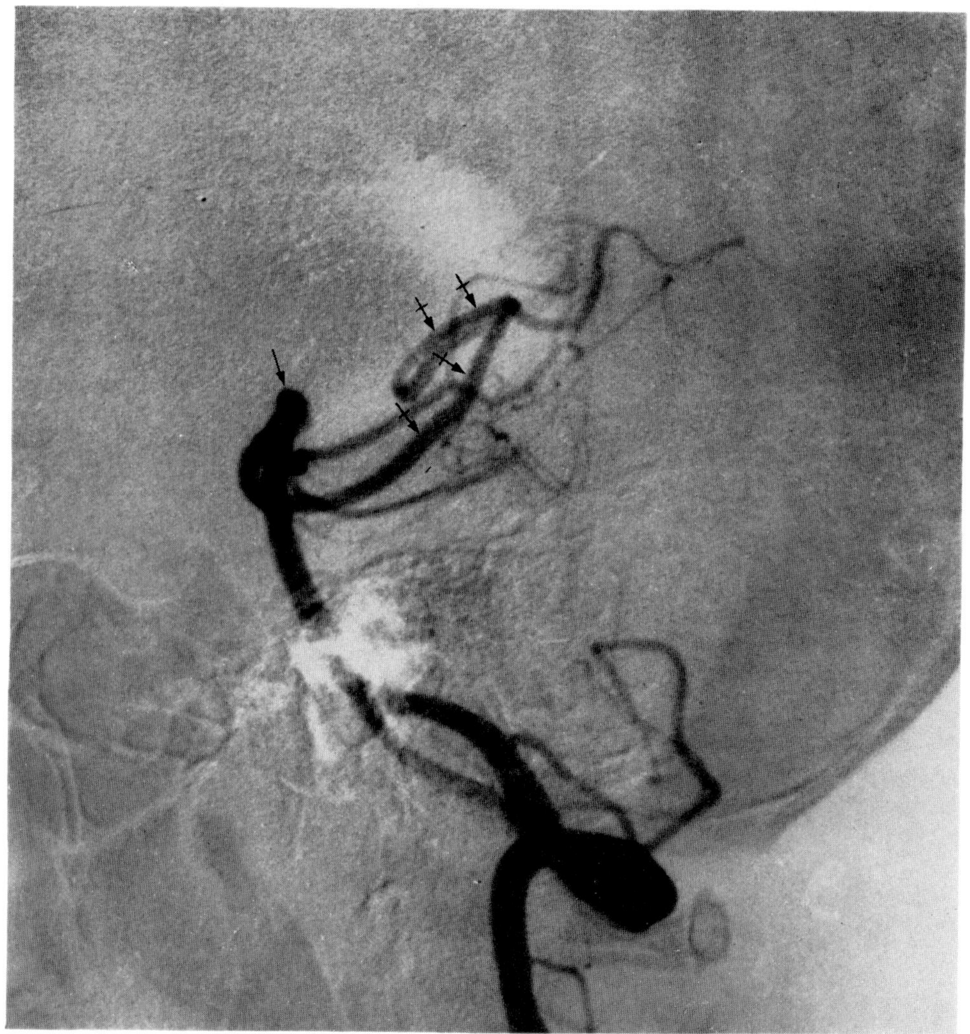

Fig. 336

Multiple Aneurysms of the Vertebrobasilar System

A 37-year-old male: Figs. 337 and 338

Fig. 337 Arterial phase in the Towne projection. There is a large 1.7 × 0.7 cm aneurysm at the anterior ambient segment of the right posterior cerebral artery (4 arrows). A small aneurysm is noted from the thalamoperforate artery (an arrowhead). There is also a fusiform aneurysm at the distal segment of the right vertebral artery (2 opposing crossed arrows).

Fig. 338 Arterial phase in the lateral projection. The aneurysm of the posterior cerebral artery is fusiform, involving a relatively long segment (3 arrows). The aneurysm of the vertebral artery is seen on end (a crossed arrow). The aneurysm of the thalamoperforate artery appears to be a fusiform aneurysm (an arrowhead).

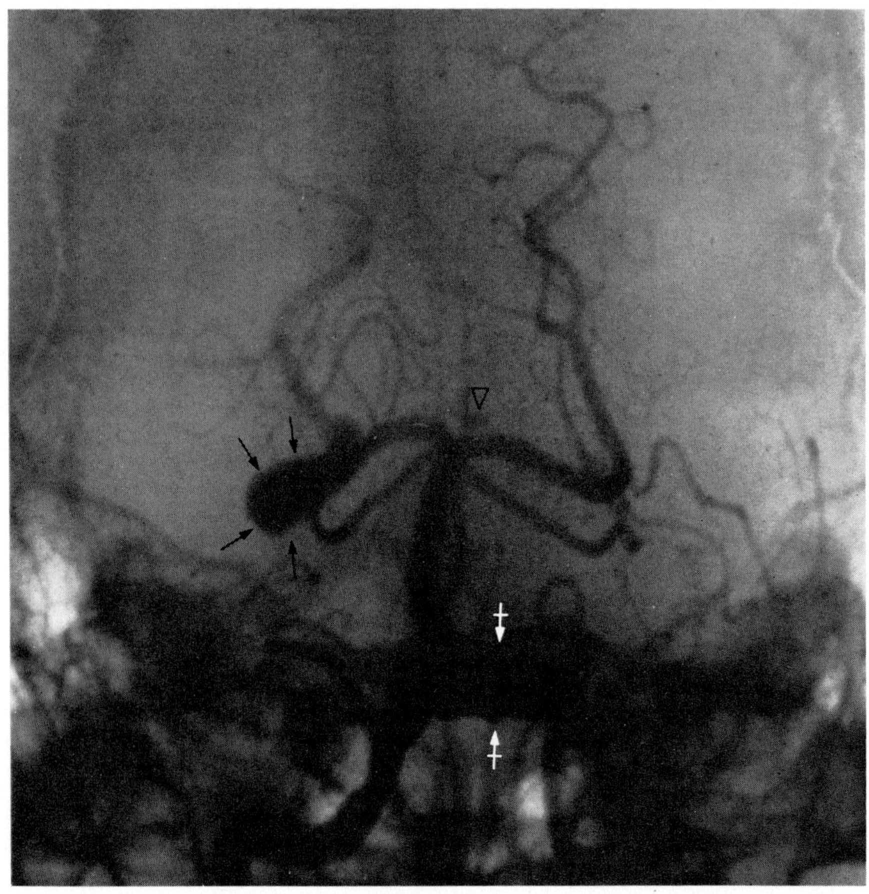

Fig. 337

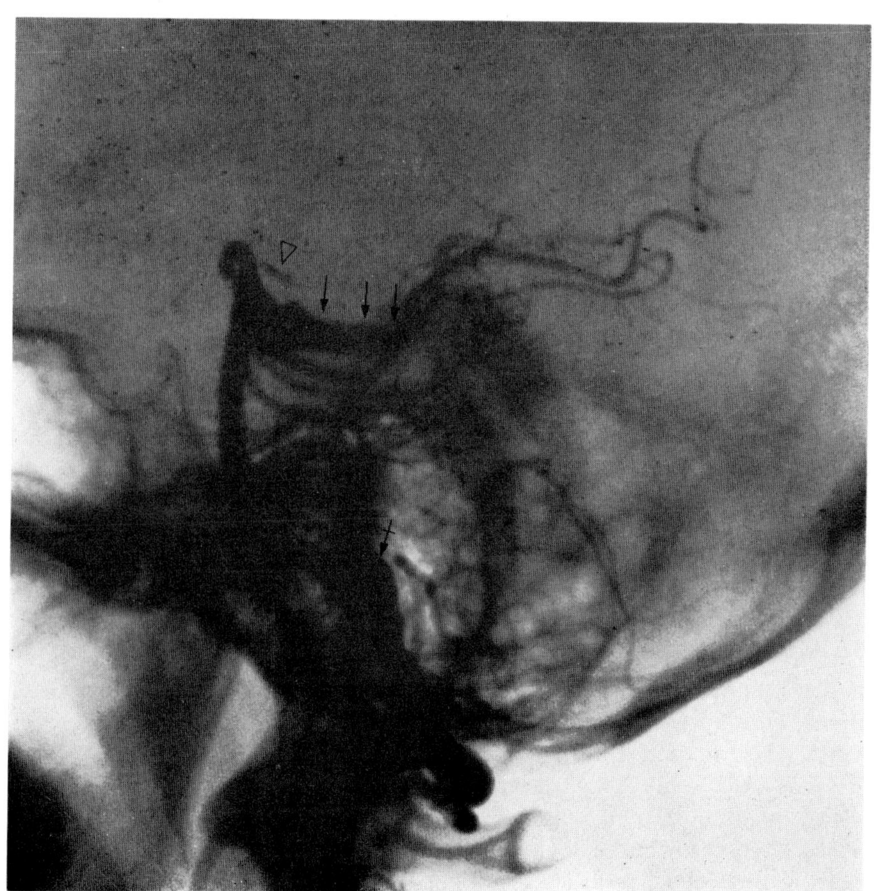

Fig. 338

VASCULAR MALFORMATION

Vascular malformations have been classified pathologically into (1) capillary teleangiectases, (2) cavernous angiomas, and (3) venous and arteriovenous malformations (Russell and Rubinstein, 1959).

Arteriovenous malformations

The arteriovenous malformations are the most common lesions characterized by pathological connections between arteries and veins. Angiographic characteristics include (1) presence of rapid shunting from the artery to the vein within a tangle of numerous abnormal vessels, (2) enlargement of the feeding arteries and (3) enlargement of the draining veins. The lesions are frequently wedge-shaped with the base at the cerebral surface and the edge pointing centrally. The value of angiography is not only in demonstration of the size and position of the altered capillaries, but also the identification of the feeding and draining vessels.

According to a review of 800 cases by Krayenbühl and Yasargil (1958), 85.7% of the arteriovenous malformations were supratentorial, 8.1% were extracranial and only 6.2% were found to be infratentorial.

Arteriovenous malformations with early oppacification of dural sinus via the meningeal arteries are frequently seen with or without association of the usual pial arteriovenous malformations. Such malformations are called dural arteriovenous malformations. Incidence of dural malformation is as high as 50% in the posterior fossa lesions, while the indidence is 21% in supratentorial malformations (Newton et al., 1969). Pure dural arteriovenous malformation without pial components is more common in the posterior fossa than in the supratentorial regions.

An arteriovenous malformation is not infrequently associated with an arterial aneurysm. The reported incidence has been 3 aneurysms in 110 patients with arteriovenous malformation (Patterson and McKissock, 1956) or 13 aneurysms in 150 patients (Cronqvist and Troupp, 1966). Such aneurysms frequently occur on an artery feeding the arteriovenous malformation. Therefore, pathogenesis of these aneurysms may be explained on the basis of early aging of the feeding arteries, or the same pathological weakness that causes the malformation.

Supratentorial arteriovenous malformation

The malformation in the occipital, posterior parietal and temporal regions receives blood supply from the branches of the posterior cerebral artery in addition to supply from the middle and anterior cerebral arteries. In the deep seated lesions of the thalamus, the basal ganglia and the lateral ventricles, the posterior choroidal arteries, the thalamoperforate arteries, and the colliculi quadrigemini and corpori geniculati arteries may play a major role in supplying the malformations. The dural arteriovenous malformations of tentorium and the posterior falx are frequently supplied by the meningohypophyseal arteries from the internal carotid arteries and meningeal branches of the external and vertebral arteries. Therefore, the supratentorial arteriovenous malformations are best studied by vertebral angiography as well as carotid angiography unless they are localized in the frontal lobe or its vicinity.

Infratentorial arteriovenous malformation

The infratentorial arteriovenous malformations are rare, the incidence being 6.2 per cent (Krayenbühl and Yasargil, 1958) to 20 % (Newton et al., 1969) of all cranial arteriovenous malformations. The feeding arteries are mostly by branches of the superior cerebellar, anterior inferior cerebellar and posterior inferior cerebellar arteries, but the meningeal branches of the vertebral artery, and external carotid arteries may become enlarged and contribute to the blood supply, especially in the dural involvement. The meningohypophyseal artery from the internal carotid artery may also participate in the blood supply in dural arteriovenous malformation.

The malformations may be small and localized or they may appear to fill the entire posterior fossa.

Other vascular malformations

The capillary teleangiectases are usually microscopic and common in the pons. They can not be demonstrated angiographically. Cavernous angiomas and venous malformations may be visualized as clusters of enlarged veins on the surface of the brain. Infratentorial lesions are rare and may be confused with the normal veins.

Arteriovenous Malformation of the Vermis

A 16-year-old male: Figs. 339–342

Fig. 339 Arterial phase in the lateral projection. There is a mesh of abnormal vessels in the vermis near the torcular (4 open arrowheads). The feeding arteries consist of the tonsillohemispheric (a crossed arrow) and vermian (an arrow) segments of the posterior inferior cerebellar artery and the vermian segment (a double-crossed arrow) of the superior cerebellar artery. Early opacification of sinus confluence or superior sagittal sinus is seen(2 closed arrowheads). There are minimal anterior displacement of the basilar artery, and arcuate stretching of the vermian segments of the superior cerebellar artery, suggesting the presence of increased intracranial pressure due to intracerebellar hemorrhage.

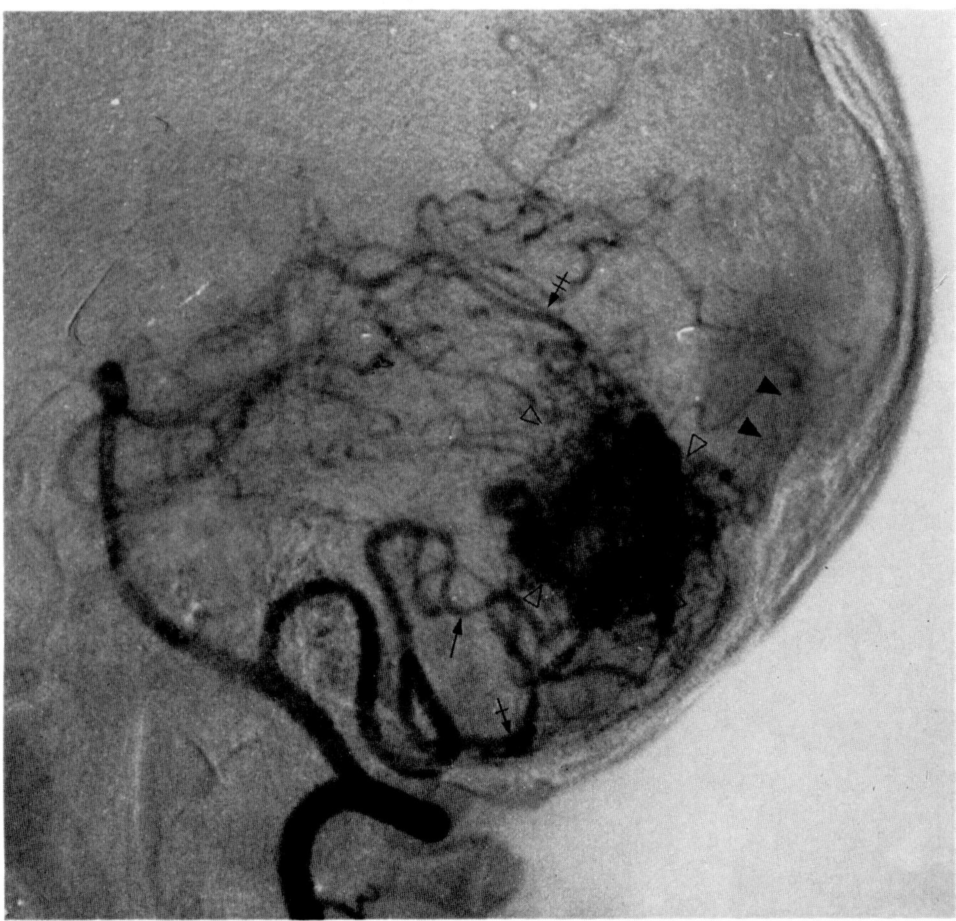

Fig. 339

Fig. 340 Late arterial phase in the lateral projection. The abnormal vessels are much denser on this phase (4 open arrowheads). The inferior vermian vein is considerably enlarged and drains into the sinus confluence (4 closed arrowheads).

Fig. 341 Arterial phase in the Towne projection. A mesh of abnormal vessels are localized in the midline (4 open arrowheads). The left posterior inferior cerebellar artery is enlarged and supplies the lesion (2 arrows).

Fig. 342 Venous phase in the Towne projection. The abnormal vessels (4 open arrowheads) drain into the petrosal vein and the superior petrosal sinus (3 crossed arrows) via the vein of the lateral recess of the fourth ventricle (2 arrows) and the inferior hemispheric vein (2 closed arrowheads). The major drainage into the sinus confluence is also demonstrated (3 double-crossed arrows).

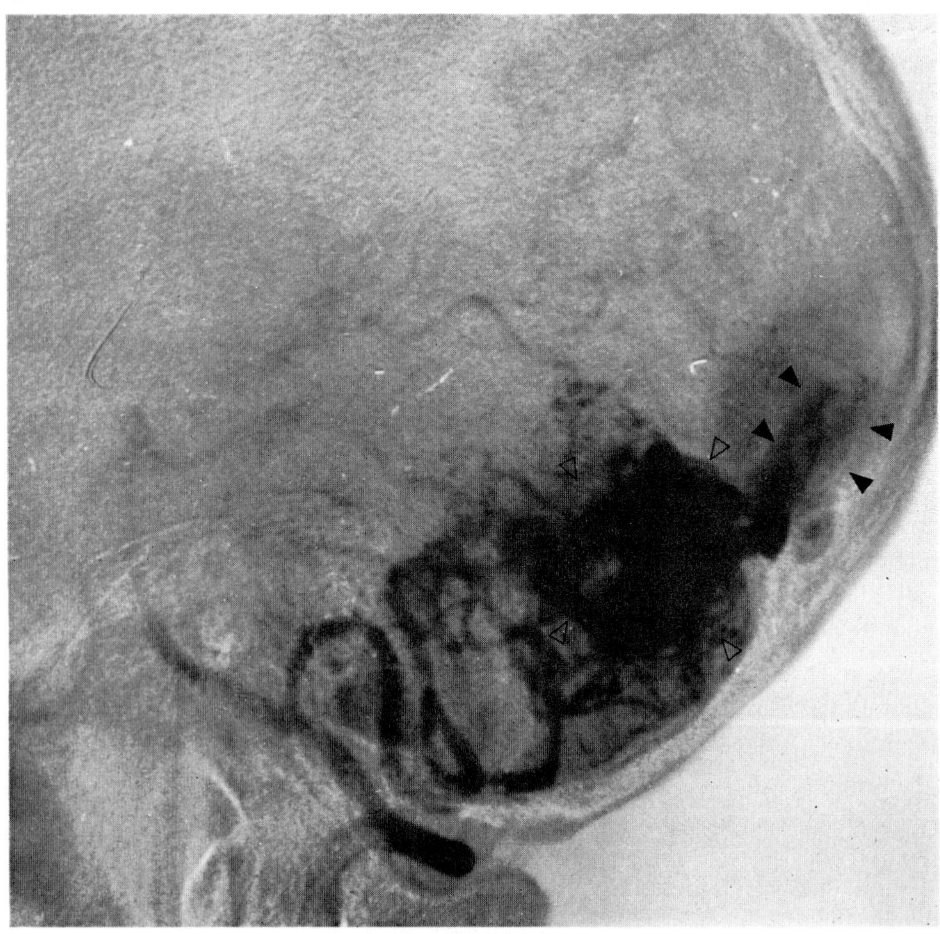

Fig. 340

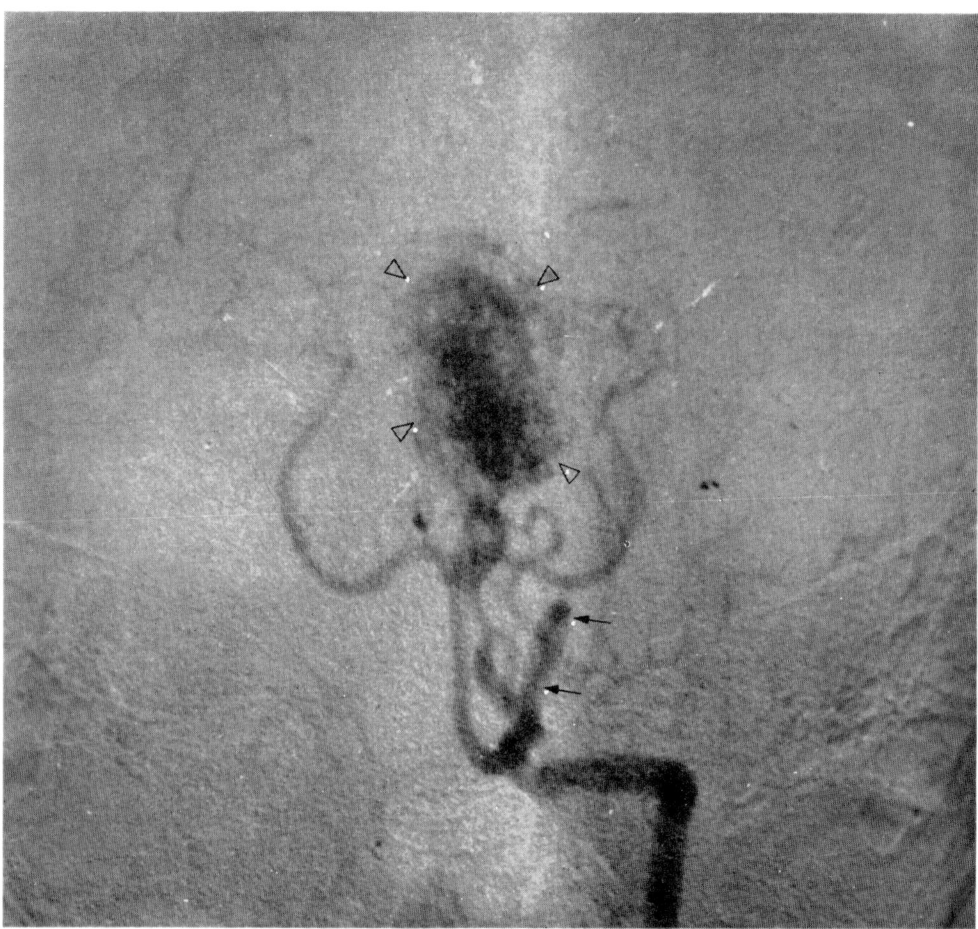

Fig. 341

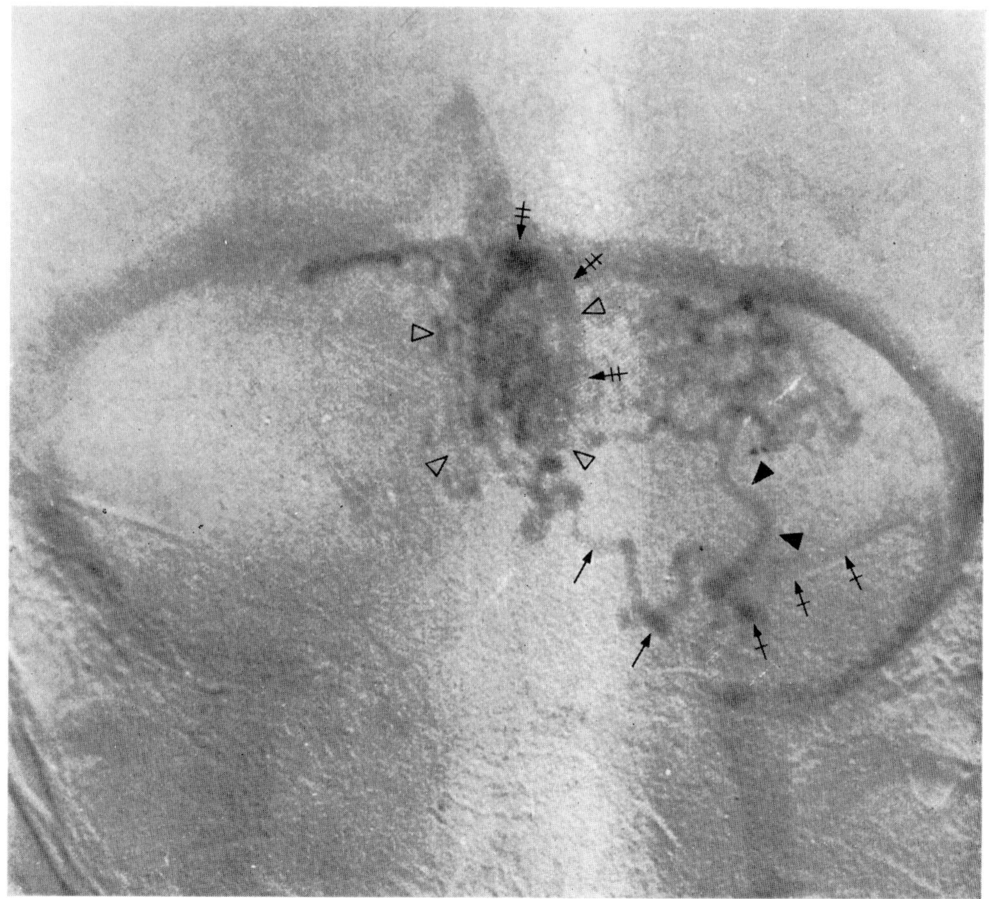

Fig. 342

Arteriovenous Malformation of the Right Cerebellar Hemisphere with an Aneurysm of the Left Superior Cerebellar Artery

A 44-year-old female: Figs. 343–346

Fig. 343 Arterial phase in the Towne projection. There is a mesh of abnormal vessels on the superior aspect of the right cerebellar hemisphere (4 arrows). The blood supply comes from the hemispheric branch of the right superior cerebellar artery, which is enlarged and has an aneurysm at its origin (2 opposing crossed arrows). There is early opacification of abnormal veins around the lesion. The major draining veins course towards the sinus confluence (2 closed arrowheads) and the petrosal vein (2 open arrowheads).

Fig. 344 Capillary phase in the Towne projection. The aneurysm (2 opposing crossed arrows) and the arteriovenous malformation (4 arrows) are seen to good advantage. The draining vein towards the sinus confluence is seen with opacification of the proximal portion of the lateral sinus (3 closed arrowheads). Another drainage is into the anastomotic lateral mesencephalic vein via the petrosal vein (3 open arrowheads).

Fig. 345 Arterial phase in the lateral projection. There appear to be two feeding arteries from the right superior cerebellar artery (2 open arrowheads). The draining vein towards the sinus confluence is seen (2 closed arrowheads) from the malformation (3 crossed arrows). The aneurysm is localized in the quadrigeminal cistern (2 opposing arrows).

Fig. 346 Venous phase in the lateral projection. The anastomotic lateral mesencephalic vein (2 closed arrowheads) is enlarged and drains into the posterior mesencephalic vein. These veins drain the lesion via the petrosal vein. The aneurysm and the malformation are indicated by 2 opposing arrows and 3 crossed arrows, respectively. Aneurysms sometimes develop in association with arteriovenous malformations.

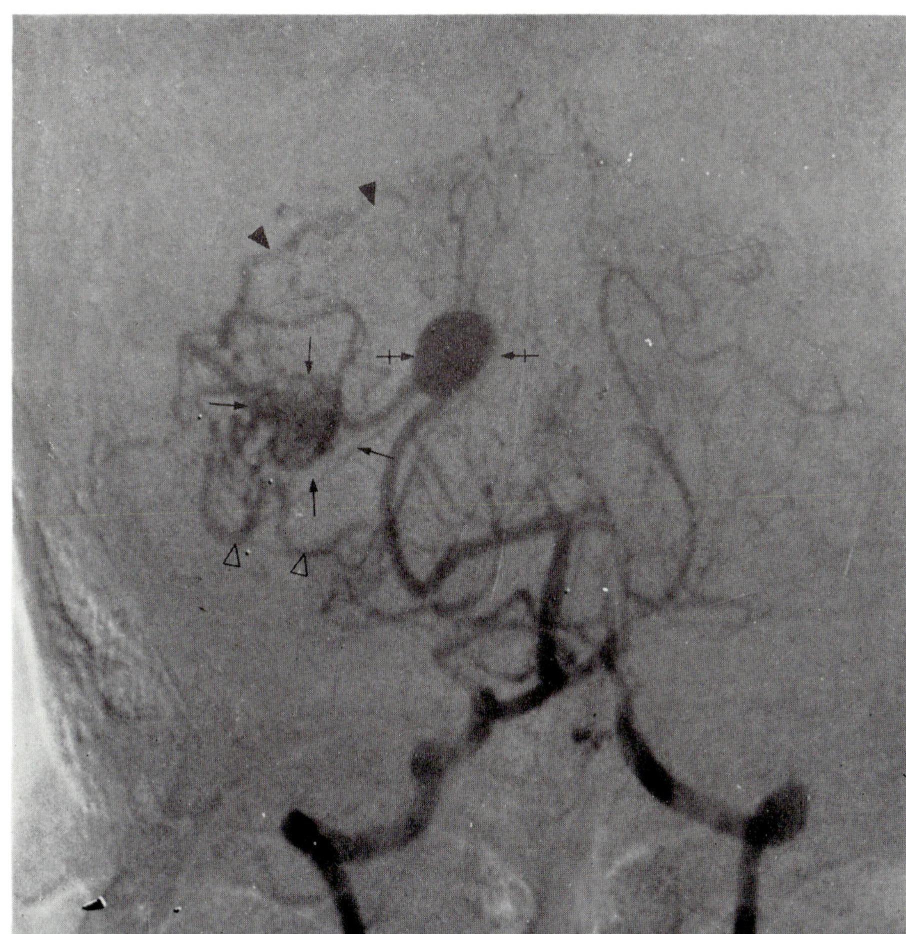

Fig. 343

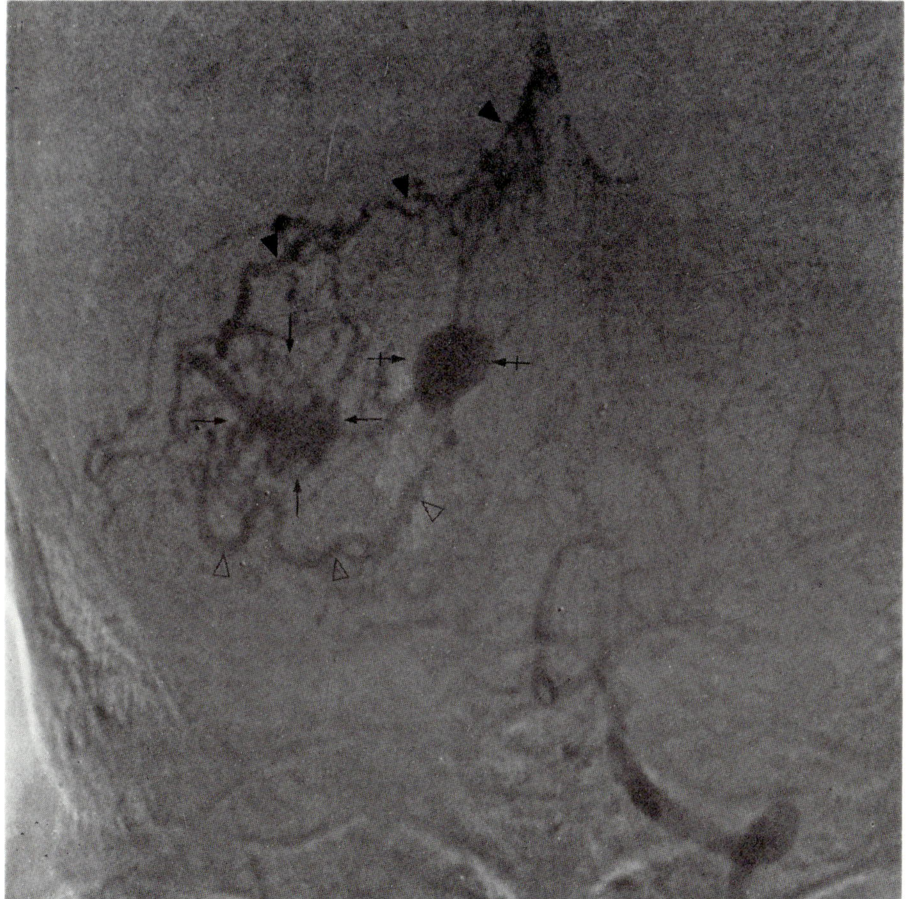

Fig. 344

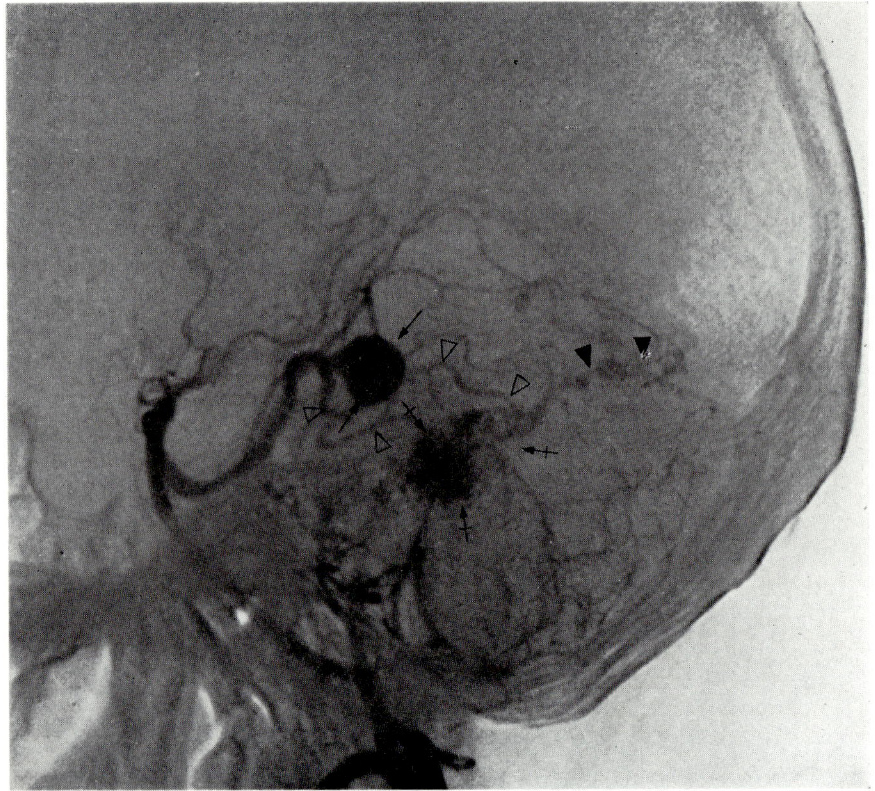

Fig. 345

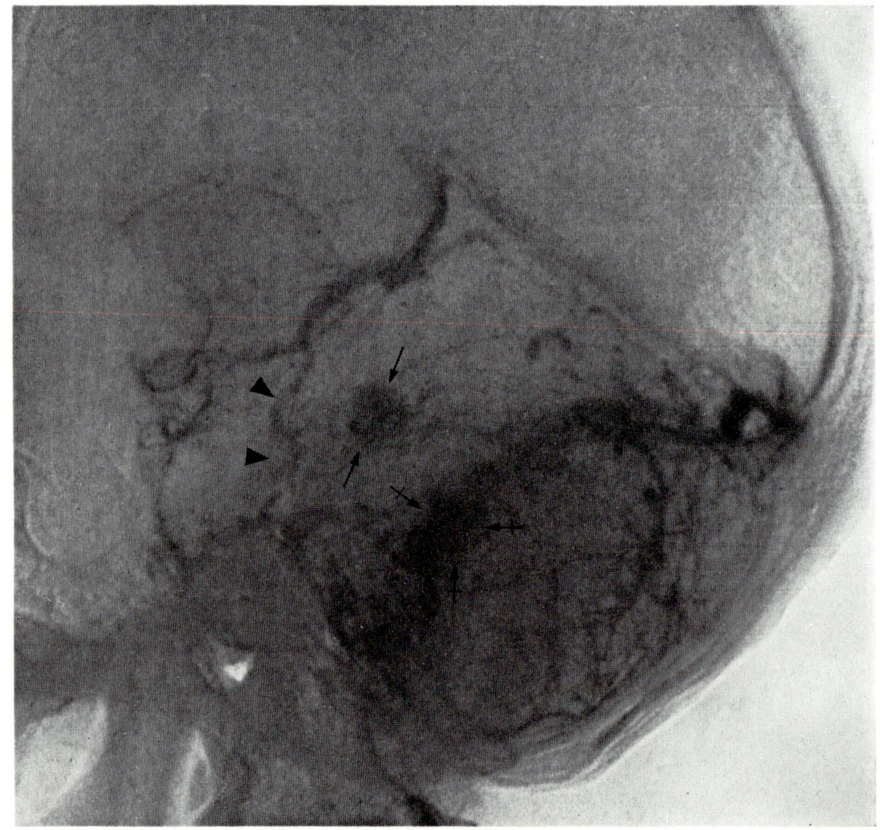

Fig. 346

Arteriovenous Malformation of the Right Superior Vermis and Cerebellar Hemisphere

A 20-year-old female: Figs. 347–351

Fig. 347 Arterial phase in the Towne projection. A large arteriovenous malformation is demonstrated near the midline (4 arrows). The blood supply is primarily from the enlarged superior cerebellar artery on the right. There is early opacification of the straight sinus (a crossed arrow).

Fig. 348 Venous phase in the Towne projection. The drainage is into the straight sinus (a crossed arrow) via an enlarged midline vein (4 arrows), probably the precentral cerebellar vein. There is also drainage into both petrosal veins via the brachial veins (2 open arrowheads).

Fig. 349 Arterial phase in the lateral projection. The malformation is localized in the superior vermis and cerebellum (4 arrows). The superior cerebellar artery is enlarged and tortuous (2 crossed arrows), entering the lesion from its posterior aspect. The proximal portion of the superior cerebellar artery is markedly enlarged and swings downwards (2 double-crossed arrows).

Fig. 350 Late arterial phase in the lateral projection. The malformation is denser because of opacification of the enlarged draining veins (4 arrows). The vein of Galen and the straight sinus are opacified early.

Fig. 351 Venous phase in the lateral projection. The enormously enlarged draining vein is probably the precentral cerebellar vein (4 arrows). There is reflux into the basal vein of Rosenthal (2 open arrowheads). The petrosal vein is also opacified (2 closed arrowheads).

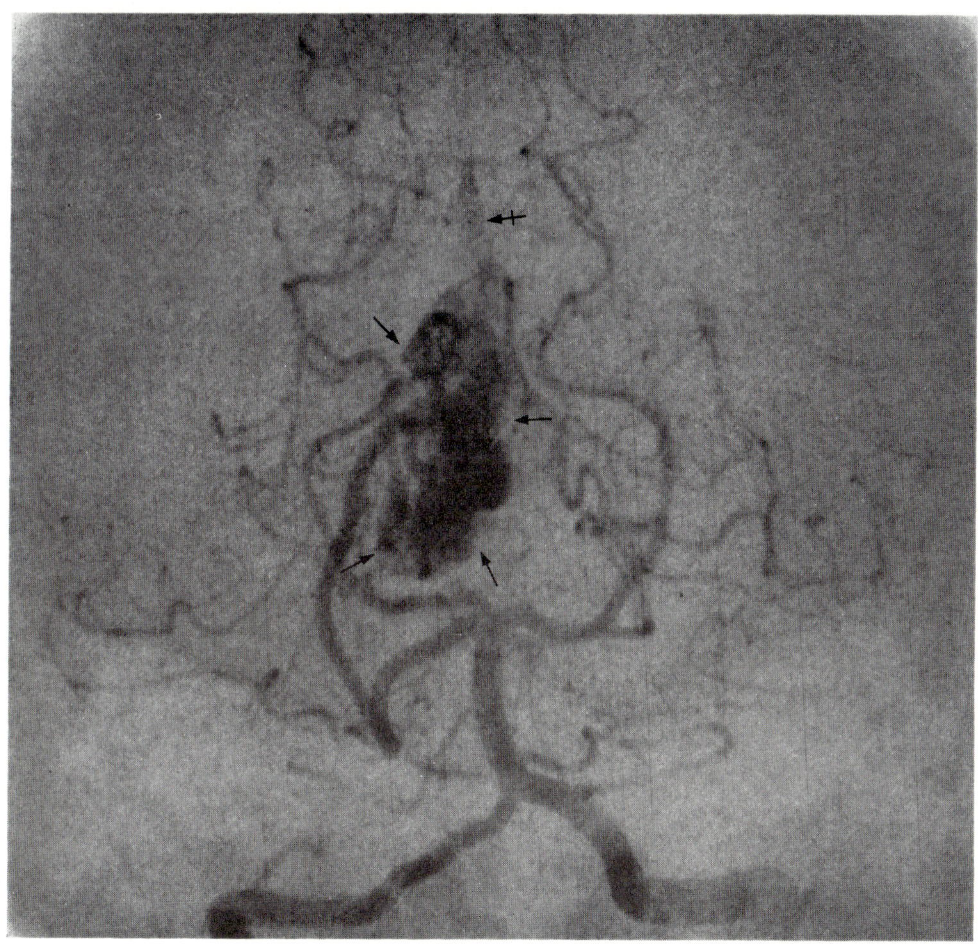

Fig. 347

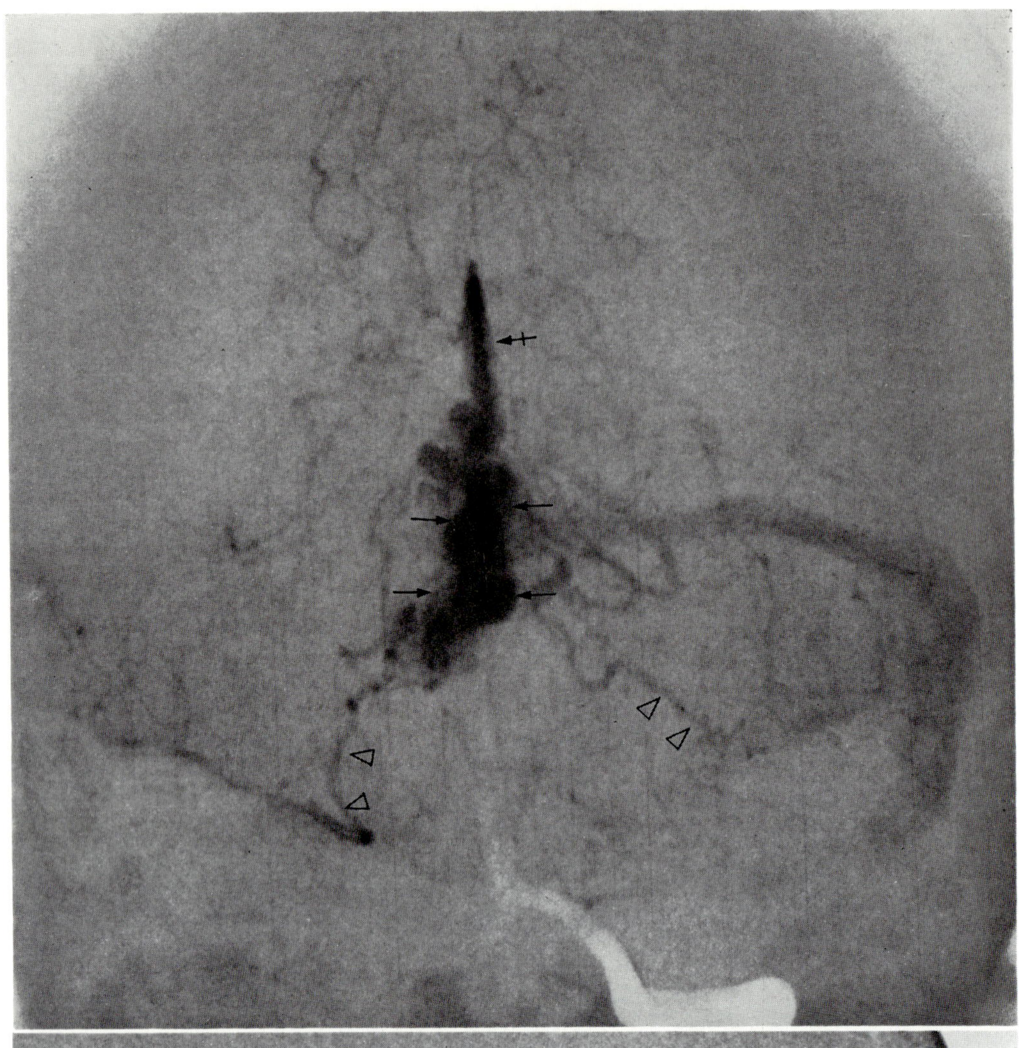

Fig. 348

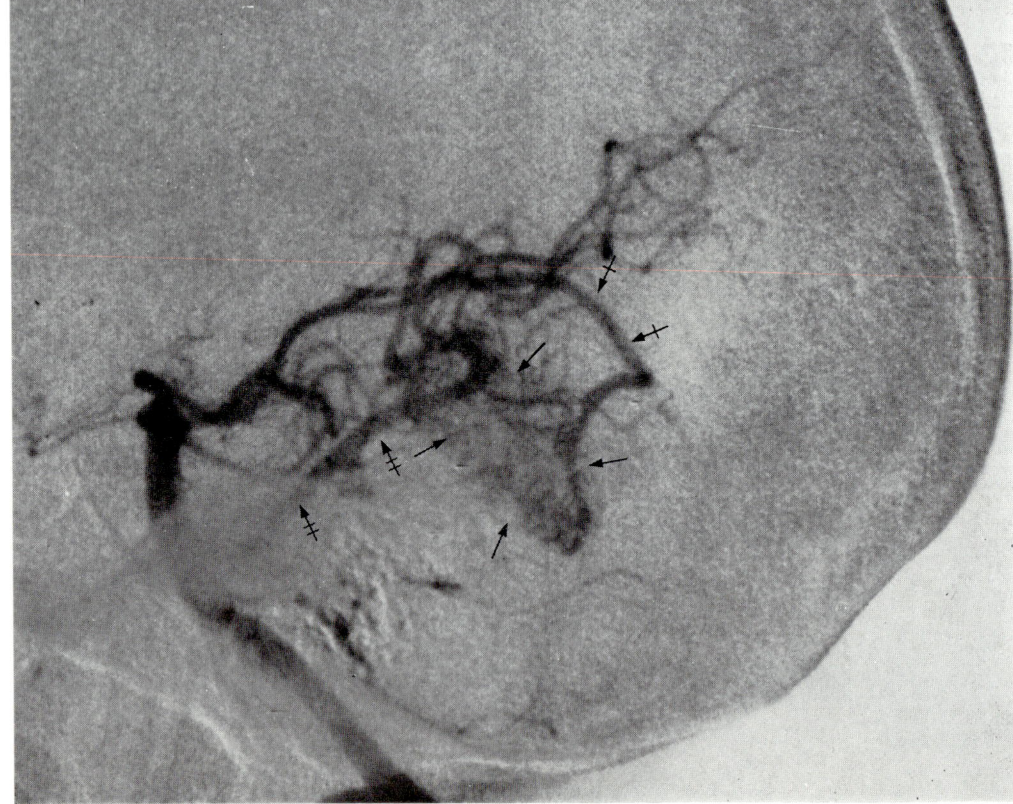

Fig. 349

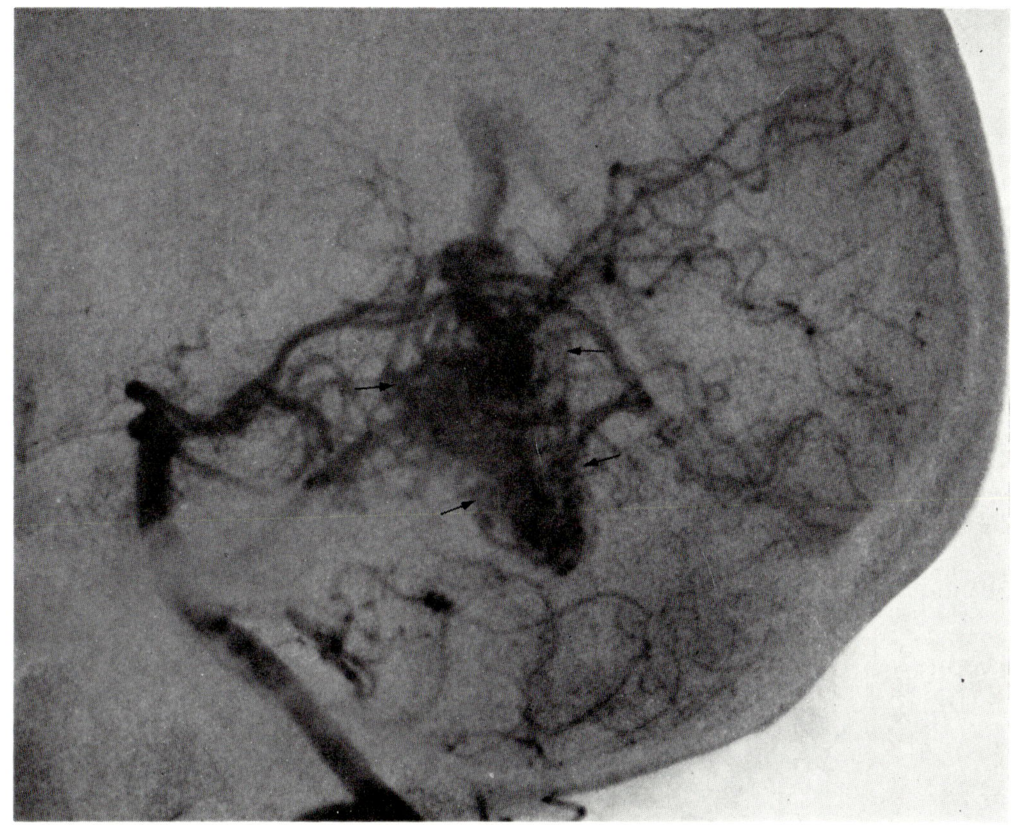

Fig. 350

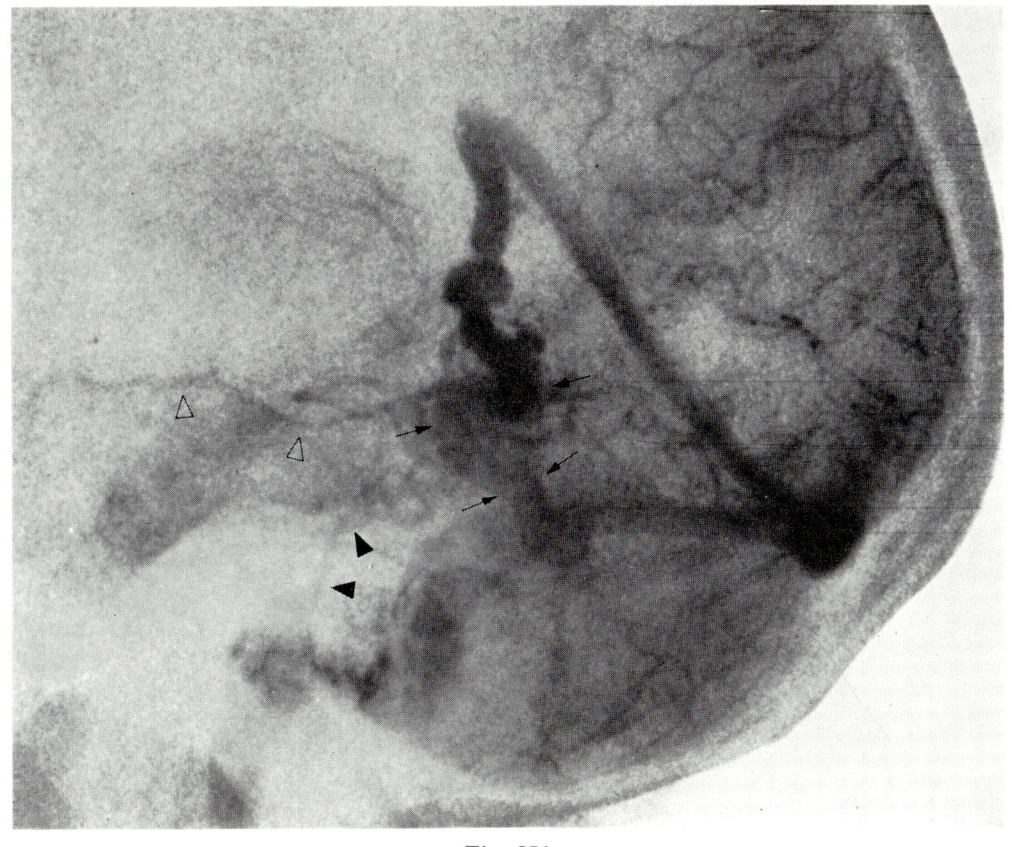

Fig. 351

Arteriovenous Malformation in the Left Cerebellopontine Angle

A 62-year-old male: Figs. 352–355

Fig. 352 Arterial phase in the Towne projection. There is a 1.2 cm cluster of abnormal vessels in the left cerebellopontine angle (3 arrows). The feeding artery cannot be identified well, but the anterior inferior cerebellar artery is considered to be the feeding artery. The drainage is in 3 ways: The superior petrosal sinus (2 open arrowheads), the lateral sinus via the lateral inferior cerebellar vein (2 closed arrowheads) and the straight sinus via the transverse pontine vein, anterior pontomesencephalic vein, and posterior mesencephalic vein (10 crossed arrows). No arterial displacement is noted.

Fig. 353 Venous phase in the Towne projection. The abnormal vessels and the draining veins are seen to good advantage (the markers are same as on Fig. 352).

Fig. 354 Arterial phase in the lateral projection. The malformation is faintly demonstrated because of the superimposing mastoids (2 arrows). The superior draining veins are seen to good advantage (see Fig. 355 for markers). The lateral inferior cerebellar vein is also shown (2 closed arrowheads).

Fig. 355 Venous phase in the lateral projection. The superior drainage consists of the transverse pontine vein (2 crossed arrows), the anterior pontomesencephalic vein (3 double-crossed arrows), the posterior mesencephalic vein and the vein of Galen (2 open arrowheads). The lateral inferior cerebellar vein drains into the lateral sinus (2 closed arrowheads).

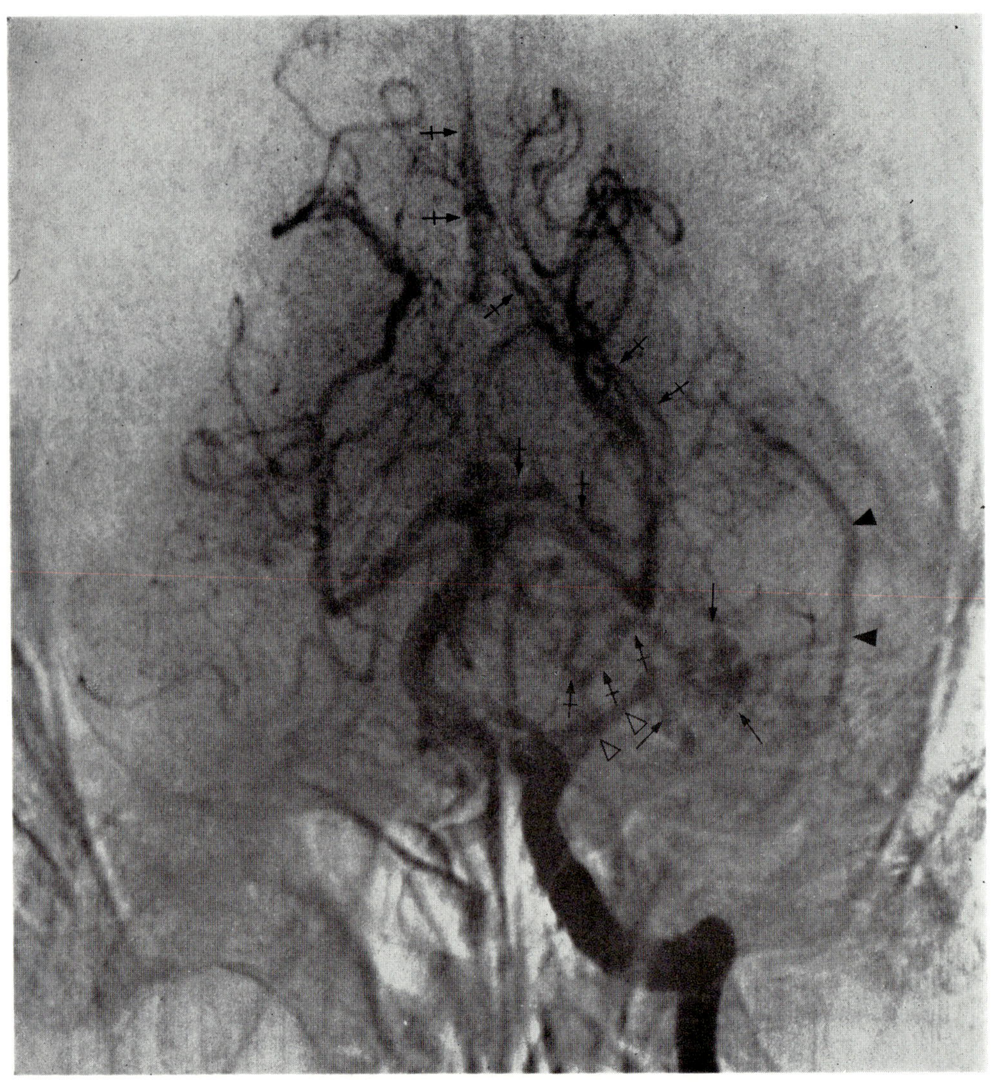

Fig. 352

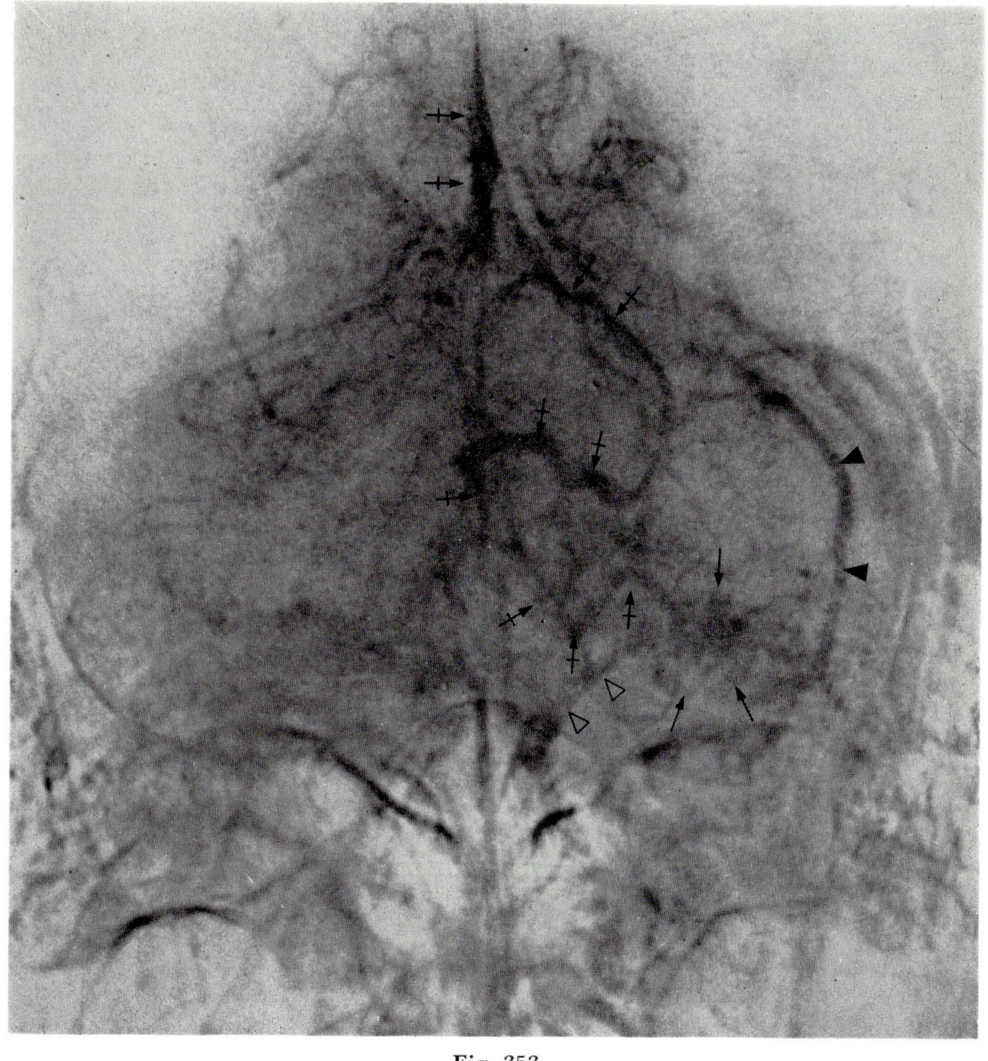

Fig. 353

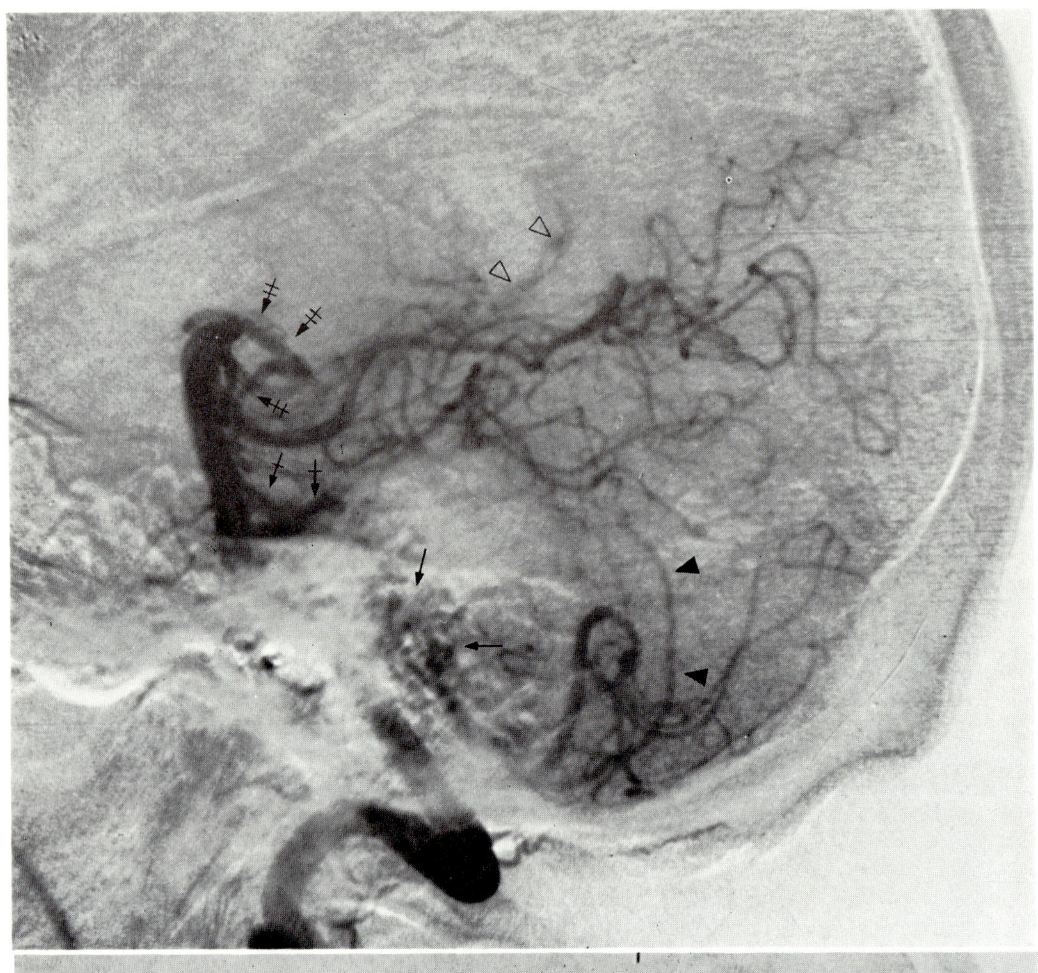

Fig. 354

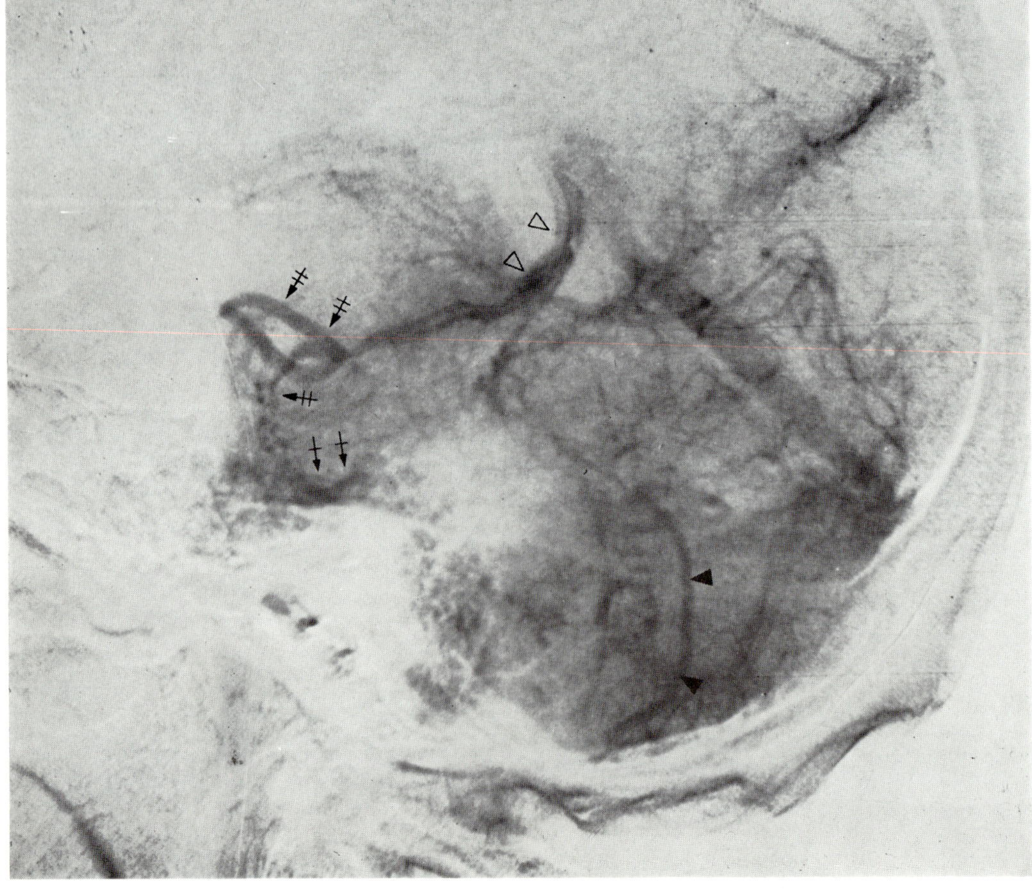

Fig. 355

Arteriovenous Malformation in the Middle Temporal Region

A 43-year-old female: Figs. 356–359

Fig. 356 Arterial phase in the Towne projection. There is a cluster of abnormal vessels superimposed over the left cerebellopontine angle (3 arrows). Since the feeding artery is the enlarged posterior temporal artery (2 crossed arrows), the lesion should be supratentorial in location. There is no arterial displacement.

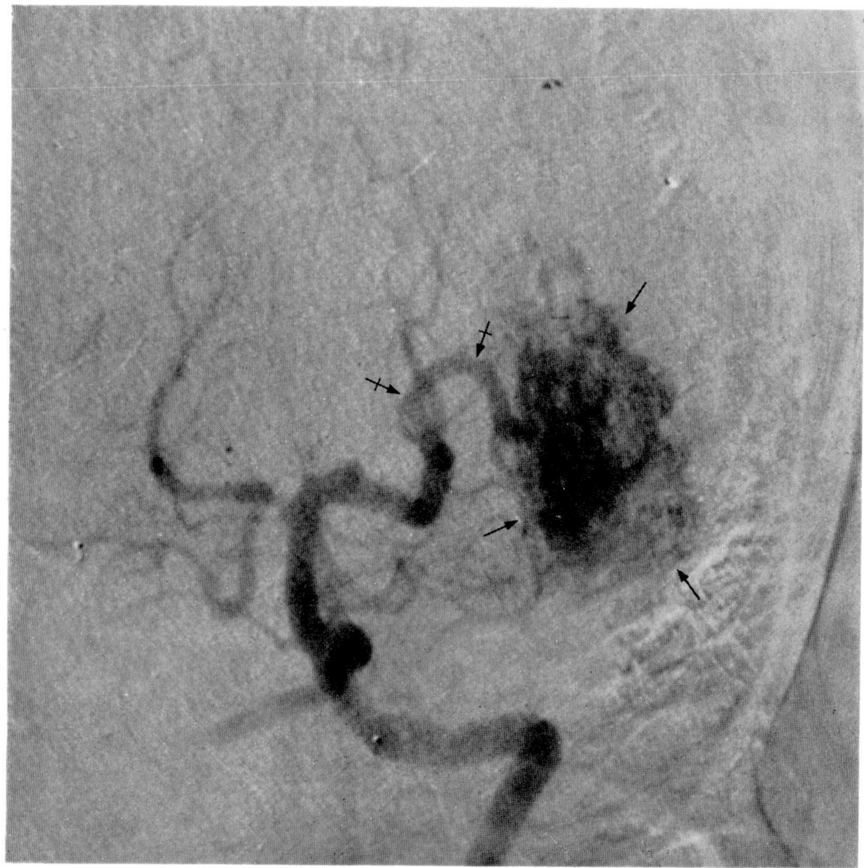

Fig. 356

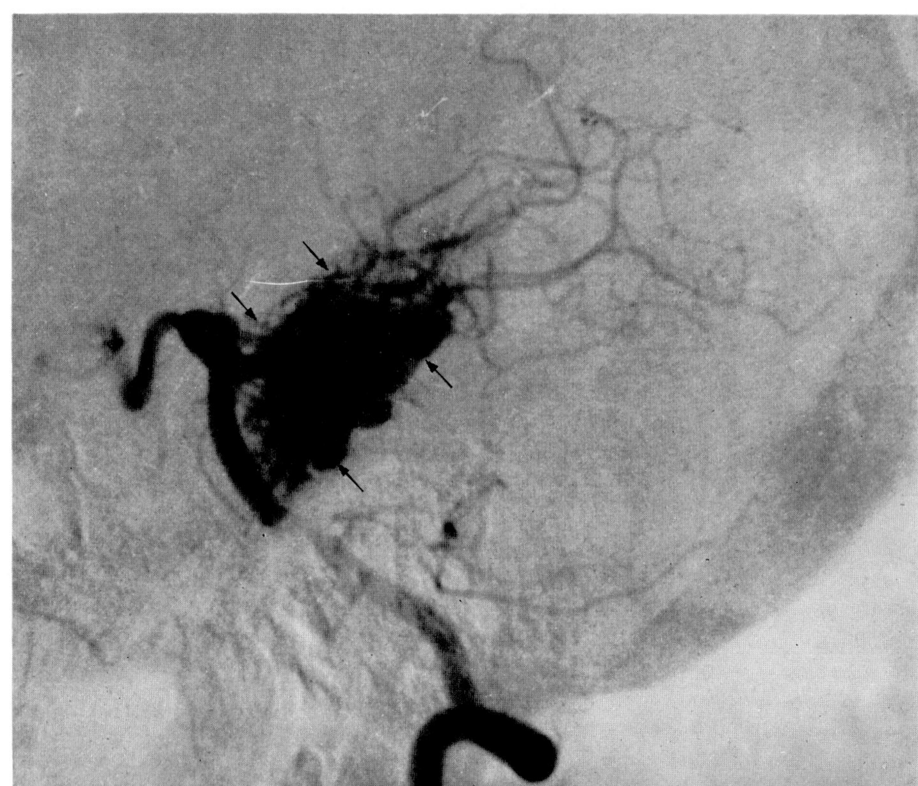

Fig. 357

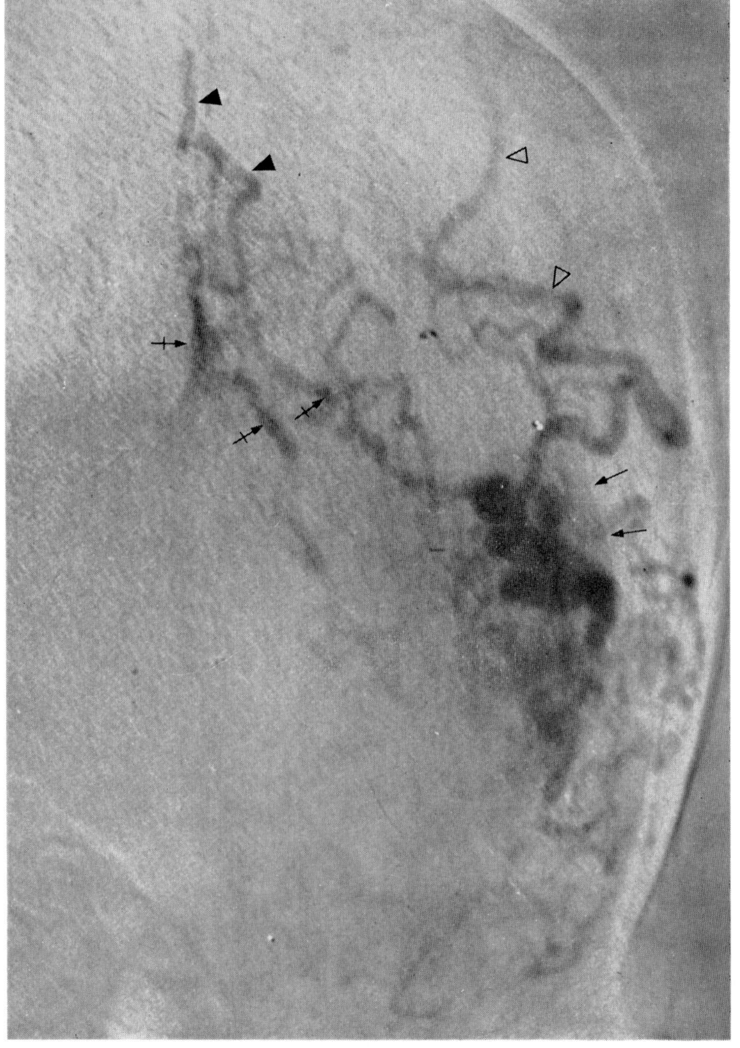

Fig. 358

Fig. 357 Arterial phase in the lateral projection. The malformation is in the middle temporal region (4 arrows), superimposed upon the upper brain stem.

Fig. 358 Venous phase in the Towne projection. There are multiple draining veins on the surface of the temporal lobe. The major drainage is into the lateral sinus directly (2 arrows) and into the straight sinus via the veins under the temporal lobe (3 crossed arrows). There is also drainage into the superior sagittal sinus via the veins over the lateral aspect of the temporal lobe (2 open arrowheads)and via the veins within the central fissure(2 closed arrowheads).

Fig. 359 Venous phase in the lateral projection. The drainage into the lateral sinus (2 arrows) and the straight sinus (2 crossed arrows) are shown to good advantage. There is an additional drainage into the superior sagittal sinus via the veins over the cerebral hemisphere (2 open arrowheads) and within the central fissure (2 closed arrowheads). There are draining veins about the parasellar area as well (2 double-crossed arrows).

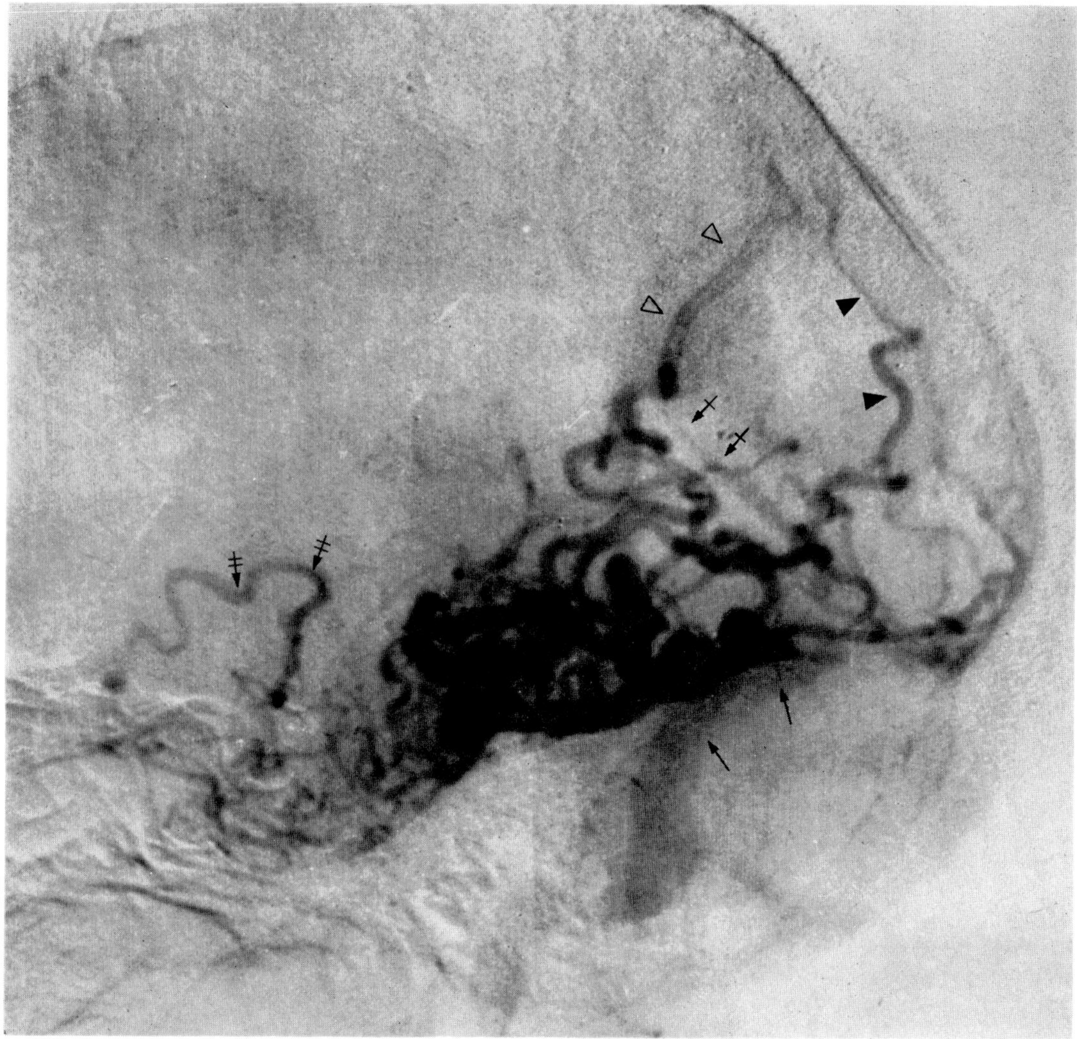

Fig. 359

Arteriovenous Malformation of the Right Posterior Temporal Region

A 19-year-old female: Figs. 360 and 361

Fig. 360 Arterial phase in the Towne projection. There is an arteriovenous malformation in the medial and inferior aspect of the posterior temporal lobe (3 arrowheads). The feeding artery is the calcarine branch of the right posterior cerebral artery (an arrow). The drainage is into the vein of Galen and the straight sinus (2 crossed arrows).

Fig. 361 Arterial phase in the lateral projection. The malformation is localized partly within the quadrigeminal cistern (3 arrowheads). The posterior meningeal artery is well shown.

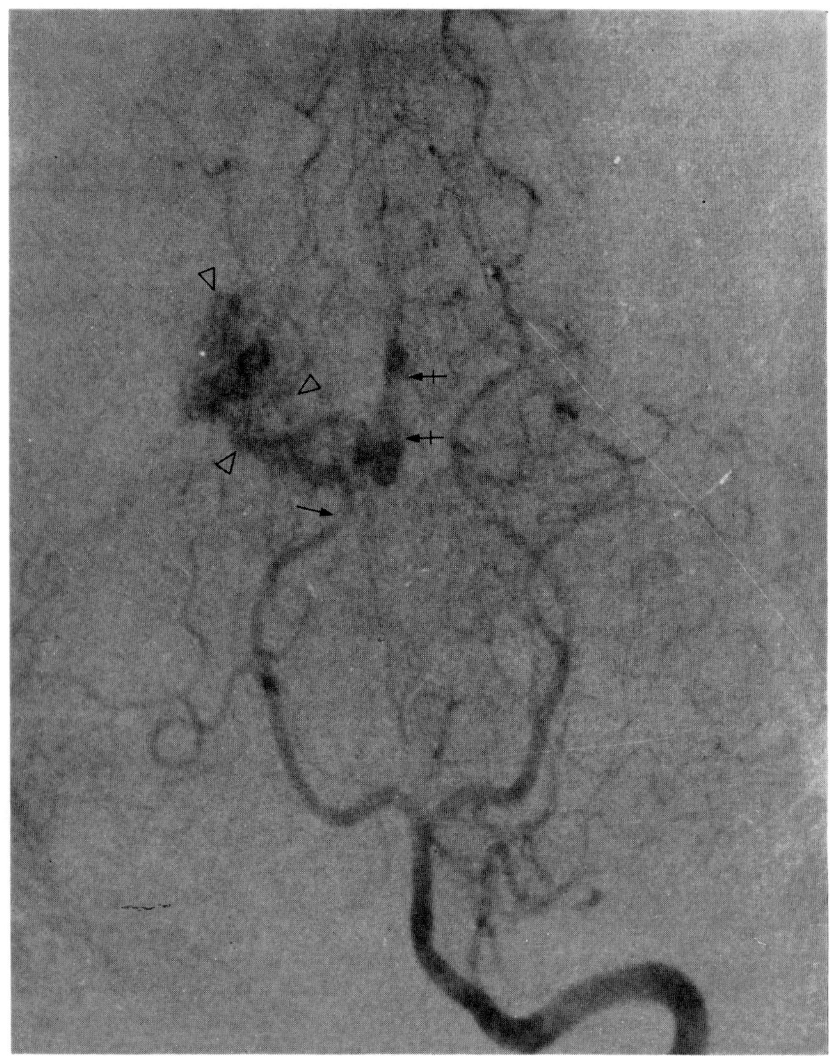

Fig. 360

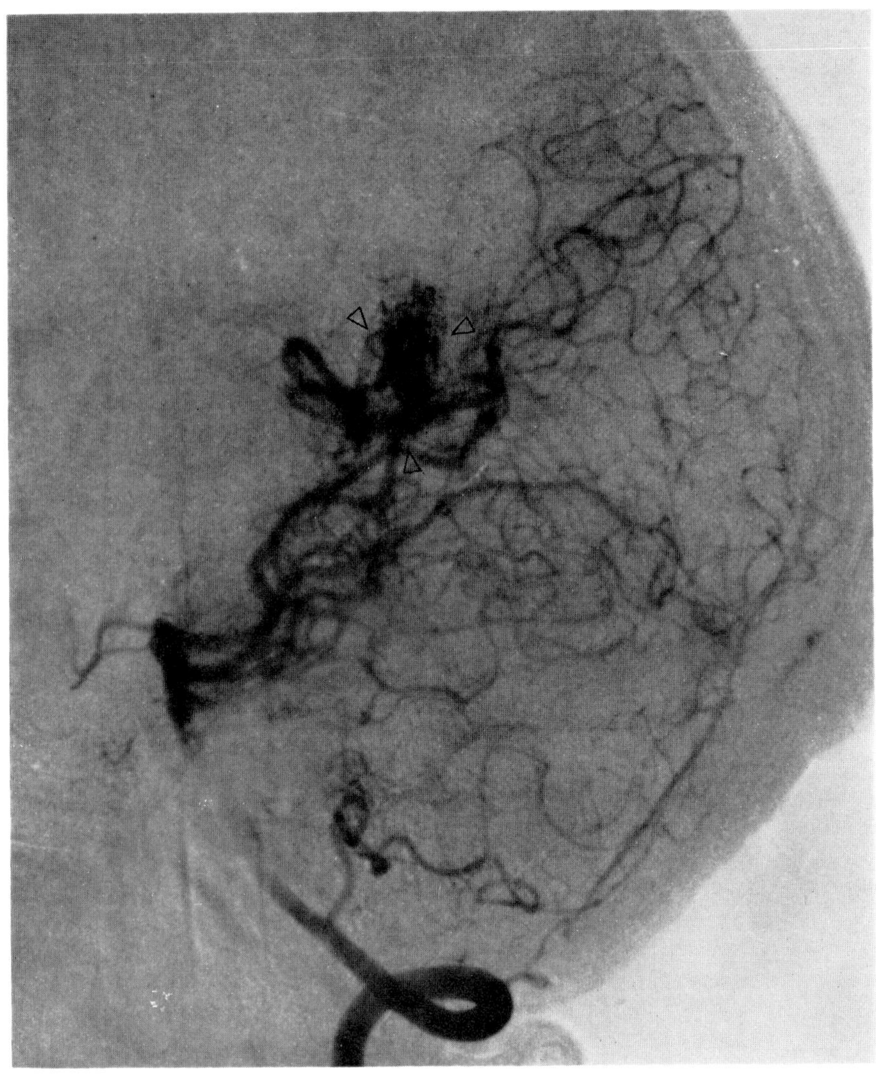

Fig. 361

Extensive Arteriovenous Malformation in the Parietal and Occipital Regions

A 20-year-old male: Figs. 362–365

Fig. 362 Arterial phase in the lateral projection. The parieto-occipital and the calcarine branches of the left posterior cerebral artery are enlarged and supply abnormal vessels in the posterior parietal and occipital lobes. The posterior choroidal and posterior pericallosal arteries also supply abnormal vessels in the splenium (4 arrows). There is no vascular displacement. Early venous filling is seen within the lesion.

Fig. 363 Arterial phase in the Towne projection. The arteriovenous malformation is identified in the medial aspect of the occipital and parietal lobes as well as in the splenium (4 arrows). There is early filling of the cortical veins (2 crossed arrows).

Fig. 364 Arterial phase of the left internal carotid angiogram in the lateral projection. There are small abnormal vessels in the sylvian fissure and the parietal lobe supplied by the sylvian segments, the callosomarginal and the pericallosal arteries.

Fig. 365 Venous phase of the left internal carotid angiogram in the lateral projection. The malformation is seen to good advantage. There is extensively enlarged anastomotic vein of Trolard draining into the superior sagittal sinus (an arrow). The superficial sylvian vein also drains the lesion (a crossed arrow). Since the straight sinus is opacified, there must be veins draining deep into the vein of Galen or internal cerebral vein (2 arrowheads).

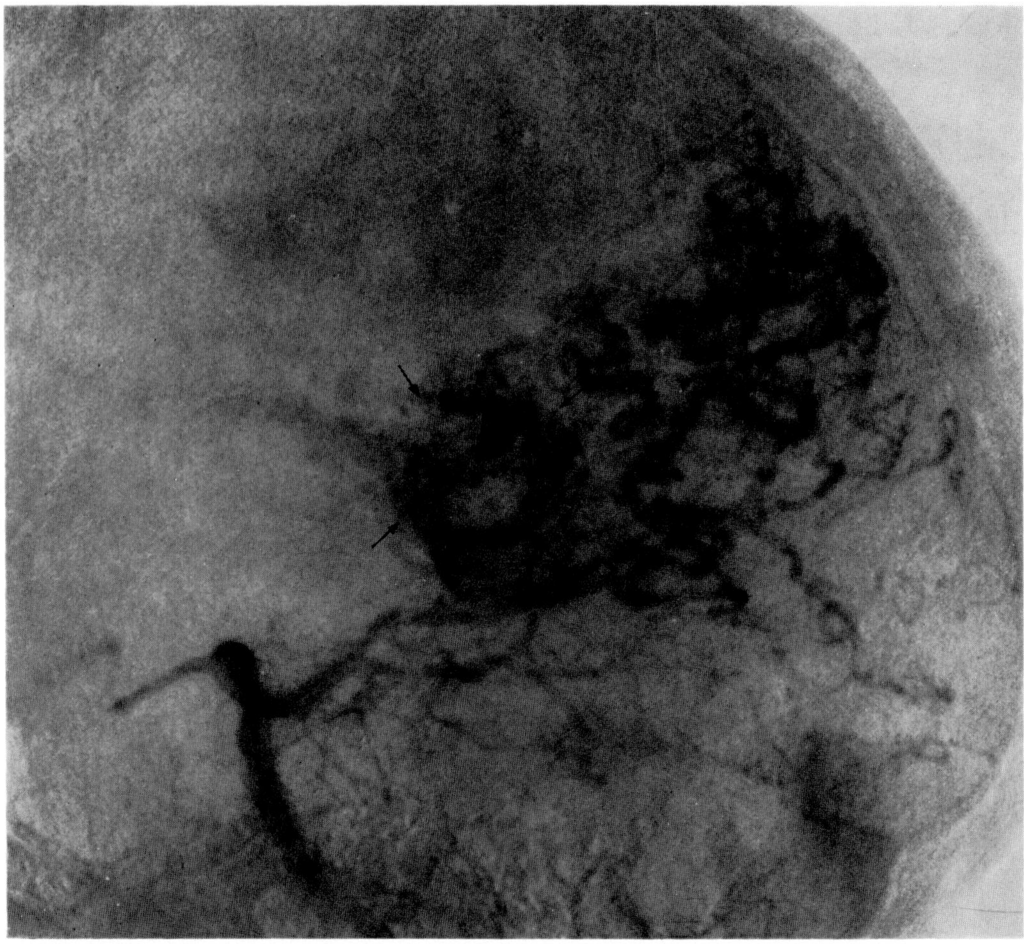

Fig. 362

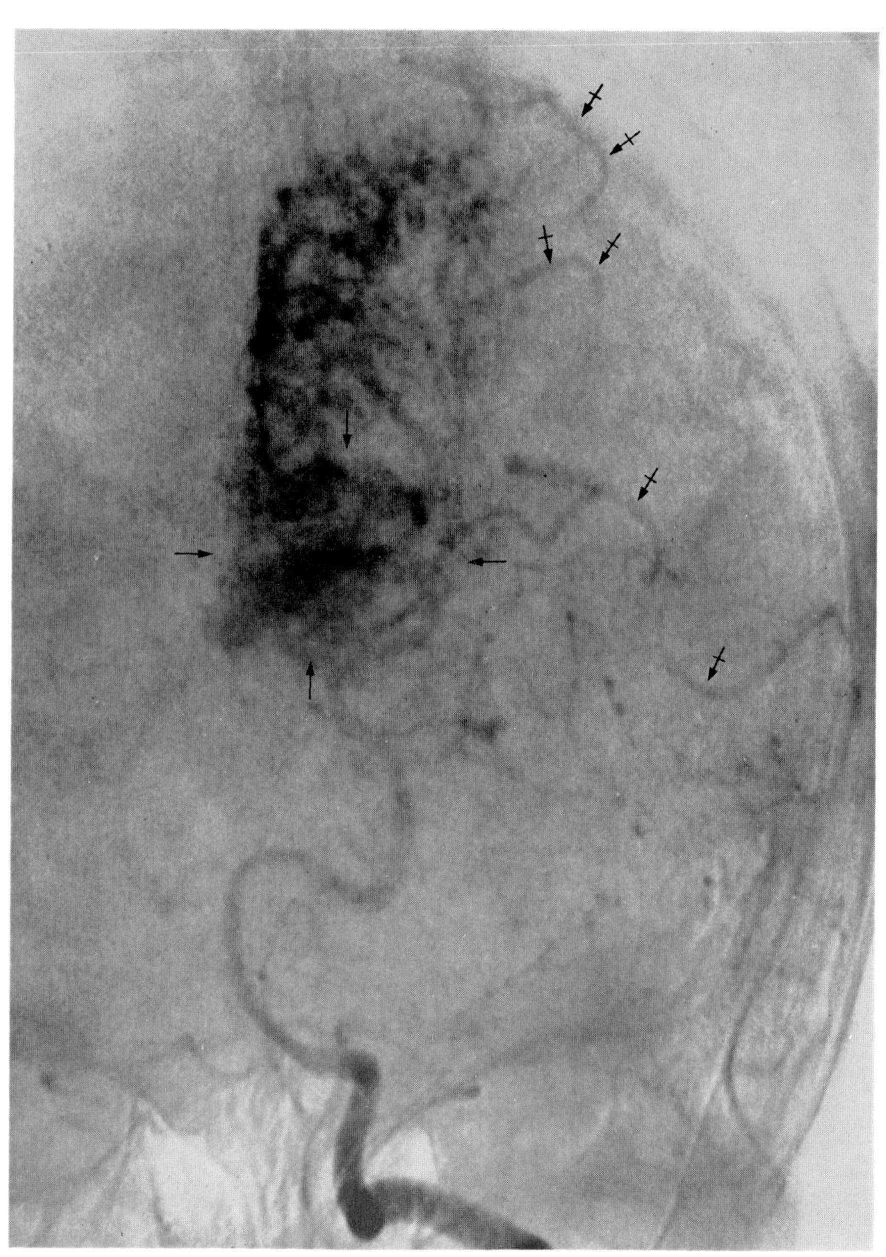

Fig. 363

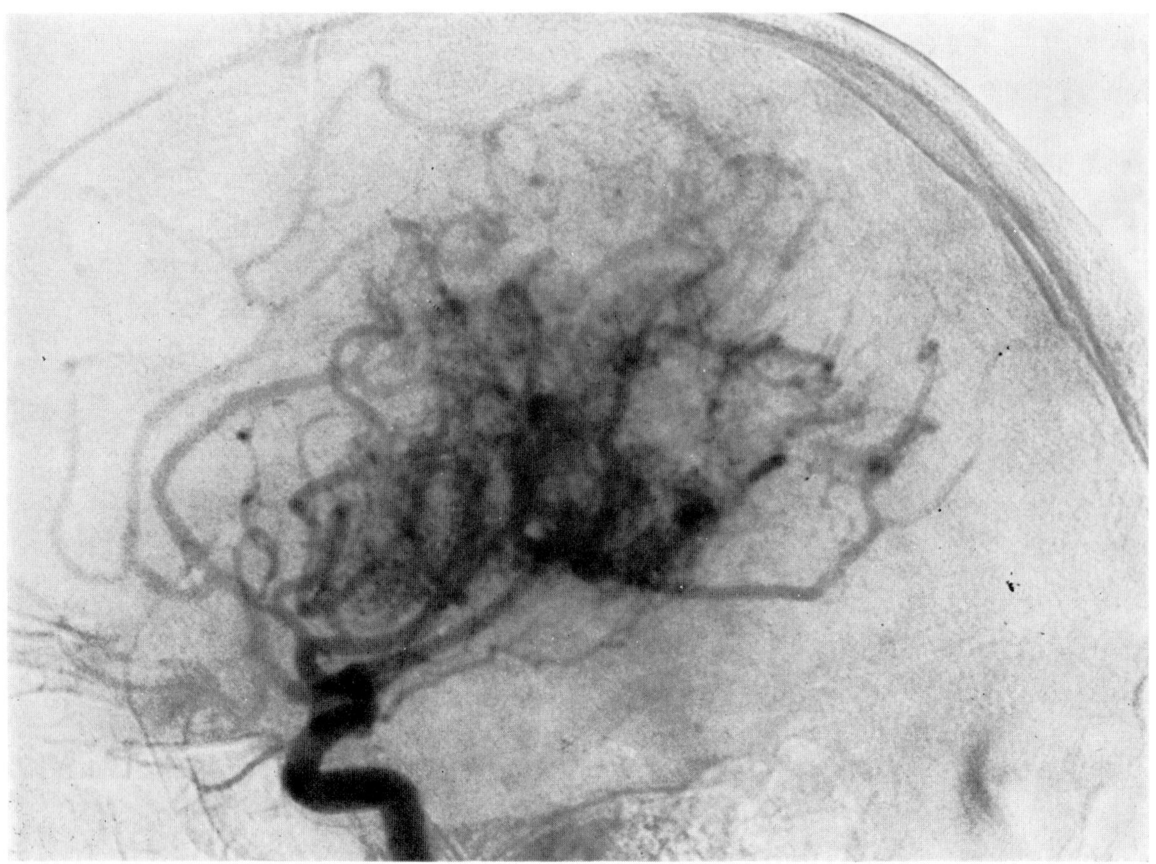

Fig. 364

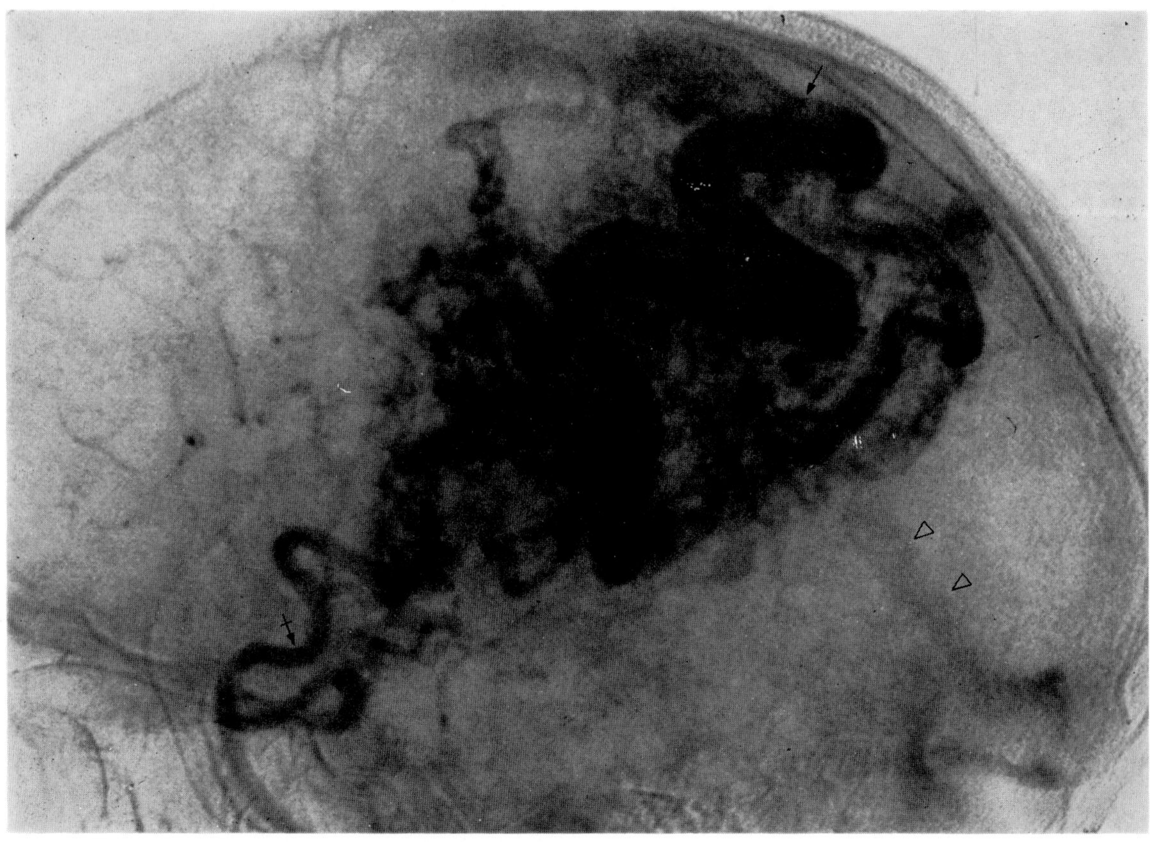

Fig. 365

Arteriovenous Malformation in the Right Diencephalon with Huge Dilatation of the Vein of Galen

An 11-year-old female: Figs. 366–370

Fig. 366 Arterial phase in the lateral projection. Arteriovenous malformation is seen in the posterior thalamus with feeding vessels from the thalamoperforate arteries and posterior choroidal arteries.

Fig. 367 Late arterial phase in the lateral projection. There is early opacification of the enormously enlarged vein of Galen (2 opposing arrows) and the straight sinus (2 opposing crossed arrows). The subependymal veins are slightly dilated and also drain the lesion (2 arrowheads). The internal cerebral vein (a double-crossed arrow) is shown to good advantage (see Fig. 370).

Fig. 368 Arterial phase in the Towne projection. The enlarged vein of Galen (2 arrows) and the straight sinus (2 opposing open arrowheads) are seen to good advantage. There is reflux of contrast media into the superior sagittal sinus (2 opposing closed arrowheads).

Fig. 369 Arterial phase of the right internal carotid angiogram in the lateral projection. The malformation is supplied by the enlarged anterior choroidal artery (an arrow) and the lenticulostriate arteries. There is early opacification of the vein of Galen and the straight sinus (2 opposing arrowheads). A cortical draining vein is also demonstrated (2 crossed arrows).

Fig. 370. Early venous phase of the right internal carotid angiogram. The enormously enlarged vein of Galen and the straight sinus are again demonstrated. The internal cerebral vein (3 arrows) and the anterior thalamic veins (an open arrowhead) are also enlarged. The subependymal veins are connected with cortical veins (2 crossed arrows), which drain into the superior sagittal sinus. There is reflux of contrast media into the distal superior sagittal sinus (2 closed arrowheads).

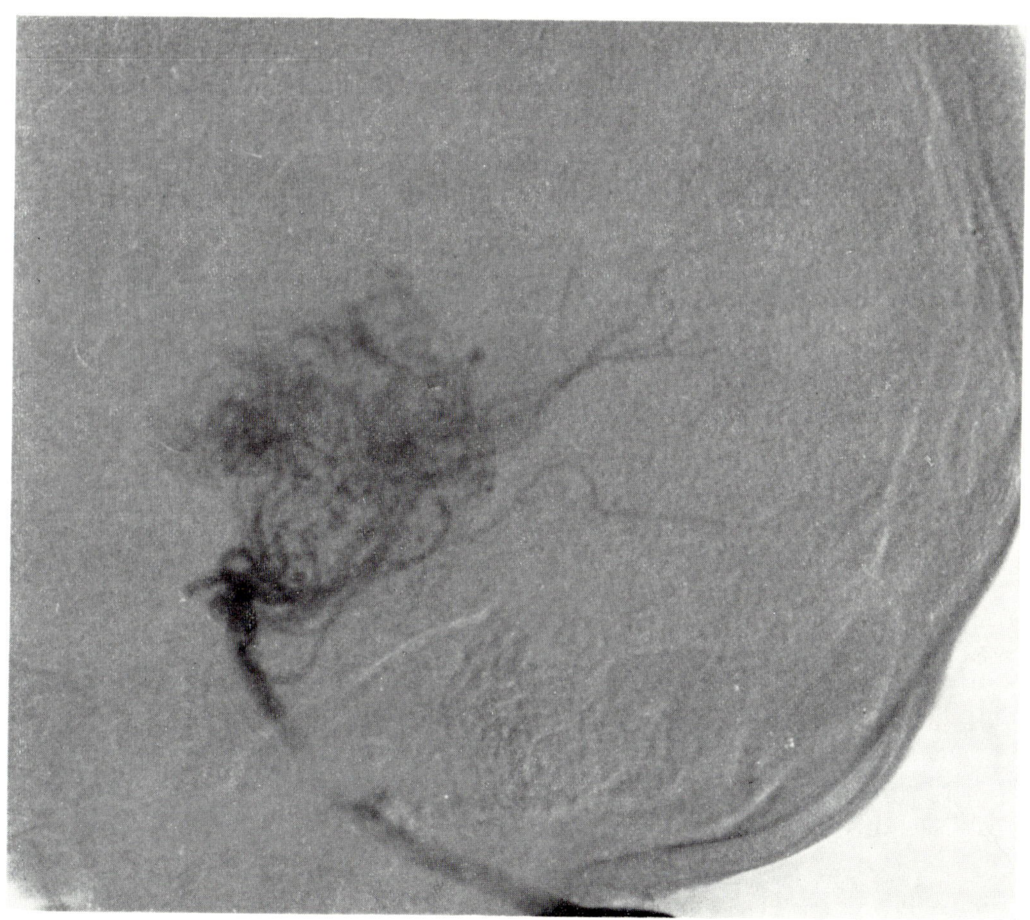

Fig. 366

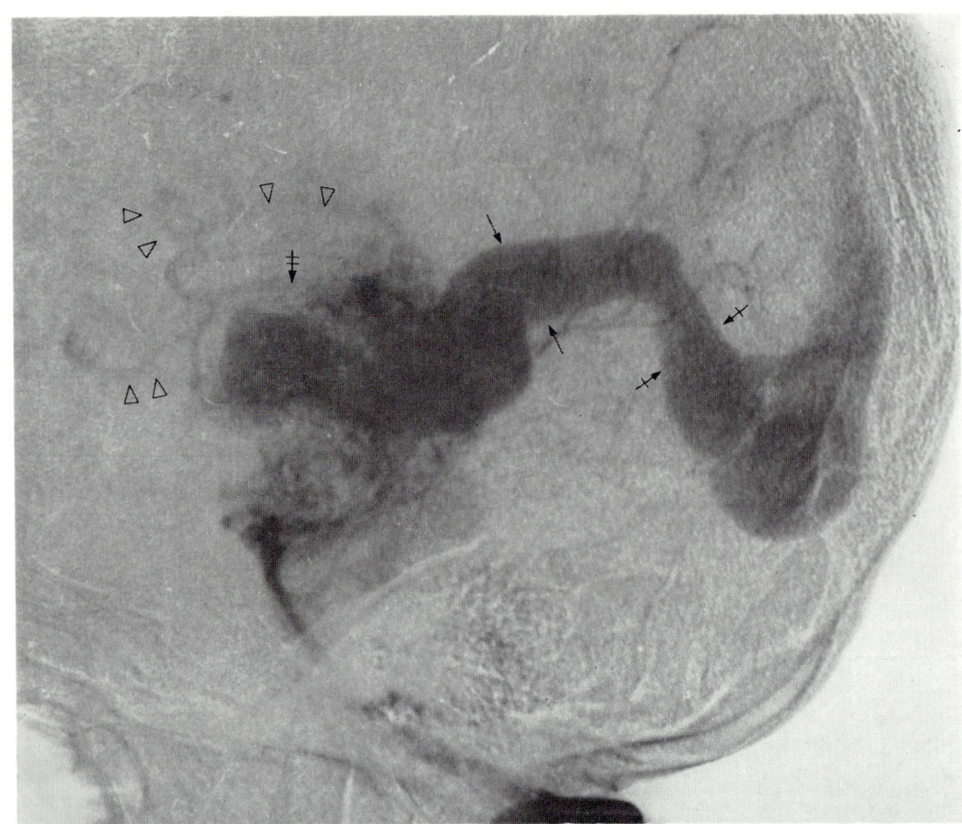

Fig. 367

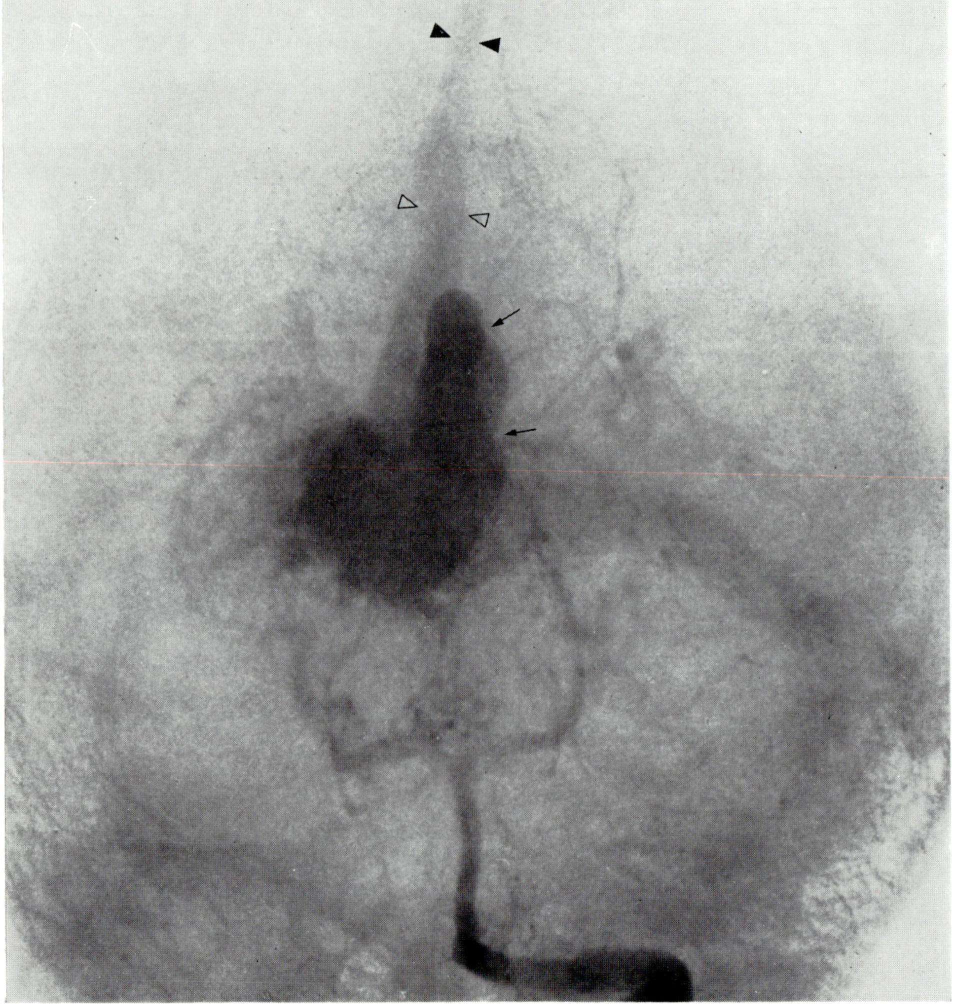

Fig. 368

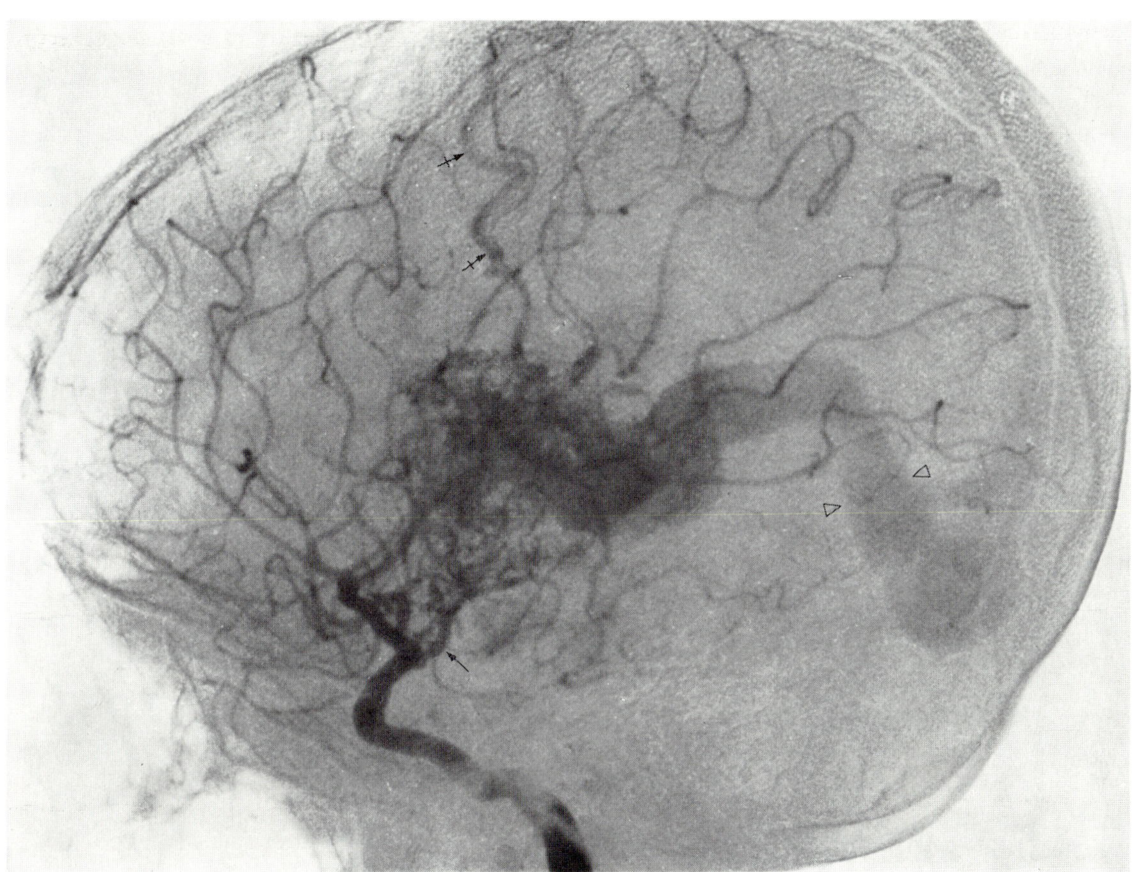

Fig. 369

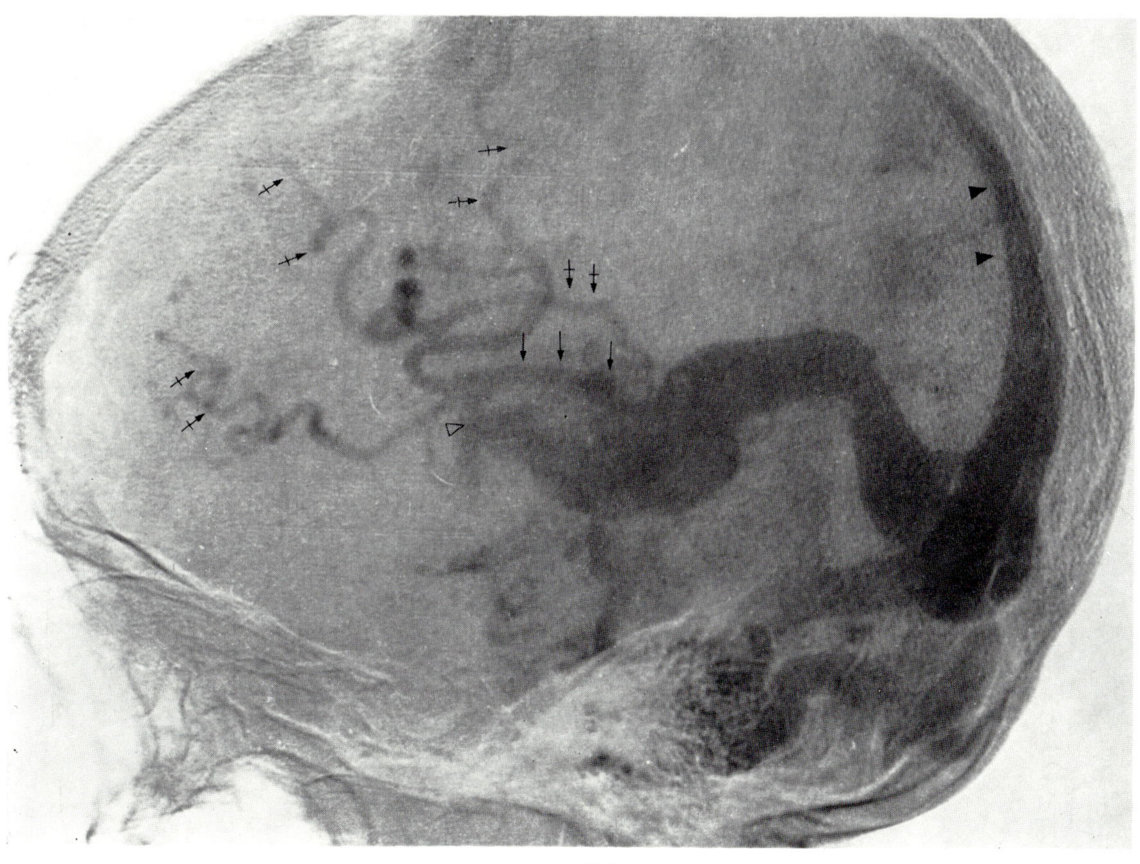

Fig. 370

Arteriovenous Malformation in the Diencephalon and Mesencephalon

A 9-year-old male: Figs. 371–376

Fig. 371 Arterial phase in the lateral projection. There is a mesh of abnormal arteries and veins in the area of the thalamus (4 arrows). The thalamoperforate arteries, the posterior choroidal arteries, and the colliculi quadrigemini and corpori geniculati arteries are all enlarged and feeding the abnormal vessels.

Fig. 372 Capillary phase. Early filling of abnormal veins is demonstrated. The superior thalamic vein (3 arrows) and the internal cerebral veins (2 crossed arrows) appear to be enlarged. The anterior pontomesencephalic vein (2 open arrowheads) and the posterior mesencephalic vein or basal vein of Rosenthal (2 closed arrowheads) also drain the lesion. The latter vein appears to drain into the straight sinus directly.

Fig. 373 Arterial phase in the Towne projection. The cluster of abnormal vessels are seen to good advantage. The lesion involves not only the thalamus (3 arrows), but also the mesencephalon (3 arrowheads).

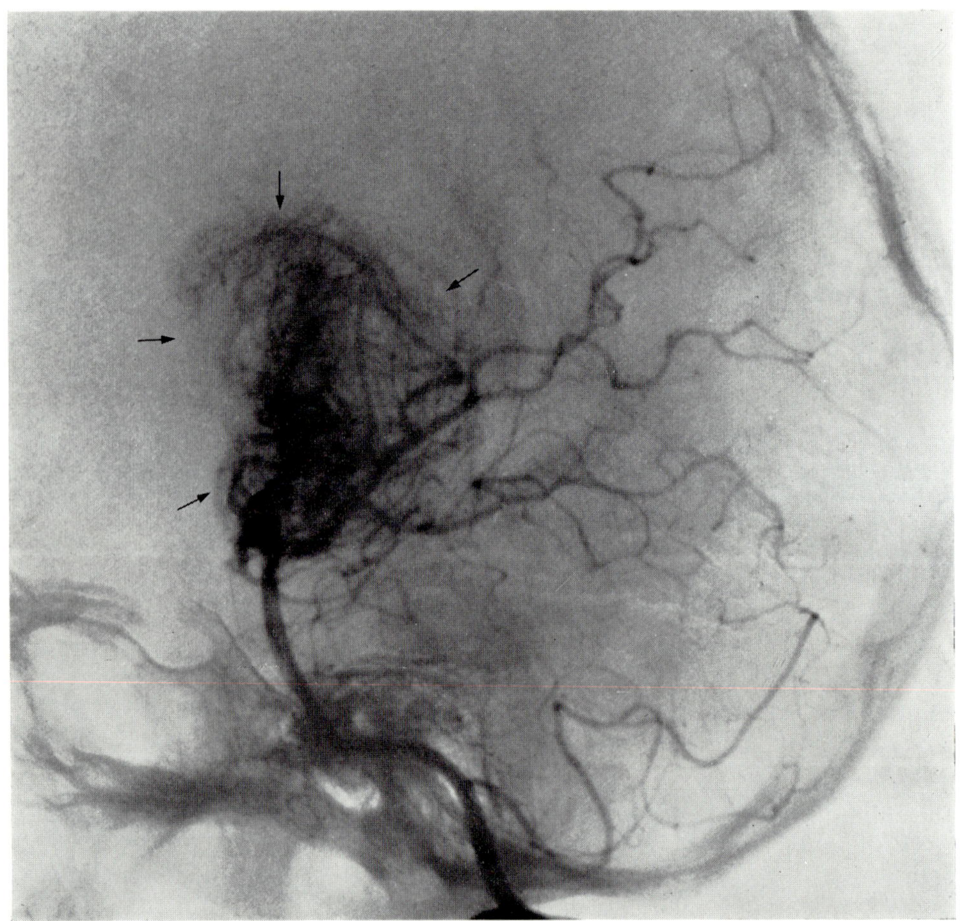

Fig. 371

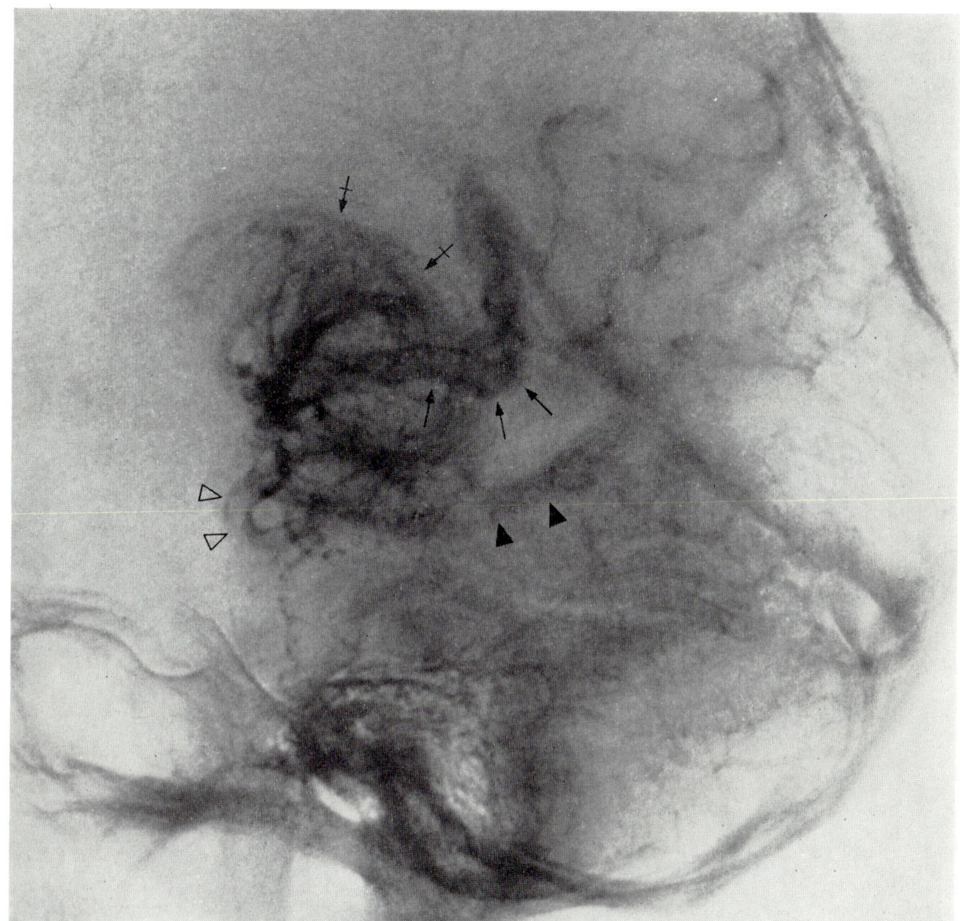

Fig. 372

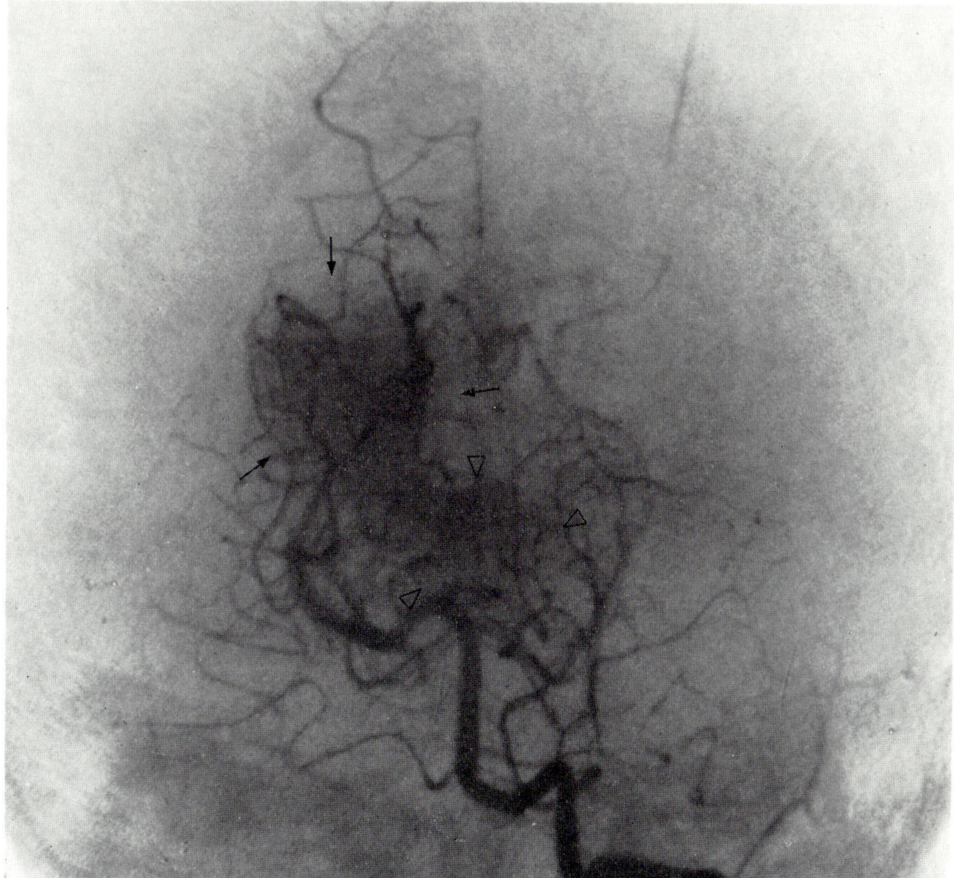

Fig. 373

Fig. 374 Capillary phase in the Towne projection. The lesion is drained via the posterior mesencephalic vein (2 arrows) and the vein of Galen and straight sinus (2 crossed arrows).

Fig. 375 Arterial phase of the left internal carotid angiogram. Abnormal vessels are supplied by the lenticulostriate arteries and the anterior choroidal artery(an arrow). The left posterior cerebral artery is also enlarged and supplies the lesion via the posterior choroidal arteries (2 opposing crossed arrows). The anterior aspect of the lesion, not demonstrated by vertebral angiography, is seen on the internal carotid angiogram.

Fig. 376 Capillary phase of the left internal carotid angiogram. The abnormal veins are shown to good advantage. The anterior thalamic (2 arrows), posterior thalamic (2 closed arrowheads) and internal cerebral vein (2 crossed arrows) are markedly enlarged and drain the lesion. The posterior mesencephalic vein or the basal vein of Rosenthal is enlarged and appears to drain into the straight sinus directly. The right internal carotid angiogram showed almost similar findings.

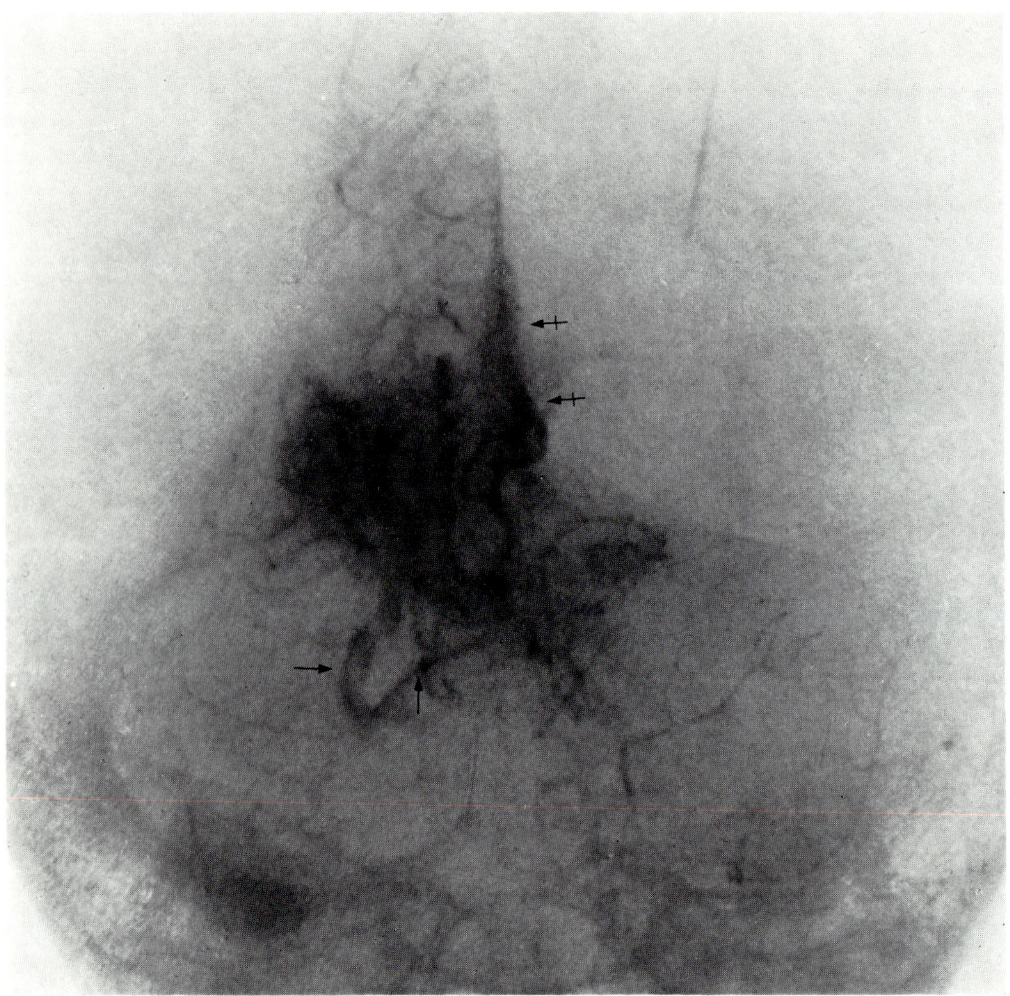

Fig. 374

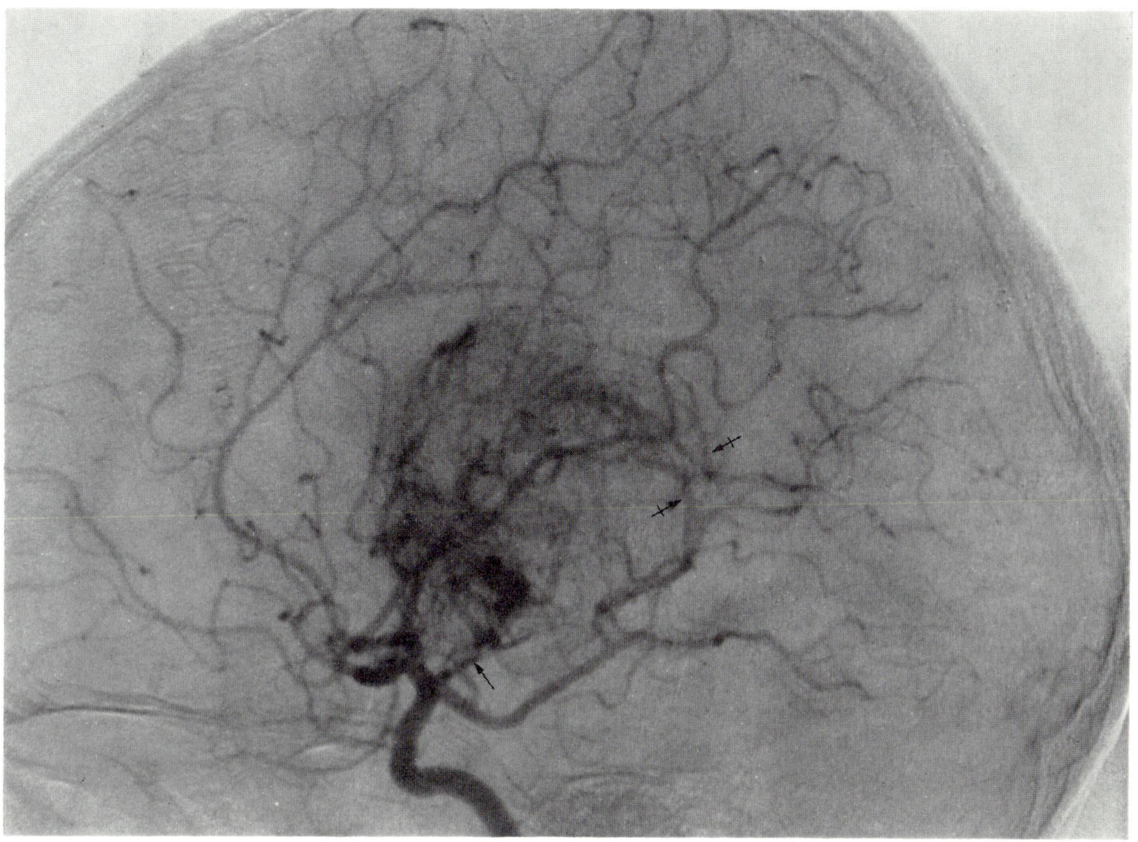

Fig. 375

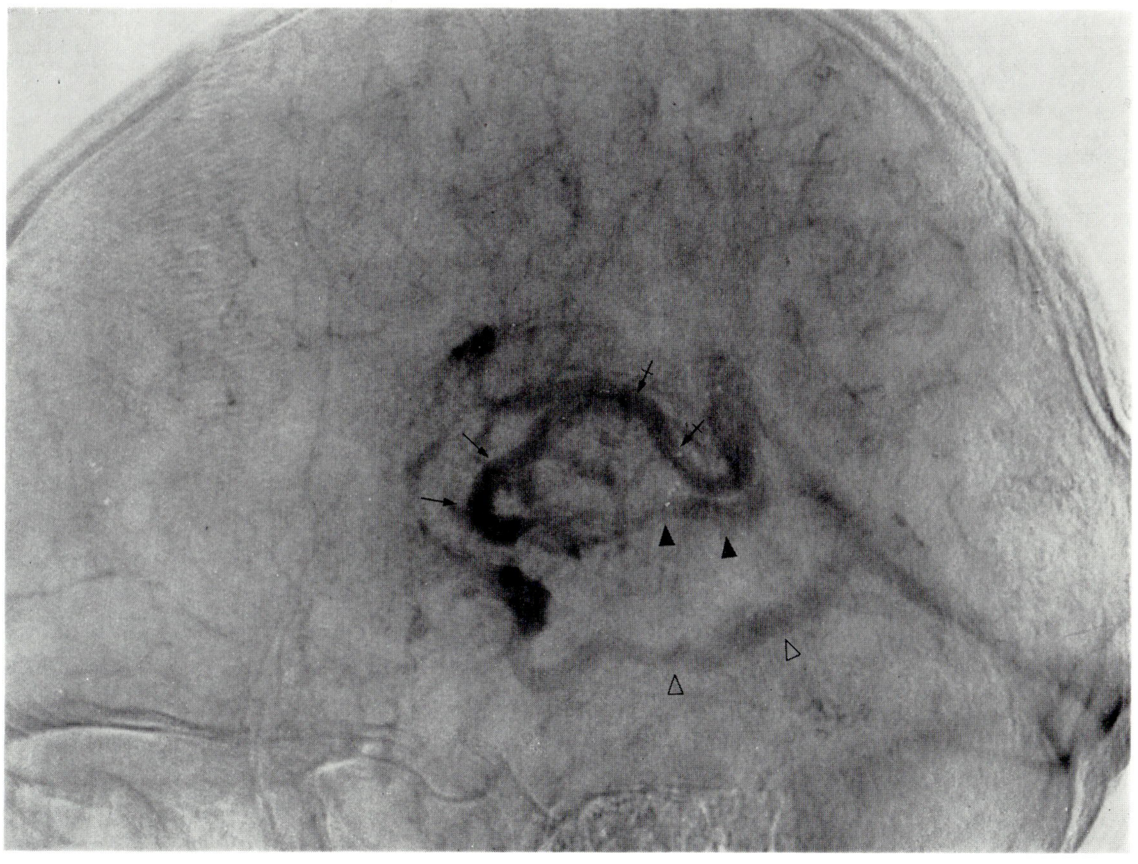

Fig. 376

ARTERIOSCLEROSIS

The angiographic features of arteriosclerosis include narrowing of the vascular lumen with thickening of the intima, "plaque formation" and dilatation and elongation of the artery. The arterial bifurcations are most frequently affected.

Dilatation and elongation can be demonstrated in any arteries of the vertebrobasilar system, but the basilar artery is most frequently and markedly affected. The diameter of the basilar artery may be widened to 4.5 mm in contrast to the greatest diameter of 4.1 mm in normal cases (Busch, 1966). The course of the basilar artery is markedly curved and tortuous with convexity toward the smaller vertebral artery. When these changes are marked, the findings are referred to as "fusiform aneurysm or dilatation" or "megadolichobasilar artery". Such elongation of the basilar artery may indent the floor of the third ventricle with compression of the aqueduct and resulting hydrocephalus. If a pneumoencephalogram is performed first, differentiation from a pontine tumor or third ventricle tumor may be difficult.

Fusiform Aneurysm of the Basilar Artery

A 51-year-old male: Figs. 377 and 378

Fig. 377 Arterial phase in the lateral projection. The basilar artery is markedly tortuous and lies adjacent to the clivus. The distal end of this artery is elongated and pointed posteriorly probably indenting the floor of the third ventricle (2 arrows). The tip of the dorsum sellae is marked with a crossed arrow. The diameter of the basilar artery is considerably widened.

Fig. 378 Arterial phase in the Towne projection. The basilar artery is markedly curved to the right. The proximal posterior cerebral artery is dilated and tortuous bilaterally. The superior cerebellar artery is tortuous as well.

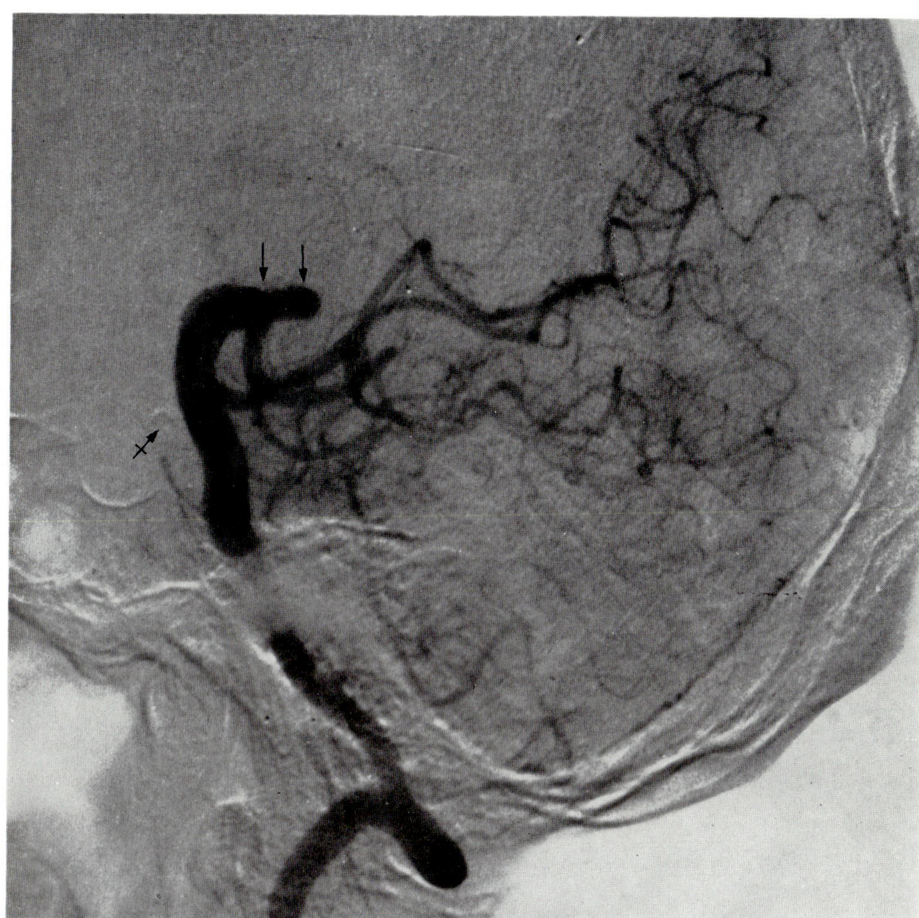

Fig. 377

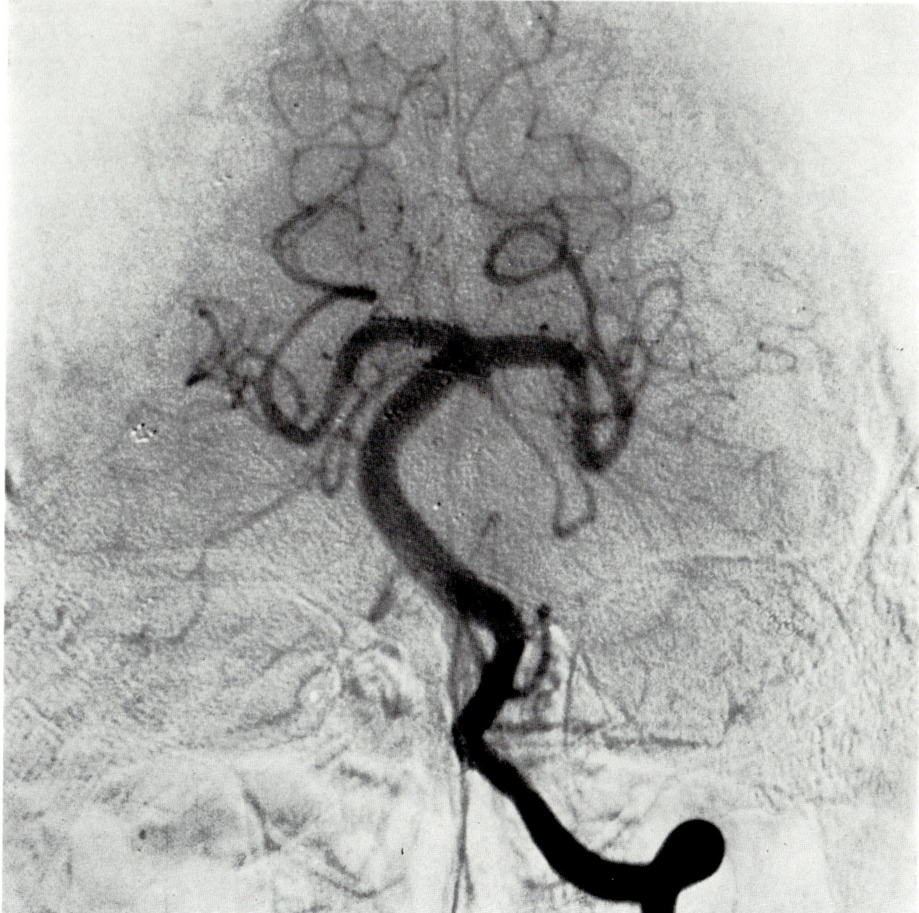

Fig. 378

Fusiform Aneurysm of the Basilar Artery

A 59-year-old male: Figs. 379 and 380

Fig. 379 Arterial phase in the lateral projection. The basilar artery is markedly widened and its diameter measures 0.6 cm. The artery courses close to the clivus. The distal portion of this artery is projected above the tip of the dorsum sellae for a distance of 2 cm. The tip of the dorsum sellae is marked with a crossed arrow. The thalamoperforate arteries show buckled appearance (2 arrows).

Fig. 380 Arterial phase in the Towne projection. The basilar and distal vertebral arteries are considerably widened. At the same time, the proximal portion of the posterior cerebral artery is dilated significantly on both sides.

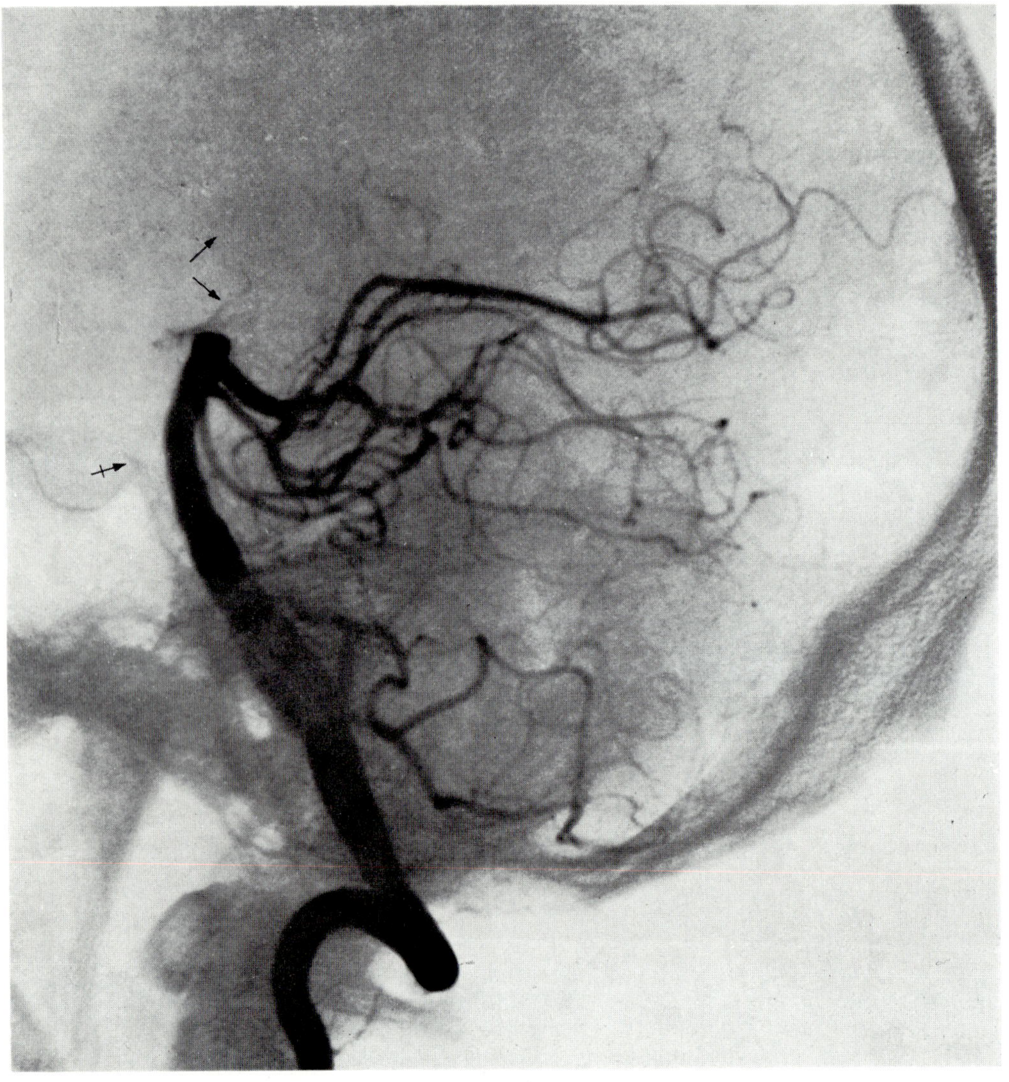

Fig. 379

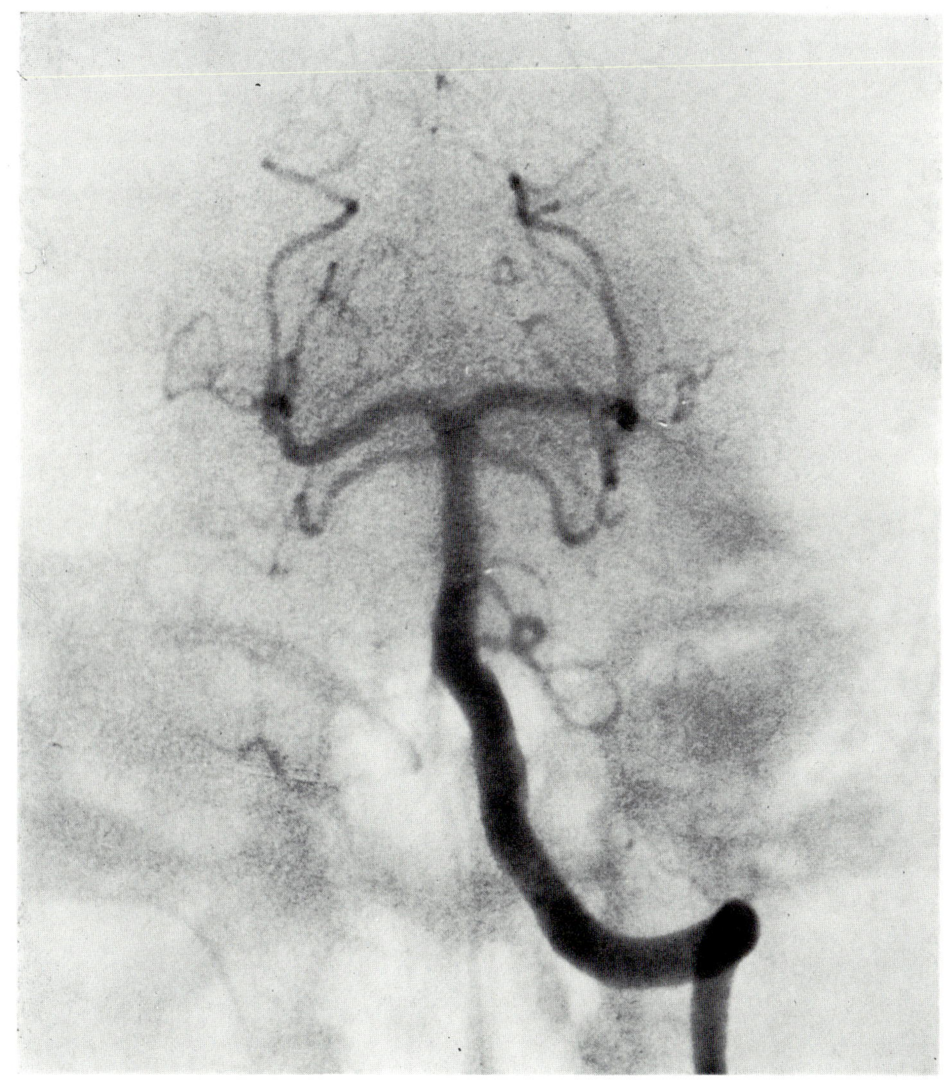

Fig. 380

STENOTIC AND OCCLUSIVE LESIONS

The etiologies of the stenotic and occlusive lesions include arteriosclerotic changes of the arteries, thrombosis, compression and inflammation of the vessels. Trauma and spasm may be responsible for these lesions.

Occlusive and stenotic lesion

Vertebral artery

The vertebral artery is frequently narrowed or occluded at the origin from the subclavian artery. Narrowing or occlusion may also be produced by compressive effect of osteophytes within the vertebral canal. In such instances, marked narrowing may be elicited by turning the head. Basilar impression may sometimes produce vertebral narrowing by compression. Thrombosis may occur at the level of the atlanto-odontoid sulcus (KRAYENBÜHL, 1955).

Not infrequently the distal vertebral artery is spastic and contrast media flow into the posterior inferior cerebellar artery without visualization of the basilar artery. This type of spasm is most frequently due to irritation of the vessels by the catheter or needles. In these instances there is usually prolonged opacification of the injected vertebral artery. This finding should not be mistaken as a distal vertebral occlusion.

Basilar artery

Thrombosis and atherosclerotic occlusion of the basilar artery are not uncommon. Occlusions frequently occur just proximal to the bifurcation of the artery. With occlusion of this artery, there is usually retrograde filling of the distal basilar artery and posterior cerebral arteries on carotid injection.

Laminar flow or partial filling of the basilar artery should not be considered as an arterial thrombosis, since non-opacified blood flows into the basilar artery from the non-injected vertebral artery. Diagnosis of the basilar artery occlusion should not be made unless there is good reflux of contrast media into the opposite vertebral artery or bilateral vertebral angiograms have been made. Collateral circulation usually develops via the posterior communicating artery or leptomeningeal pathways.

Posterior cerebral arteries

For the diagnosis of an occlusion of this artery, bilateral carotid and vertebral angiograms should be performed, since the posterior cerebral artery is oppacified by the internal carotid artery in 30 per cent. In the presence of occlusion of the artery, there develops extensive leptomeningeal collateral circulation from the middle and anterior cerebral arteries. The posterior pericallosal artery may play a significant role in formation of collateral circulation.

Cerebellar arteries

Thrombosis of the posterior inferior cerebellar artery is a well known syndrome. Angiographic diagnosis is considerably difficult, since this artery may originate as a branch of the anterior inferior cerebellar artery. The superior cerebellar artery is rarely occluded or thrombosed. Surgical occlusion or atherosclerotic occlusion of the anterior inferior cerebellar artery is a definite clinical entity (ADAMS, 1943; ATKINSON, 1949), but its angiographic demonstration has seldom been made.

In the presence of an occlusion of a cerebellar artery, multiple collaterals develop from the remaining cerebellar arteries.

Collateral circulation

In the presence of occlusions, there develop multiple collateral networks as follows:

Intracranial:

(A) Leptomeningeal collaterals
Posterior cerebral a.—middle cerebral a.
Posterior choroidal a.—anterior choroidal a.
Thalamoperforate a.—lenticulostriate a.
Posterior pericallosal a.—pericallosal a. (anterior cerebral)
Collaterals between cerebellar arteries
Collaterals between superior cerebellar and posterior cerebral arteries
(B) Transdural collateral (Rete mirabile)
Meningeal a. 1)–6)—posterior cerebral artery directly or via middle cerebral, anterior cerebral and internal carotid artery

1) middle meningeal a.
2) meningeal branches of the occipital a.
3) posterior meningeal branches of the ascending pharyngeal a.
4) meningohypophyseal a.
5) meningeal branches of the ophthalmic a.
6) anterior and posterior meningeal branches of the vertebral a.

(C) Collateralls via circle of Willis

Extracranial:

1) Vertebral a.—muscular branches—occipital a.
2) Vertebral a.—spinal a.—vertebral a.
3) Vertebral a.—mucular branches—thyrocervical a. and costocervical a.—subclavian a.
4) Subclavian steal

Multiple progressive intracranial occlusions (TAVERAS, 1969)

This syndrome in children and young adults was originally reported in the Japanese (KUDO, 1968; NISHIMOTO, 1968), but later proved that the disease is not confined to the Japanese (TAVERAS, 1969; GALLIGIONI, et al., 1971). The etiology of this condition is unknown and the disease is more frequently seen in females.

There are 4 main angiographic features of this syndrome: (1) Localized narrowing of the internal carotid artery at the bifurcation, including anterior cerebral, middle cerebral arteries and frequently involving the posterior cerebral, and basilar arteries; (2) Extensive collateral development of a network of fine vessels in the region of the basal ganglia and upper brain stem, primarily consisting of perforating branches from the circle of Willis and its adjacent arteries; (3) Marked development of rete mirabile collaterals (transdural external-internal carotid anastomosis); and (4) Development of the leptomeningeal collaterals from the basilar artery and posterior cerebral arteries.

Vertebral angiography is always indicated in this condition, since the posterior cerebral and basilar arteries are frequently involved and the abnormal vascular network is fed by the branches of the posterior cerebral artery. In addition, the meningeal branches of the vertebral artery frequently supply the transdural anastomosis.

Occlusion of the Distal Vertebral Artery Secondary to Arteritis

A 23-year-old female: Figs. 381 and 382

Fig. 381 Arterial phase of the left vertebral angiogram. There is occlusion of a short segment of the distal vertebral artery within the costotransverse foramen of the first and second vertebrae (2 arrows). Collaterals, consisting of multiple muscular branches, reconstitute the vertebral artery with visualization of the basilar, posterior cerebral and internal carotid arteries. There is filling of the carotid siphon via the collaterals from the external carotid artery (a crossed arrow).

Fig. 382 Arterial phase of the right common carotid angiogram. The internal carotid artery (an arrow) and the external carotid artery (a crossed arrow) are occluded just above the bifurcation. The lingual (2 open arrowheads) and submandibular (2 double-crossed arrows) arteries reconstitute the internal maxillary artery (a closed arrowhead), which in turn sends collaterals to the internal carotid artery. Similar changes were noted on the left common carotid angiogram.

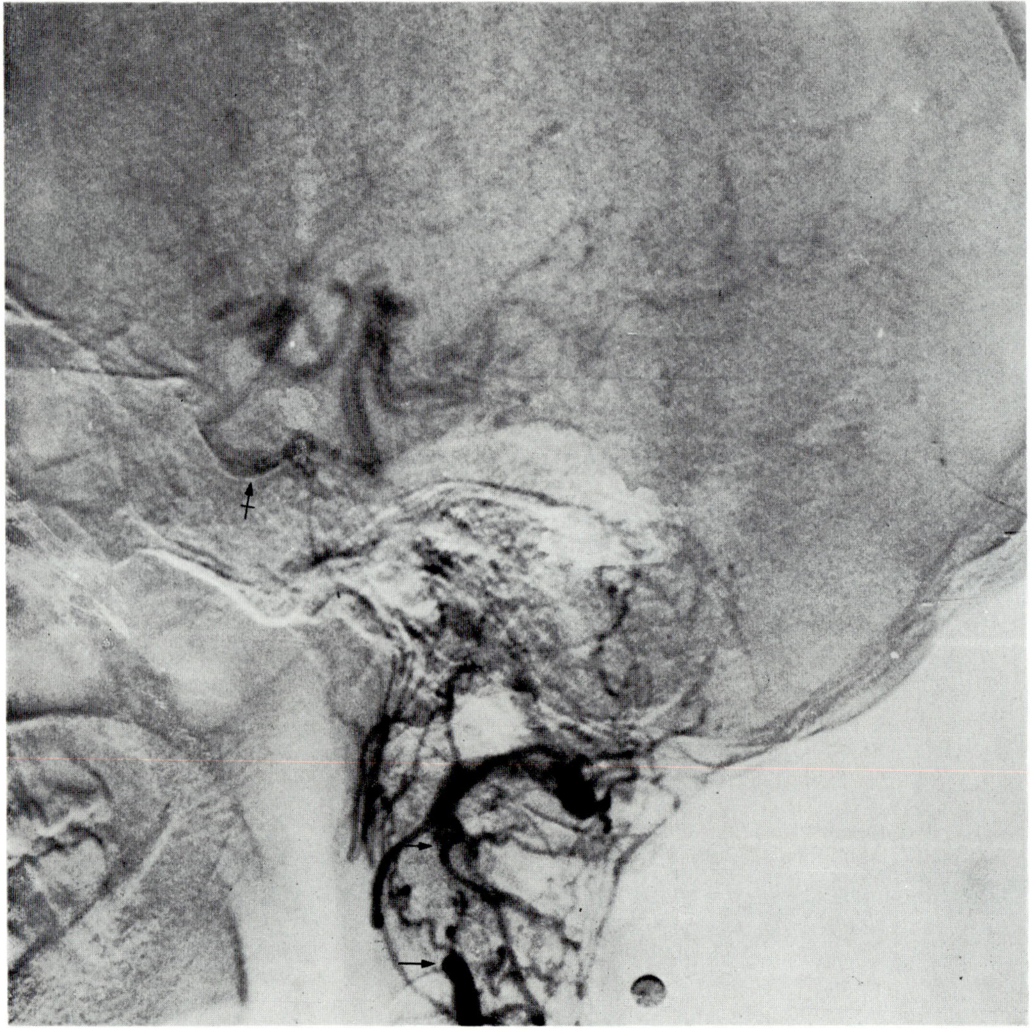

Fig. 381

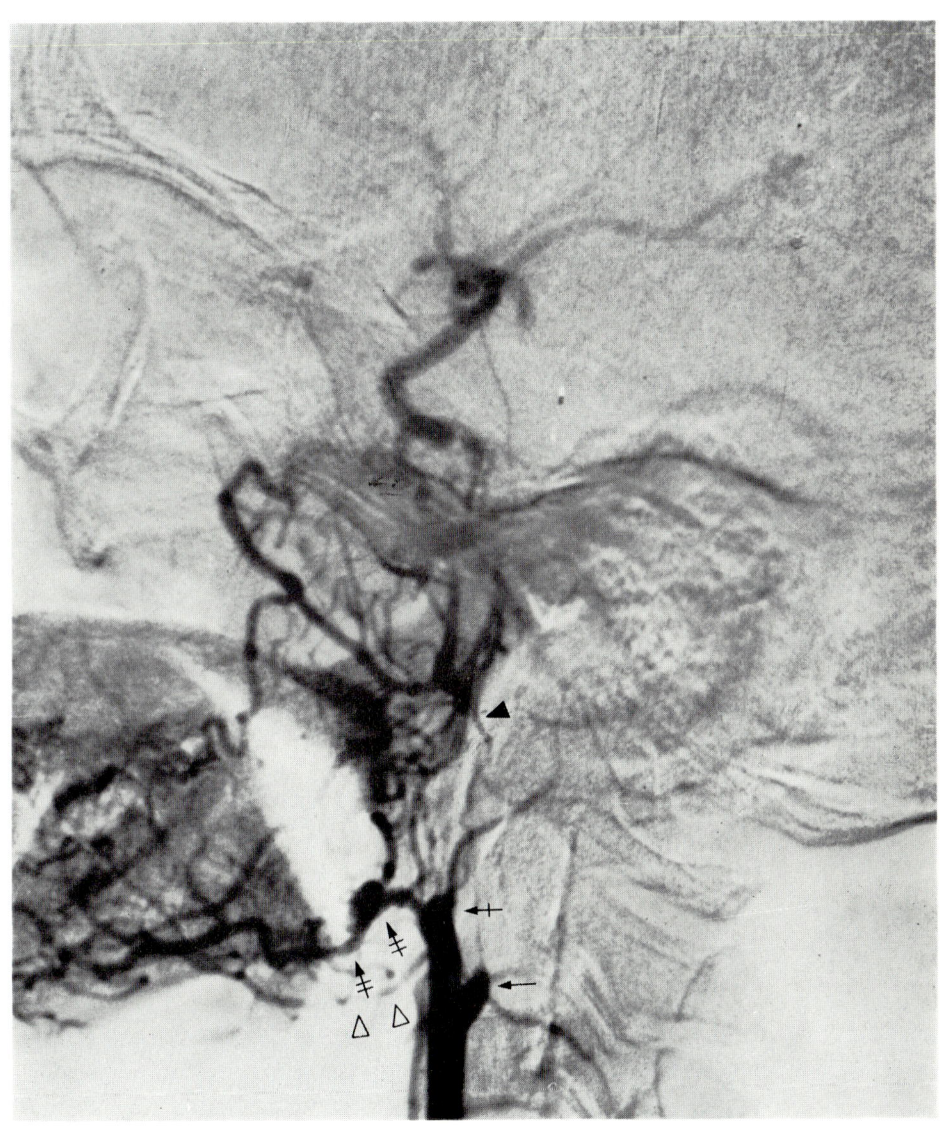

Fig. 382

Transient Stenosis of the Left Vertebral Artery with Rotation of the Head to the Right

A 33-year-old male: Figs. 383–385

Fig. 383 Left vertebral angiogram in the anteroposterior projection. The course of the distal extracranial vertebral artery is anomalous in association with fusion and deformity of the atlas and axis. There is no stenosis of the distal vertebral artery.

Fig. 384 Left vertebral angiogram with rotation of the head to the right in the supine position. There is marked stenosis of the left vertebral artery between the atlas and the occipital bone (an arrow). A fenestration of the right vertebral artery is demonstrated (2 crossed arrows).

Fig. 385 Right vertebral angiogram with rotation of the head to the right in the supine position. There is good reflux of contrast media into the left vertebral artery, which shows stenosis at the same segment (an arrow).

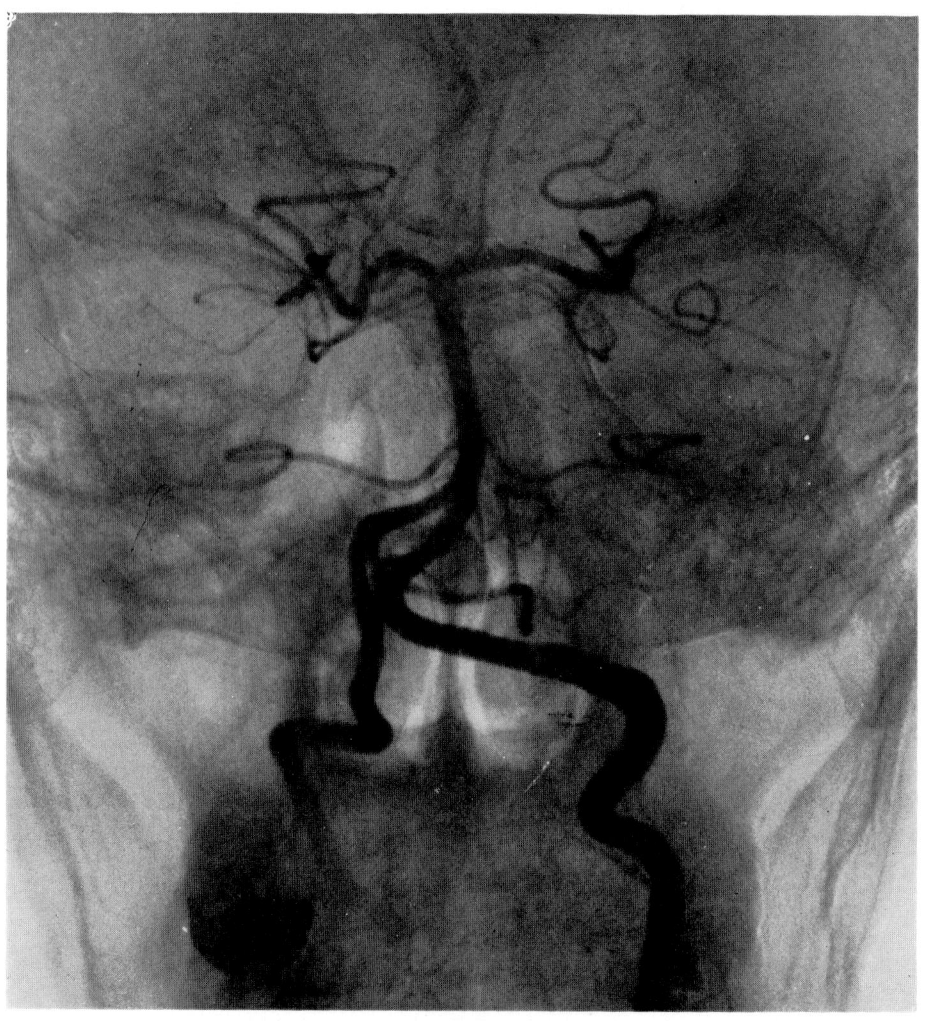

Fig. 383

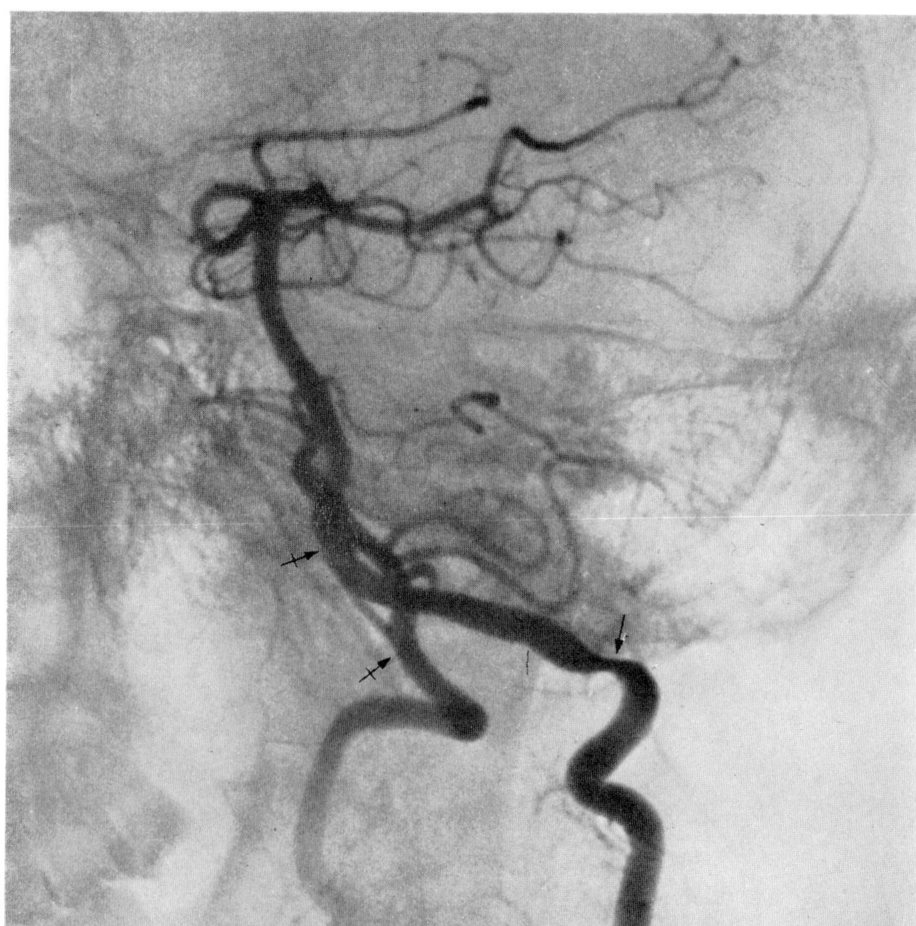

Fig. 384

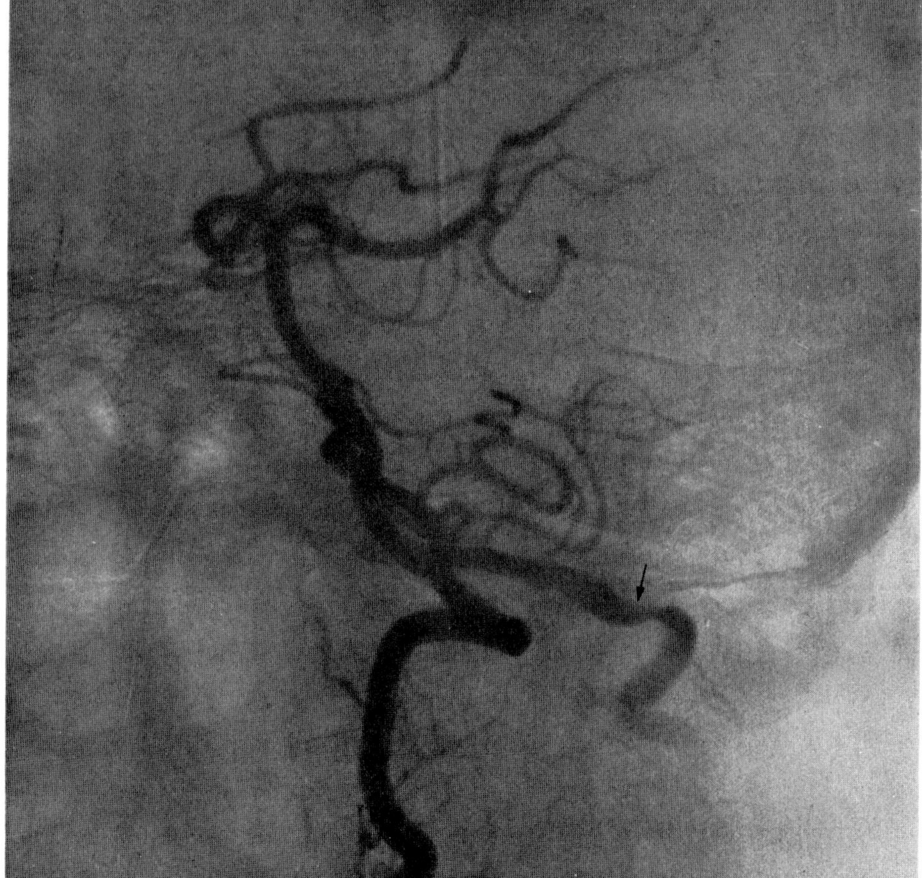

Fig. 385

Occlusion of the Left Posterior Inferior Cerebellar Artery and Stenosis of the Anterior Inferior Cerebellar Artery

A 66-year-old male: Figs. 386 and 387 (Through the courtesy of Dr. YAMAGUCHI, Akita Research Institute of Brain and Blood Vessels, Akita)

Fig. 386 Arterial phase in the Towne projection. The distal vertebral, basilar and posterior cerebral arteries are tortuous and dilated. The left posterior inferior cerebellar artery is not visualized. This was thought to represent occlusion from its origin, considering the clinical findings. There is poor visualization of the anterior inferior cerebellar artery, which probably indicates stenosis at its origin (3 arrows). The left superior cerebellar artery is also stenotic at its origin (2 crossed arrows).

Fig. 387 Arterial phase in the lateral projection. The basilar artery is elongated and projecting into the interpeduncular cistern. The tip of dorsum sellae is marked with an arrow. Only one anterior inferior cerebellar artery and its branches are visualized.

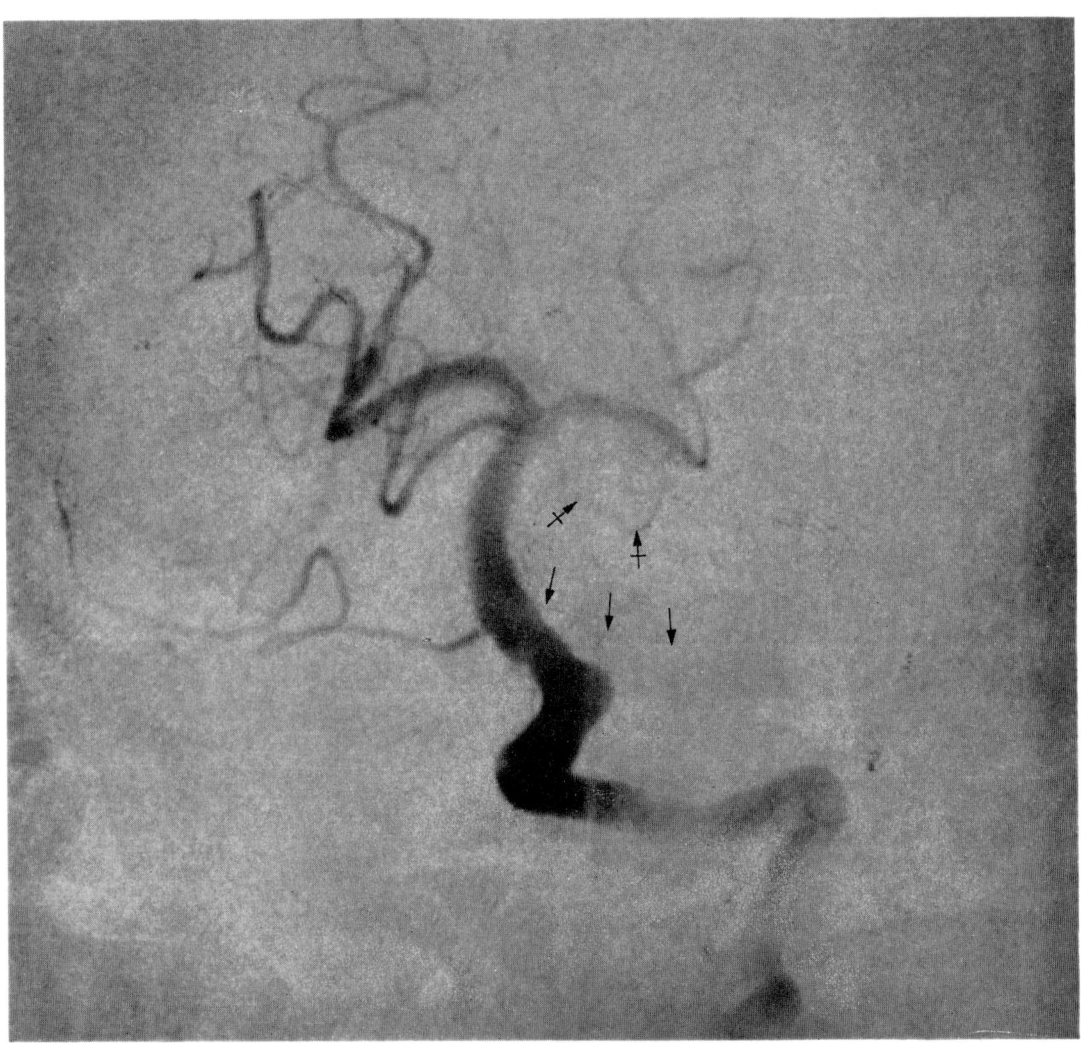

Fig. 386

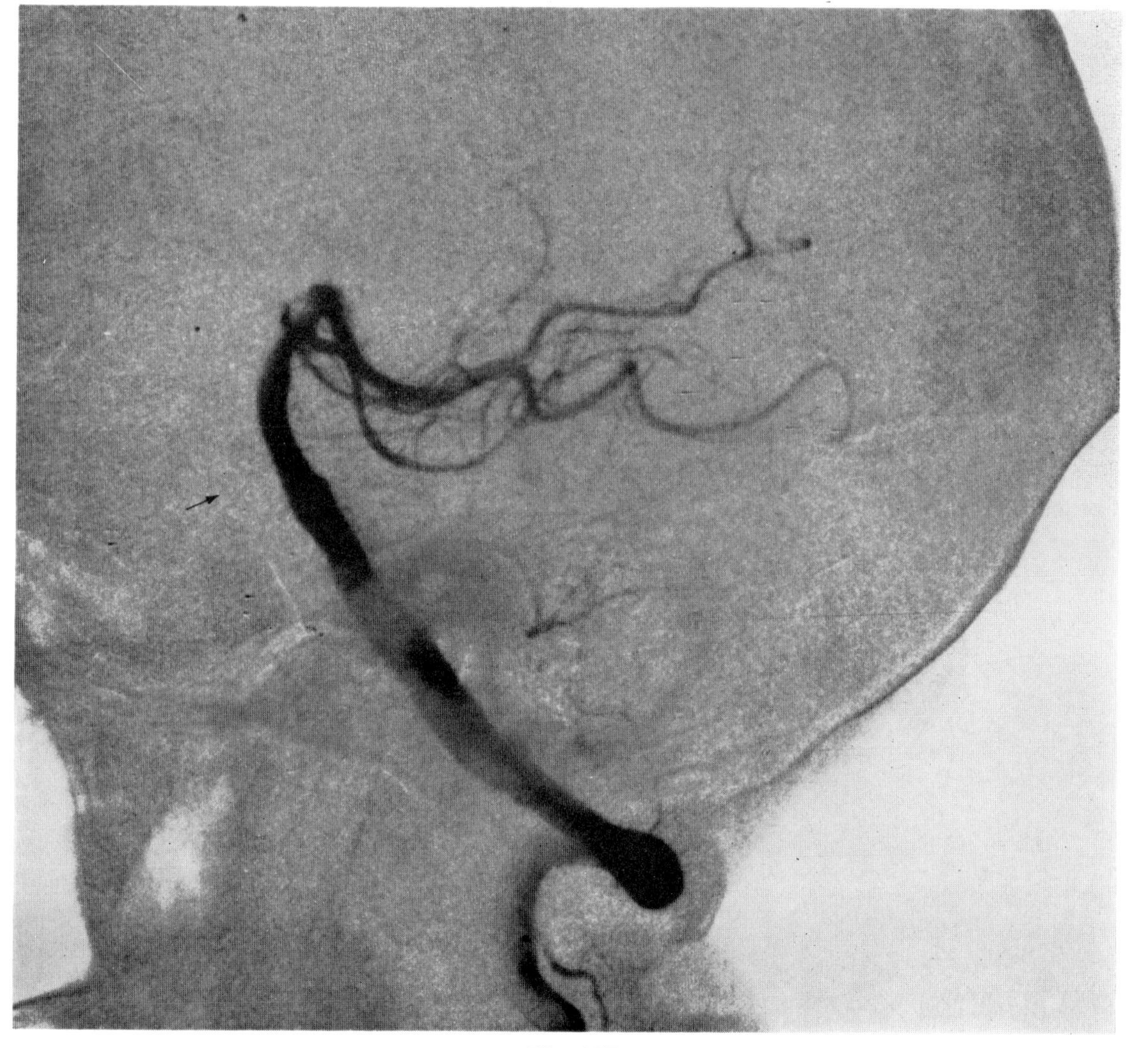

Fig. 387

Occlusion of the Basilar Artery with Cerebellar Leptomeningeal Collaterals

A 15-year-old male: Figs. 388–390 (Through the courtesy of Dr. YAMAGUCHI, Research Institute of Brain and Blood Vessels, Akita)

Fig. 388 Arterial phase in the Towne projection. There is occlusion of the basilar artery just distal to the origin of the anterior inferior cerebellar artery (an arrow). The posterior inferior cerebellar artery arises from the anterior inferior cerebellar artery bilaterally.

Fig. 389 Arterial phase in the lateral projection. There are diffuse leptomeningeal collaterals from the posterior inferior cerebellar artery to the superior cerebellar arteries (arrowheads).

Fig. 390 Capillary phase in the lateral projection. The anterior culminate and vermian segments of the superior cerebellar artery are reconstituted by the leptomeningeal collaterals (arrows) together with the hemispheric branches (2 crossed arrows).

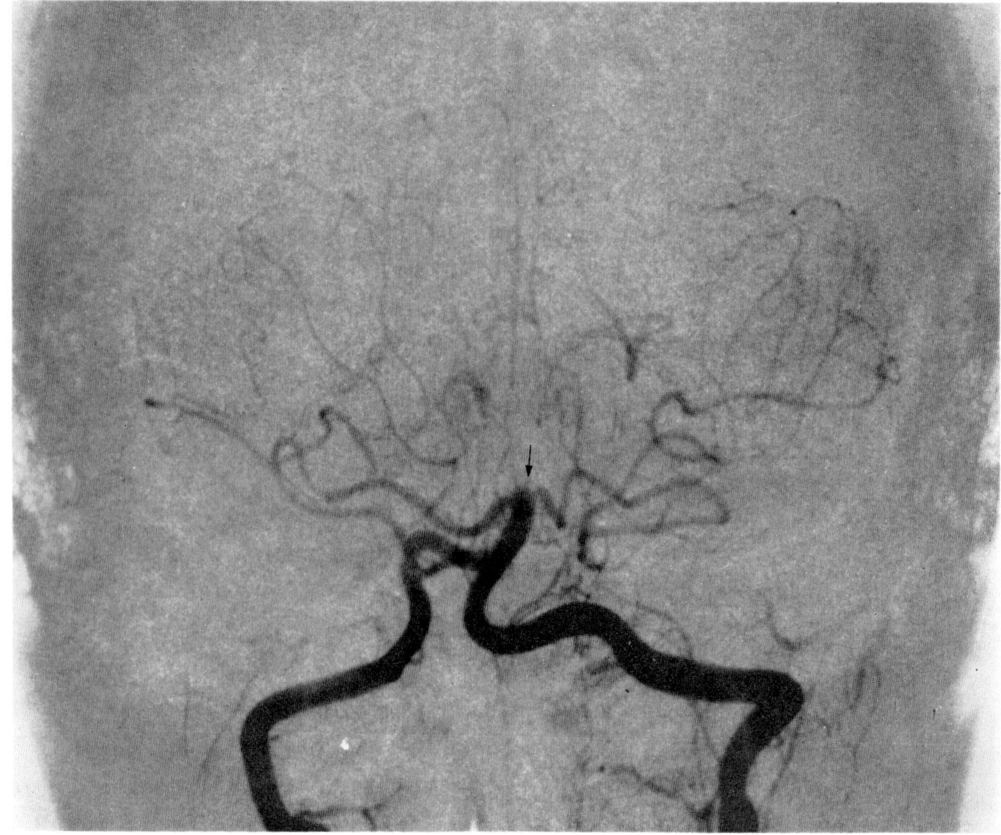

Fig. 388

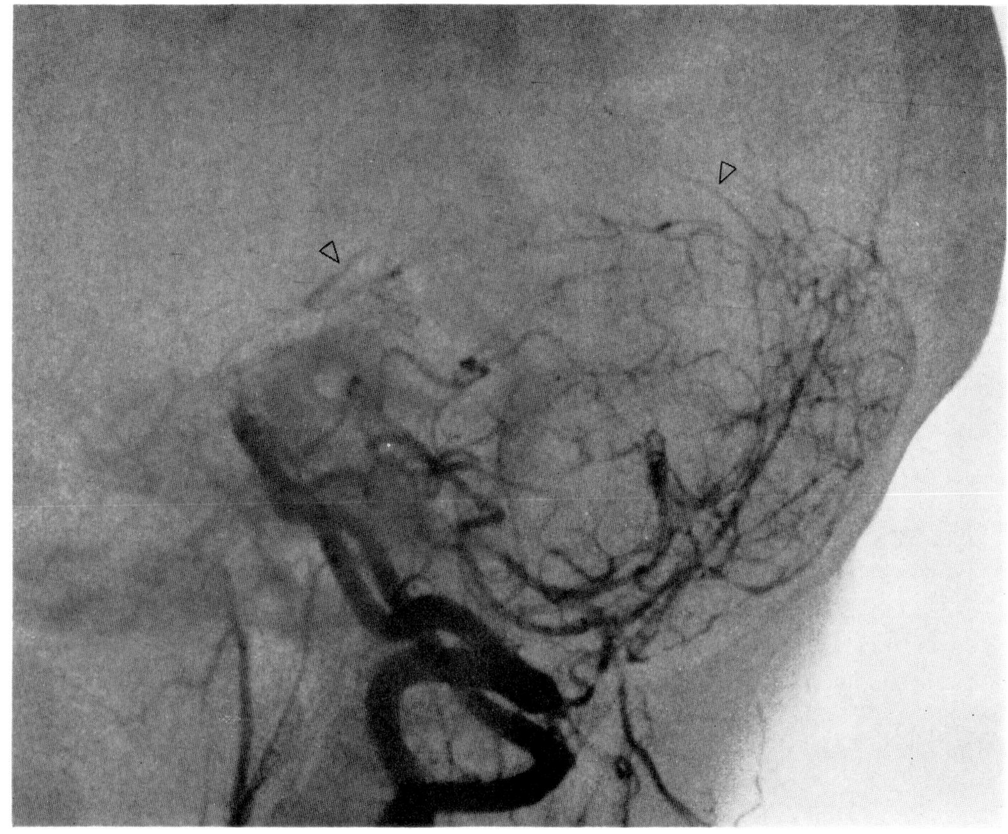

Fig. 389

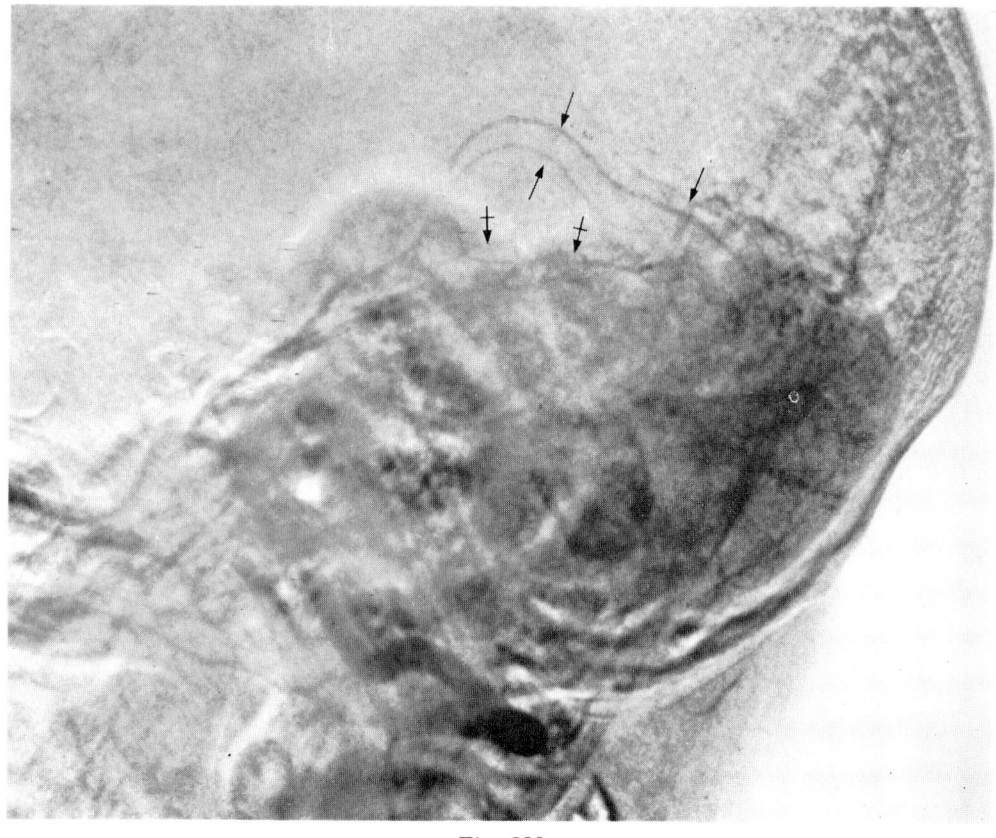

Fig. 390

Occlusion of the Right Posterior Cerebral Artery

A 49-year-old female: Fig. 391 (Through the courtesy of Dr. YAMAGUCHI, Research Institute of Brain and Blood Vessels, Akita)

Fig. 391 Arterial phase in the Towne projection. There is occlusion of the ambient segment of the right posterior cerebral artery (an arrow). There is no significant collateral development.

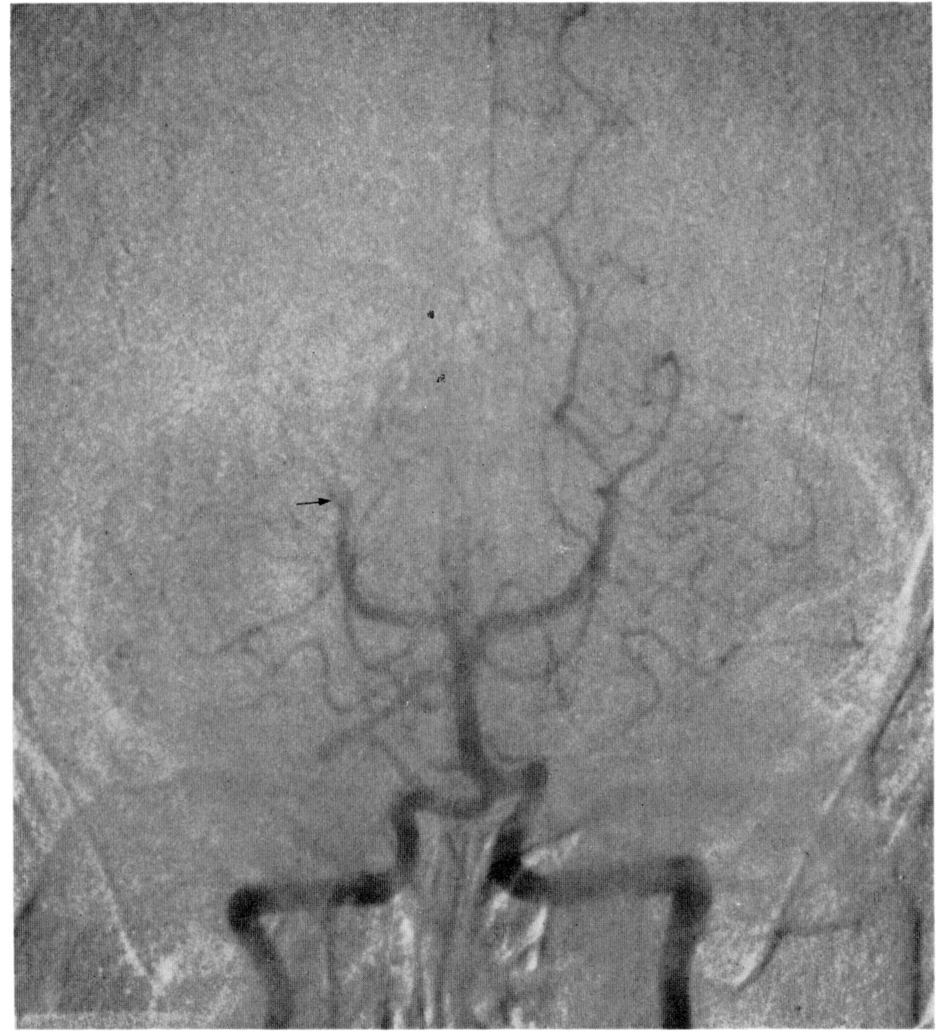

Fig. 391

Occlusion of the Left Posterior Cerebral Artery

A 44-year-old male: Fig. 392

Fig. 392 Arterial phase in the Towne projection. There is a one cm occluded segment of the left posterior cerebral artery at its ambient segment (2 arrows). The collaterals reconstitute the distal posterior cerebral artery. Although the posterior temporal and calcarine arteries are visualized, the flow distal to the occluded segment appears to be delayed (a crossed arrow). Collateral development is minimal to the occipital and temporal lobes.

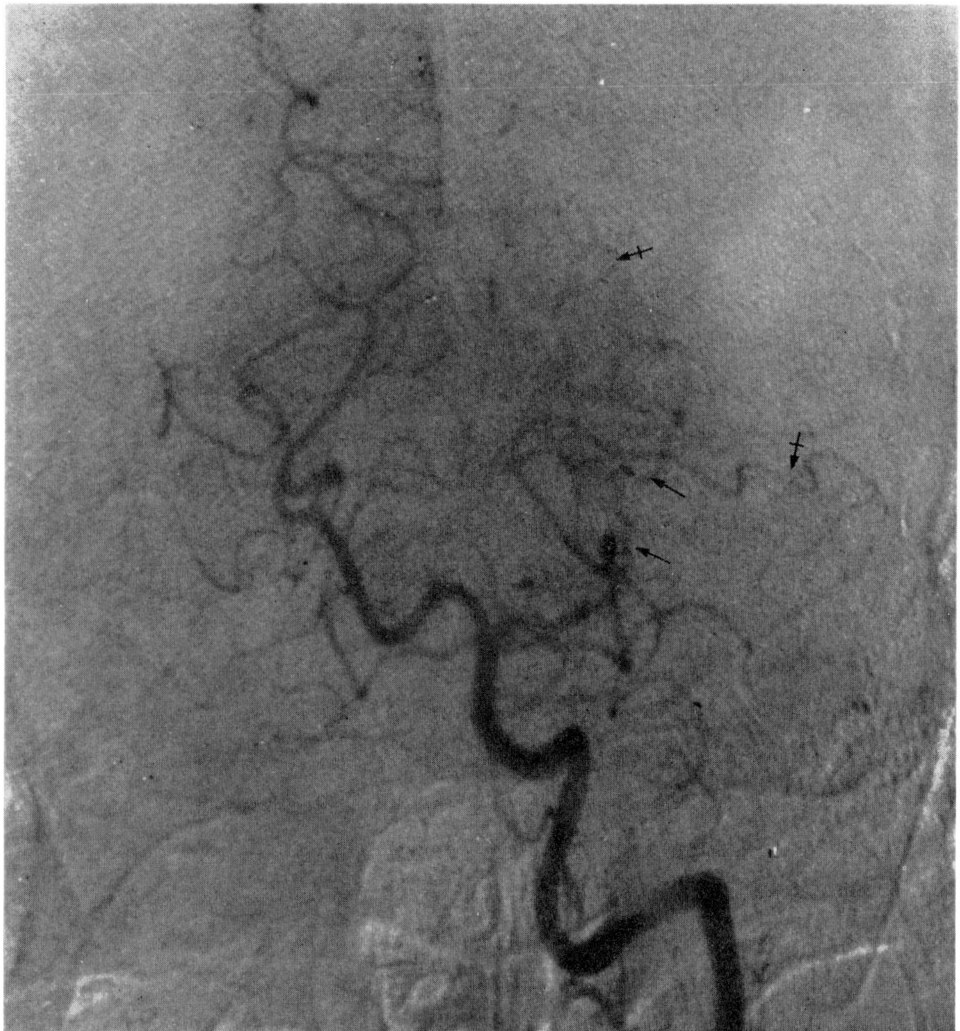

Fig. 392

Complete Occlusion of the Bilateral Internal Carotid Arteries just above the Common Carotid Bifurcation with Extensive Collaterals from the Vertebrobasilar System

A 45-year-old male: Figs. 393 and 394

Fig. 393 Arterial phase in the lateral projection. The anterior and middle cerebral arteries are filled via the posterior communicating arteries and small dilated arterial branches in the base of the brain (5 arrows). There is development of leptomeningeal collaterals between the posterior cerebral and pericallosal arteries (2 crossed arrows).

Fig. 394 Arterial phase in the anteroposterior projection. Leptomeningeal collaterals are present from the posterior cerebral artery to the middle cerebral artery (arrows) and to the pericallosal artery (2 crossed arrows). Profuse fine collaterals are also seen at the base of the brain (arrowheads).

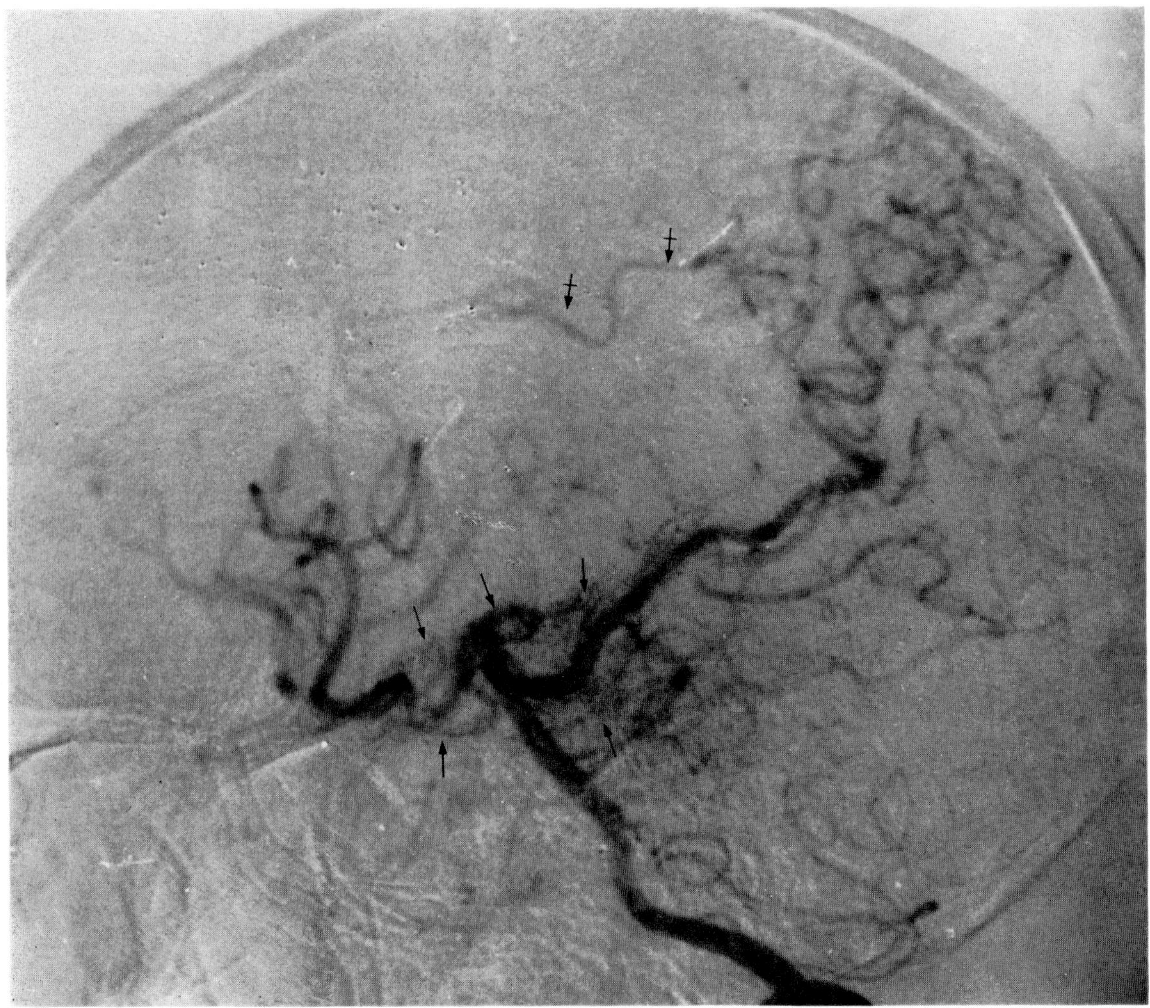

Fig. 393

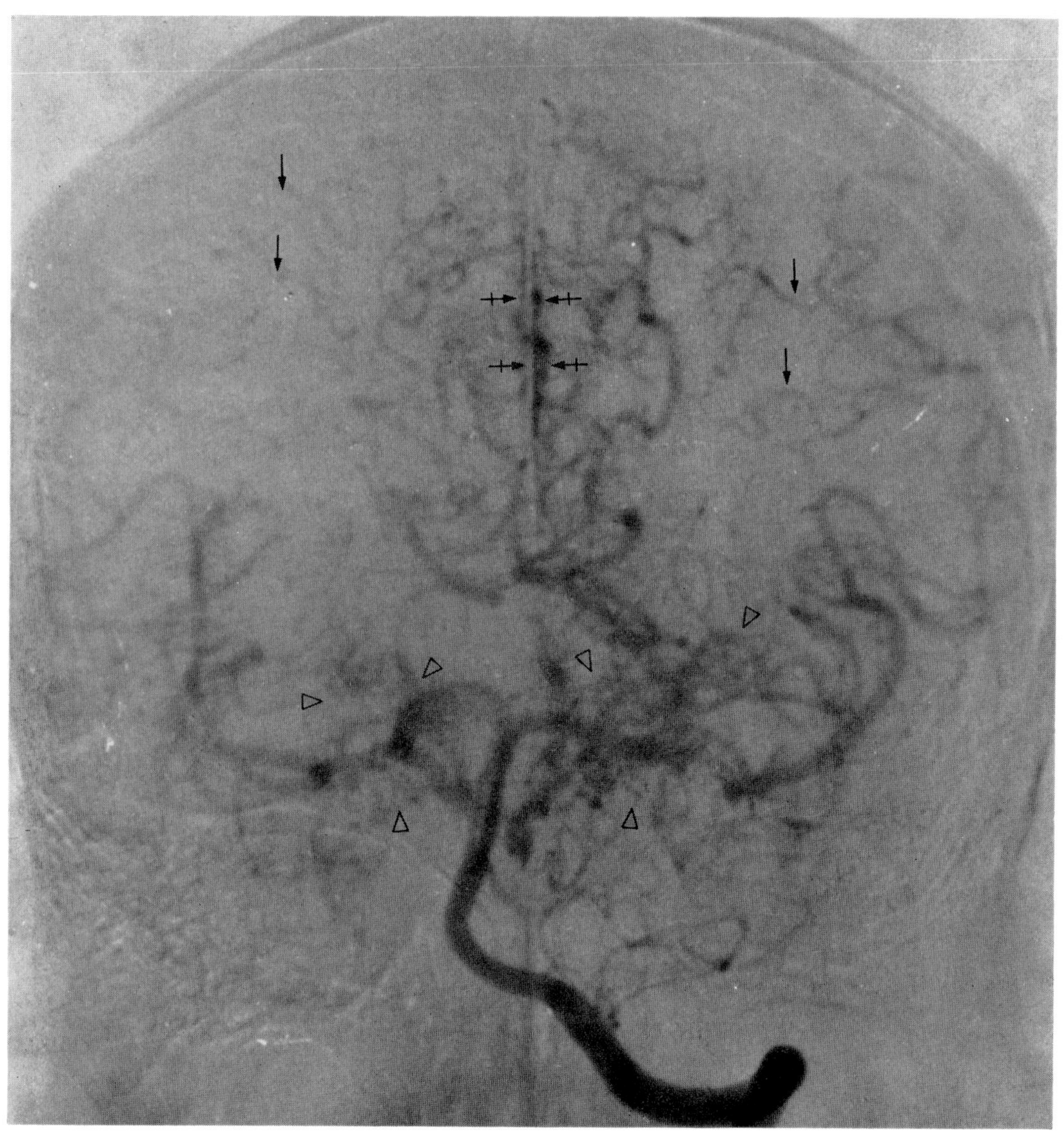

Fig. 394

Multiple Progressive Intracranial Occlusions

A 7-year-old female: Figs. 395–398

Fig. 395 Arterial phase in the lateral projection. There is extensive collateral development of fine vessels in the region of the basal ganglia, which primarily consists of the thalamoperforate, posterior choroidal, lenticulostriate and anterior choroidal arteries. The colliculi quadrigemini artery probably participates in the collateral development. The left anterior and middle cerebral arteries are reconstituted by these collaterals and by the posterior communicating arteries.

Fig. 396 Arterial phase in the Towne projection. The reconstitution of the right middle and anterior cerebral artery is poor from the vertebrobasilar system compared with the left middle and anterior cerebral arteries.

Fig. 397 Arterial phase of the left common carotid angiogram. The supraclinoid portion of the internal carotid artery is completely occluded (an arrowhead). There are rete mirabile collaterals from the anterior ethmoidal (an arrow) and posterior ethmoidal (2 opposing arrows) arteries of the ophthalmic artery as well as from the anterior (a crossed arrow) and posterior (2 crossed arrows) branches of the middle meningeal artery. The anterior cerebral artery is faintly reconstituted.

Fig. 398 Arterial phase of the right common carotid angiogram. The supraclinoid portion of the internal carotid artery is occluded (an open arrowhead). The rete mirabile collaterals are formed from the anterior falx (an arrow), anterior ethmoidal (2 arrows) and posterior ethmoidal (3 arrows) arteries of the ophthalmic artery. The ophthalmic artery is enlarged. The anterior (a crossed arrow) and posterior (2 crossed arrows) branches of the middle meningeal artery are slightly dilated for formation of collaterals. The meningohypophyseal artery is also dilated (closed arrowheads).

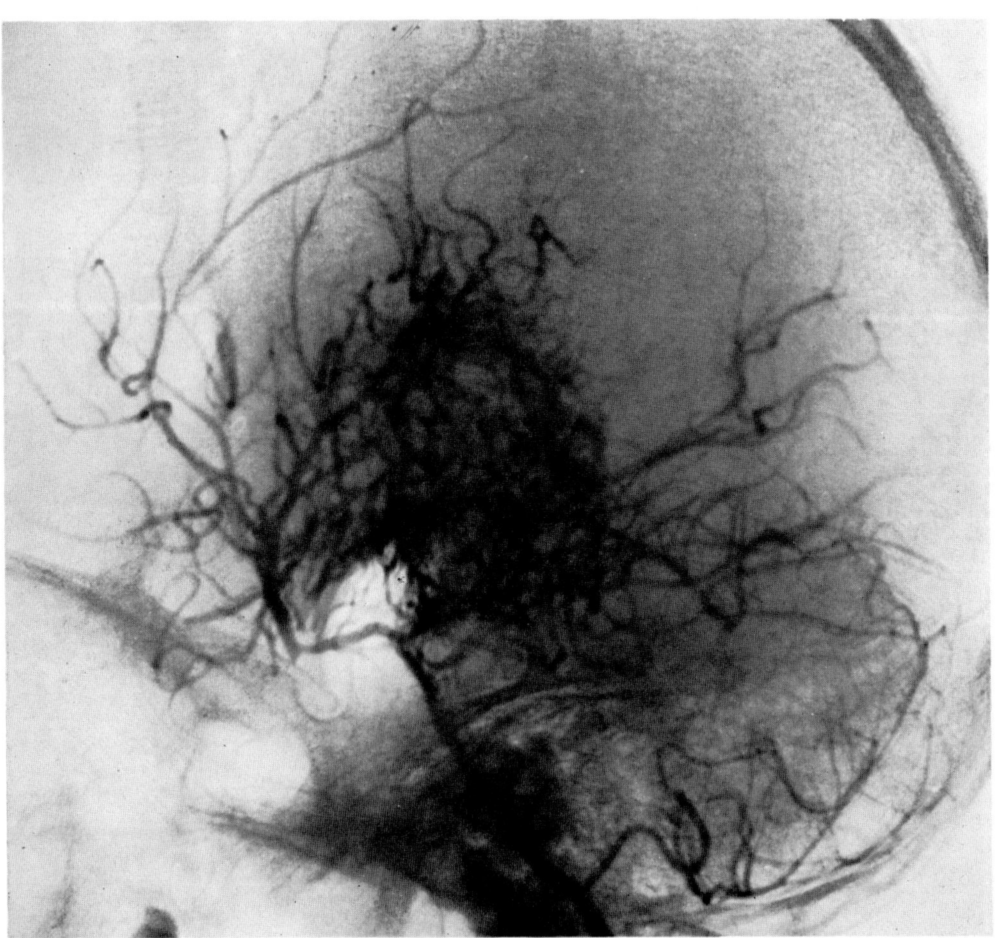

Fig. 395

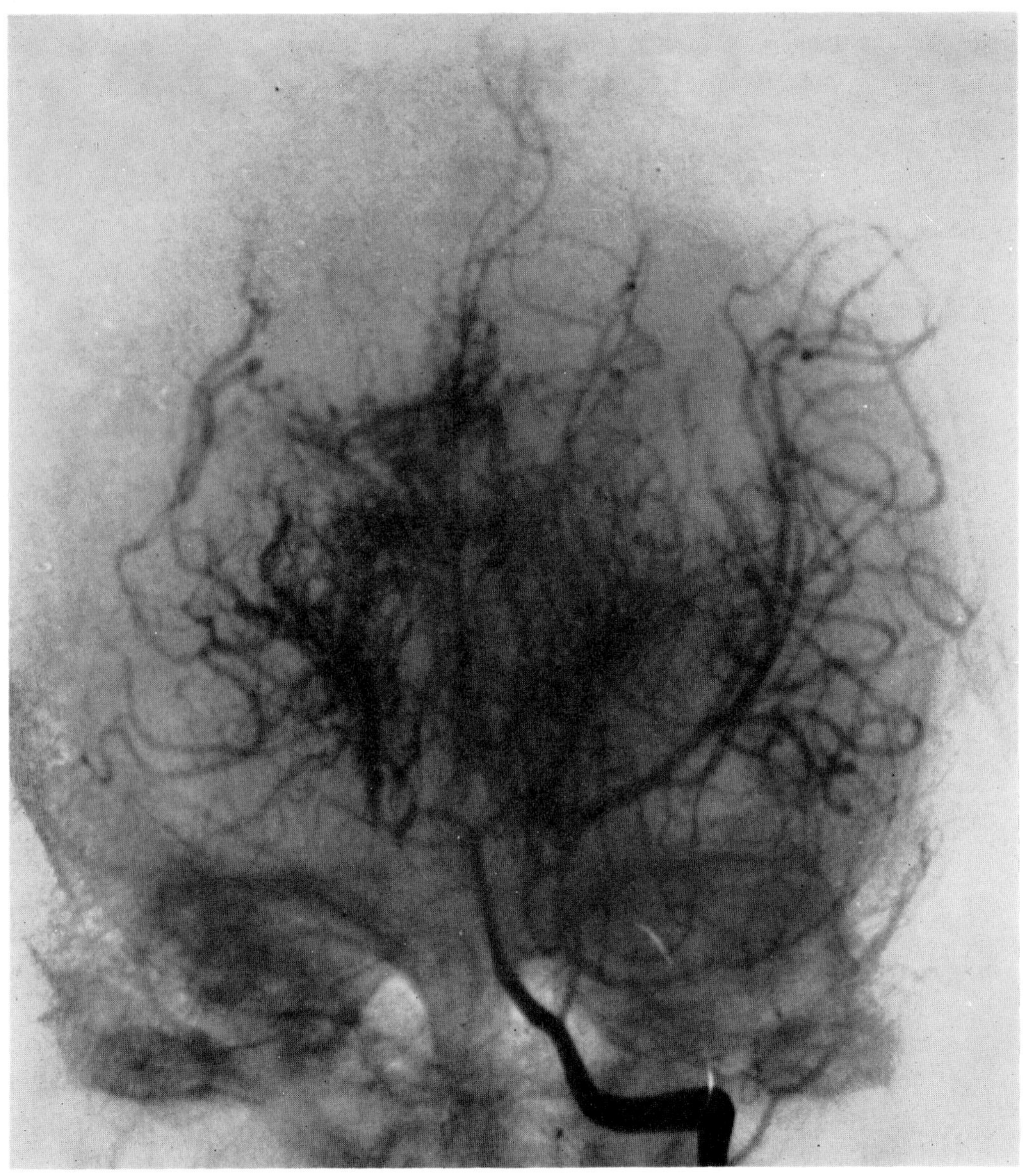

Fig. 396

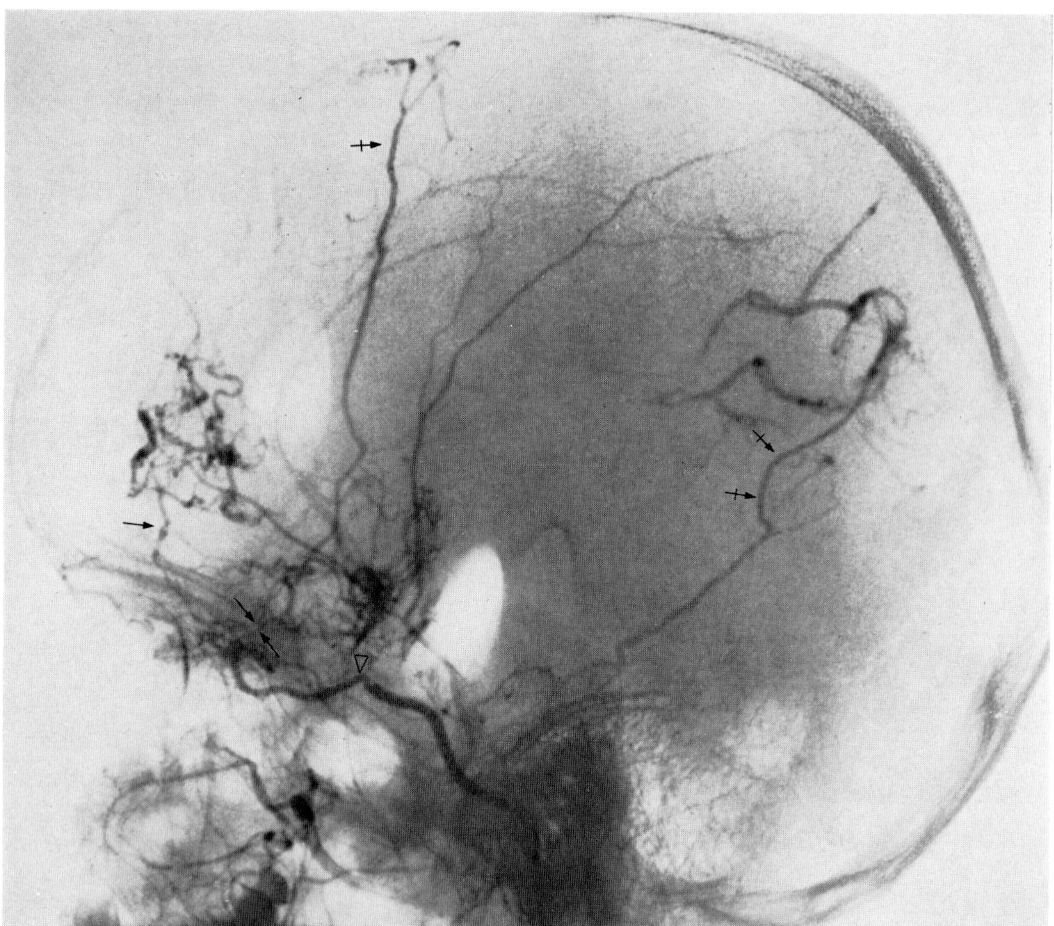

Fig. 397

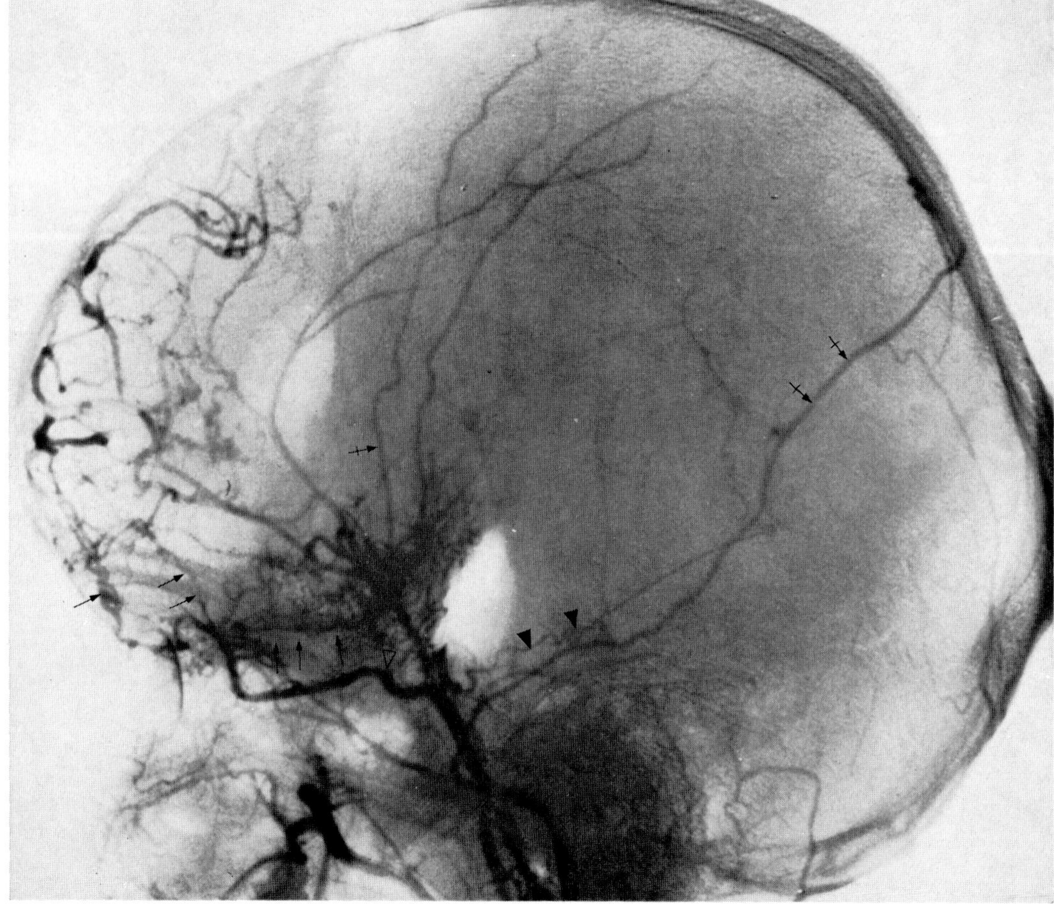

Fig. 398

Multiple Progressive Intracranial Occlusions

A 9-year-old female: Figs. 399 and 400

Fig. 399 Arterial phase in the lateral projection. The collaterals are formed by the thalamoperforate (2 arrows), posterior choroidal (2 crossed arrows), posterior pericallosal (2 open arrowheads) and posterior communicating arteries (2 closed arrowheads) to reconstitute the middle and anterior cerebral arteries. There are leptomeningeal collaterals from the posterior cerebral to the middle cerebral arteries. The collateral network in the basal ganglia is not marked in this case.

Fig. 400 Arterial phase in the Towne projection. Reconstitution of the middle cerebral artery is primarily from the posterior communicating artery. On the carotid angiograms, there was complete occlusion of the supraclinoid portion of both internal carotid arteries. There were extensive rete mirabile collaterals.

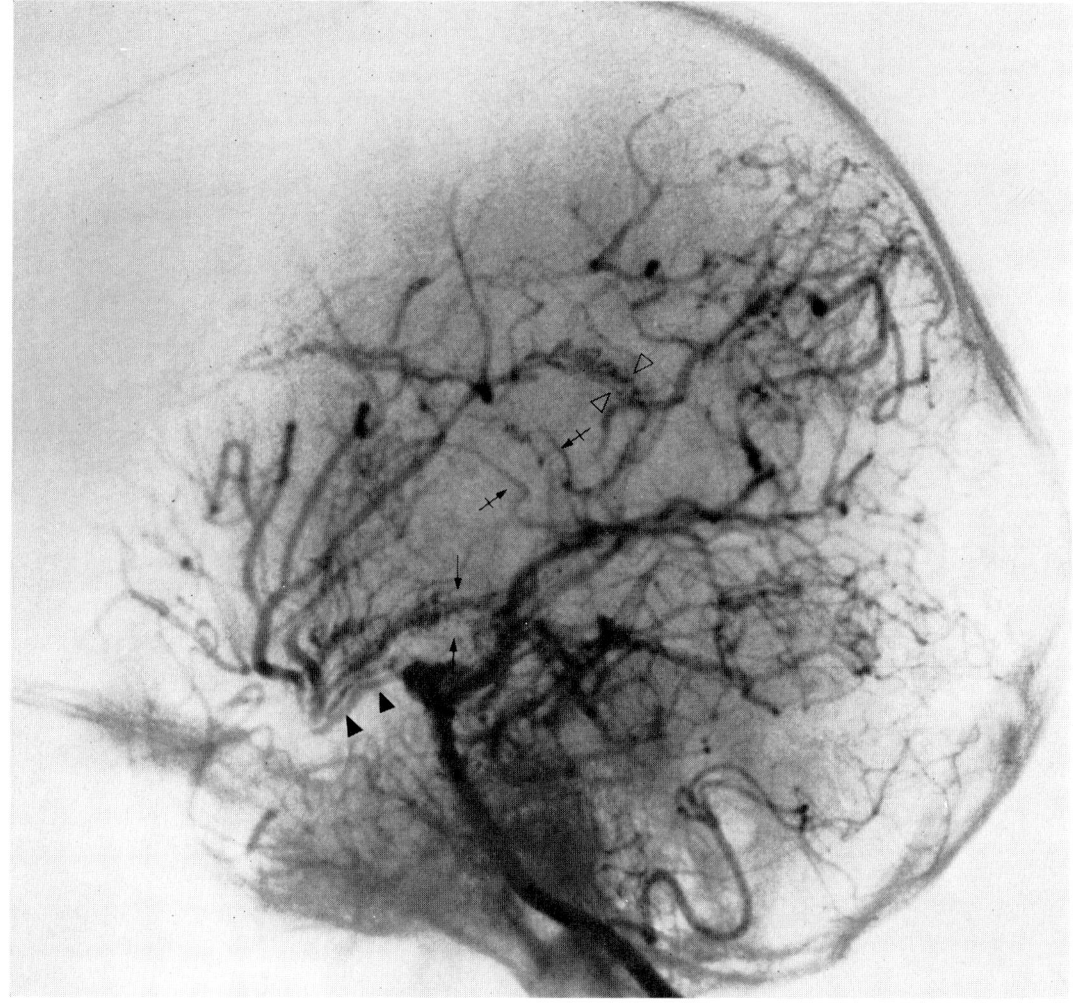

Fig. 399

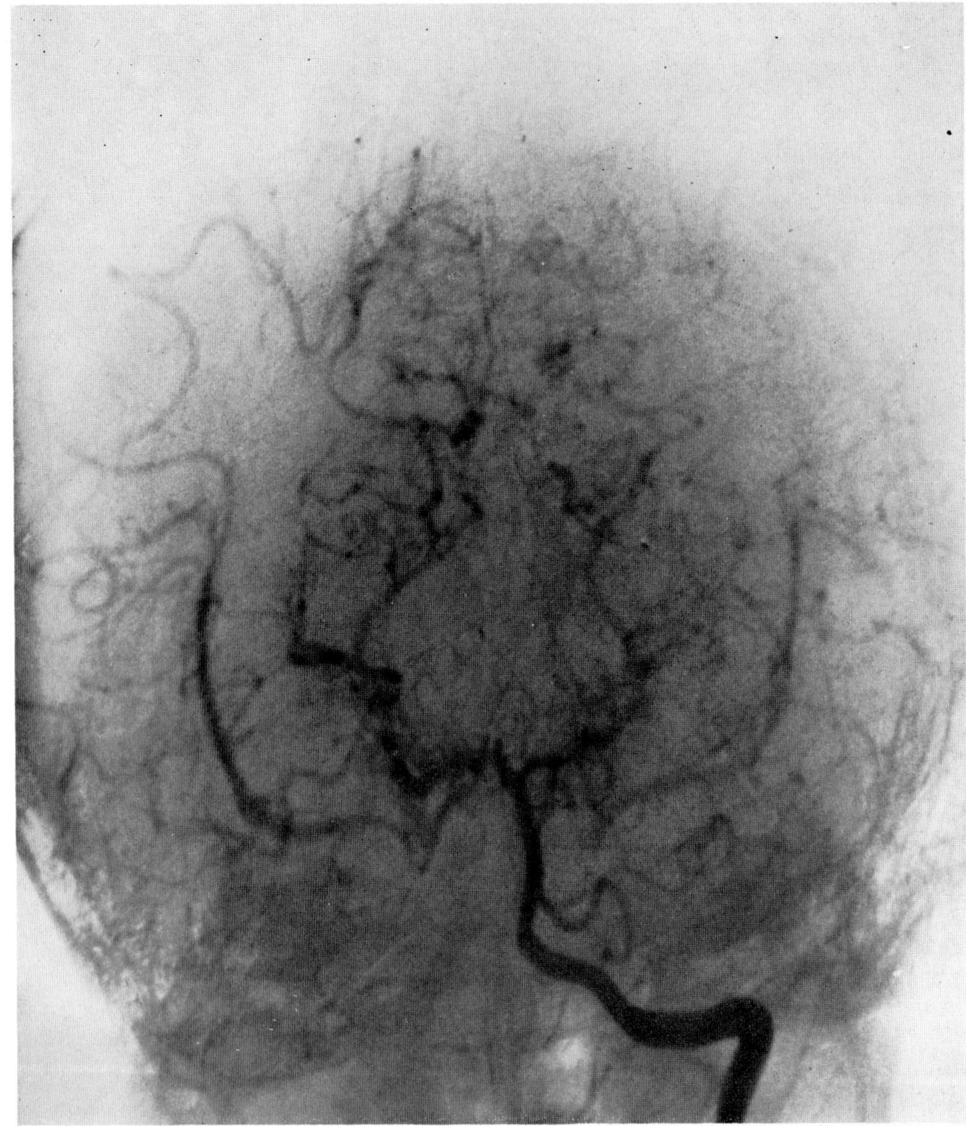

Fig. 400

Multiple Progressive Intracranial Occlusions

An 8-year-old male: Figs. 401–404

Fig. 401 Arterial phase in the lateral projection. There is development of a network of fine vessels in the region of the basal ganglia. The thalamoperforate, posterior pericallosal, posterior choroidal and lenticulostriate arteries participate in formation of this network. The posterior communicating artery is not demonstrated in this case. The proximal segment of the posterior cerebral artery is occluded (an arrow) with reconstitution of the distal segment (2 crossed arrows).

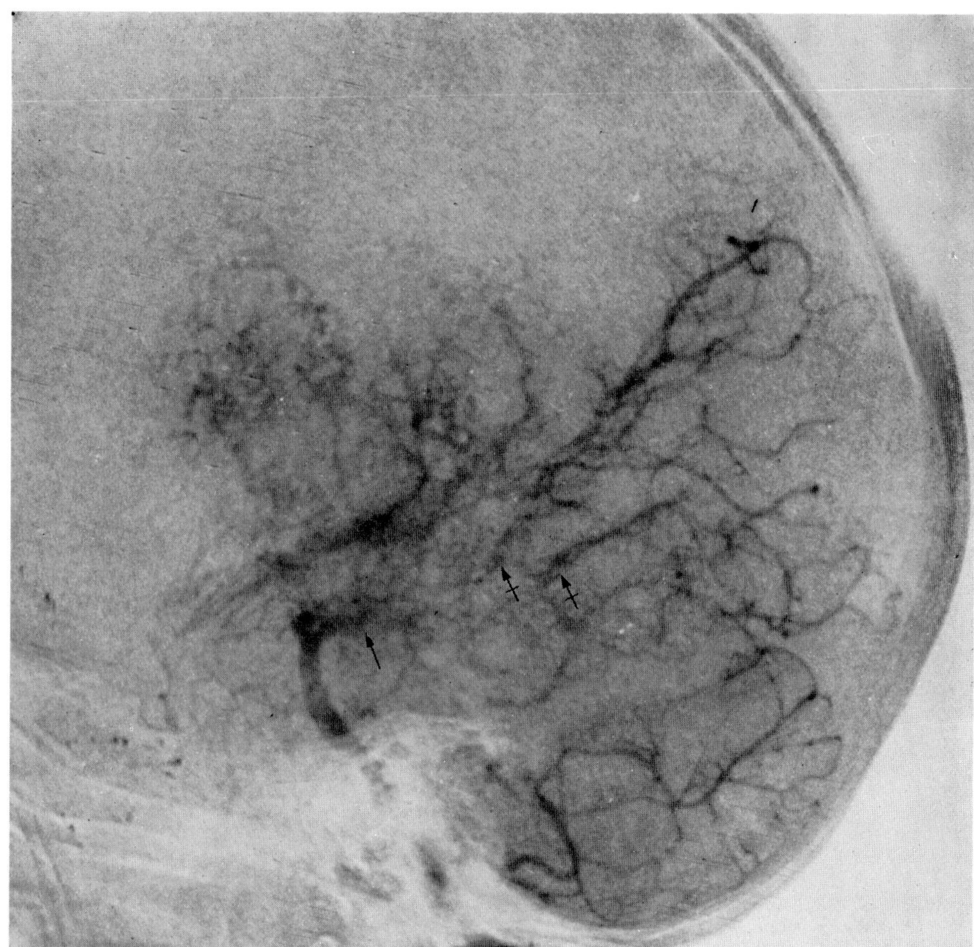

Fig. 401

Fig. 402 Arterial phase in the Towne projection. The collateral developments are observed to good advantage. The left posterior cerebral artery is occluded (an arrow) and reconstituted (a crossed arrow). The medial posterior choroidal artery is enlarged and demonstrated well (2 arrowheads).

Fig. 403 Arterial phase of the left common carotid angiogram in the lateral projection. The supraclinoid portion of the internal carotid artery is occluded (an arrow) with reconstitution of the anterior cerebral artery from the multiple unnamed collaterals (3 open arrowheads) and the posterior ethmoidal artery of the ophthalmic artery (2 closed arrowheads). The anterior falx artery is slightly enlarged (2 crossed arrows). A rete mirabile is formed by the posterior branch of the middle meningeal artery (3 arrows).

Fig. 404 Arterial phase of the right common carotid angiogram. The supraclinoid portion of the internal carotid artery is occluded and reconstituted by multiple unnamed collaterals (3 open arrowheads), and the anterior (2 crossed arrows) and the posterior (2 closed arrowheads) ethmoidal arteries of the ophthalmic artery. The posterior branch of the middle cerebral artery is supplied by a rete mirabile collateral of the middle meningeal artery (2 arrows).

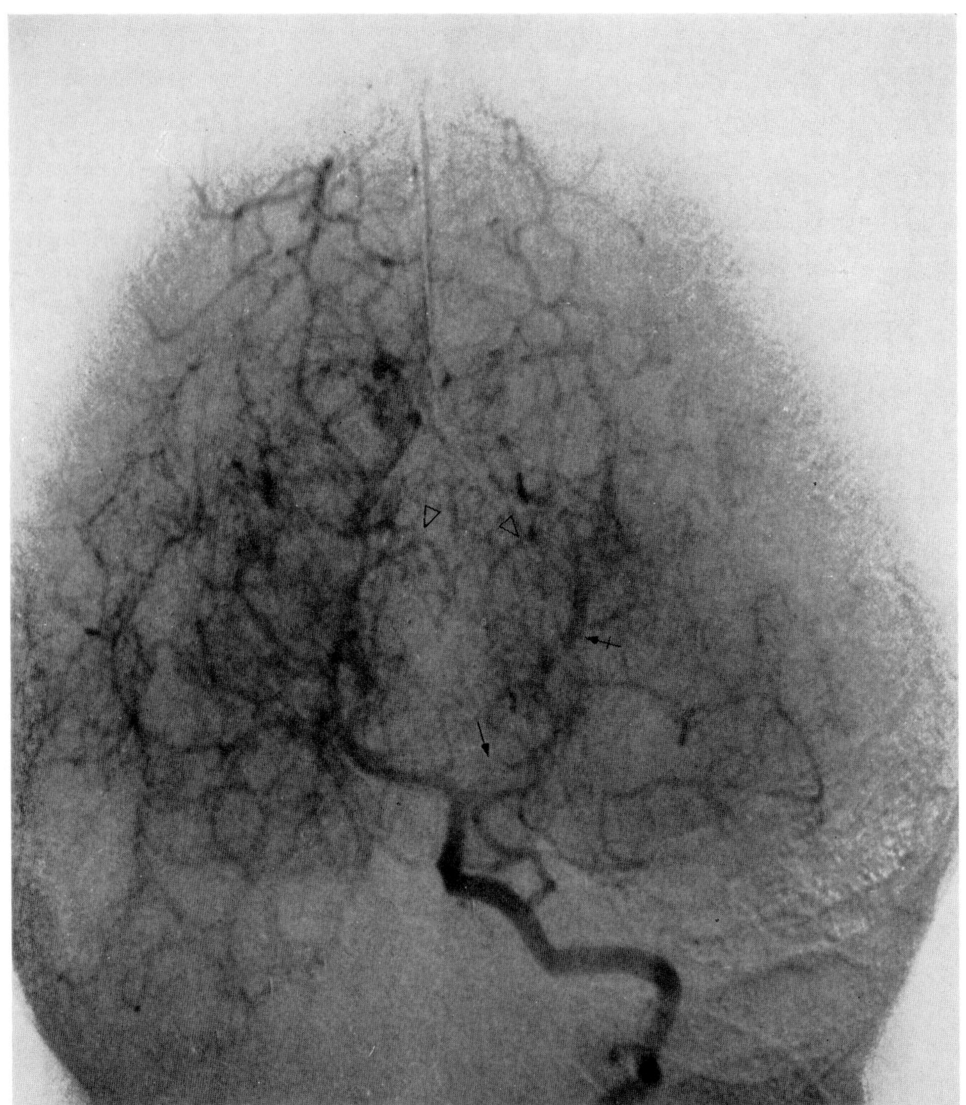

Fig. 402

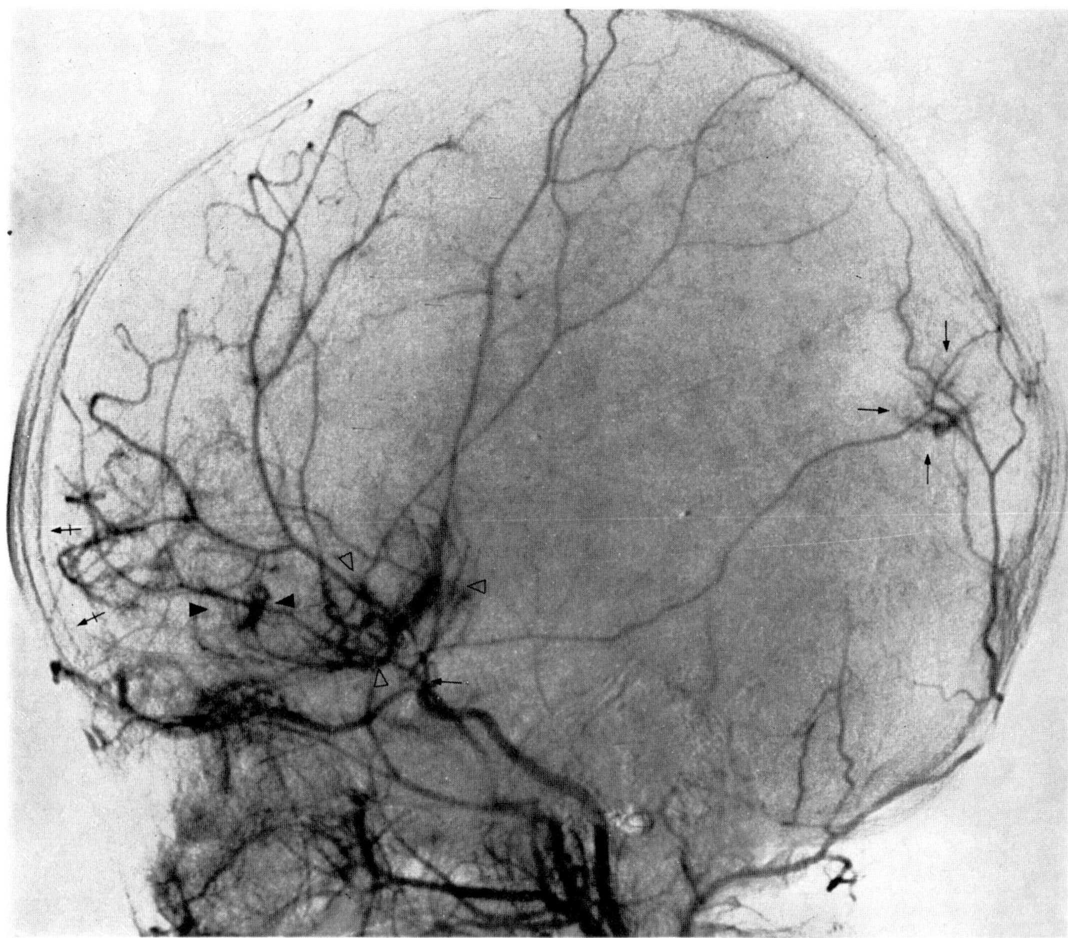

Fig. 403

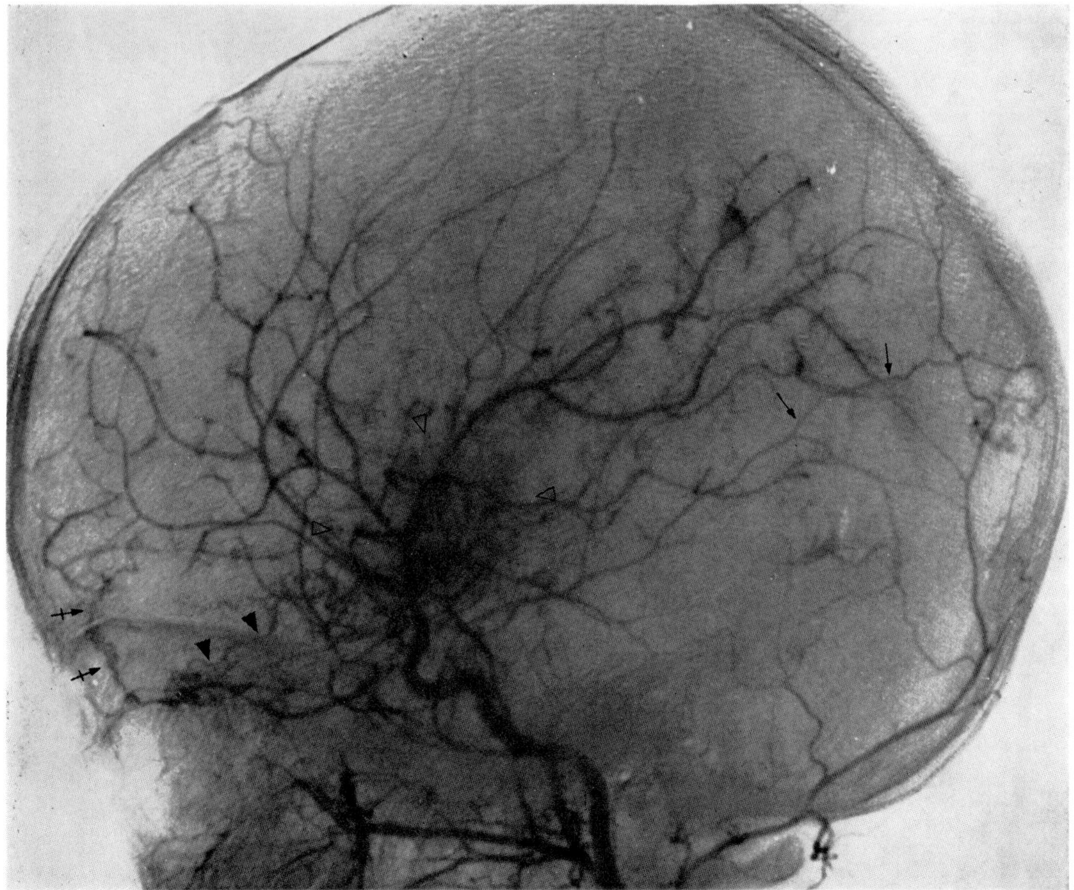

Fig. 404

Multiple Progressive Intracranial Occlusions

A 2-year-old female: Figs. 405–407

Fig. 405 Arterial phase in the lateral projection. There is an extensive network of fine vessels in the basal ganglia. Both posterior cerebral arteries are occluded with reconstitution of the right posterior cerebral artery (2 arrows).

Fig. 406 Capillary phase in the lateral projection. There is reconstitution of the distal segments of middle (2 crossed arrows) and posterior cerebral arteries (2 arrows).

Fig. 407 Arterial phase in the Towne projection. The collateral network with reconstitution of the right posterior cerebral artery is demonstrated to good advantage (2 arrows). There is visualization of the occipital artery via the muscular branches and a communicating vessel (2 crossed arrows).

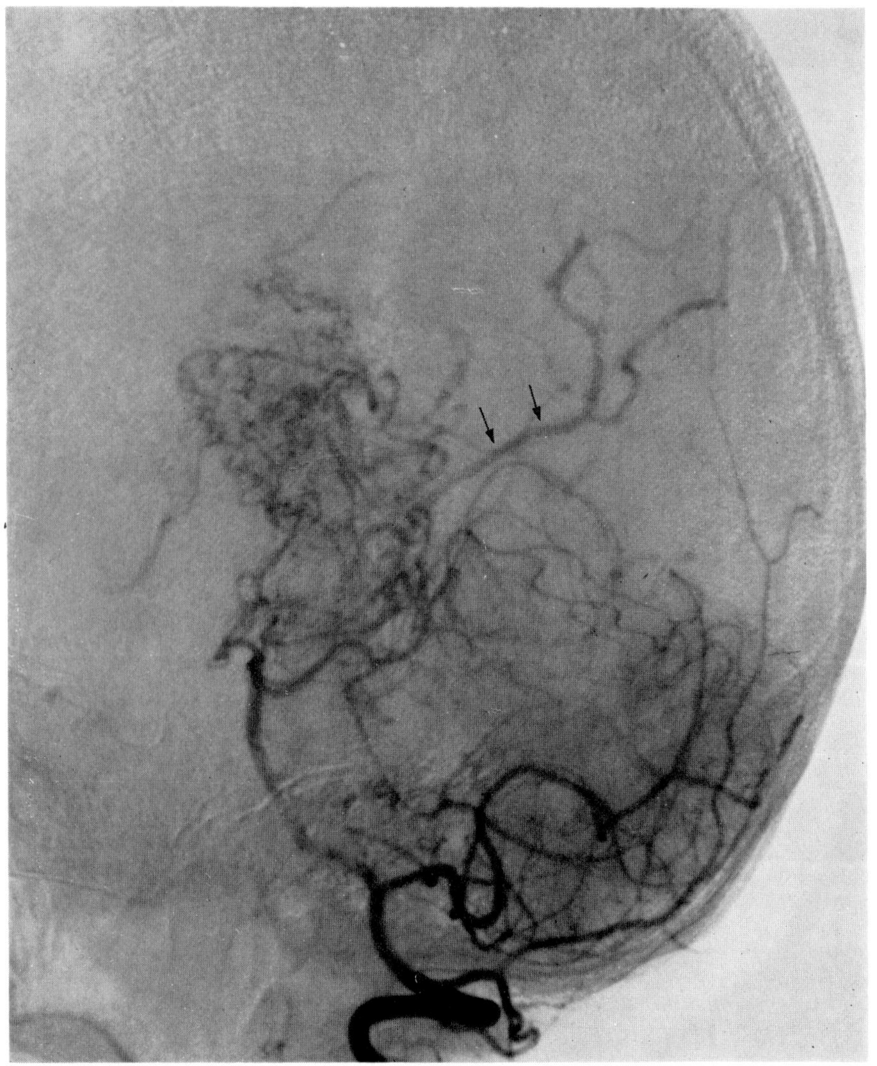

Fig. 405

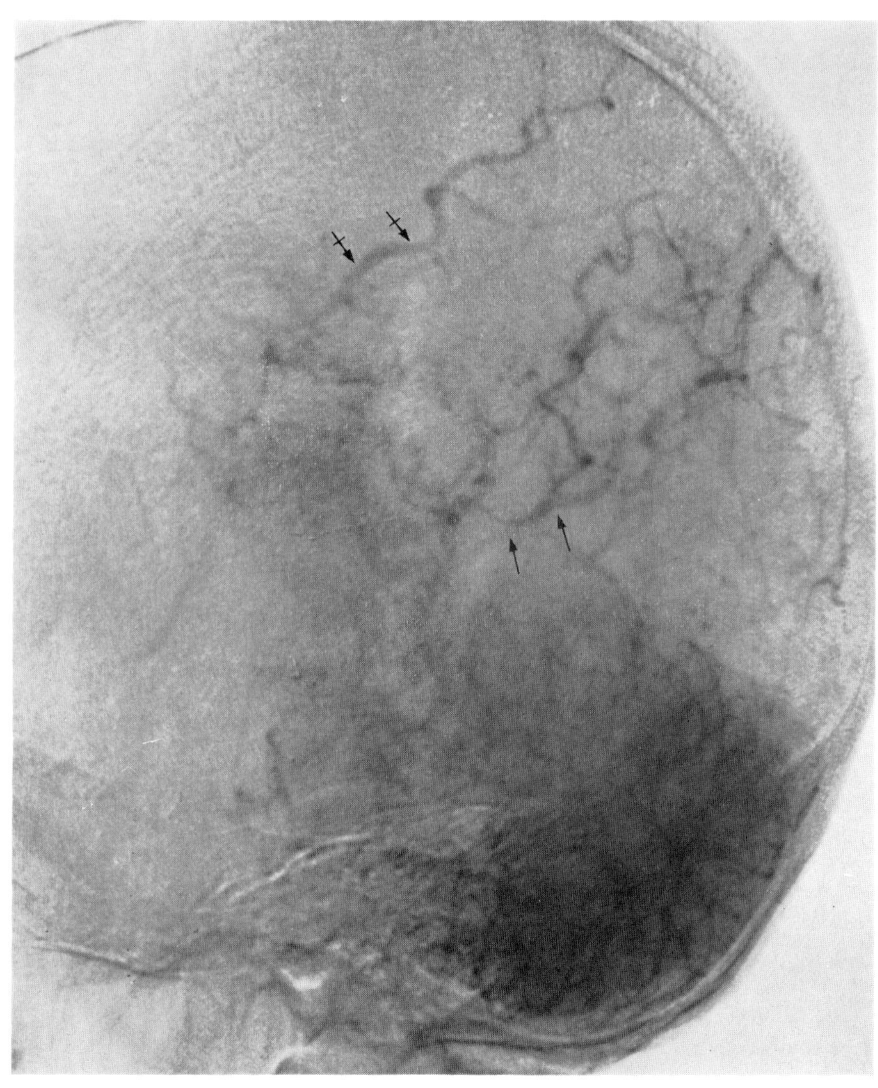

Fig. 406

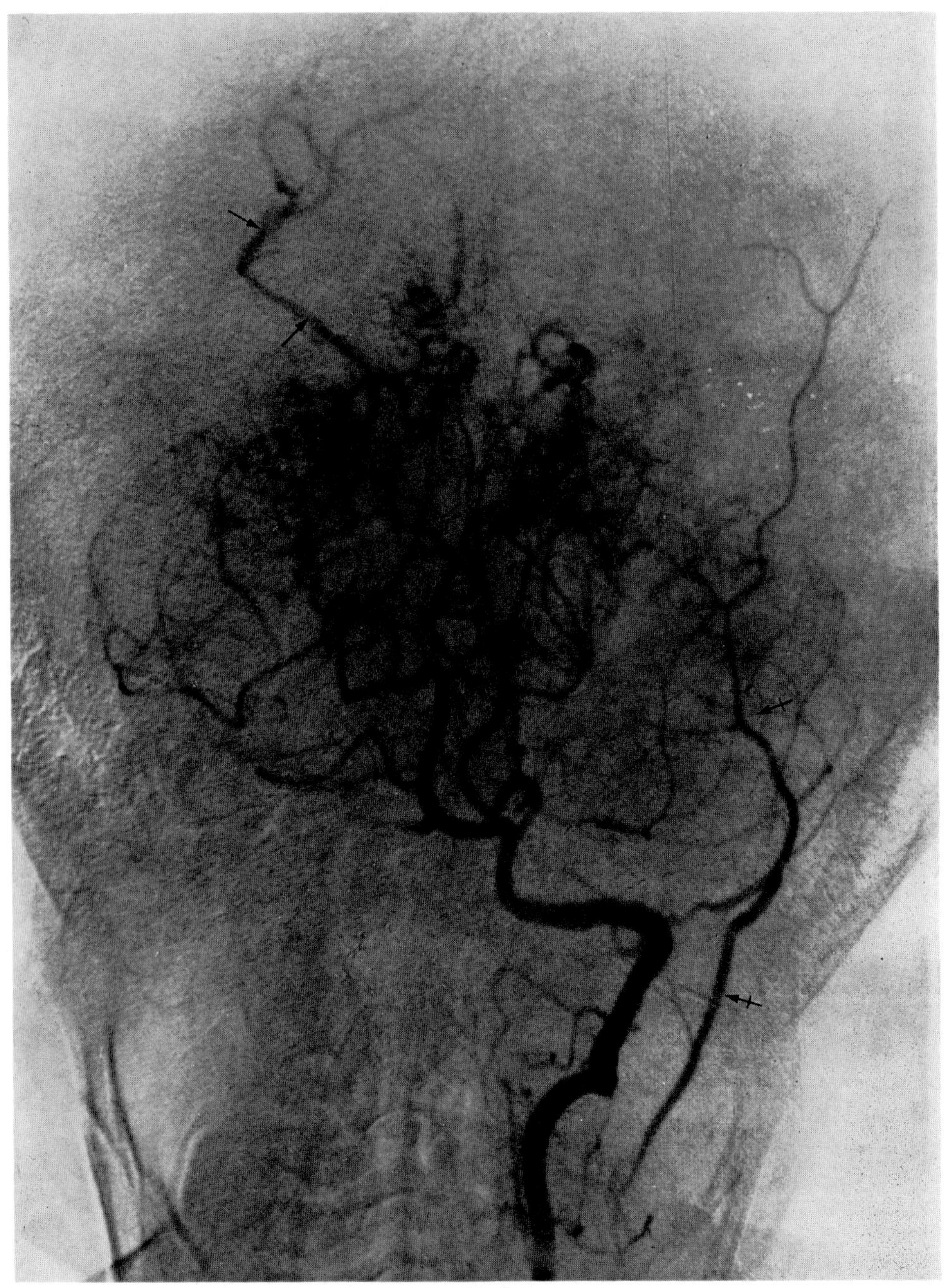

Fig. 407

INTRACEREBRAL HEMORRHAGE

Angiographic findings of hemorrhages in the cerebellum or pons are those of avascular space-taking lesions in the cerebellum and pons, which have been discussed in the sections of intracranial tumors. Aneurysms and arteriovenous malformations may be demonstrated as the source of bleeding. Extravasation of contrast media may be demonstrated.

Infratentorial hemorrhage occurs in the brain stem and the cerebellar hemisphere. The intracerebellar hemorrhage develops near the dentate nucleus and frequently ruptures into the fourth ventricle. Therefore, intracerebellar hemorrhage usually shows angiographic findings of a posterior fossa mass without evidence of midline shift. Intracerebellar hemorrhage with marked lateral extension reveals midline shift on vertebral angiograms. Extravasation of contrast media may also be observed if angiography is performed during active bleeding. Hemorrhage into the brain stem shows angiographic findings similar to a brain stem tumor.

Intracerebellar Hemorrhage

A 50-year-old female: Figs. 408–411 (Through the courtesy of Dr. Yamaguchi, Research Institute of Brain and Blood Vessels, Akita)

Fig. 408 Arterial phase in the lateral projection. The basilar artery is compressed against the clivus and the quadrigeminal, ambient and the superior culminate segments of the superior cerebellar artery are markedly displaced superiorly in an arcuate fashion (3 crossed arrows). There is extravasation of contrast media superimposed over the fourth ventricle (an arrow). The posterior inferior cerebellar artery is displaced anteriorly and downwards with angulation of the supratonsillar segment (an arrowhead). These findings suggest a large mass in the cerebellar hemisphere with hemorrhage.

Fig. 409 Venous phase in the lateral projection. The anterior pontomesencephalic vein is displaced against the clivus (2 crossed arrows). The precentral cerebellar vein is displaced anteriorly (2 closed arrowheads), and the superior vermian vein is displaced in the superior direction (2 open arrowheads). There is marked downward dislocation of the inferior vermian vein (3 arrows). Extravasation of contrast media is again seen (an arrow).

Fig. 410 Arterial phase in the Towne projection. The basilar artery is shifted to the left of the midline. The vermian branches of the left posterior inferior cerebellar artery are also displaced across the midline (2 arrows).

Fig. 411 Venous phase in the Towne projection. There is poor visualization of the posterior fossa veins on the right.

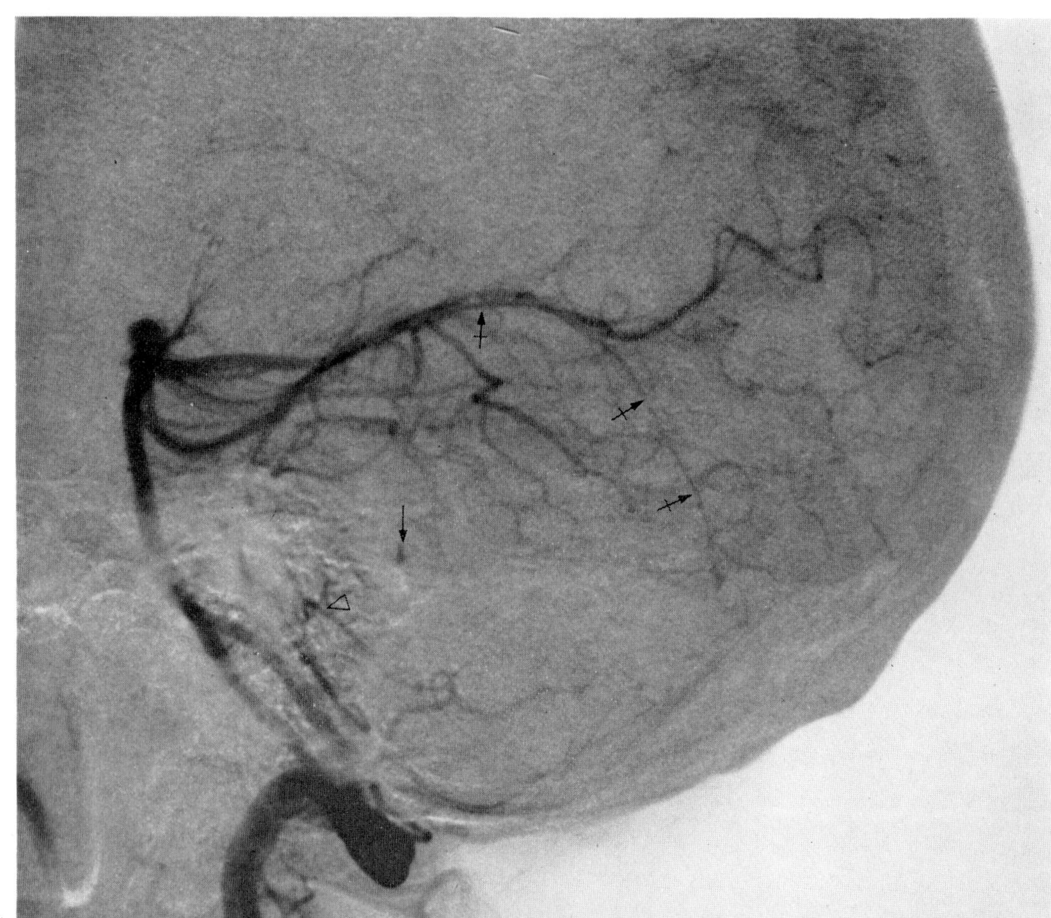

Fig. 408

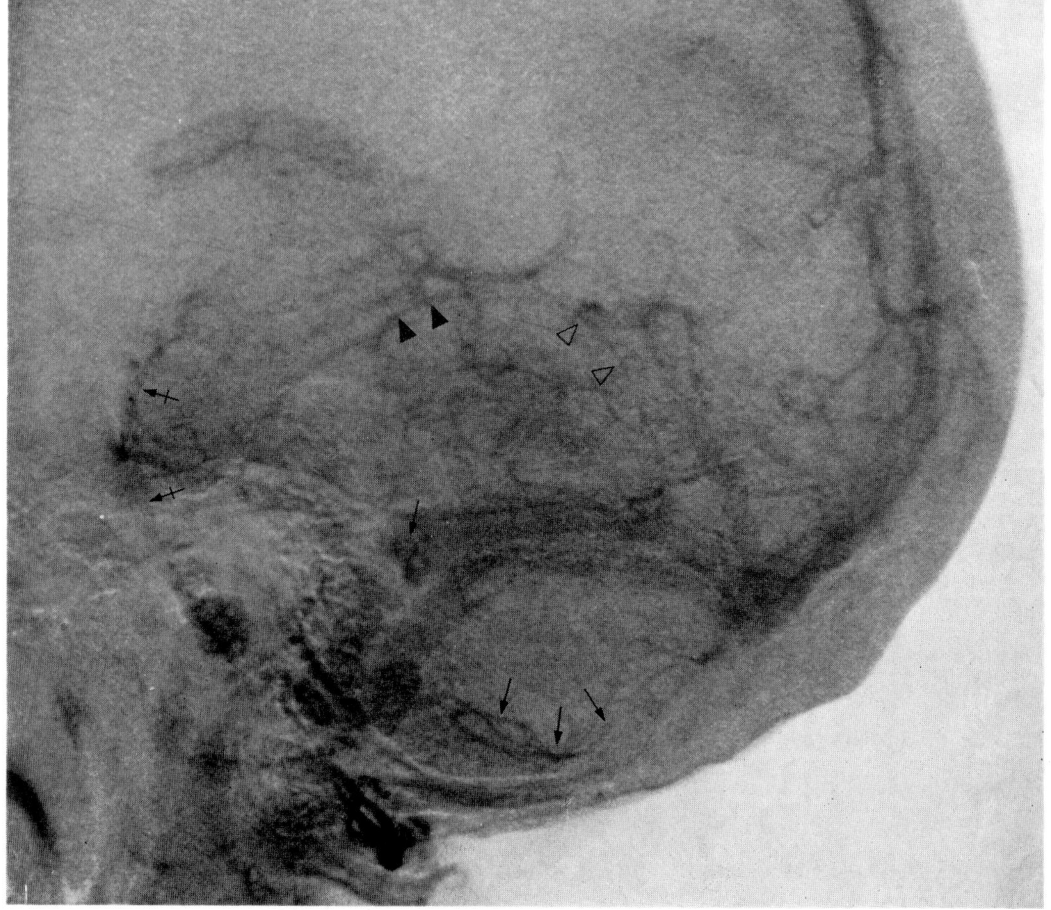

Fig. 409

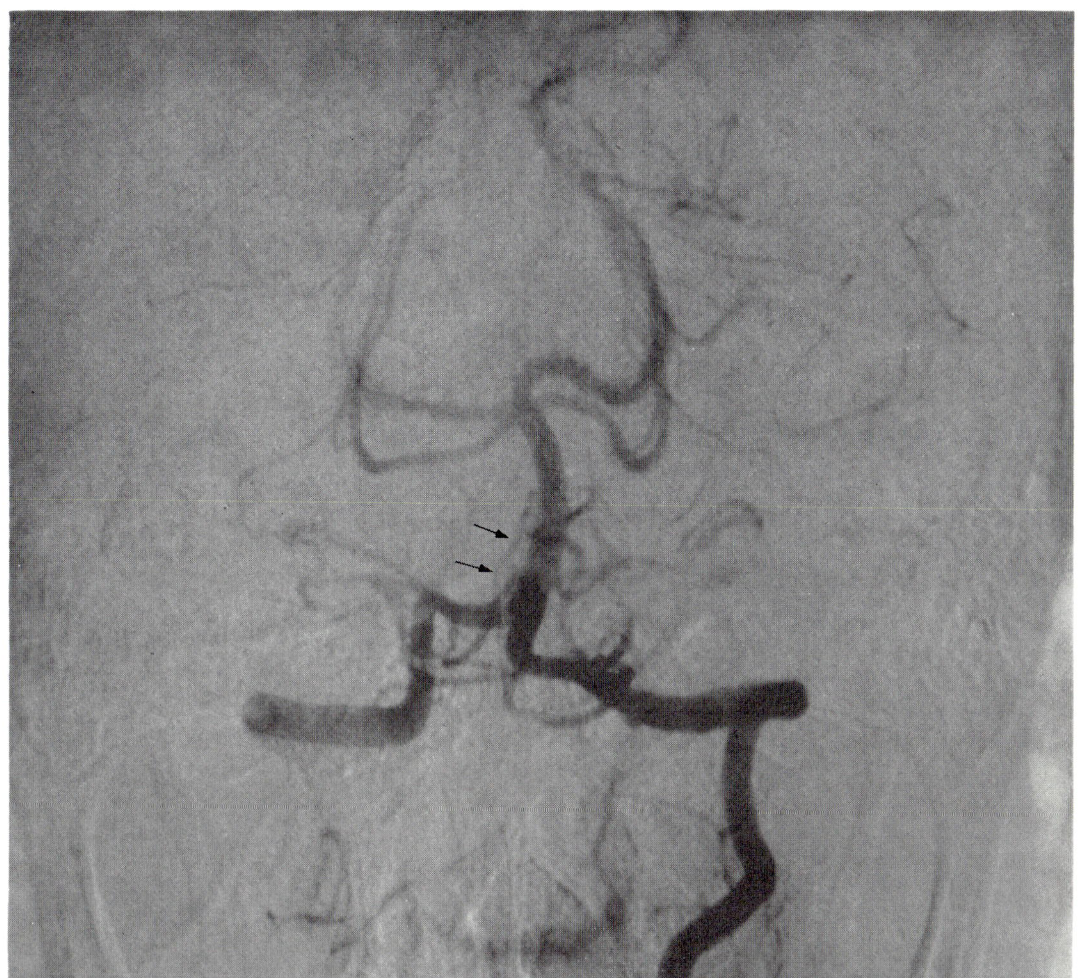

Fig. 410

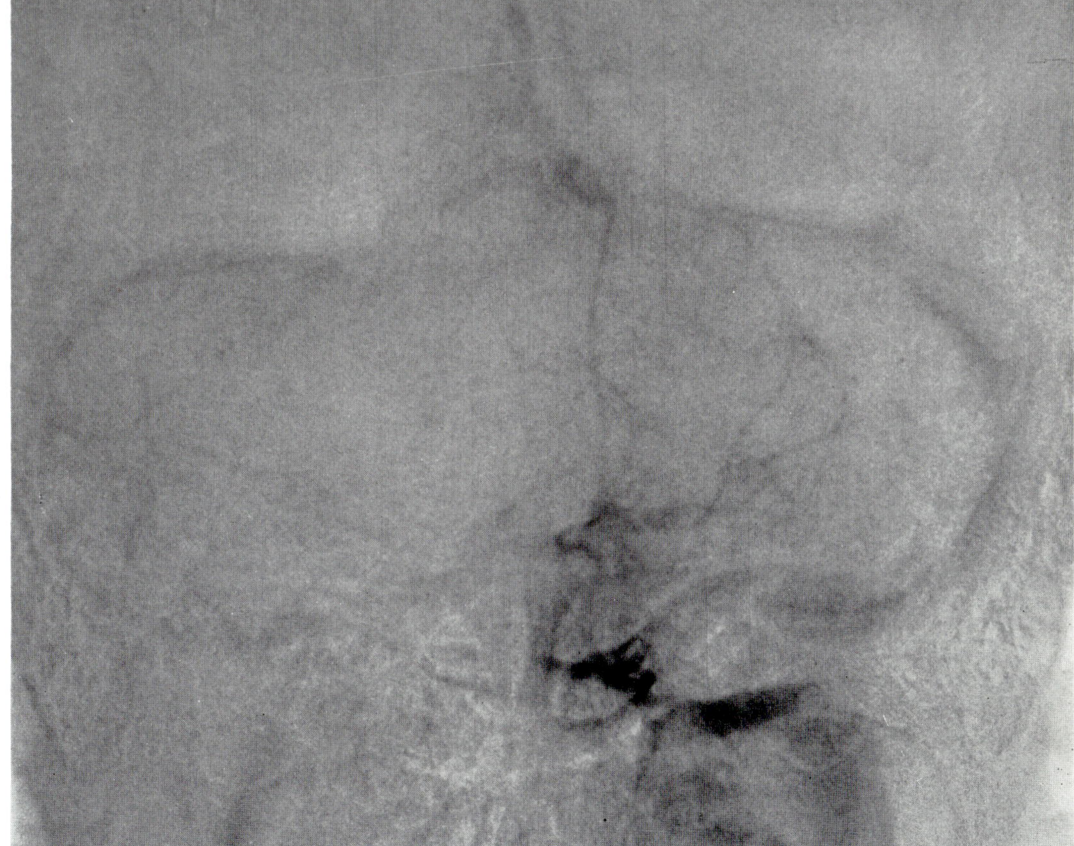

Fig. 411

Hemorrhage into the Upper Brain Stem

A 44-year-old male: Figs. 412 and 413 (Through the Courtesy of Dr. YAMAGUCHI, Research Institute of the Brain and Blood Vessels, Akita)

Fig. 412 Arterial phase in the lateral projection. The basilar artery is compressed against the clivus. The medial posterior choroidal artery is displaced backwards in an arcuate fashion (2 arrows). The lateral posterior choroidal artery is straightened, suggesting lateral displacement of this artery (2 crossed arrows).

Fig. 413 Venous phase in the lateral projection. The pontine segment of the anterior pontomesencephalic vein is displaced anteriorly (2 arrows) and the precentral cerebellar vein is displaced backwards (2 crossed arrows). All the angiographic findings point to a mass lesion in the midbrain and upper pons.

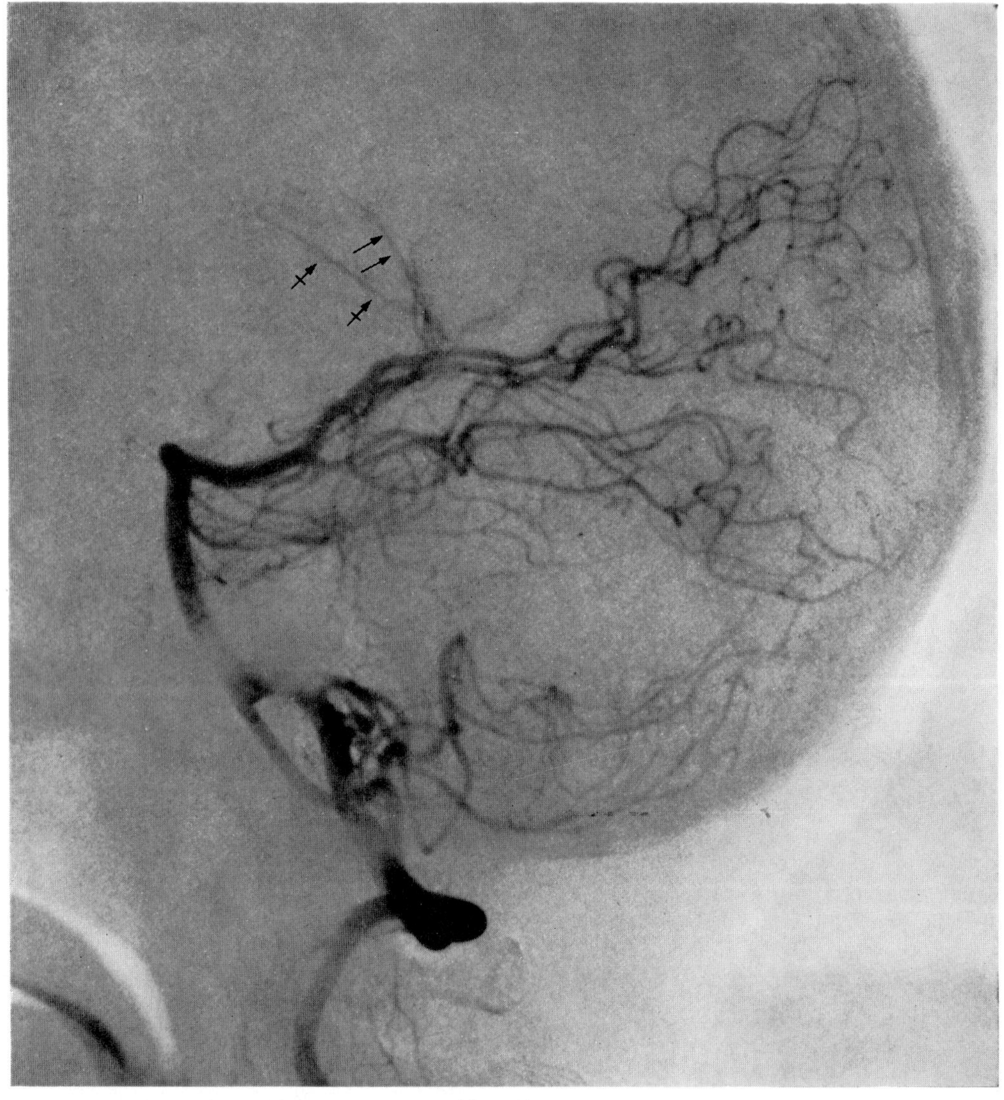

Fig. 412

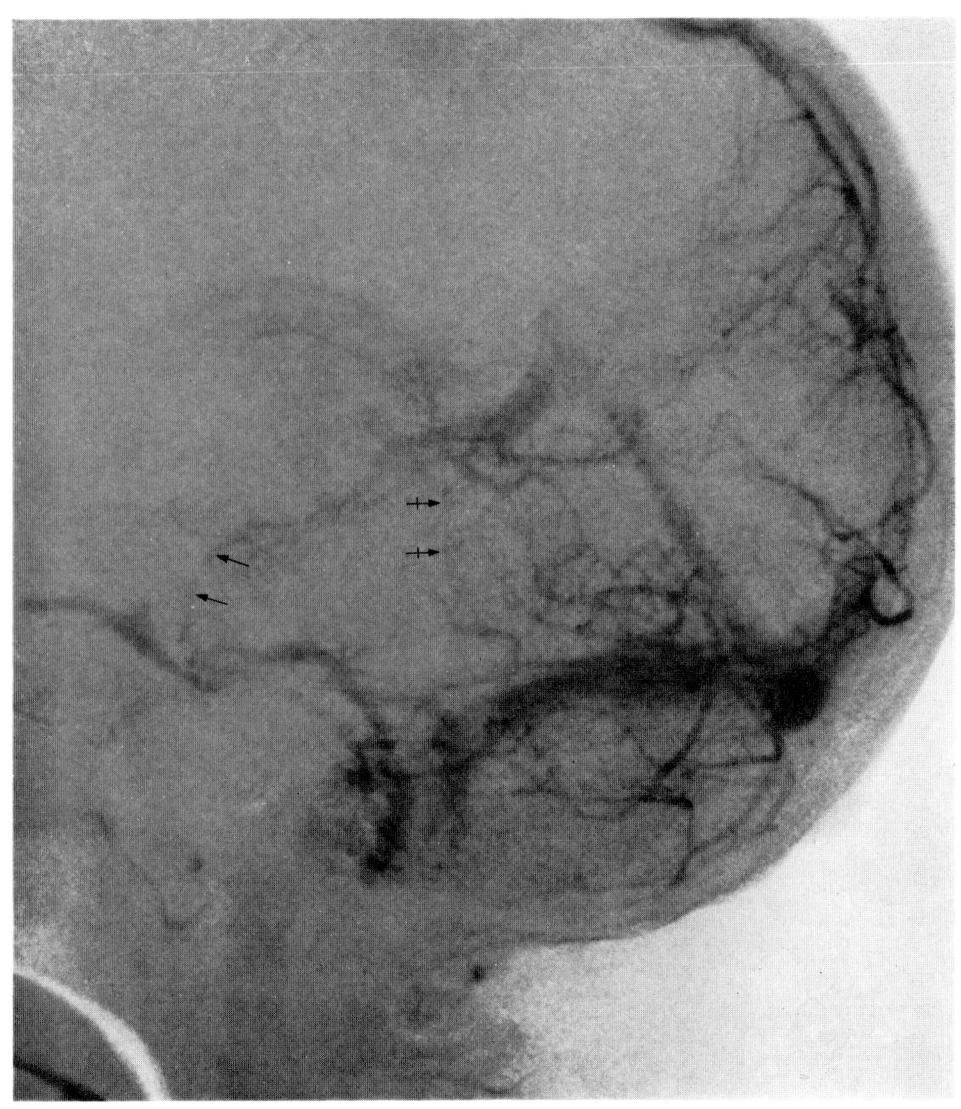

Fig. 413

Hemorrhage into the Lower Pons and Medulla due to Head Trauma

A 15-year-old male: Figs. 414 and 415

Fig. 414 Arterial phase in the lateral projection. The basilar and intracranial vertebral arteries are compressed against the clivus (3 arrows). The posterior medullary and the supratonsillar segments of the posterior inferior cerebellar arteries are displaced posteriorly with angulation of the supratonsillar segment (3 crossed arrows). The anterior and lateral medullary segments are stretched around the brain stem (3 arrowheads). The findings suggest a large mass lesion in the lower brain stem and medulla.

Fig. 415 Arterial phase in the Towne projection. The basilar artery is markedly spastic and elongated with displacement to the left (2 arrows).

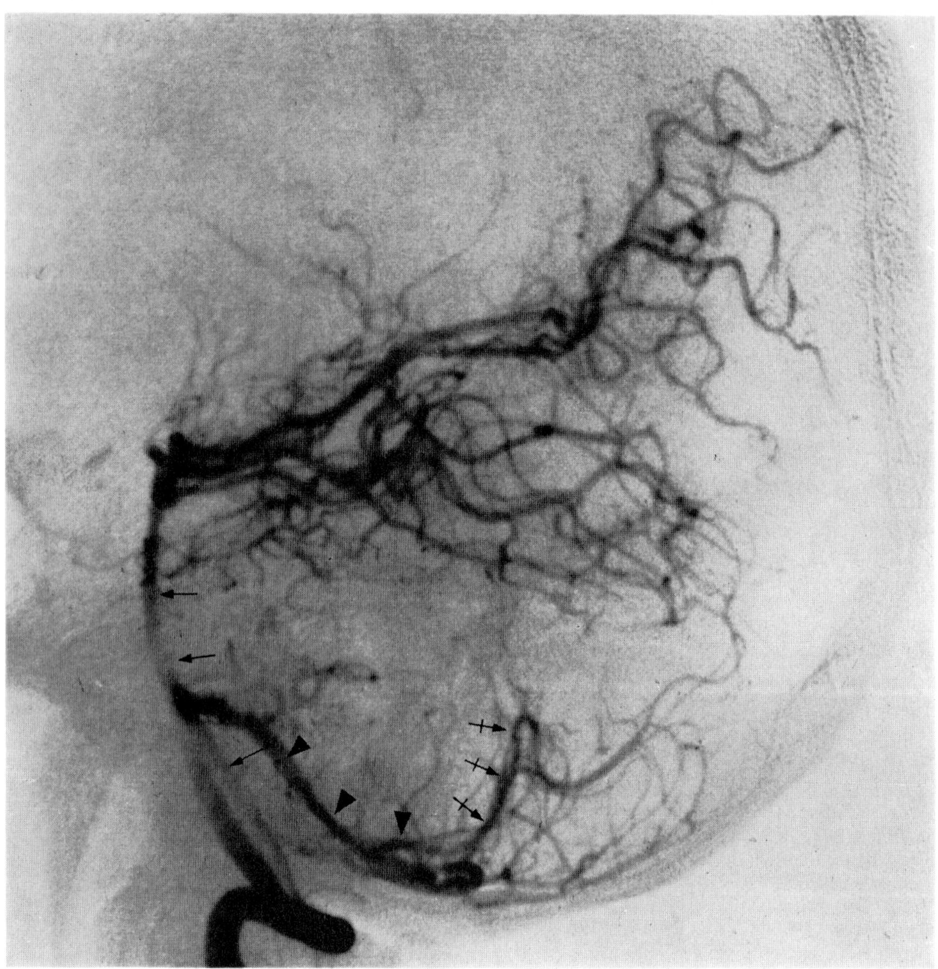

Fig. 414

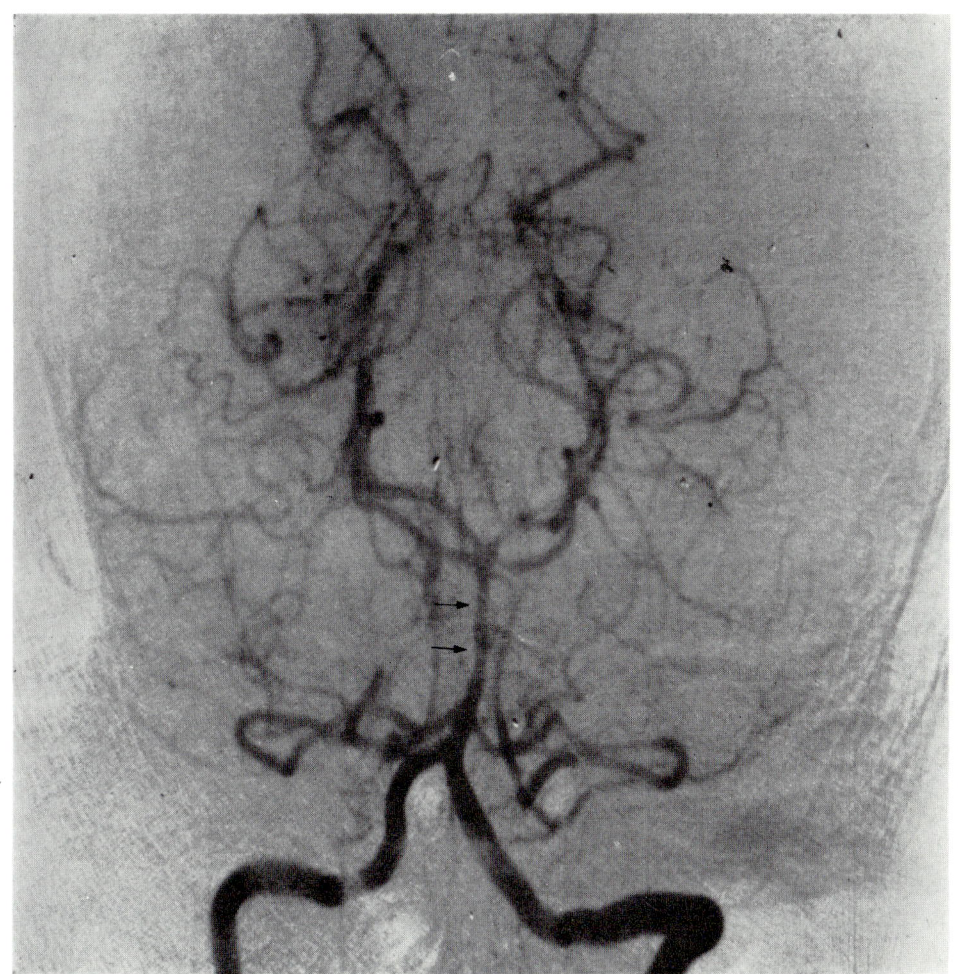

Fig. 415

Occipital Hematoma due to a Rupture of a Small Aneurysm of the Calcarine Artery

A 26-year-old male: Figs. 416–418

Fig. 416 Arterial phase in the lateral projection. The parieto-occipital artery is superiorly stretched in an arcuate fashion (3 arrows) with inferior displacement of a branch of the calcarine artery (2 open arrowheads), suggesting an avascular space-occupying lesion in the occipital lobe. There is a 3 mm aneurysm in the anterior portion of the avascular mass (a crossed arrow). The proximal posterior cerebral artery is slightly elevated (2 closed arrowheads).

Fig. 417 Venous phase in the lateral projection. The cortical veins of the occipital lobe are visualized poorly. Two veins are stretched in an arcuate fashion (3 arrows; 3 crossed arrows), suggesting an occipital mass.

Fig. 418 Arterial phase in the Towne projection. The parieto-occipital artery is displaced laterally in an arcuate fashion (5 arrows). The aneurysm (a crossed arrow) appears to arise from the calcarine artery (2 arrowheads).

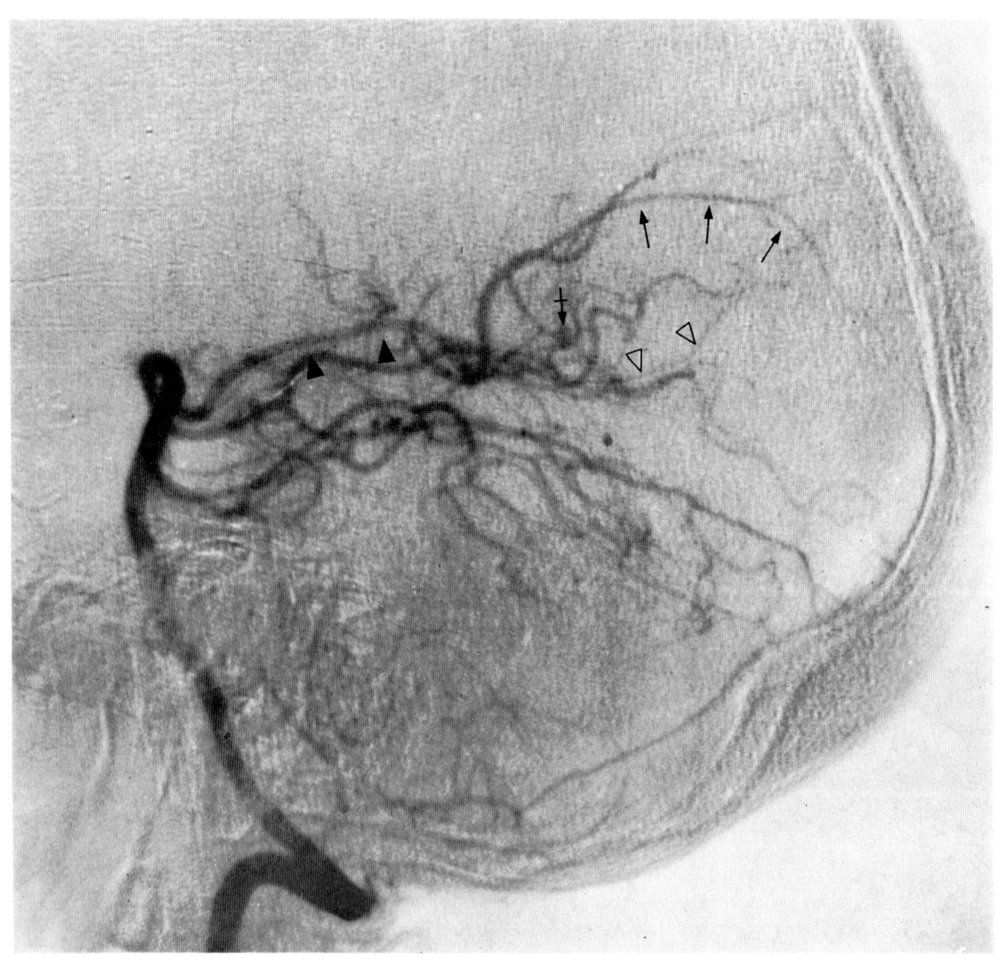

Fig. 416

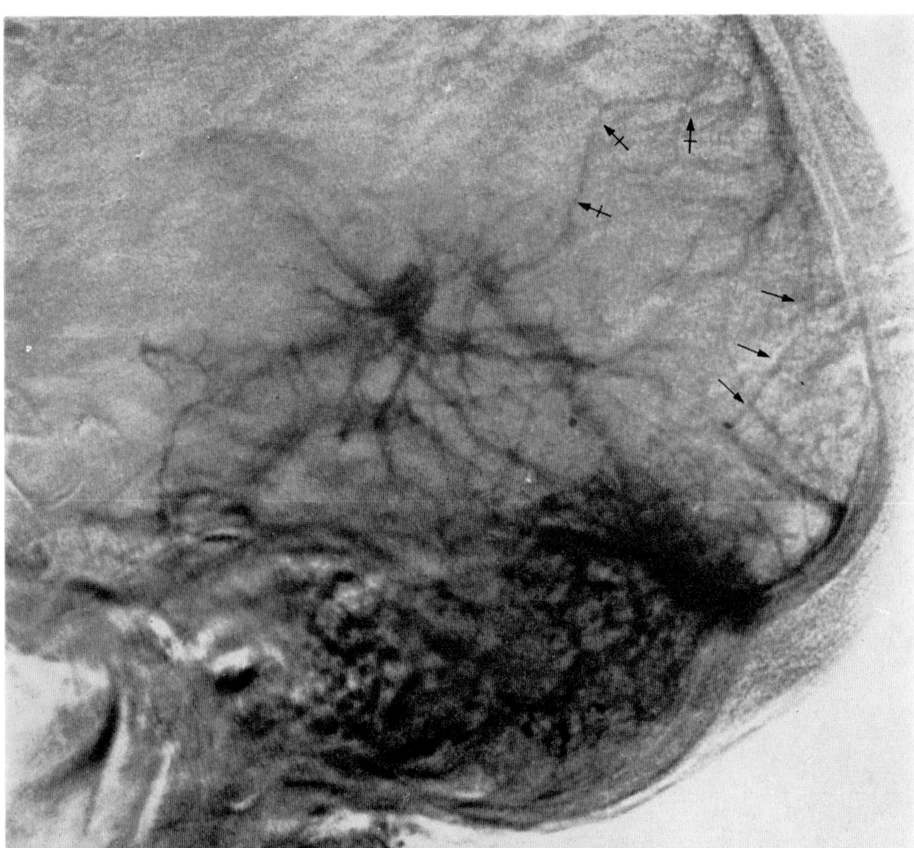

Fig. 417

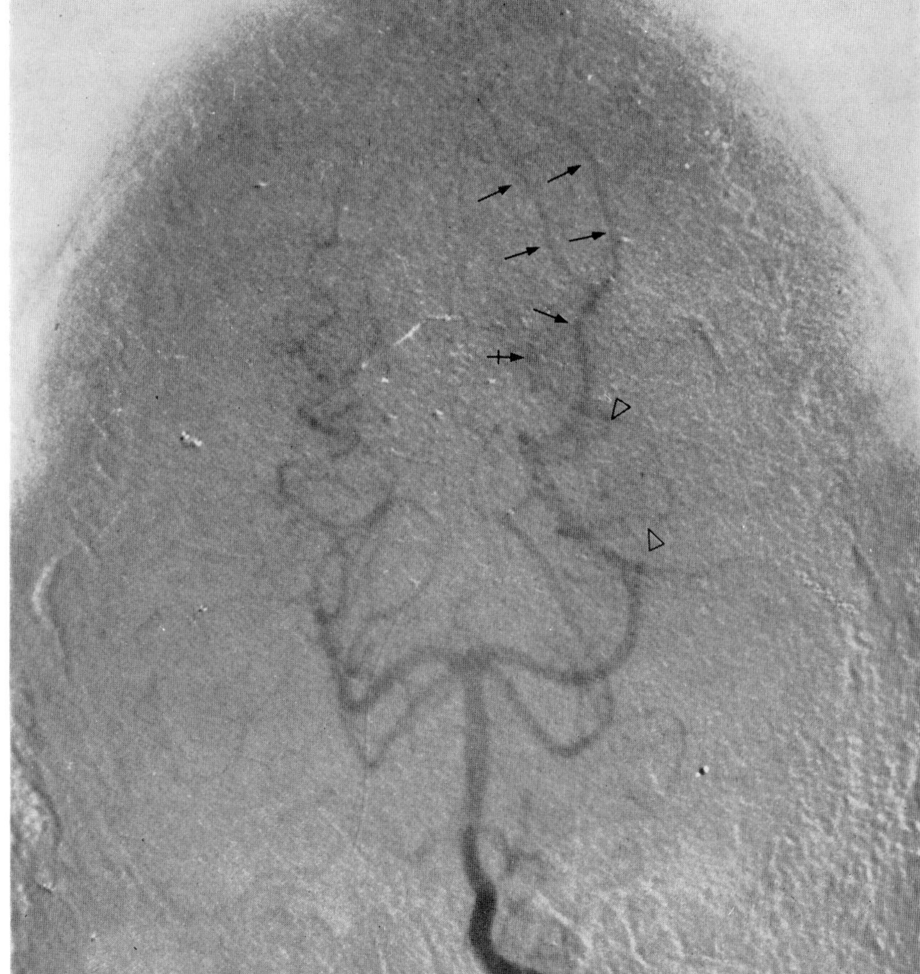

Fig. 418

9

Miscellaneous Diseases

DEVELOPMENTAL ANOMALIES OF THE ARTERIES

Basilar artery

Since the basilar artery is formed by union of a pair of the longitudinal neural arteries, there may develop partial or complete non-union of the longitudinal neural arteries. Partial non-union remains as longitudinal septum, fenestration or high junction of the vertebral arteries. In complete non-union, there develops complete doubling of the basilar artery.

Formation of the septum in the basilar artery is uncommon with incidence of 3 per 1,000 autopsies (Busch, 1966). Incidence of fenestration is 5.26 per cent of 291 dissected brains by Wollschlaeger et al. (1967), or 4 out of 84 dissected brains by Adachi (1928). Complete doubling of the basilar artery has been reported in a few cases by Krayenbühl and Yasargil (1958) and Adachi (1928) in autopsy material and one case each by Fielas (1962) and Handa et al. (1968) in their clinical materials.

Vertebral artery

Fenestration or partial duplication of the vertebral arteries has also been reported as a rare condition. This anomaly involves the intracranial vertebral artery or the distal extracranial vertebral artery. Embryologically, the vertebral artery is formed by anastomoses between the successive cervical segmental arteries arising from the primitive dorsal aortae. The proximal ends of the segmental arteries are subsequently obliterated, forming a primitive vertebral artery. It is possible that two anastomoses develop between adjacent segments, forming a bypass or fenestration. The intracranial fenestration has been considered to be a remnant of the first segmental artery and the extracranial fenestration is formed by excessive anastomoses between the distal ends of the successive segmental arteries.

This anomaly is quite rare and reported only by the Japanese authors (Takahashi et al., 1970; Maki et al., 1969; Handa et al., 1968).

Clinical significance of vertebral fenestration is its frequent association with other congenital anomalies such as cerebral aneurysms, arteriovenous malformations, or other congenital tumors.

Carotid-basilar anastomosis

Carotid basilar anastomoses may exist at 4 levels as a result of the persistence of some embryological arteries. According to Padget (1944), there are anastomotic channels in a 4 mm embryo between the longitudinal neural arteries (the primitive basilar artery) and the primitive internal carotid arteries at 4 different levels: the primitive trigeminal artery, the primitive otic artery, the primitive hypoglossal artery and the first cervical intersegmental artery. These primitive arteries normally disappear as there develop arteries such as the posterior communicating, basilar and vertebral arteries. One of these primitive arteries persists in cases with carotid basilar anastomosis.

It should be noted that these anastomoses are usually demonstrated by carotid angiography. For demonstration with vertebral angiography, the ipsilateral carotid artery should be compressed.

Persistent primitive trigeminal artery

This artery originates just proximal to the intercaver nous portion of the internal carotid artery and joins the distal portion of the basilar artery.

The incidence of this anomaly is 0.5 to 2 per cent of anatomical studies and 0.1 to 0.5 per cent of carotid angiograms (Krayenbühl and Yasargil, 1968).

Persistent primitive acoustic artery

This anomaly is extremely rare. The artery arises from the intrapetrosal portion of the internal carotid artery and joins the middle portion of the basilar artery.

Persistent hypoglossal artery

This artery communicates the cervical portion of the internal carotid artery with the vertebral artery by way of the hypoglossal canal. This anomaly is quite rare and its incidence is 1 or 2 cases in 2,207 to 7,382 examinations (WIEDENMANN et al. 1959; EADIE et al., 1964; FUKUI and KITAMURA, 1969).

Persistent proatlantal intersegmental artery

This artery arises from the internal carotid artery at the level of the third to the fifth cervical vertebra and joins the distal vertebral artery after passing through the foramen magnum. This anomaly is sometimes excluded from the discussion of the carotid-basilar anastomosis.

Association with other intracranial diseases

The carotid-basilar anastomoses are frequently associated with intracranial aneurysms and arteriovenous malformations (LIE, 1968). In addition, there is frequent association with intracranial tumors (PASSERINI et al., 1962).

Fenestration of the Basilar Artery

A 24-year-old male: Fig. 419

Fig. 419 Arterial phase in the Towne projection. There are two basilar arteries which are connected at their proximal (2 opposing arrows) and distal (a crossed arrow) ends, indicating fenestration of the basilar artery. The distal portion of the left posterior cerebral artery is not shown because of blood flow from the posterior communicating artery. The right vertebral artery is hypoplastic.

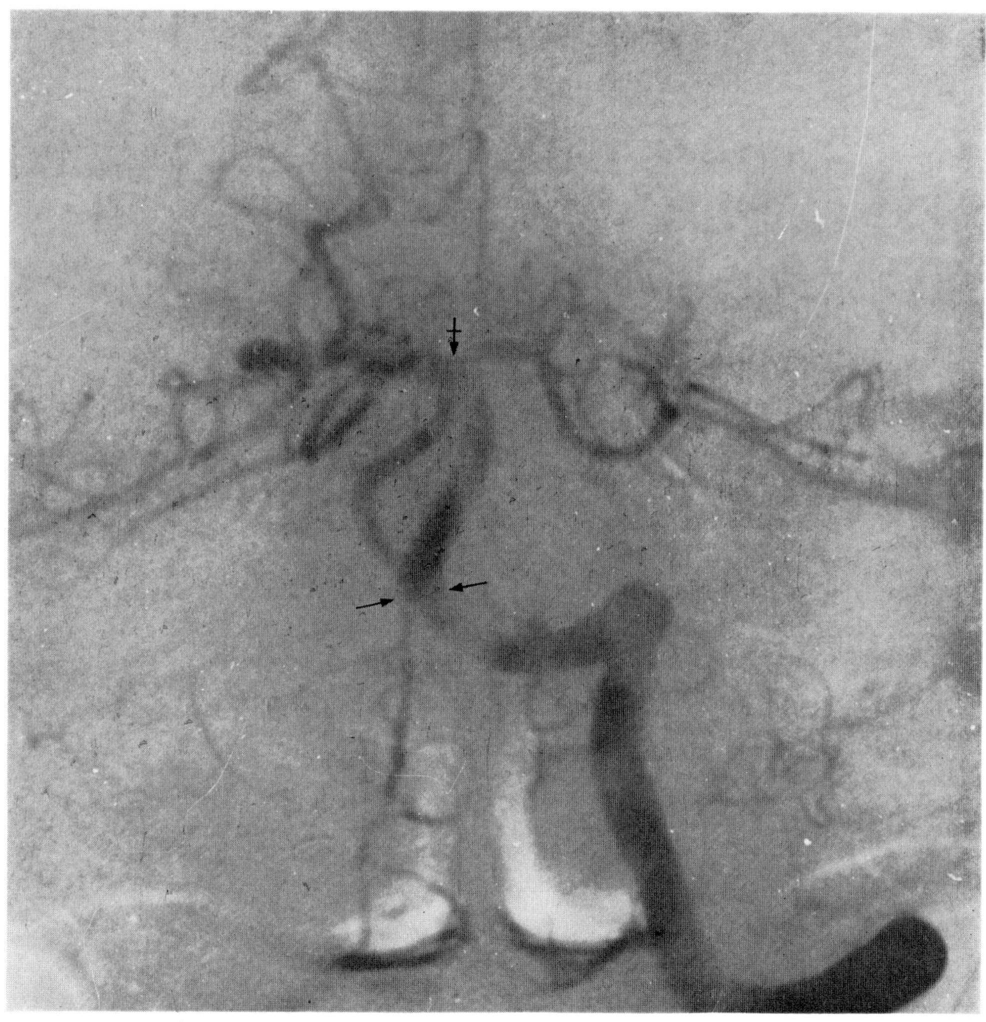

Fig. 419

Fenestration of the Basilar Artery

A 32-year-old male: Fig. 420

Fig. 420 Arterial phase in the Towne projection. There is a small window in the middle portion of the basilar artery with fusiform dilatation of this segment (2 opposing arrows). This is a fenestration of the basilar artery.

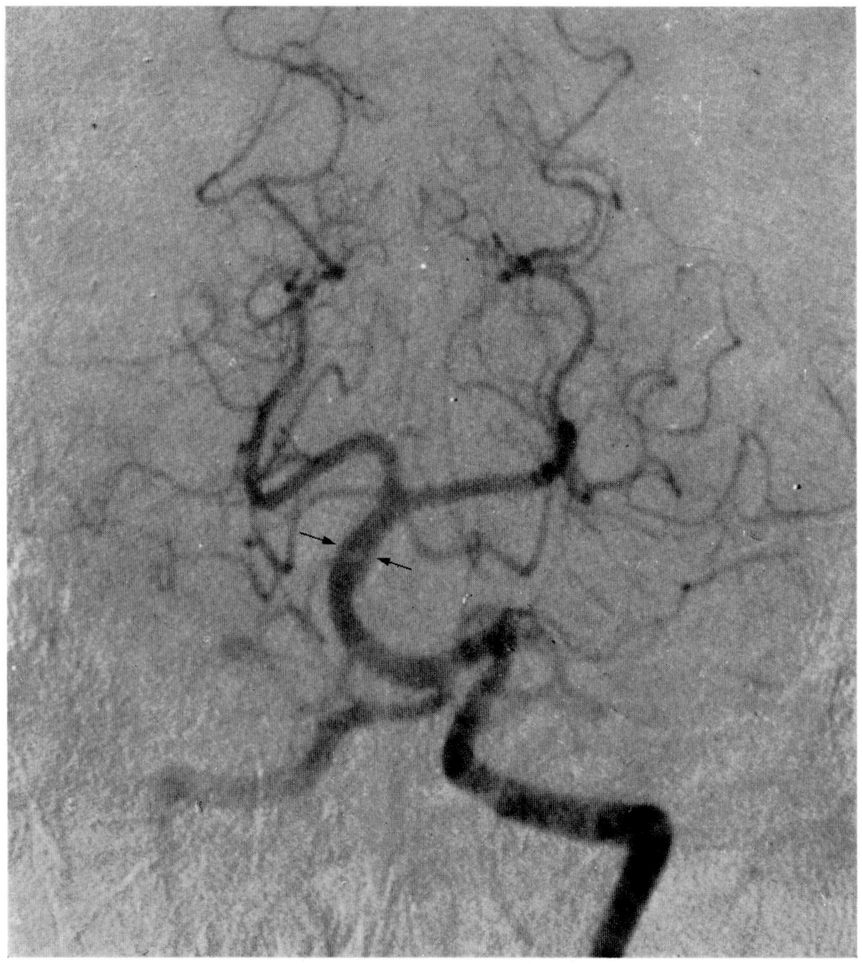

Fig. 420

Short Basilar Artery with High Junction of the Vertebral Arteries

A 37-year-old male: Figs. 421 and 422

Fig. 421 Arterial phase in the anteroposterior projection. There is high junction of the vertebral arteries (2 opposing arrows). The anterior and posterior inferior cerebellar arteries arise from the distal vertebral artery as a common trunk. Superimposition of the intracranial vertebral arteries is observed.

Fig. 422 Arterial phase in the lateral projection. There is high junction of the vertebral arteries (an arrow). The basilar artery is short. The course of the extracranial vertebral artery is anomalous with associated anomalies of the upper cervical vertebrae.

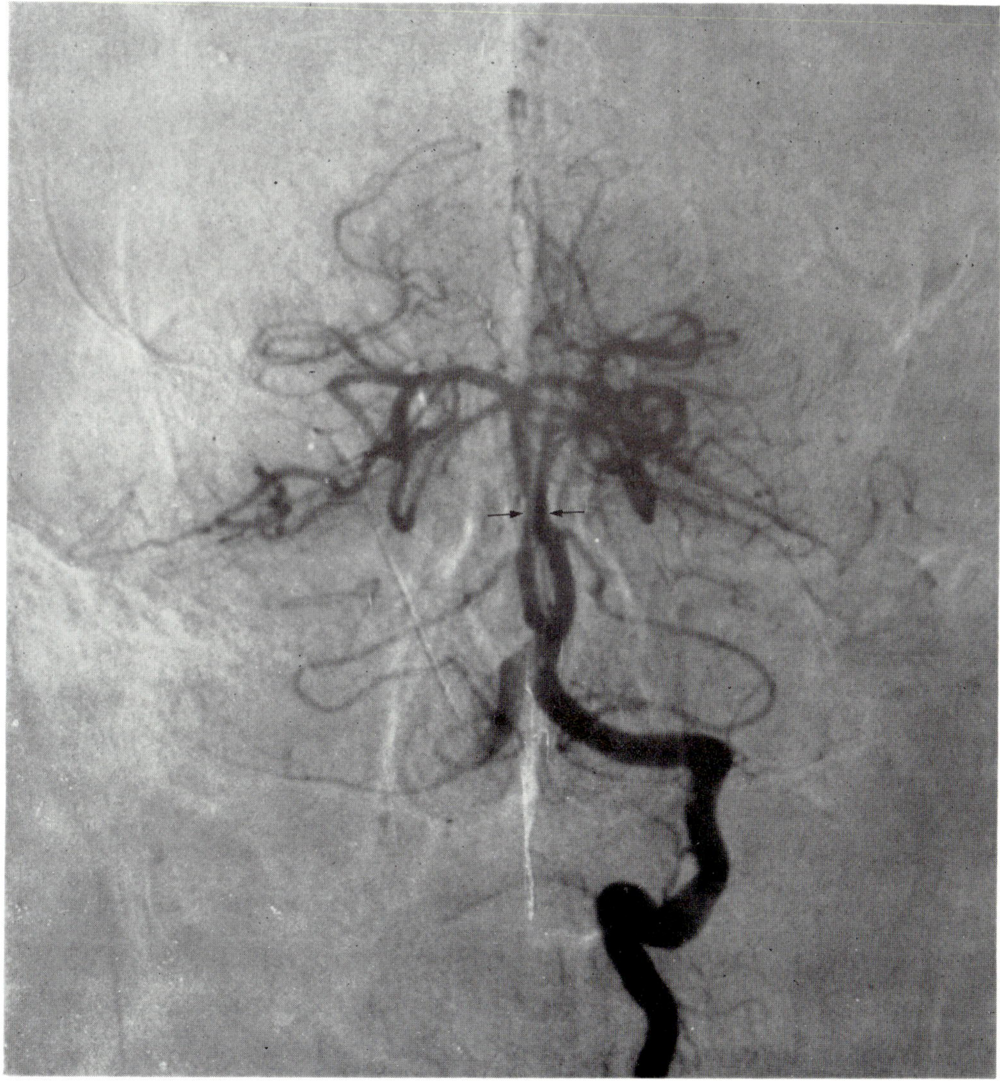

Fig. 421

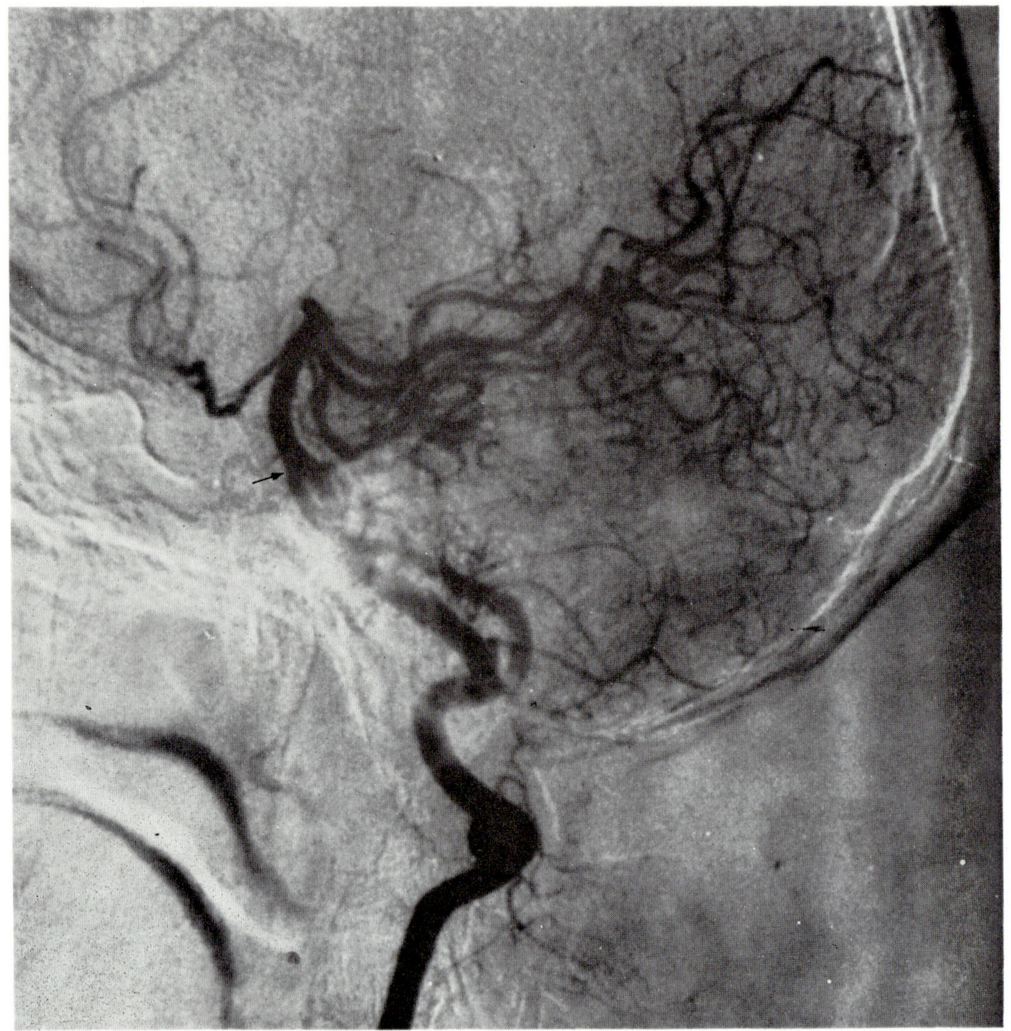

Fig. 422

Fenestration of the Extracranial Vertebral Artery with Occlusion of Bilateral Posterior Cerebral Arteries

A 26-year-old male: Figs. 423 and 424

Fig. 423 Arterial phase in the Towne projection. There is partial duplication or fenestration of the distal extracranial vertebral artery. The anomalous artery begins at the level of the atlanto-axial joint and ends at the lower margin of the atlas (2 arrows). The anomalous artery is larger than the left vertebral artery (2 crossed arrows) and appears to course within the spinal canal. The ambient segment of the posterior cerebral artery is occluded on both sides (arrowheads).

Fig. 424 Arterial phase in the lateral projection. The course of the anomalous artery is well observed within the spinal canal (2 arrows). The true left vertebral artery courses normally (2 crossed arrows). The posterior cerebral arteries are occluded with formation of multiple collateral vessels (arrowheads).

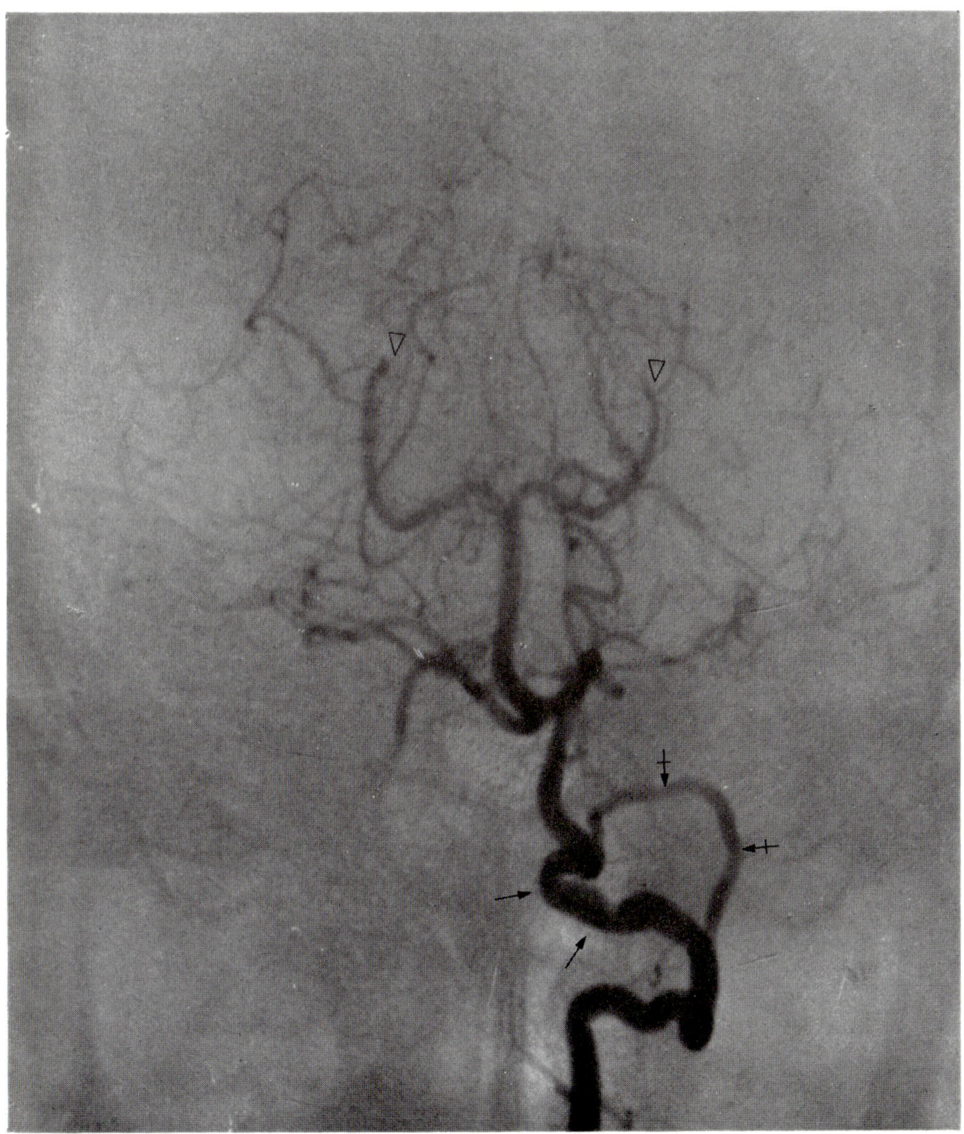

Fig. 423

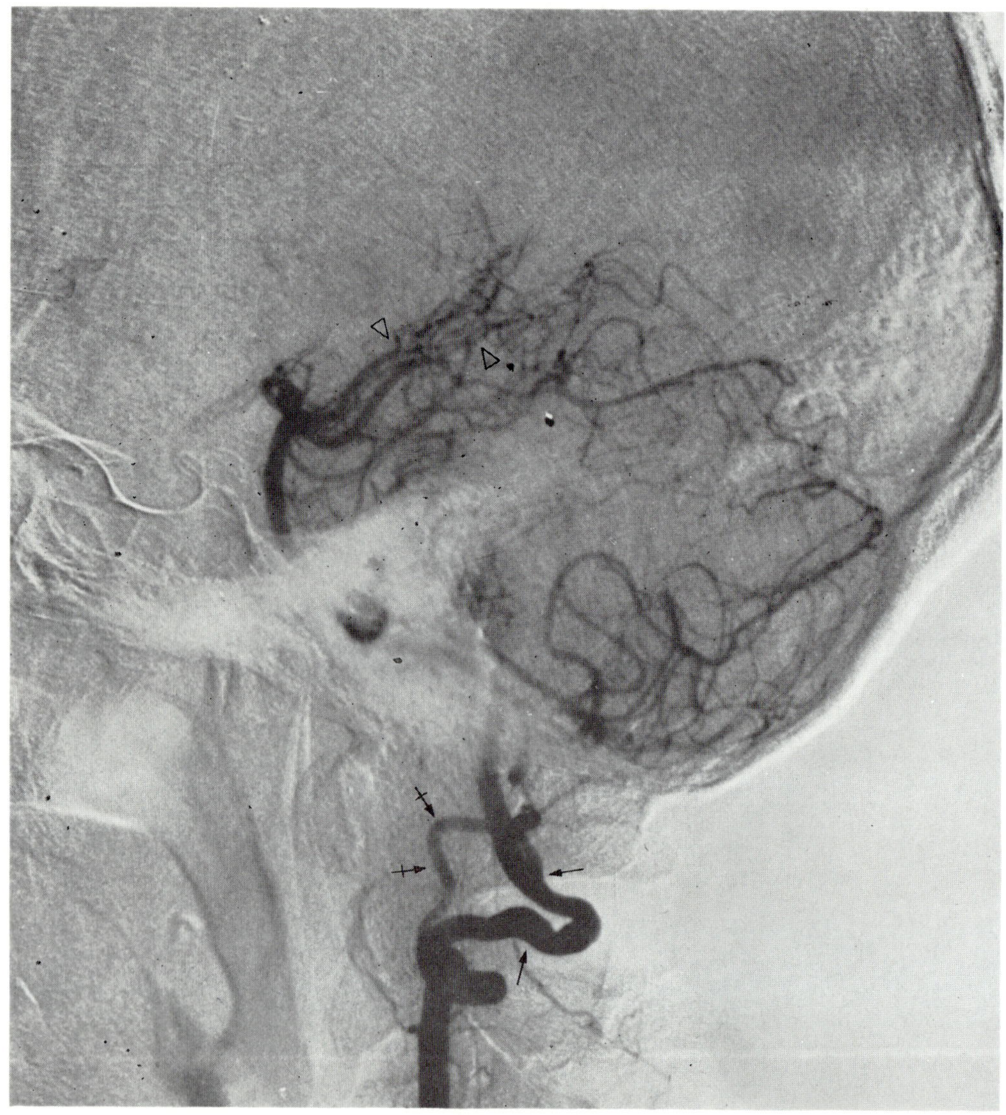

Fig. 424

Fenestration of the Intracranial Vertebral Artery

A 33-year-old male: Figs. 425 and 426

Fig. 425 Right vertebral angiogram in the anteroposterior projection. The course of the distal vertebral artery is anomalous on both sides in association with anomalies of the upper cervical vertebrae. There is duplication of the distal portion of the right vertebral artery (2 arrows).

Fig. 426 Right vertebral angiogram with horizontal X-ray. The patient was in the supine position with rotation of the head to the right. The fenestration of the intracranial vertebral artery is well shown (2 arrows). There is minimal reflux of contrast media into the left vertebral artery (2 crossed arrows).

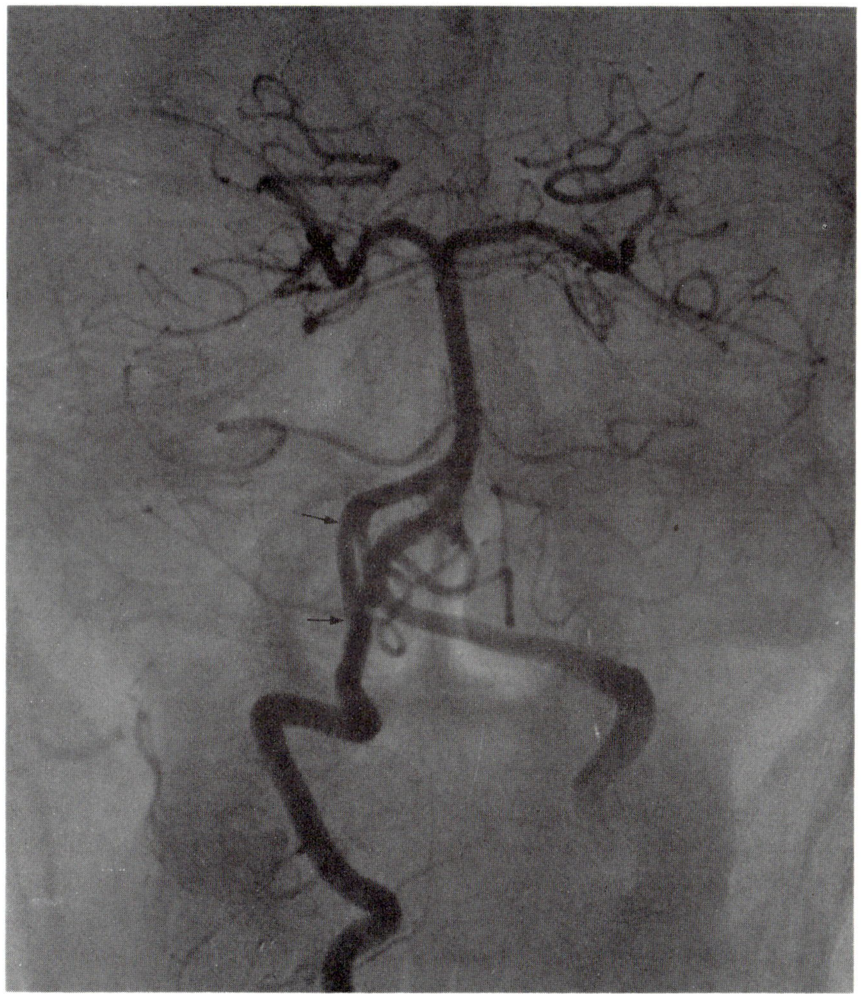

Fig. 425

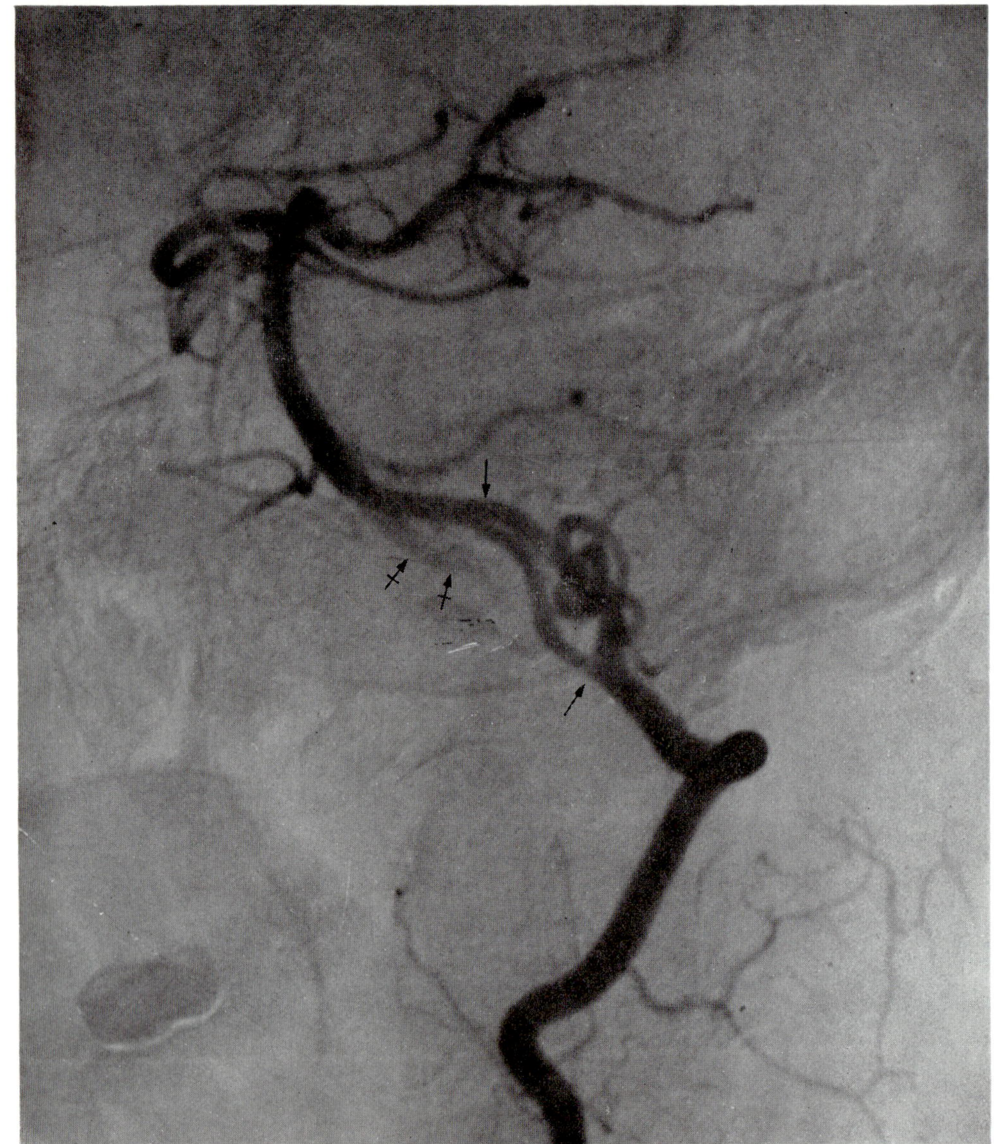

Fig. 426

Persistent Hypoglossal Artery with Hypoplastic Vertebral Arteries

A 20-year-old female: Figs. 427–430

Fig. 427 Left common carotid angiogram in the lateral projection. The persistent hypoglossal artery arises from the internal carotid artery at the level of the third cervical vertebra (an arrow). It courses upwards and continues as the basilar artery after passing through the hypoglossal canal (2 crossed arrows).

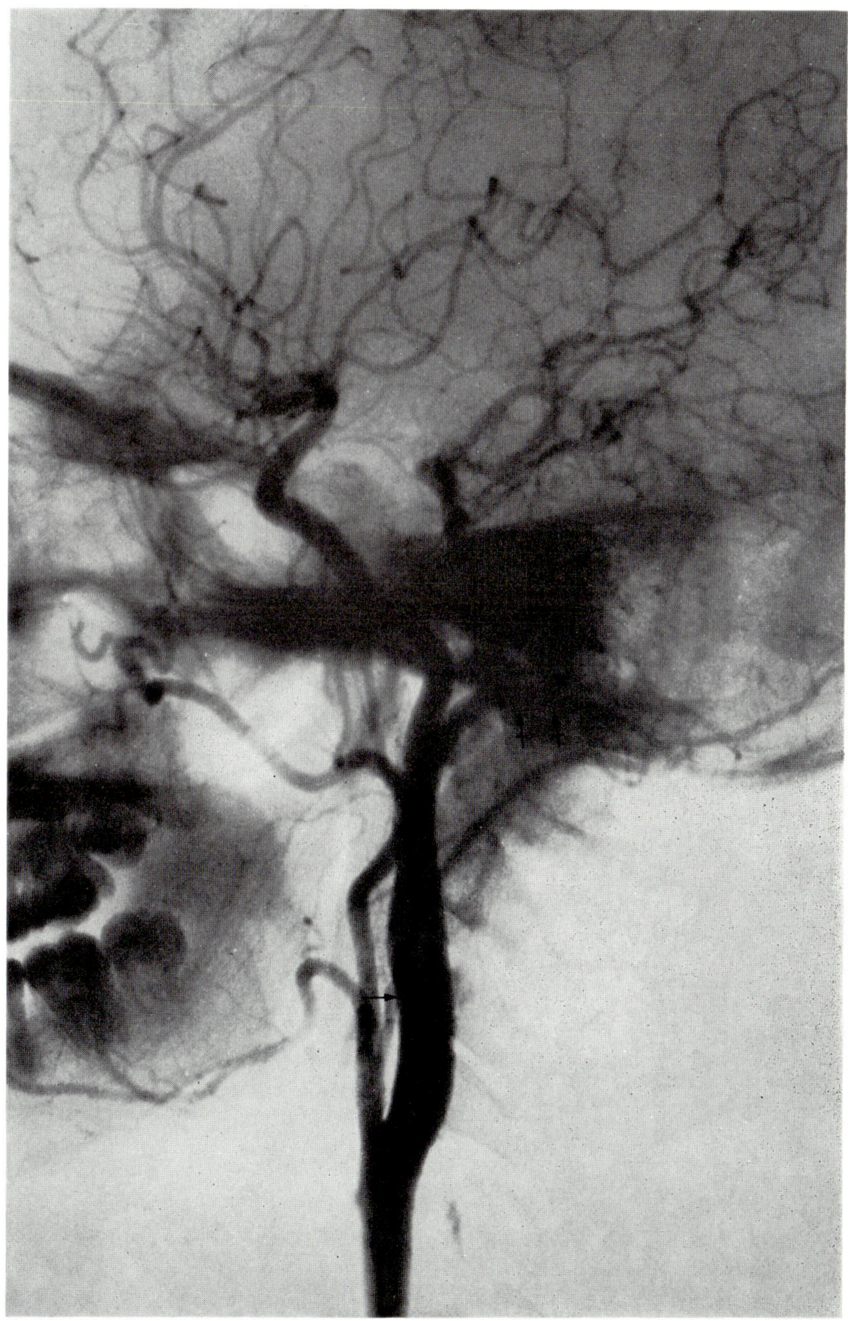

Fig. 427

Fig. 428 Left common carotid angiogram in the anteroposterior projection. The origin of the persistent hypoglossal artery is marked with an arrow together with the course at the hypoglossal canal (a crossed arrow).

Fig. 429 Left subclavian angiogram in the anteroposterior projection. The left vertebral artery is markedly hypoplastic (2 arrows).

Fig. 430 Right subclavian angiogram in the anteroposterior projection. The right vertebral artery is also hypoplastic (2 arrows). The right common carotid artery and its branches were normal.

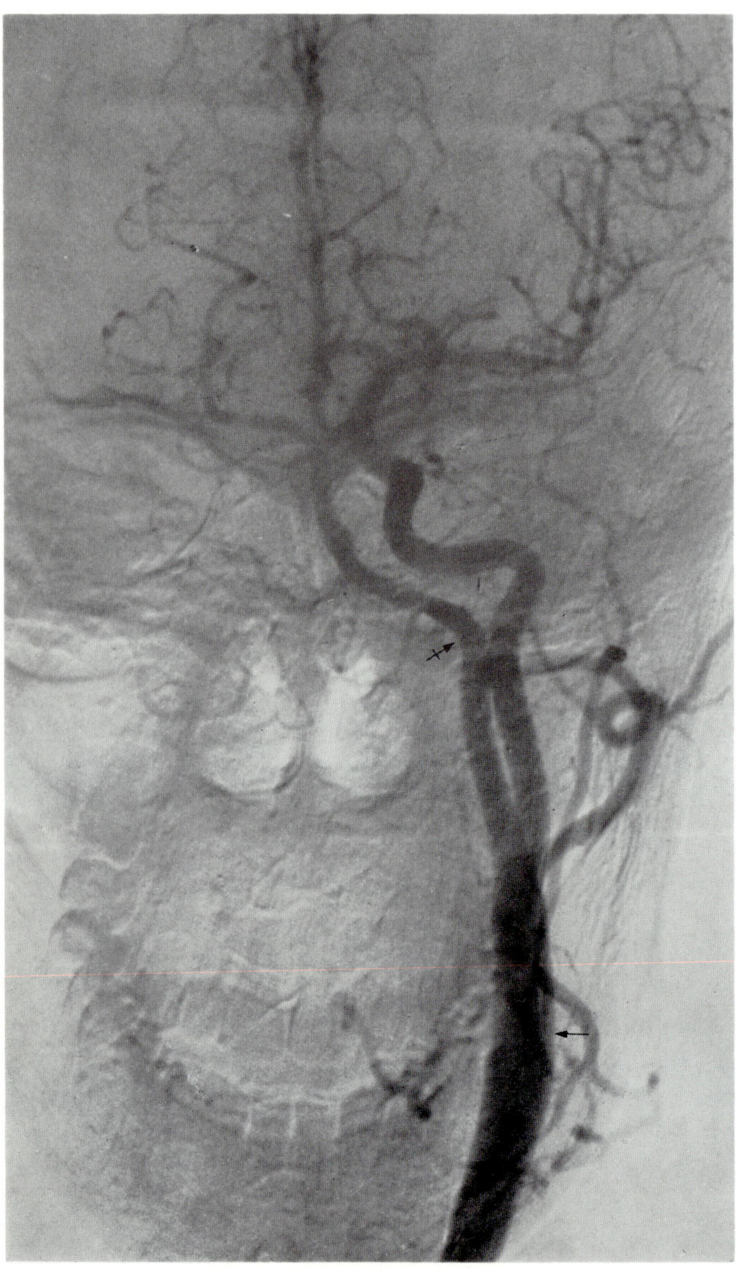

Fig. 428

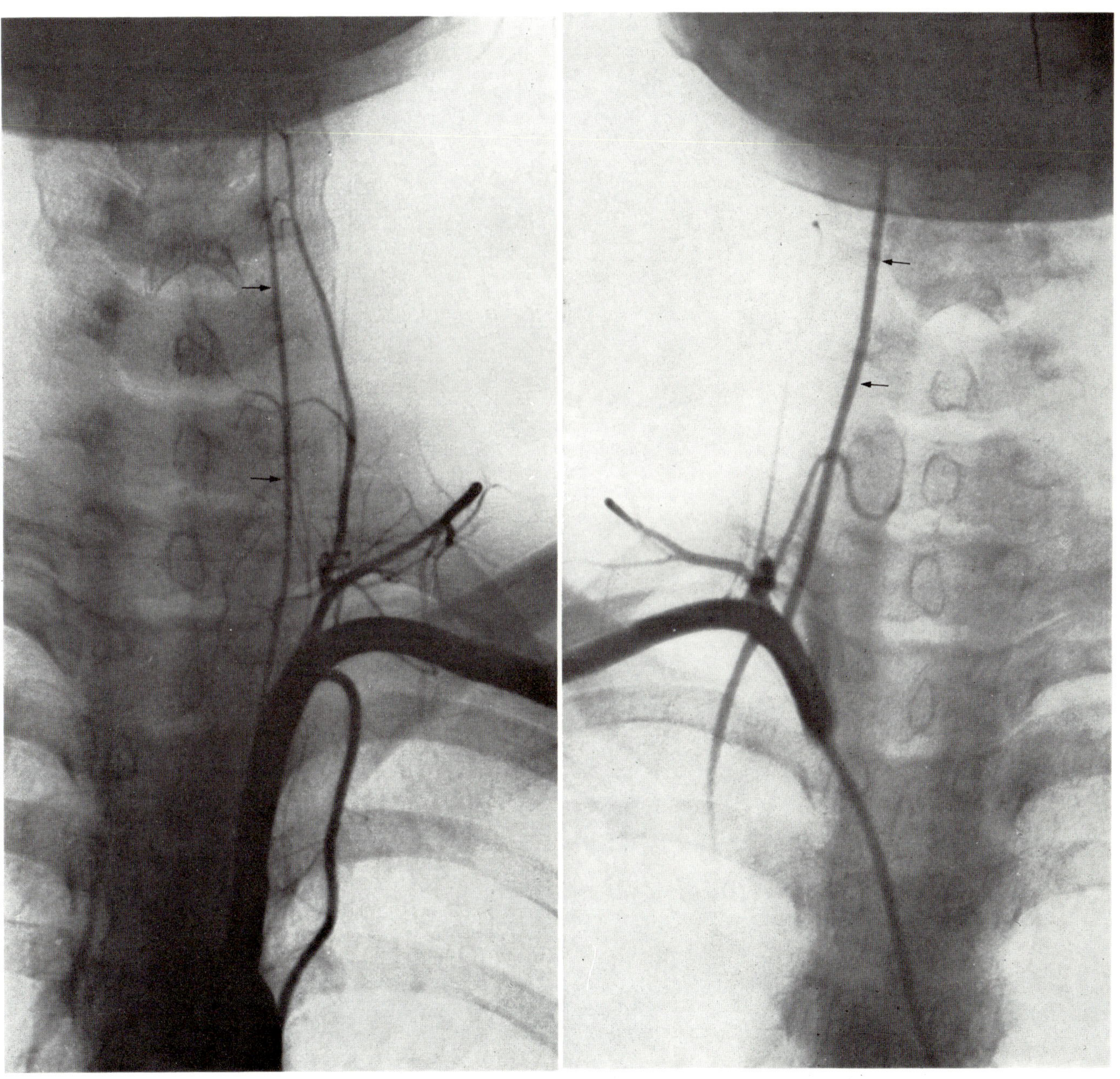

Fig. 429 Fig. 430

CONGENITAL ANOMALIES OF THE CEREBELLUM AND ADJACENT STRUCTURES

Congenital anomalies occur in the cerebellum, skull, cervical vertebrae and soft tissues. Vertebral angiography is infrequently indicated in these conditions.

The most common anomalies of the cerebellum may be Arnold-Chiari malformation and Dandy-Walker syndrome, in which the caudal loop of the posterior inferior cerebellar artery is displaced below the foramen magnum. There are various anomalies of the cervical vertebrae in association with anomalies of the occipital bone such as atlanto-axial dislocation, occipitalization of the atlas and Klippel-Feil syndrome. With these anomalies of the bones, there are usually associated anomalies in the course and caliber of the vertebral arteries.

Klippel-Feil Syndrome with Occipitalization of the Atlas

A 29-year-old female: Figs. 431–434

Fig. 431 Left vertebral angiogram in the anteroposterior projection. The third segment of the vertebral artery swings medially in association with the marked scoliosis and fusion of C_1, C_2 and C_3 (2 arrows). There is a fenestration of the basilar artery (a crossed arrow). The posterior inferior cerebellar artery is displaced inferiorly.

Fig. 432 Left vertebral angiogram in the lateral projection. The third segment is kinked between the atlas and axis (2 arrows). The basilar artery is displaced posteriorly secondary to atrophy of the brain stem. The tonsillohemispheric branch and caudal loop is displaced to the level of the foramen magnum (2 crossed arrows). The clivus is marked with 2 arrowheads.

Fig. 433 Right vertebral angiogram in the anteroposterior projection. There is considerable lateral sweep of the third segment of the right vertebral artery (an arrow).

Fig. 434 Right vertebral angiogram in the lateral projection. The third segment courses posteriorly (an arrow) and the fourth segment is redundant in association with the bony anomalies (a crossed arrow).

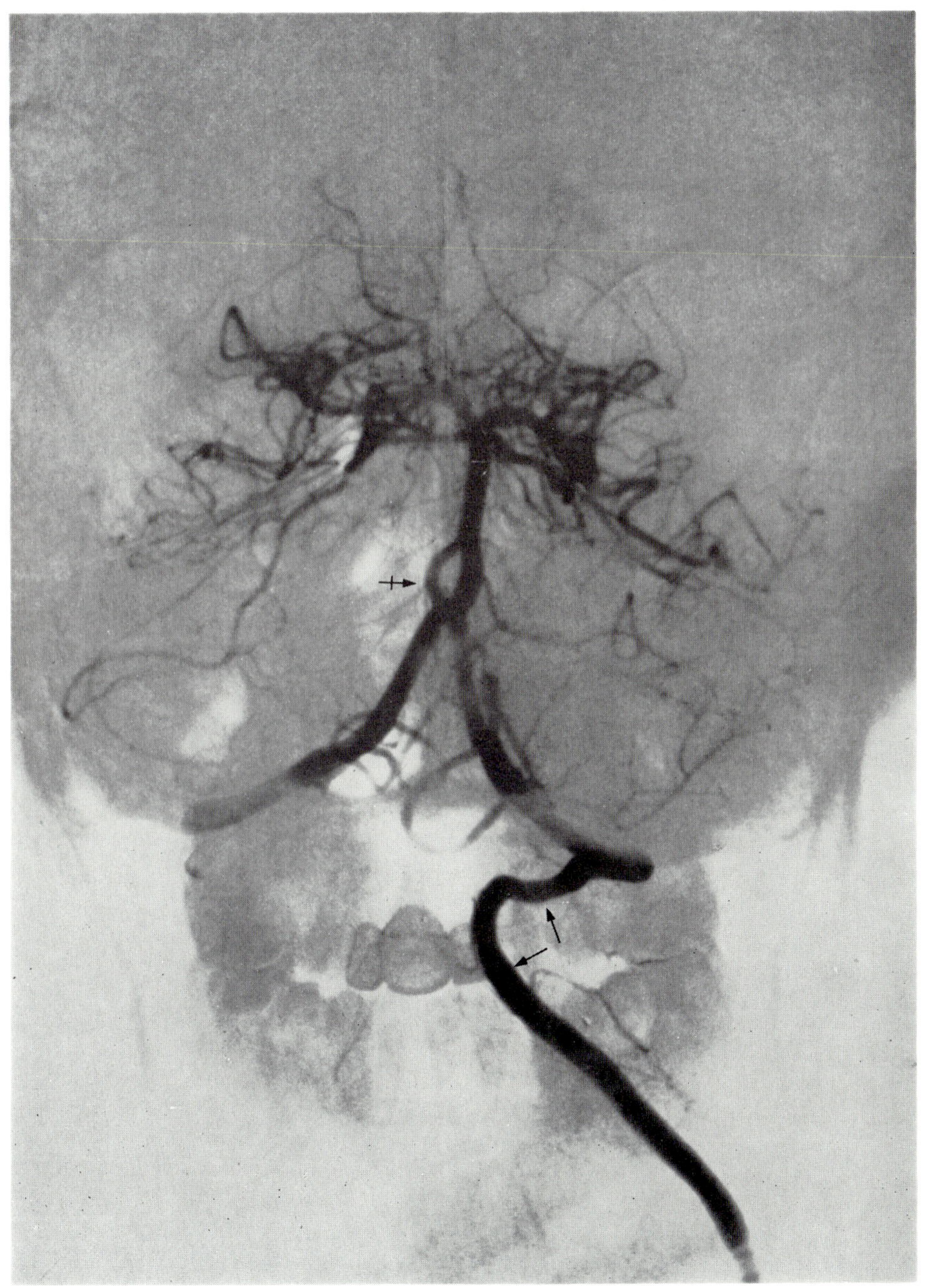

Fig. 431

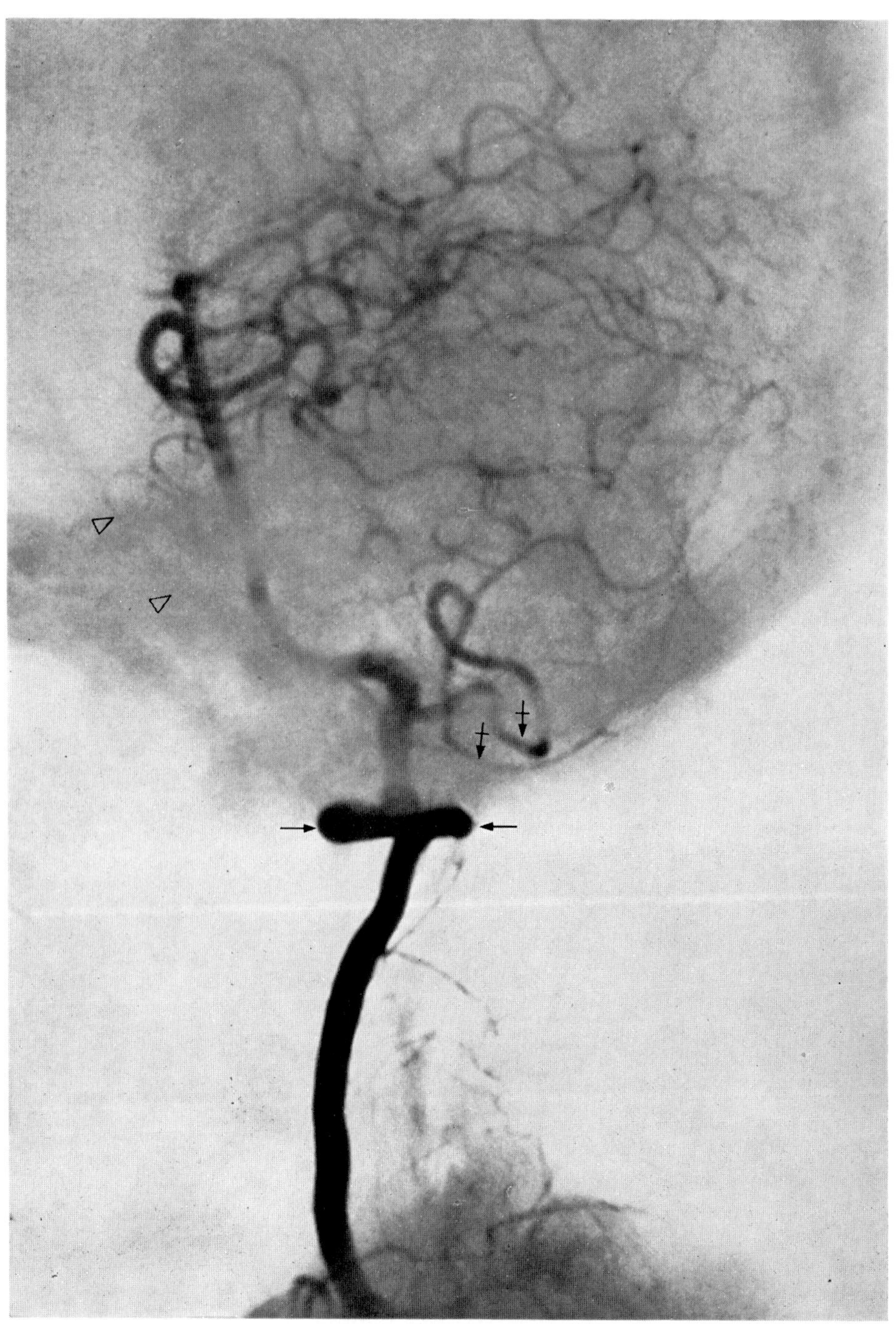

Fig. 432

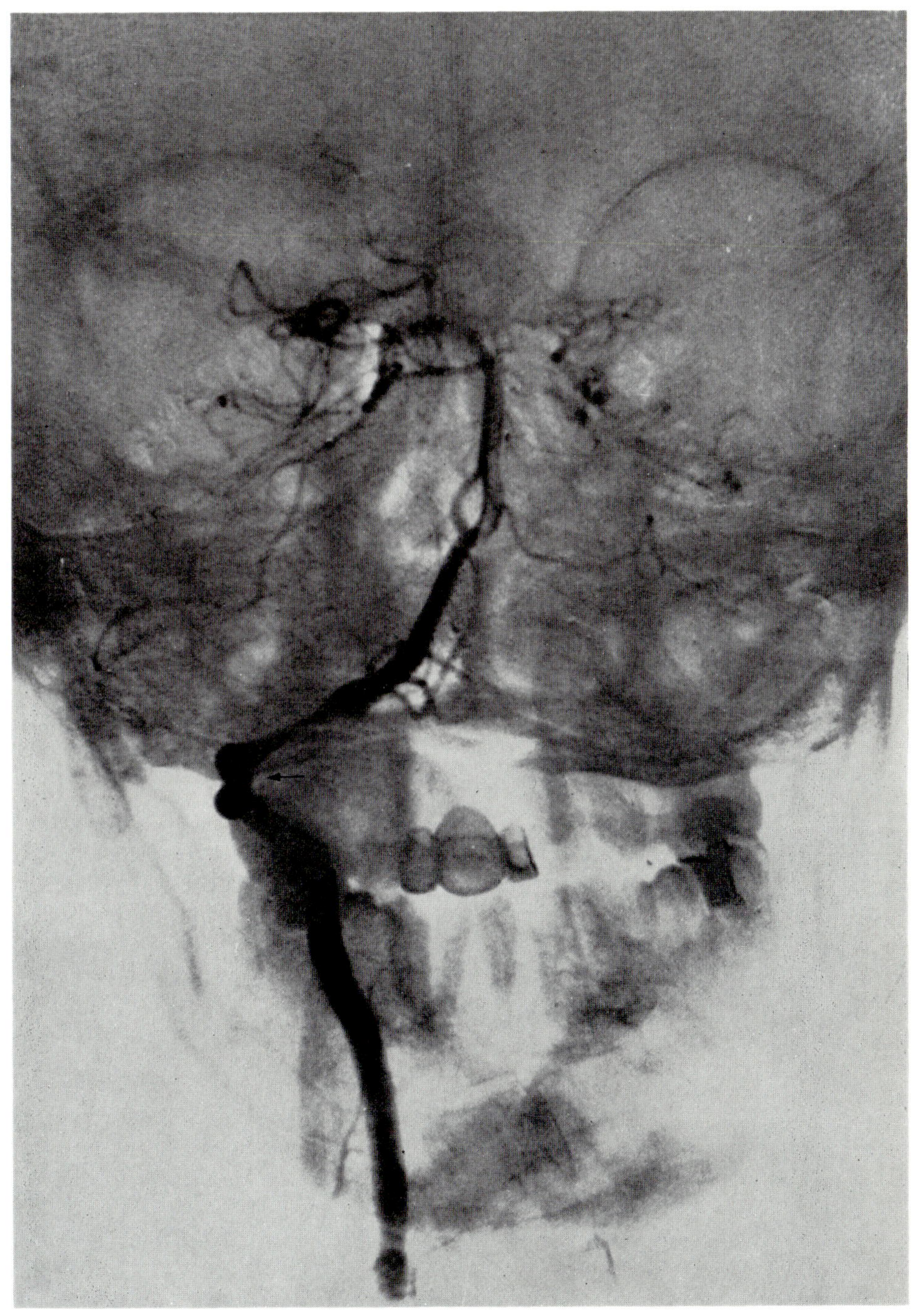

Fig. 433

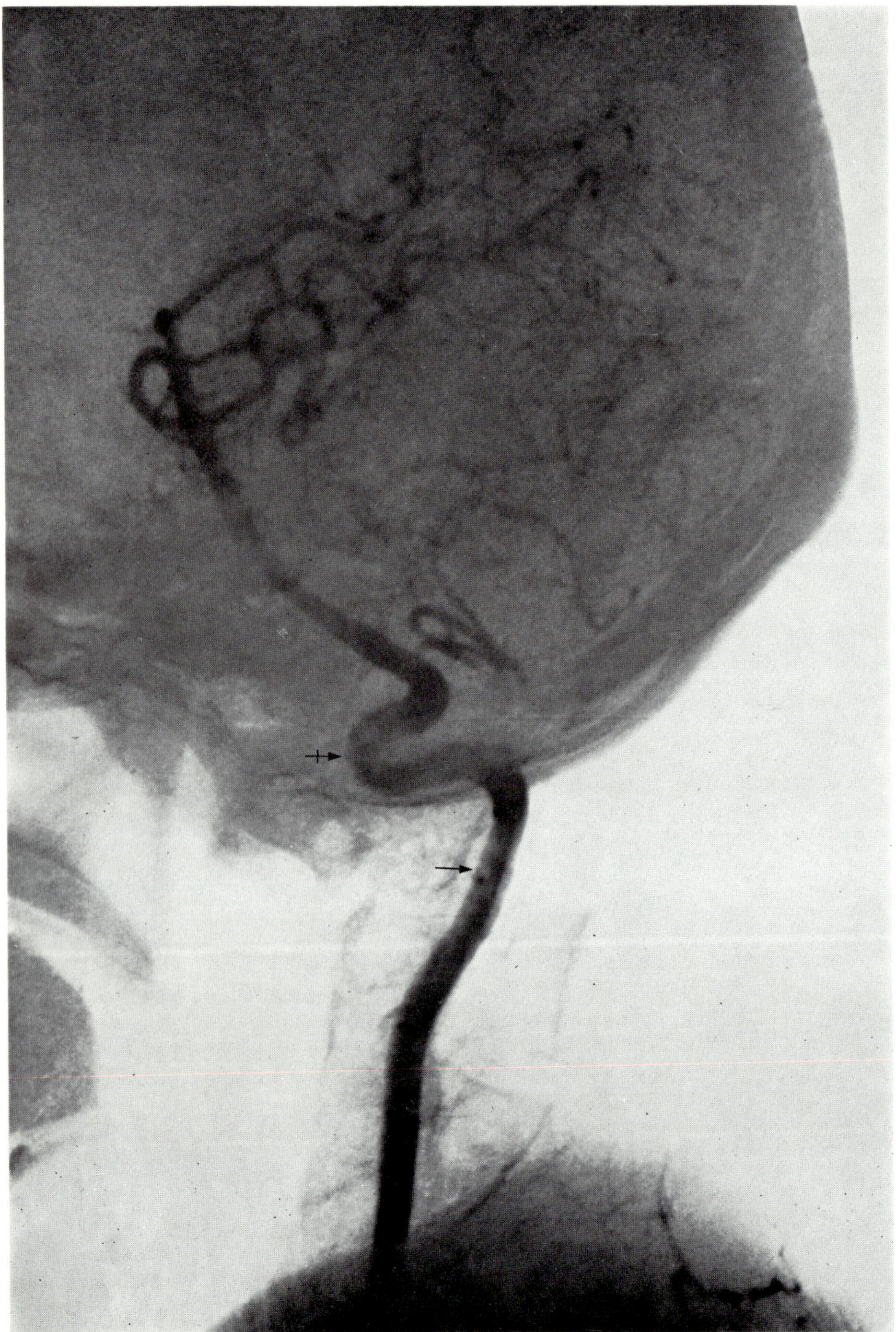

Fig. 434

SPINAL TUMORS

The most common intraspinal lesion diagnosed by vertebral angiography is spinal cord hemangioblastoma. The tumor usually shows homogeneous stain identical to those described in the cases associated with cerebellar lesions. No rapid shunting from the arteries to the veins is usually demonstrable. Arterial supply is from the anterior and posterior spinal arteries as well as from the muscular branches of the vertebral artery, thyrocervical trunk and external carotid artery.

Intramedullary gliomas may show irregular tumor vessels. Intradural, extramedullary tumors, such as meningiomas and neurinomas, may also reveal tumor vessels supplied by the spinal arteries and muscular branches. Tumor vessels are infrequently demonstrated in the extradural tumors such as metastatic tumors, malignant lymphoma and neurinoma of the cervical nerves.

Extra- and Intradural Neurinoma Arising from the Cervical Nerve Root

A 23-year-old male: Figs. 435 and 436

Fig. 435 Arterial phase in the lateral projection. Irregular tumor vessels are noted in an area of 1.5×1.0 cm at the second cervical vertebra (3 arrows). A feeding artery is demonstrated (a crossed arrow).

Fig. 436 Arterial phase in the anteroposterior projection. The tumor vessels (3 arrows) and the feeding artery (a crossed arrow) are demonstrated to good advantage.

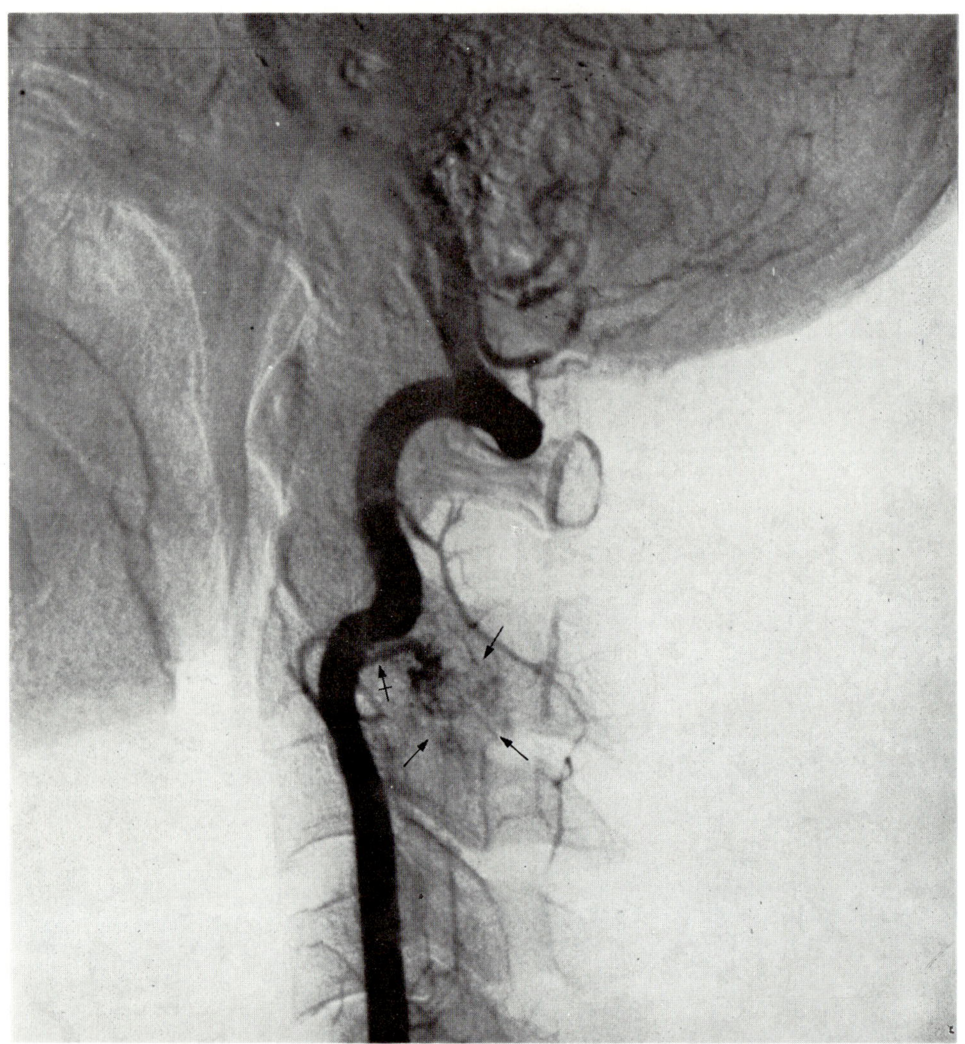

Fig. 435

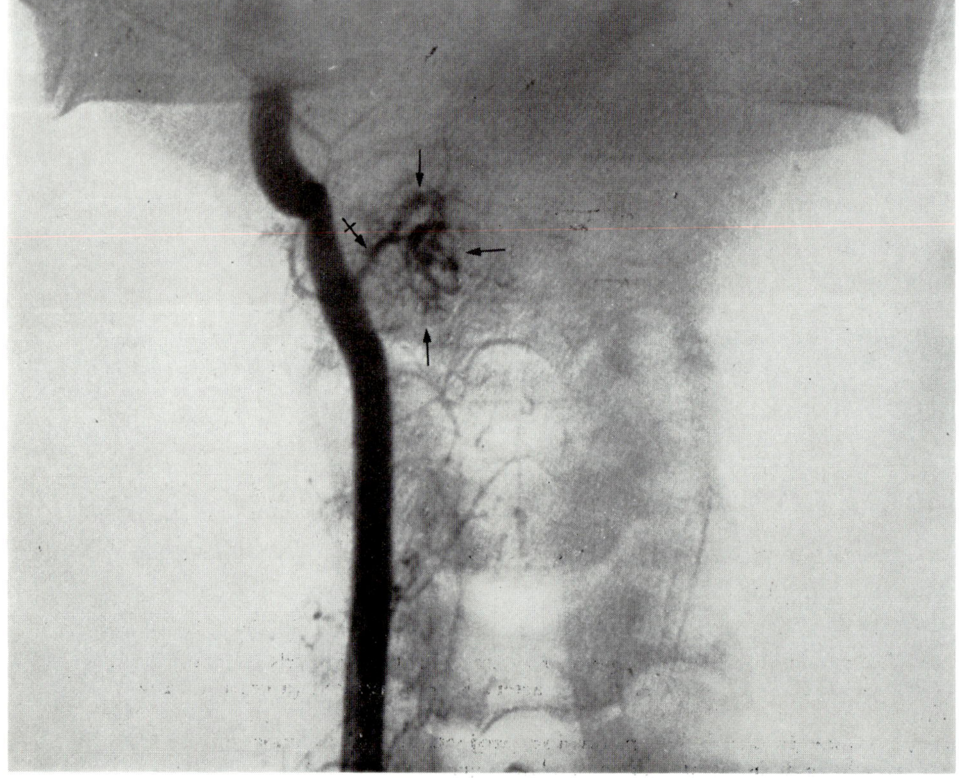

Fig. 436

SPINAL ARTERIOVENOUS MALFORMATIONS

Arteriovenous malformations of the cervical spinal cord are supplied by the anterior and posterior spinal arteries as well as muscular branches of the vertebral artery, thyrocervical trunk and the costocervical trunk. The lesions usually consist of conglomerates of individual vessels and no tumor stains or tumor vessels are observed. Rapid arteriovenous shunt may or may not be present.

Infrequently, the arteriovenous malformation in the cervical cord is supplied by the artery of Adamkiewicz.

Cervical Arteriovenous Malformation

A 26-year-old male: Figs. 437–439

Fig. 437 Arterial phase in the lateral projection. There are conglomerates of minute vessels posterior to the axis (3 arrows), which are supplied by the enlarged anterior spinal artery (an arrowhead) and the muscular branches of the vertebral artery.

Fig. 438 Late arterial phase in the lateral projection. The lesion is drained by two enlarged veins (a crossed arrow and an arrow).

Fig. 439 Capillary phase in the lateral projection. The veins in the lesion as well as the draining vein are well demonstrated. The draining vein drains into the inferior vermian vein (2 arrows) by way of the foramen magnum (an arrowhead).

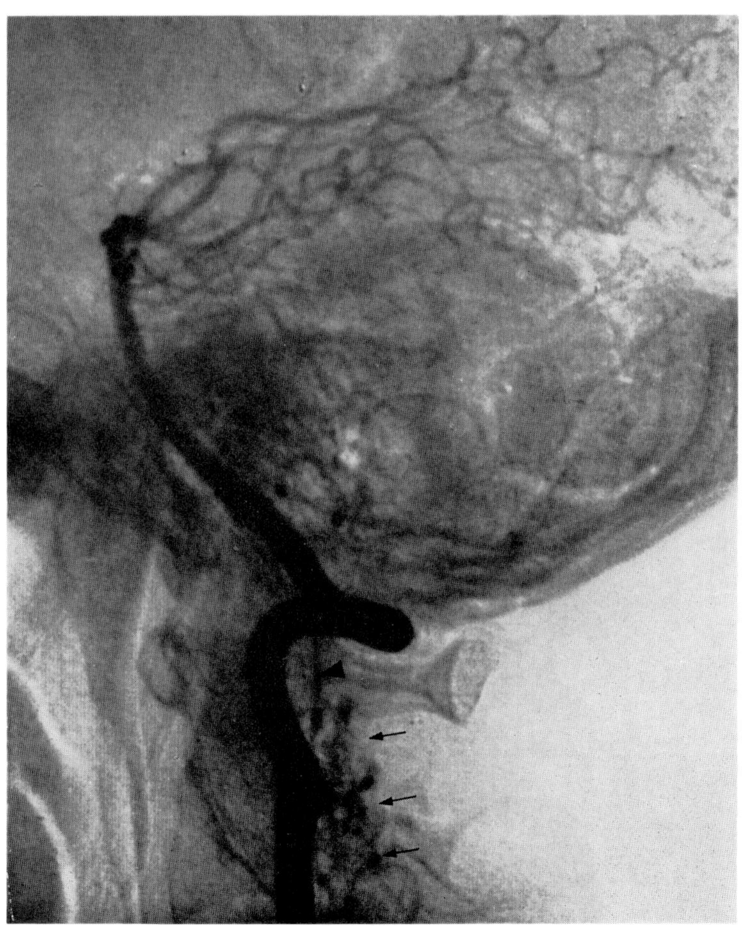

Fig. 437

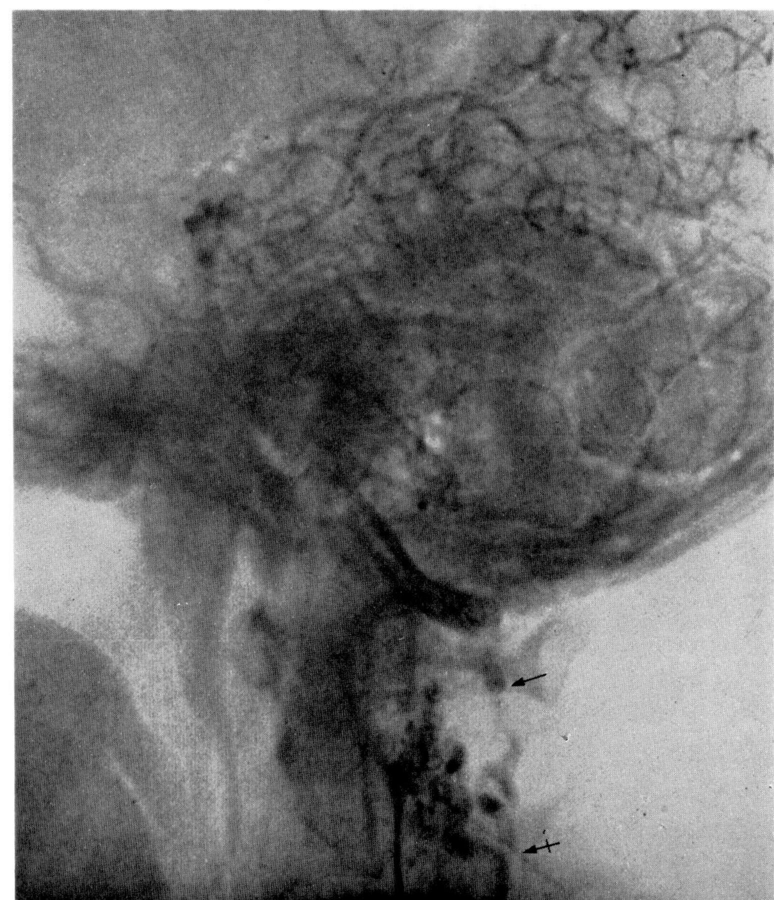

Fig. 438

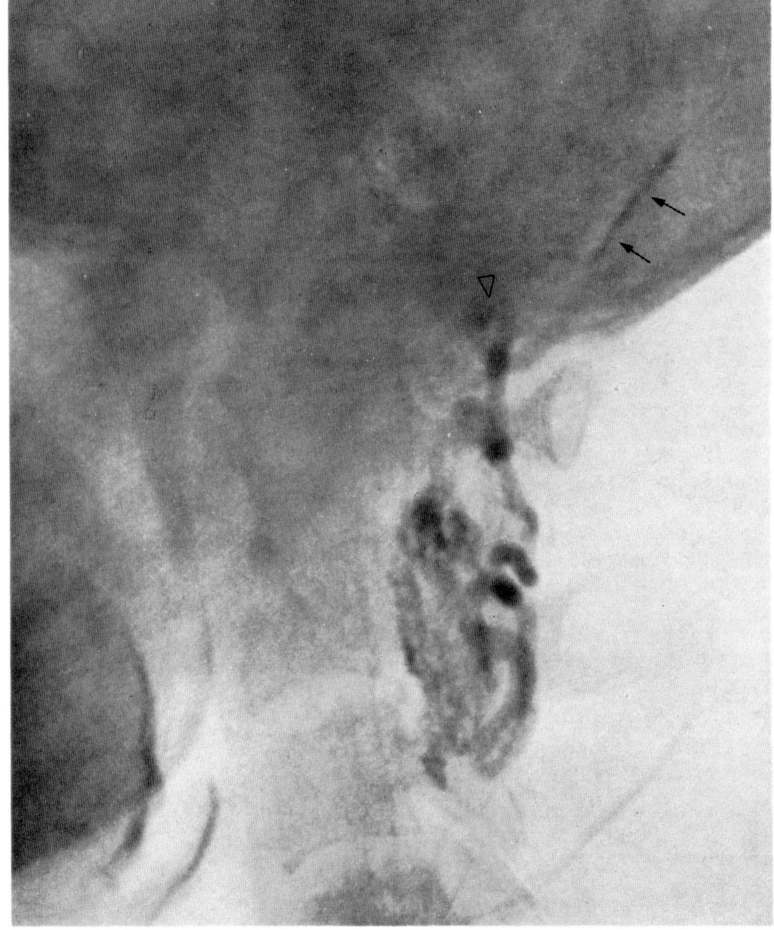

Fig. 439

References

Chapters 1, 2 and 3

Abbott, K. H., Gay, J. R., and Goodall, R. J.: Clinical complications of cerebral angiography. J. Neurosurg., 9: 247–258, 1952.

Ameli, N. O.: Practical method of vertebral angiography. Br. J. Surg., 39: 327–330, 1952.

Amplatz, K., and Harner, R.: A new subclavian artery catheterization technique: Preliminary report. Radiology, 78: 963–966, 1962.

Amundsen, P., Dietrichson, P., Enge, I., and Williamson, R.: Cerebral angiography by catheterization: Complications and side effects. Acta Radiol. (Diagn.), 1: 164–172, 1963.

Barbieri, P. L., and Verdechia, G. D.: Vertebral arteriography by percutaneous puncture of the subclavian artery. Acta Radiol., 48: 444–448, 1957.

Bergquist, E., Bergström, K., Hugosson, R., and Jorulf, H.: Complicated arteriovenous fistula after vertebral angiography. Neuroradiology, 2: 170–175, 1971.

Bonte, G., Riff, G., and Spy, E.: Angiographie vertébrale par cathétérisme rétrograde fémoral. Acta Radiol., 50: 67–76, 1958.

Brinker, R. A., and Skucas, J.: Routine cerebral angiography by the femoral catheter approach. Am. J. Roentgenol., 115: 27–34, 1972.

Chase, N., Hass, W. K., and Ransohoff, J.: Modified method for percutaneous brachial angiography. Arch. Neurol., 8: 632–639, 1963.

Chynn, K-Y.: Simplified subtraction technique. Am. J. Roentgenol., 95: 970–975, 1965.

Collins, W. F., Slade, H. W., and Lockhart, W. G.: Brachial vertebral angiography in adults. J. Neurosurg., 14: 466–468, 1957.

Cronqvist, S.: Vertebral catheterization via the femoral artery. Acta Radiol., 55: 113–118, 1961.

Cronqvist, S., Efsing, H. O., and Palacios, E.: Embolic complications in cerebral angiography with the catheter technique. Acta Radiol. (Diagn.), 10: 97–107, 1970.

Ederli, A., Sassaroli, S., and Spaccarelli, G.: Vertebral angiography as a cause of necrosis of the cervical spinal cord. Br. J. Radiol., 35: 261–264, 1962.

Eiken, M., and Cormsen, J.: Complications of carotid angiography in acute cerebrovascular conditions. Acta med. scand., 172: 151–161, 1962.

Feild, J. R., Lee, L., and McBurney, R. F.: Complications of 1000 brachial arteriograms. J. Neurosurg., 36: 324–332, 1972.

Feild, J. R., Robertson, J. T., and DeSaussure, R. L., Jr.: Complications of cerebral angiography in 2000 consecutive cases. J. Neurosurg., 19: 775–781, 1962.

Gerhardt, P. und Oldenkott, P.: Ergebnisse der Schicht-Angiographie der Hinteren Schädelgrube. Acta Radiol., 13: 94–96, 1972.

Gensini, G. G., and Ecker, A.: Percutaneous aortocerebral angiography; A diagnostic and physiologic method. Radiology, 75: 885–893, 1960.

Gibson, R. D.: Complications of cerebral angiography: Catheter technique. Aust. Radiol., 15: 117–122, 1971.

Glickman, M. G., Gletne, J. S., and Mainzer, F.: The basal projection in cerebral angiography. Radiology, 98: 611–618, 1971.

Gonsette, R., and Andre-Balisaux, G.: A study of capillary and venous phases of vertebral arteriography using a new contrast medium (Vasombrix 32). Neuroradiology, 1: 101–106, 1970.

Gould, P. L., Peyton, W. T., and French, L. A.: Vertebral angiography by retrograde injection of the brachial artery. J. Neurosurg., 12: 369–374, 1955.

Guinto, F. C., Jr., and Radcliffe, W. B.: Percutaneous catheterization of the femoral artery in infants, using a scalp vein needle. Radiology, 102: 408, 1972.

Hanafee, W.: Axillary artery approach to carotid, vertebral, abdominal aorta, and coronary angiography. Radiology, 81: 559–567, 1963.

Hauge, T.: Catheter vertebral angiography. Acta Radiol., Suppl. 109: 1–129, 1954.

Howieson, J., and Megison, L. C., Jr.: Complications of vertebral artery catheterization. Radiology, 91: 1109–1111,1968.

Jamieson, K. G.: Vertebral arteriovenous fistula caused by angiography needle: Report of a case. J. Neurosurg., 23: 620–621, 1965.

Kaplan, A. D., and Walker, A. E.: Complications of cerebral angiography. Neurology, 4: 643, 1954.

Krayenbühl, H. A., and Yasargil, M. G.: Cerebral Angiography. 2nd ed., Butterworth & Co. Ltd., London, 1968.

Kricheff, I. I., and Chase, N. E.: Evaluation of complication rates of meglumine diatrizoate and meglumine iothalamate in cerebral angiography. Am. J. Roentgenol., 101: 220–223, 1967.

Kuhn, R. A.: Brachial cerebral angiography. J. Neurosurg., 17: 955–971, 1960.

Lester, J.: Arteriovenous fistula after percutaneous vertebral angiography. Acta Radiol. (Diagn.), 5: 337–340, 1966.

Lester, J., and Klee, A.: Complications of 337 percutaneous vertebral angiographies. Acta Neurol. Scand., 41: 301–314, 1965.

Lindgren, E.: Percutaneous angiography of the vertebral artery. Acta Radiol., 33: 389–490, 1950.

Lindgren, E.: Another method of vertebral angiography. Acta Radiol., 46:257–261, 1956.

Maslowski, H. A.: Vertebral angiography: Percutaneous lateral atlanto-occipital method. Br. J. Surg., 43: 1–8, 1955.

Mones, R.: Vertebral angiography: An analysis of 106 cases. Radiology, 76: 230–236, 1961.

Moniz, E.: L'encéphalographie artérielle, son importance dans la localisation des tumeurs cérébrales. Rev. neurol., 34: 72–89, 1927.

Moniz, E., and Alves, A.: L'importance diagnostique de l'atériographie de la fosse postérieure. Rev. neurol., 2: 91–96, 1933.

Moniz, E., Pinto, A., and Alves, A.: Artériographie du cervelet et des autres organes de la fosse postérieure. Bull. Acad. méd., 109: 758–760, 1933.

Newton, T. H.: The axillary artery approach to arteriography of the aorta and its branches. Am. J. Roentgenol., 89: 275–283, 1963.

Newton, T. H., and Darroch, J.: Vertebral arteriovenous fistula complicating vertebral angiography. Acta Radiol. (Diagn.), 5: 428–440, 1966.

Newton, T. H., and Gooding C. A.: Catheter techniques in pediatric cerebral angiography. Am. J. Roentgenol., 104: 63–65, 1968.

Newton, T. H., Kramer, R. A., and Mani, J. R.: Catheter technic in vertebral arteriography. Radiology, 87: 691–695, 1966.

Oldenkott, P., and Gerhardt, P.: Angio-tomography of the posterior fossa. Neuroradiology, 2: 212–215, 1971.

Olsson, O.: Vertebral angiography. Acta Radiol., 40: 103–107, 1953.

Palmieri, A.: ECG changes in vertebral angiography by puncture and retrograde injection of the brachial artery. Acta Radiol., 12: 769–775, 1972.

Perret, G.: Diagnostic value and complications of carotid and vertebral angiography. Acta Radiol. (Diagn.), 5: 453–457, 1966.

Perret, G., and Nishioka, H.: Report on the cooperative study of intracranial aneurysms and subarachnoid hemorrhage. J. Neurosurg., 25: 98–114, 1966.

Pribrum, H. F. W.: Complications of angiography in cerebrovascular disease. Radiology, 85: 33–37, 1965.

Pygott, F., and Hutton, C. F.: Vertebral arteriography by percutaneous brachial artery catheterization. Br. J. Radiol., 32: 114–119, 1959.

Radner, S.: Intracranial angiography via the vertebral artery: Preliminary report of a new technique. Acta Radiol., 28: 838–842, 1947.

Radner, S.: Vertebral angiography by catheterization: New method employed in 222 cases. Acta Radiol., Suppl. 87: 1–134, 1951.

Raskind, R., Weiss, S. R., Wermuth, R., and Reed, W. A.: Complications of cerebral angiography: Preliminary report of 432 examinations. Angiology, 21: 447–450, 1970.

Riddervold, H. O., and Craddock, W. E.: An improved technique for selective femorocerebral angiography. Radiology, 101: 701–702, 1971.

Ruggiero, G., Thibaut, A. et al.: L'artériographie vertébrale dans le diagnostic neuro-chirurgical. Acta Radiol., 50: 365–380, 1958.

Salamon, G. M., Combalbert, A., Raybaud, C., and Gonzalez, J.: An angiographic study of meningiomas of the posterior fossa. J. Neurosurg., 35: 731–741, 1971.

Sano, K. Vertebral angiography. Brain Nerve, 2: 28–37, 1950.

Scatliff, J. H., Mishkin, M. M., and Hyde. I.: Vertebral arteriography: An evaluation of methods. Radiology, 85: 14–22, 1965.

Schechter, M. M. and de Gutiérrez-Mahoney, C. G.: The evolution of vertebral angiography. Neuroradiology, 5: 157–164, 1973.

Scott, M., Murtagh, Fr., Lapayowker, M., and Baird, R. M.: Vertebral, basilar and carotid angiography by injection of brachial artery: A cannula (non-catheter) technique. Am. J. Roentgenol., 90: 546–553, 1963.

Seldinger, S. I.: Catheter replacement of the needle in percutaneous arteriography: A new technique. Acta Radiol., 39: 368–376, 1953.

Sheldon, P. A. W.: A special needle for percutaneous vertebral angiography. Br. J. Radiol., 29: 231–232, 1956.

Shimidzu, K.: Beiträge zur Arteriographie des Gehirns: Einfache percutane Methode. Arch. f. klin. Chir., 188: 295–316, 1937.

Sjögren, S. E.: Percutaneous vertebral angiography: A review of 250 cases. Acta Radiol., 40: 113–127, 1953.

Sjöqvist, O.: Arteriographische Darstellung der Gefässe der hinteren Schädelgrube. Chirurg., 10: 377–380, 1938.

Steinberg, I., and Evans, J. A.: Technique of intravenous carotid and vertebral arteriography. Am. J. Roentgenol., 85: 1138–1145, 1961.

Sugar, O., Holden, L. B., and Powell, C. B.: Vertebral angiography. Am. J. Roentgenol., 61: 166–182, 1949.

Sutton, D., and Hoare, R. D.: Percutaneous vertebral arteriography. Br. J. Radiol., 24: 589–597, 1951.

Swann, G. F.: Vertebral arteriography using the Sheldon needle and modifications of it. Br. J. Radiol., 31: 23, 1958.

Takahashi, K.: Die percutane Arteriographie der Arteria vertebralis und ihrer Versorgungsgebiete. Arch. f. Psychiatr., 111: 373–379, 1940.

Takahashi, M., and Kawanami, H.: Femoral catheter techniques in cerebral angiography: An analysis of 422 examinations. Br. J. Radiol., 43: 771–775, 1970.

Takahashi, M., and Kawanami, H.: Catheter cerebral angiography in children: Analysis of 67 examinations. Clin. Radiol., 22: 308–311, 1971.

Takahashi, M., and Kawanami, H.: Complications of catheter cerebral angiography: An analysis of 500 examinations. Acta Radiol., 13: 248–258, 1972.

Takahashi, M., Wilson, G., and Hanafee, W.: Diagnostic value of catheter vertebral angiography: Review of 250 examinations. Acta Radiol. (Diagn.), 9: 1–9, 1969.

Takahashi, M., Wilson, G., and Hanafee, W.: Catheter vertebral angiography: A review of 300 examinations. J. Neurosurg., 30: 722–731, 1969.

Tatelman, M., and Sheehan, S.: Total vertebral-basilar arteriography via transbrachial catheterization. Radiology, 78: 919–929, 1962.

Taveras, J. M., and Wood, E. H.: Diagnostic Neuroradiology. Williams & Wilkins Co., Baltimore, 1964.

Wallman, H., and Wickbom, I.: Electronic subtraction. Acta Radiol. (Diagn.), 5: 562–569, 1966.

Westcott, J. L., and Taylor, P. T.: Transaxillary selective four-vessel arteriography. Radiology, 104: 277–281, 1972.

Wishart, D. L.: Complications in vertebral angiography as compared to non-vertebral cerebral angiography in 447 studies. Am. J. Roentgenol., 113: 527–537, 1971.

Ziedses des Plantes, B. G.: Subtraktion. G. Thieme Verlag, Stuttgart, 1961, p. 72.

Ziedses des Plantes, B. G.: Application of the roentgenographic subtraction method in neuroradiology. Acta Radiol. (Diagn.), 1: 961–966, 1963.

Chapter 4

Atkinson, W. J.: The anterior inferior cerebellar artery: Its variations, pontine distribution, and significance in the surgery of cerebello-pontine angle tumors. J. Neurol. Neurosurg. Psychiat., 12: 137–151, 1949.

Ben-Amor, M., and Billewicz, O.: The posterior cerebral vein. Neuroradiology, 1: 179–182, 1971.

Ben-Amor, M., Marion, Ch., and Heldt, N.: Normal and pathological radioanatomy of the superior choroid vein. Neuroradiology, 3: 16–19, 1971.

Billewicz, O., and Heldt, N.: The visualization of the anterior spinal artery and its blood-stream direction during brachial vertebral angiography. Neuroradiology, 2: 46–51, 1971.

Bories, J., Rosier, J., and Fredy, D.: Some technical considerations on the opacification of capillaries and veins in vertebral angiography (In connection with the so-called spasm of the vertebral artery). Neuroradiology, 1: 82–87, 1970.

Bradac, G. B.: The Ponto-mesencephalic veins (radio-anatomical study). Neuroradiology, 1: 52–57, 1970.

Bradac, G. B., Holdorff, B., and Simon, R. S.: Aspects of the venous drainage of the pons and the mesencephalon. Neuroradiology, 3: 102–108, 1971.

Bull, J., and Kozlowski, P.: The angiographic pattern of the petrosal veins in the normal and pathological. Neuroradiology, 1: 20–26, 1971.

Busch, W.: Beitrag zur Morphologie und Pathologie der Arteria basialis (Untersuchungsergebnisse bei 1,000 Gehirnen). Arch. f. Psychiat. u. Zeitshrif. f. d. Neurol., 208: 326–344, 1966.

Dor, P., and Salamon, G.: The arterioles and capillaries of the brain stem and cerebellum: A microangiographic study. Neuroradiology, 1: 27–29, 1970.

Economos, D., and Prosalentis, A.: L'artére cérébelleuse supèrieure dans les tumeurs de la fosse posterieure. Acta Radiol. (Diagn.), 1: 267–277, 1963.

Frugoni, P., Nori, A., Galligioni, F., and Giammusso, V.: A particular angiographic sign in meningiomas of the tentorium: The artery of Bernasconi and Cassinari. Neurochirurgia, 2: 142–152, 1959.

Gabrielsen, T. O., and Amundsen, P.: The pontine arteries in vertebral angiography. Am. J. Roentgenol., 106: 296–302, 1969.

Galloway, J. R., and Greitz, T.: The medial and lateral choroid arteries; An anatomic and roentgenographic study. Acta Radiol., 53: 353–366, 1960.

Galloway, J. R., Greitz, T., and Sjögren, S. E.: Vertebral angiography in the diagnosis of ventricular dilatation. Acta Radiol. (Diagn.), 2: 321–333, 1964.

Giudicelli, G., and Salamon, G.: The veins of the thalamus. Neuroradiology, 1: 92–98, 1971.

Gray, H., and Goss, C. M.: Anatomy of the Human Body. 28th ed. Lea & Febiger, Philadelphia, 1966.

Greitz, T., and Lindgren, E.: Cerebral angiography. *In* Abrams (ed.): Angiography. Vol. 1. Little & Brown, Boston, 1971.

Greitz, T., and Sjögren S. E.: The posterior inferior cerebellar artery. Acta Radiol., 1: 284–297, 1963.

Handa, H., Handa, J., and Tazumi, M.: Tentorial branch of the internal carotid artery (arteria tentorii): Report of three cases. Am. J. Roentgenol., 98: 595–598, 1966.

Hara, K., and Fujino, Y.: The thalamoperforate artery. Acta Radiol. (Diagn.), 5: 192–200, 1966.

Hassler, O.: Deep cerebral venous system in man: A microangiographic study on its areas of drainage and its anastomoses with the superficial cerebral veins. Neurology, 16: 505–511, 1966.

Hassler, O.: Arterial pattern of human brain stem: Normal appearance and deformation in expanding supratentorial conditions. Neurology, 17: 368–375, 1967.

Huang, Y. P., and Wolf, B. S.: Veins of the white matter of the cerebral hemispheres (The medullary veins): Diagnostic importance in carotid angiography. Am. J. Roentgenol., 92: 739, 1964.

Huang, Y. P., and Wolf, B. S.: The veins of the posterior fossa: Superior or Galenic draining group. Am. J. Roentgenol., 95: 808–821, 1965.

Huang, Y. P., and Wolf, B. S.: Precentral cerebellar vein in angiography. Acta Radiol. (Diagn.), 5: 250–262, 1966.

Huang, Y. P., and Wolf, B.S.: The vein of the lateral recess of the fourth ventricle and its tributaries. Am. J. Roentgenol., 101: 1–21, 1967.

Huang, Y. P., and Wolf, B. S.: Angiographic features of fourth ventricle tumors with special reference to the posterior inferior cerebellar artery. Am. J. Roentgenol., 107: 543–564, 1969.

Huang, Y. P., and Wolf, B. S.: Differential diagnosis of fourth ventricle tumors from brain stem tumors in angiography. Neuroradiology, 1: 4–19, 1971.

Huang, Y. P., Wolf, B. S., Antin, S. P., and Okudera, T.: The veins of the posterior fossa: Anterior or petrosal draining group. Am. J. Roentgenol., 104: 36–56, 1968.

Huang, Y. P., Wolf, B. S., and Okudera, T.: Angiographic anatomy of the inferior vermian vein of the cerebellum. Acta Radiol. (Diagn.), 9: 327–344, 1969.

Johanson, C.: The central veins and deep dural sinuses of the brain; An anatomical and angiographic study. Acta Radiol., Suppl., 107: 1–184, 1954.

Kaplan, H. A., and Ford, D. H.: The Brain Vascular System. Elsevier Publishing Co., Amsterdam, 1966.

Khilnani, M., and Silverstein, A.: Displacement of the superior cerebellar artery: A means of distinguishing intra- and extra-axial posterior fossa masses by vertebral arteriography. Arch. Neurol., 8: 502–505, 1963.

Krayenbühl, H., and Yasargil, M. G.: Die vaskulären Erkrankungen in Gebiete der Arteria Vertebralis und Arteria Basialis: Eine anatomische und pathologische, klinische und neuroradiologische Studie. Fortschr. Röntgenstr., Suppl., 80, 1957.

Lofgren, F. O.: Vertebral angiography in the diagnosis of tumors in the pineal region. Acta Radiol., 50: 108–124, 1958.

Mani, R. L., and Newton, T. H.: The superior cerebellar artery: Arteriographic changes in the diagnosis of posterior fossa lesions. Radiology, 92: 1281–1287, 1969.

Mani, R. L., Newton, T. H., and Glickman, M. G.: The superior cerebellar artery: An anatomic-roentgenographic correlation. Radiology, 91: 1102–1108, 1968.

Margolis, M. T. and Newton, T. H.: Borderlands of the normal and abnormal posterior inferior cerebellar artery. Acta Radiol., 13: 163–176, 1972.

Margolis, M.T., Newton, T. H., and Hyot,, W. F.: Cortical branches of the posterior cerebral artery. Anatomic-radiologic correlation. Neuroradiology, 2: 127–135, 1971.

Matsubara, T., and Nomura, T.: A sign of cerebral ventricular dilatation observed in carotid phlebograms. Am. J. Roentgenol., 84: 93–95, 1960.

Megret, M.: A landmark for the choroidal arteries of the fourth ventricle-branches of the posterior inferior cerebellar artery. Neuroradiology, 5: 85–90, 1973.

Möller, A.: Selective postmortem angiography of the posterior fossa: Technical considerations. Acta Radiol., 12: 401–409, 1972.

Mori, O., Hirasawa, K., Ogawa, T., and Mori, M.: Textbook of Anatomy. 8th ed., Vol. 2., Kanehara Shuppan, Ltd., Tokyo, 1964.

Netter, F. H.: Nervous System. Vol. I of the Ciba Collection of Medical Illustrations. 6th ed., Ciba Pharmaceutical Company, New York, 1964.

Padget, D. H.: Development of cranial venous system in man, from viewpoint of comparative anatomy. Contrib. Embryol., 36: 79–140, 1957.

Pernkopf, E.: Topographische Anatomie des Menschen. Vol. 1., Urban & Schwarzenberg, München-Berlin, 1960.

Perese, D. M.: Superficial veins of the brain from a surgical point of view. J. Neurosurg., 17: 402–412, 1960.

Potts, D. G., and Taveras, J. M.: Differential diagnosis of space-occupying lesions in the region of the thalamus by cerebral angiography. Acta Radiol. (Diagn.), 1: 373–384, 1963.

Rauber-Kopsch, F.: Lehrbuch der Anatomie des Menschen. Bd. II., Georg Thieme Verlag, Leipzig, 1948.

Rosa, M., and Viale, G. L.: Diagnostic value of vertebral phlebogram. Neuroradiology, 1: 147–150, 1971.

Smaltino, F., Bernini, F. P., and Elefante, R.: Normal and pathological findings of the angiographic examination of the internal auditory artery. Neuroradiology, 2: 216–222, 1971.

Stephens R. B., and Stilwell, D. L.: Arteries and Veins of the Human Brain. Charles C Thomas, Springfield, Illinois, 1969.

Sunderland, S.: The arterial relations of the internal auditory meatus. Brain, 68: 23–27, 1945.

Takahashi, M., and Okudera, T.: The choroid plexus and the choroid vein of the lateral ventricle: Their angiographic appearance and clinical significance. Radiology, 103: 113–120, 1972.

Takahashi, M., Okudera, T., Fukui, M., and Kitamura, K.: The choroidal and nodular branches of the posterior inferior cerebellar artery: Their value in the diagnosis of medulloblastomas. Radiology, 103: 347-351, 1972.

Takahashi, M., Okudera, T., Tanaka, M., Kitamura, K., and Yonemasu, Y.: Angiographic diagnosis of cerebellar medulloblastomas: Evaluation with pre- and postoperative vertebral angiographies. Am. J. Roentgenol., 118: 622–632, 1973.

Takahashi, M., Wilson, G., and Hanafee, W.: The significance of the petrosal vein in the diagnosis of cerebellopontine angle tumors. Radiology, 89: 834–840, 1967.

Takahashi, M., Wilson, G., and Hanafee, W.: The anterior inferior cerebellar artery: Its radiographic anatomy and significance in the diagnosis of extra-axial tumors of the posterior fossa. Radiology, 90: 281–287, 1968.

Wackenheim, A.: Some views regarding the diagnostic value of the veins of the posterior fossa. Neuroradiology, 3: 75–76, 1971.

Wackenheim, A., and Ben-Amor, M.: Phlebographic location of the inferior vermis. Neuroradiology, 3: 12–15, 1971.

Wackenheim, A., and Braun, J. P.: Angiography of the Mesencephalon: Normal and pathological findings. Springer-Verlag, Berlin-Heidelberg-New York, 1970.

Wackenheim, A., Heldt, N., and Ben-Amor, M.: Variations in the drainage of the lateral mesencephalic vein. Neuroradiology, 2: 154–161, 1971.

Watt, J. C., and McKillop, A. N.: Relation of arteries to roots of nerves in posterior cranial fossa in man. Arch. Surg., 30: 336–345, 1935.

Westberg, G.: Arteries of the basal ganglia. Acta Radiol. (Diagn.), 5: 581–596, 1966.

Wolf, B. S., and Huang, Y. P.: The subependymal veins of the lateral ventricles. Amer. J. Roentgenol., 91: 406–426, 1964.

Wolf, B. S., Huang, Y. P., and Newman, C. M.: The lateral anastomotic mesencephalic vein and other variations in drainage of the basal cerebral vein. Am. J. Roentgenol., 89: 411–422, 1963.

Wolf, B. S., Newman, C. M., and Khilnani, M. T.: The posterior inferior cerebellar artery on vertebral angiography. Am. J. Roentgenol., 87: 322–337, 1962.

Chapters 5, 6 and 7

Azambuja, N., Lindgren, E., and Sjögren, S. E.: Tentorial herniations. I. Anatomy. II. Pneumoencephalography. III. Angiography. Acta Radiol., 46: 215–241, 1956.

Braun, J. P. et Wackenheim, A.: Phlébographie mésencéphalique dans les tumeurs du tronc cérébral. Acta Radiol., 13: 45–53, 1972.

Bull, J., and Kozlowski, P.: The angiographic pattern of the petrosal veins in the normal and pathological. Neuroradiology, 1: 20–26, 1971.

Castellanos, F., and Ruggiero, G.: Meningiomas of the posterior fossa. Acta Radiol., Suppl., 104, 1953.

Columella, F., and Papo, I.: Vertebral angiography in supratentorial expansive processes. Acta Radiol., 46: 178, 1956.

Cushing, H.: Intracranial Tumors. Charles C Thomas, Springfield, Illinois, 1932.

David, M., Bernard-Weil, E., and Dilenge, D.: Les tumeurs de la glande pineale. Ann. Endocrinol., 24: 287–330, 1963.

Dechaume, J. P., Bochu, M., Michel, D., Joyeux, O., Bret, Ph., and Barbeau, P.: Pathological tumour circulation: A study of 50 cases by retrograde brachial vertebral angiography. Neuroradiology, 1: 151–154, 1970.

Decker, K.: The displacement of the posterior cerebral artery in vertebral angiograms. Acta Radiol., 40: 91–95, 1953.

Dilenge, D., and David, M.: L'opacification des arteres thalamique au cours de l'angiographie vertebrale. Neurochirurgie, 11: 511–518, 1965.

Economos, D., and Prosalentis, A.: L'artère cérébelleuse supérieure dans les tumeurs de la fosse postérieure. Acta Radiol., 1: 267–277, 1963.

Epstein, B. S., Epstein, J. A., and Carras, R.: Extension of posterior fossa tumors, particularly intraventricular fourth ventricle tumors, into the upper cervical spinal canal. Am. J. Roentgenol., 110: 31–38, 1970.

Fokes, E. C., and Earle, K. M.: Ependymomas: Clinical and pathological aspects. J. Neurosurg., 30: 585–594, 1969.

Frugoni, P., Nori, A., Galligioni, F., and Giammusso, V.: A particular angiographic sign in meningiomas of the tentorium: The artery of Bernasconi and Cassinari. Neurochirurgia, 2: 142–152, 1959.

Galligioni, F., Bernardi, R., Pellone, M., and Iraci, G.: The veins of the posterior cranial fossa: An angiographic study under pathologic conditions. Am. J. Roentgenol., 110: 39–49, 1970.

GALLOWAY, J. R., AND GREITZ, T.: The medial and lateral choroid arteries: An anatomic and roentgenographic study. Acta Radiol., 53: 353–366, 1960.

GALLOWAY, J. R., GREITZ, T., AND SJÖGREN, S. E.: Vertebral angiography in the diagnosis of ventricular dilatation. Acta Radiol. (Diagn.), 2: 321–333, 1964.

GIUDICELLI, G., AND SALAMON, G.: The veins of the thalamus. Neuroradiology, 1: 92–98, 1970.

GLICKMAN, M. G., AND SHOLKOFF, S. D.: Posterior displacement of the basilar artery by intrinsic pontine tumors. Am. J. Roentgenol., 112: 276–280, 1971.

GOREE, J. A., AND DUKES, H. T.: The angiographic differential diagnosis between the vascularized malignant glioma and the intracranial arteriovenous malformation. Am. J. Roentgenol., 90: 512–521, 1933.

GOREE, J. A., TINDALL, G. T., AND ODOM, G. L.: Percutaneous retrograde brachial angiography in the diagnosis of acoustic neurinoma: Results in 4 cases. Am. J. Roentgenol., 92: 829–835, 1964.

GREITZ, T.: Tumours of the quadrigeminal plate and adjacent structures. Acta Radiol., 12: 513–538, 1972.

GREITZ, T., AND SJÖGREN, S. E.: The posterior inferior cerebellar artery. Acta Radiol., 1: 284–297, 1963.

HARA, K., AND FUJINO, Y.: The thalamoperforate artery. Acta Radiol. (Diagn.), 5: 192–200, 1966.

HAUGE, T.: Catheter vertebral angiography. Acta Radiol., Suppl., 109, 1954.

HUANG, Y. P., AND WOLF, B. S.: Angiographic features of unilateral hydrocephalus of obstructive nature. Am. J. Roentgenol., 92: 792–810, 1964.

HUANG, Y. P., AND WOLF, B. S.: Angiographic features of fourth ventricle tumors with special reference to the posterior inferior cerebellar artery. Am. J. Roentgenol., 107: 543–564, 1969.

HUANG, Y. P., AND WOLF, B. S.: Angiographic features of brain stem tumors and differential diagnosis from fourth ventricle tumors. Am. J. Roentgenol., 110: 1–30, 1970.

HUANG, Y. P., AND WOLF, B. S.: Differential diagnosis of fourth ventricle tumors from brain stem tumors in angiography. Neuroradiology, 1: 4–19, 1971.

HUANG, Y. P., WOLF, B. S., ANTIN, S. P., OKUDERA, T., AND KIM, I. H.: Angiographic features of aqueductal stenosis. Amer. J. Roentgenol., 104: 90–108, 1968.

JEFFERSON, A., AND SHELDON, P.: Transtentrorial herniation of the brain as revealed by the displacement of arteries. Acta Radiol., 46: 480–497, 1956.

KHILNANI, M., AND SILVERSTEIN, A.: Displacement of the superior cerebellar artery: A means of distinguishing intra- and extra-axial posterior fossa masses by vertebral arteriography. Arch. Neurol., Chicago, 8: 502–505, 1963.

KRAYENBÜHL, H., AND YASARGIL, M. G.: Die vaskularen Erkrankungen im Gebiet der Arteria Vertebralis and Arteria Basilaris; Eine anatomische und pathologische, klinische und neuroradiologische Studie. Fortschr. Röntgenstr., Suppl., 80, 1957.

KURU, Y., HARA, K., SHIGA, H., AND FUJINO, Y.: Arterial midline shift in the posterior fossa. Neuroradiology, 1: 188–194, 1970.

LEHMANN, R.: Venenbilder Bei Akustikusneurinomen. Acta Radiol., 13: 150–156, 1972.

LINDGREN, E., AND SJÖGREN, S. E.: Tentorial herniations. Acta Radiol., 46: 215, 1956.

LÖFGREN, F. O.: Vertebral angiography in the diagnosis of hydrocephalus and differentiation between stenosis of the aqueduct and cerebellar tumour. Acta Radiol., 46: 186–194, 1956.

LÖFGREN, F. O.: Vertebral angiography in the diagnosis of tumors in the pineal region. Acta Radiol., 50: 124–180, 1958.

MANI, R. L., NEWTON, T. H., AND GLICKMAN, M. G.: The superior cerebellar artery: An anatomic-roentgenographic correlation. Radiology, 91: 1102–1108, 1968.

MARGOLIS, M. T., AND NEWTON, T. H.: An angiographic sign of cerebellar tonsillar herniation. Neuroradiology, 2: 3–8, 1971.

MATSON, D. D.: Neurosurgery of Infancy and Childhood (second ed.). Charles C Thomas Springfield, Illinois, 1969.

MONES, R.: Vertebral angiography: An analysis of 106 cases. Radiology, 76: 230–236, 1961.

NADJMI, M., ENGELHARDT, F., JENSEN, H. P., GRUSS, P., UND MÜLLER, H. A.: Zur Diagnose der Lindau-Tumoren im Retrograden Brachialisangiogram. Fortschr. Röntgenstr., 116: 190–198, 1972.

OLSSON, O.: Vertebral angiography in the diagnosis of acoustic nerve tumours. Acta Radiol., 39: 265–272, 1953.

OLSSON, O.: Vertebral angiography in cerebellar haemangioma. Acta Radiol., 40: 9–16, 1953.

PADGET, D. H.: Development of cranial venous system in man, from viewpoint of comparative anatomy. Contrib. Embryol., 36: 79–140, 1957.

PEETERS, F. L. M.: The vertebral angiogram in patients with tumours in or near the midline. Neuroradiology, 5: 53–58, 1973.

REIGH, E. E., AND NELSON, M.: Posterior fossa subdural hematoma with secondary hydrocephalus: Report of case and review of the literature. J. Neurosurg., 19: 346–348, 1962.

REIGH, E. E., AND O'CONNELL, T. J.: Extradural hematoma of the posterior fossa with concomitant supratentorial subdural hematoma: Report of a case and review of the literature. J. Neurosurg., 19: 359–364, 1962.

ROSA, M., AND VIALE, G. L.: Diagnostic value of vertebral phlebogram. Neuroradiology, 1: 147–150, 1970.

SAVOIARDO, M., AND LEMAY, M.: Diagnosis of posterior fossa lesions by angiography. Br. J. Radiol., 43: 291–302, 1970.

SEEGER, J. F., AND GABRIELSEN, T. O.: Angiography of eccentric brain stem tumors. Radiology, 105: 343–351, 1972.

SKUCAS, J., AND BRINKER, R. A.: Cerebellar hemangioblastoma with a tentorial artery supply: Report of a case. Neuroradiology, 3: 113–115, 1971.

STATTIN, S.: Significance of some angiographic signs of intracranial meningiomas. Acta Radiol. (Diagn.), 5: 530–535, 1966.

SUTTON, D.: Radiologic aspects of pontine gliomata. Acta Radiol., Stockh., 40: 234, 1953.

TAKAHASHI, M., AND KAWANAMI, H.: Catheter cerebral angiography in children: Analysis of 67 examinations. Clin. Radiol., 22: 308–311, 1971.

TAKAHASHI, M., AND OKUDERA, T.: The choroid plexus and the choroid vein of the lateral ventricle: Their angiographic appearance and clinical significance. Radiology, 103: 113–120, 1972.

TAKAHASHI, M., OKUDERA, T., FUKUI, M., AND KITAMURA, K.: The choroidal and nodular branches of the posterior inferior cerebellar artery: Their value in the diagnosis of medulloblastomas. Radiology, 103: 347–351, 1972.

TAKAHASHI, M., OKUDERA, T., TANAKA, M., KITAMURA, K., AND YONEMASU, Y.: Angiographic diagnosis of cerebellar medulloblastomas: Evaluation of pre- and postoperative vertebral angiographies. Am. J. Roentgenol., 118: 622–632, 1973.

Takahashi, M., Okudera, T., Tomonaga, M., and Kitamura, K.: Angiographic diagnosis of acoustic neurinomas: Analysis of 30 lesions. Neuroradiology, 2: 191–200, 1971.

Takahashi, M., Wilson, G., and Hanafee, W.: The significance of the petrosal vein in the diagnosis of cerebellopontine angle tumors. Radiology, 89: 834–840, 1967.

Takahashi, M., Wilson, G., and Hanafee, W.: The anterior inferior cerebellar artery: Its radiographic anatomy and significance in the diagnosis of extra-axial tumors of the posterior fossa. Radiology, 90: 281–287, 1968.

Takahashi, M., Wilson, G., and Hanafee, W.: Catheter vertebral angiography: A review of 300 examinations. J. Neurosurg., 30: 722–731, 1969.

Taveras, J. M., and Wood, E. H.: Diagnostic Neuroradiology. The Williams & Wilkins Co., Baltimore, 1964.

Tönnis, W., Brandt, P., and Walter, W.: The roentgenological diagnosis of tumors of the corpus callosum: With a contribution to the normal roentgenological anatomy of the anterior cerebral artery. J. Neurosurg., 17: 183–196, 1960.

Tristan, T. A., and Hodges, P. J.: Meningiomas of the posterior cranial fossa. Radiology, 70: 1, 1958.

Wackenheim, A., and Ben-Amor, M.: Arteriovenous separation of the prepontine vessels as a sign of intrapontine tumour. Neuroradiology, 3: 77–79, 1971.

Wilner, H. I., Navarro, E., Eisenbrey, A. B., and Gracias, V.: The inferior vermian veins as a useful adjunct in the differentiation of brain stem tumors from midline cerebellar masses. Am. J. Roentgenol., 118: 605–616, 1973.

Wolf, B. S., and Huang, Y. P.: The subependymal veins of the lateral ventricles. Am. J. Roentgenol., 91: 406–426, 1964.

Wolf, B. S., Newman, C. M., and Khilnani, M. T.: The posterior inferior cerebellar artery on vertebral angiography. Am. J. Roentgenol., 87: 322–337, 1962.

Wolpert, S. M.: Angiography in posterior fossa tumors of infancy and childfood. Am. J. Roentgenol., 112: 296–305, 1971.

Yasargil, M. G.: Die Vertebralisangiographie: Ihre Bedeutung fur die Diagnose der Tumoren. Acta neurochir., Suppl., 9: 1–108, 1962.

Zatz, L. M., Hanberg, J. W., Gifford, D., and Belza, J.: The diagnosis of tumors of the splenium of the corpus callosum. Am. J. Roentgenol., 101: 130–140, 1967.

Zülch, K. J.: Brain Tumors: Their Biology and Pathology. Springer-Verlag New York Inc., New York, U.S.A., 1965.

Chapters 8 and 9

Adachi, B.: Arteriensystem der Japaner. Kaiserlich-Japanischen Universität zu Kyoto, Kyoto, Japan. Vol. 1, 1928.

Adams, R. D.: Occlusion of the anterior inferior cerebellar artery. Arch. Neurol. Psychiatr., 49: 765–770, 1943.

Aronson, H., Shafey, S., and Gargano, F.: Intracerebellar haematoma. J. Neurol. Neurosurg. Psychiat., 28: 442–444, 1965.

Baker, H. L., Jr.: Angiographic investigation of cerebrovascular insufficiency. Radiology, 77: 399–405, 1961.

Benson, D. F., and Tomlinson, E. B.: Hemiplegic syndrome of the posterior cerebral artery. Stroke, 2: 559–564, 1971.

Biemond, A.: Thrombosis of the basilar artery and the vascularization of the brain stem. Brain, 74: 300–317, 1951.

Bigelow, N. H.: Multiple intracranial arterial aneurysms: An analysis of their significance. Arch. Neurol. Psychiat., Chicago, 73: 76–99, 1955.

Bryc, S., and Wójcik, Z.: Angiographic estimation of the size and site of the lateral and fourth ventricles. Acta Radiol., 13: 54–57, 1972.

Bull, J. W. D., Marshall, J., and Shaw, D. A.: Cerebral angiography in the diagnosis of the acute stroke. Lancet, 1: 562–565, 1960.

Bull, J. W. D.: Use and limitations of angiography in the diagnosis of vascular lesions of the brain. Neurology, 11: 80–85, 1961.

Bull, J. W. D.: Contribution of radiology to the study of intracranial aneurysms. Br. Med. J., 2: 1701–1708, 1962.

Burns, J. B., Hoffman, J. C., and Brylski, J. R.: Posterior inferior cerebellar artery in fourth ventricular dilatation. Acta Radiol., 13: 58–65, 1972.

Bücheler, E., und Käufer, C.: Karotis- und Vertebralisangiographie beim Hirntod. Acta Radiol., 13: 301–311, 1972.

Ciminello, V. J., and Sachs, E. Jr.: Arteriovenous malformations of the posterior fossa. J. Neurosurg., 19: 602–604, 1962.

Cronqvist, S.: Total angiography in evaluation of cerebrovascular disease: A correlative study of aorto-cervical and selective cerebral angiography. Br. J. Radiol., 39: 805–810, 1966.

Cronqvist, S.: Regional cerebral blood flow and angiography in apoplexy. Acta Radiol. (Diagn.), 7: 521–534, 1968.

Cronqvist, S., and Troupp, H.: Intracranial arteriovenous malformation and arterial aneurysm in the same patient. Acta Neurol. Scand., 42: 307–316, 1966.

Debrun, G., and Chartres, A.: Infra- and supratentorial arteriovenous malformations. A general review. About 2 cases of spontaneous supratentorial arteriovenous malformation of the dura. Neuroradiology, 3: 184–192, 1972.

DeSaussure, R. L., Hunter, S. E., and Robertson, J. T.: Saccular aneurysms of the posterior fossa. J. Neurosurg., 15: 385–391, 1958.

DiChiro, G., and Doppman, J. L.: Differential angiographic features of hemangioblastomas and arteriovenous malformations of the spinal cord. Radiology, 93: 25–30, 1969.

DiChiro, G., Doppman, J., and Ommaya, A. K.: Selective arteriography of arteriovenous aneurysms of spinal cord. Radiology, 88: 1065–1077, 1967.

Doppman, J. L., DiChiro, G., and Ommaya, A. L.: Selective Arteriography of the Spinal Cord. Warren H. Green, Inc, St. Louis, Missouri, 1969.

Eadie, M. J., Jamieson, K. G., and Lennon, E. A.: Persistent carotid-basilar-anatomosis (18 personal cases). J. Neurol. Sci., 1: 501–511, 1964.

Echlin, F. A.: Spasm of basilar and vertebral arteries caused by experimental subarachnoid hemorrhage. J. Neurosurg., 22: 1–11, 1965.

Ferris, E. J., Gabriele, O. F., Hipona, F. A., and Shapiro, J. H.: Early venous filling in cranial angiography. Radiology, 90: 553–557, 1968.

Fields, W. S., Bruetman, M. E., and Weibel, J.: Collateral Circulation of the Brain. The Williams & Wilkins Company, Baltimore, 1965, pp. 183–207.

Fukui, M., and Kitamura, K.: Persistent primitive hypoglossal artery: A case report and review and analysis of 34cases reported in the literature. Clinical Neurol., 9: 421–428, 1969.

Gabrielsen, T. O., and Seeger, J. F.: Vertebral angiography in the diagnosis of intraspinal masses in upper cervical region. Neuroradiology, 5: 7–12, 1973.

Galligioni, F., Andrioli, G. C., Marin, G., Briani, S., and Iraci, G.: Hypoplasia of the internal carotid artery associated with cerebral pseudoangiomatosis: Report of 4 cases. Am. J. Roentgenol., 112: 251–262, 1971.

Goodhart, S. P., and Davison, C.: Syndrome of posterior inferior and anterior inferior cerebellar arteries and their branches. Arch. Neurol. Psychiat., 35: 501–524, 1936.

Handa, H., Handa, J., and Koyama, T.: Agenesis of the corpus callosum associated with multiple developmental anomalies of the cerebral arteries. Brain Nerve, 20: 317–326, 1968.

Handa, J., and Handa, H.: Progressive cerebral arterial occlusive disease: Analysis of 27 cases. Neuroradiology, 3: 119–133, 1972.

Hinck, V.C., Hopkins, C.E., and Savara, B.S.: Diagnostic criteria of basilar impression. Radiology, 76: 572–585, 1961.

Hoare, R. D.: Arteriovenous aneurysm of the posterior fossa. Acta Radiol., 40: 96–102, 1953.

Huk, W., and Klinger, M.: The diagnosis of cervical spinal angioblastomas. Neuroradiology, 5: 174–177, 1973.

Hutchinson, N. A., and Miller, J. D. R.: Persistent proatlantal artery. J. Neurol. Neurosurg. Psychiat., 33: 524–527, 1970.

Jamieson, K. G.: Aneurysms of the vertebrobasilar system: Surgical intervention in 19 cases. J. Neurosurg., 21: 781–797, 1964.

Jones, R. R., and Wetzel, N.: Bilateral carotid vertebrobasilar rete mirabile: Case report. J. Neurosurg., 33: 581–586, 1970.

Kannel, W. D.: Current status of the epidemiology of brain infarction associated with occlusive arterial disease. Stroke, 2: 295–318, 1971.

Klaus, E., und Urbánek, K.: Zur Frage der Angiographischen Vertebralisbefunde bei der Basilären Impression. Fortschr. Röntgenstr., 116: 378–385, 1972.

Koch, R. L., and Glickman, M. G.: The angiographic diagnosis of extradural hematoma of the posterior fossa. Am. J. Roentgenol., 112: 289–295, 1971.

Kowada, M., Yamaguchi, K., and Takahashi, H.: Fenestration of the vertebral artery with a review of 23 cases in Japan. Radiology, 103: 343–346, 1972.

Kramer, R. A., and Eckman, P. B.: Hemifacial spasm associated with redundancy of the vertebral artery. Am. J. Roentgenol., 115: 133–136, 1972.

Krayenbühl, H., and Siebenmann, R.: Small vascular malformations as a cause of primary intracerebral hemorrhage. J. Neurosurg., 22: 7–20, 1965.

Kudo, T.: Spontaneous occlusion of the circle of Willis: A disease apparently confined to Japanese. Neurology, 18: 485–496, 1968.

Leape, L. L., and Palacios, E.: Acute traumatic vertebral arteriovenous fistula. Ann. Surg., 174: 908–910, 1971.

Lee, K. F., and Hodes, P. J.: Intracranial ischemic lesions. Radiol. Clin. North Am., 5: 363–393, 1967.

Leslie, E. V., and Alker, G. J., Jr.: Multiple progressive intracranial arterial occlusions. Acta Radiol., 13: 157–162, 1972.

Lhermitte, F., Gautier, J. C., Poirier, J., and Tyrer, J. H.: Hypoplasia of the internal carotid artery. Neurology, 18: 439–446, 1968.

Lie, T. A.: Primitive Hypoglossal Artery in Congenital Anomalies of the Carotid Arteries. Excerpta Medica, Amsterdam, 1968.

Liebeskind, A., Chinichian, A., and Schechter, M. M.: The moving embolus seen during serial cerebral angiography. Stroke, 2: 440–443, 1971.

Liliequist, B.: Capillary phase in cerebral angiography. Acta Radiol. (Diagn.), 6: 113–125, 1967.

Lin, J. P., and Kricheff, I. I.: Angiographic investigation of cerebral aneurysms: Technical aspects. Radiology, 105: 69–76, 1972.

Locksley, H. B.: Report on the cooperative study of intracranial aneurysms and subarachnoid hemorrhage. Sec. 5, Part II, Natural history of subarachnoid hemorrhage, intracranial aneurysms and arteriovenous malformations. J. Neurosurg., 25: 321–368, 1966.

Logue, V., and Monckton, G.: Posterior fossa angiomas: A clinical presentation of nine cases. Brain, 77: 252–273, 1954.

Loop, J. W., White, L. E., Jr., and Shaw, C. M.: Traumatic occlusion of the basilar artery within a clivus fracture. Radiology, 83: 36–41, 1964.

Maki, Y., Horie, T., and Nakada, Y.: Angiographical studies on the cases of obstructive disease with abnormal vascular network. The Journal of Chiba Medical Society, 44: 272–277, 1968.

Maki, Y., Watanabe, M., Nakada, Y., Ono, Y., and Shirai S.: Angiographic demonstration of vertebral artery. Clin. Neurology, 9: 199–204, 1969.

McDonald, C. A., and Korb, M.: Intracranial aneurysms. Arch. Neurol. Psychiat., Chicago, 42: 298–328, 1939.

McKissock, W., Richardson, A., and Walsh, L.: Spontaneous cerebellar haemorrhage: A study of 34 consecutive cases treated surgically. Brain, 83: 1–9, 1960.

McKissock, W., Richardson, A., Walsh, L., and Owen, E.: Multiple intracranial aneurysms. Lancet, 1: 623–626, 1964.

Mitterwallner, F. von: Variationsstatistische Untersuchungen an den basalen Hirngefässen. Acta Anat., 24: 51–88, 1955.

Moossy, J.: Cerebral infarcts and the lesions of intracranial and extracranial atherosclerosis. Arch. Neurol., 14: 124-128, 1966.

Müller, R., Greitz, T., Liliequist, B., and Hellström, L.: Aortocervical angiography in occlusive cerebrovascular disease. Neurology, 14: 136–146, 1964.

Newton, T. H., Adams, J. E., and Wylie, E. J.: Arteriography of cerebrovascular occlusive disease. New Eng. J. Med., 270: 14–18, 1964.

Nishimoto, A., and Takeuchi, S.: Abnormal cerebrovascullar network related to the internal carotid arteries. J. Neurosurg. 29: 255–260, 1968.

Padget, D. H.: Cranial venous system in man in reference to development, adult configuration, and relation to the arteries. Am. J. Anat., 98: 307–355, 1956.

Passerini, A., and Tagliabue, G.: Aneurysms of the vertebrobasilar system. Radiol. clin. biol., 35: 257–273, 1966.

Paterson, J. H., and McKissock, W.: Clinical survey of intracranial angiomas with special reference to their mode of progression and surgical treatment. Brain, 74: 233–265, 1956.

Pecker, J., Simon, J., Guy, G., and Henry, J. F.: Nishimoto's disease: Significance of its angiographic appearances. Neuroradiology, 5: 223–230, 1973.

Perret, G., and Nishioka, H.: Report on the cooperative study of intracranial aneurysms and subarachnoid hemorrhage. Section IV. Cerebral angiography. An analysis of the diagnostic value and complications of carotid and vertebral angiography in 5,484 patients. J. Neurosurg., 25: 98–114, 1966.

Perret, G., and Nishioka, H.: Report on the cooperative study of intracranial aneurysms and subarachnoid hemorrhage. Section VI. Arteriovenous malformations. An analysis of 545 cases of cranio-cerebral arteriovenous malformations and fistulae reported to the cooperative study. J. Neurosurg., 25: 467–490, 1966.

PICARD, L., ANDRÉ, J. M., RENARD, M., MONTAUT, J., ET TRIDON, P.: Réseau admirable carotidien humain: Problémes étiologiques et nosologiques. Acta Radiol., 13: 205–219, 1972.

RICHTER, R. H.: Collaterals between the external carotid artery and the vertebral artery in cases of thrombosis of the internal carotid artery. Acta Radiol., 40: 108–112, 1953.

RING, B. A.: The Neglected Cause of Stroke. W. H. Green, Inc., St. Louis, 1969.

RING B. A., AND WADDINGTON, M. M.: The neglected cause of stroke: Intracranial occlusion of the small arteries. Radiology, 88: 924–929, 1967.

RUSSELL, D. S., AND RUBINSTEIN, L. J.: Pathology of Tumors of the Nervous System. Edward Arnold, Ltd., London, 1959.

SCHECHTER, M. M., AND ZINGESSER, L. H.: The radiology of basilar thrombosis. Radiology, 85: 23–32, 1965.

SIGHTS, W. P., JR.: Incarceration of the basilar artery in a fracture of the clivus. J. Neurosurg., 22: 588–591, 1968.

SOLÉ-LLENAS, J., AND PLANAS, M.: Occipital-vertebral anastomosis in a case of middle cerebral artery occlusion. Neuroradiology, 1: 88–91, 1971.

SPATZ, E. L., AND BULL, J. W. D.: Vertebral arteriography in the study of subarachnoid hemorrhage. J. Neurosurg., 14: 543–547, 1957.

STEHBENS, W. E.: Pathology of the Cerebral Blood Vessels. The C. V. Mosby Company, St. Louis, 1972.

STEIN, B. M., MCCORMICK, W. F., RODRIGUEZ, J. N., AND TAVERAS, J. M.: Radiography of atheromatous disease involving the extracranial arteries as seen at postmortem. Acta Radiol. (Diagn.), 1: 455–467, 1963.

SZDZUY, D., AND LEHMANN, R.: Persistent trigeminal artery in vertebral angiography. Neuroradiology, 2: 100–101, 1971.

TAKAHASHI, M., KAWANAMI, H., WATANABE, N., AND MATSUOKA, S.: Fenestration of the extracranial vertebral artery. Radiology, 96: 359–360, 1970.

TAVERAS, J. M.: Angiographic observations in occlusive cerebrovascular disease. Neurology, 11: 86–90, 1961.

TAVERAS, J. M.: Multiple progressive intracranial arterial occlusions: A syndrome of children and young adults. Am. J. Roentgenol., 106: 235–268, 1969.

TAVERAS, J. M., GILSON, J. M., DAVIS, D. O., KILGORE, B., and RUNBAUGH, C. L.: Angiography in cerebral infarction. Radiology, 93: 549–558, 1969.

VERBIEST, H.: Arteriovenous aneurysms of the posterior fossa: Analysis of six cases. Acta Neurol. Chir., 9: 171–195, 1961.

VERBIEST, H.: Arterial and arteriovenous aneurysms of the posterior fossa. Psychiat. Neurol. Neurochir., 65: 329–369, 1962.

WACKENHEIM, A.: Asymétrie de la face et des artéres vertébrales: Á propos d'un cas de persistance unilatérale de l'artére hypoglosse. Acta Radiol., 13: 268–271, 1972.

WEIBEL, J., AND FIELDS, W. S.: Atlas of Arteriography in Occlusive Cerebrovascular Disease. G. Thieme Verlag, Stuttgart, 1969.

WEIDNER, W., CRANDALL, P., HANAFEE, W., AND TOMIYASU, U.: Collateral circulation in the posterior fossa via leptomeningeal anastomoses. Am. J. Roentgenol., 95: 831–836, 1965.

WEIDNER, W., HANAFEE, W., AND MARKHAM, C. H.: Intracranial collateral circulation via leptomeningeal and rete mirabile anastomoses. Neurology, 15: 39–48, 1965.

WICKBOM, I.: Angiography of the carotid artery. Acta Radiol., Suppl., 72, 1948.

WIEDENMANN, O., AND HIPP, E.: Abnorme Kommunikation zwischen dem Versorgungs-gebiet der Arteria carotis interna und der Arteria basilaris (Karotido-basilare Anastomosen). Fortschr. Röntogenstr., 91: 350–365, 1959.

WOLLSCHLAEGER, G., WOLLSCHLAEGER, P. B., LUCAS, F. V., ET AL.: Experience and result with postmortem cerebral angiography performed as routine procedure of the autopsy. Am. J. Roentgenol., 101: 68–87, 1967.

WOLPERT, S. M., HALLER, J. S., AND RABE, E. F.: The value of angiography in the Dandy-Walker syndrome and posterior fossa extra-axial cysts. Am. J. Roentgenol., 109: 261–272, 1970.

YAMAGUCHI, K., UEMURA, K., AND TAKAHASHI, H.: Angiographic study in cerebral infarction, especially related to the timing of examination. Nipp. Act. Radiol., 31: 1090–1099, 1971.

YAMAGUCHI, K., UEMURA, K., TAKAHASHI, H., KOWADA, M., AND KUTSUZAWA, T.: Intracerebral leakage of contrast medium in apoplexy. Br. J. Radiol., 44: 689–691, 1971.

YAMAGUCHI, K., UEMURA, K., TAKAHASHI, H., KUTSUZAWA, T., AND KOWADA, M.: Early venous filling in cerebral infarction and hemorrhage. Nipp. Act. Radiol., 31: 183–193, 1971.

Name Index

Subject Index

Q

R

S

T

U

V